3rd International Symposium on Orbital Disorders

Proceedings of the
3rd International Symposium
on Orbital Disorders
Amsterdam, September 5-7, 1977

edited by

The Orbital Centre of the Amsterdam University Eye Hospital
The Netherlands Ophthalmic Research Institute
The Netherlands Ophthalmological Society
The New York Eye and Ear Infirmary

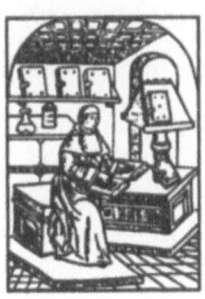

Dr. W. Junk bv Publishers – The Hague/Boston/London 1978

ISBN-13: 978-94-009-9980-0   e-ISBN-13: 978-94-009-9978-7
DOI: 10.1007/978-94-009-9978-7
© Dr. W Junk bv Publishers 1978
Softcover reprint of the hardcover 1st edition 1978

CONTENTS

Radiography vascular

Radiology C.T.

Technetium scan

Trauma and trauma surgery

Inflammations

Orbital tumors

Endocrine disorders

Vascular disorders

Reconstructive surgery

Medical therapy

Radiotherapy

Miscellaneous

LIST OF PARTICIPANTS

Austria
Antlanger, H., Schwesternweg 7, 5020 Salzburg
Casagranda, R., Weiserstrasse, Salzburg
Glensluckner, W., W. Hentholzstrasse 7, Salzburg
Hausman, N., Lük. Krankenhaus, A-6800 Feldkirch

Belgium
Brihaye-van Geertruyden; M., 13 Rue Vergote, Bruxelles
Castermans, A., Bd. de la Constitution 66, 4000 Liège
Cornelis, G., Naamsestraat 137, Leuven
Evens, L., Lakenselaan, 1090 Bruxelles
François, J., De Pintelaan 135, 9000 Gent
Garsse, A. von, University of Liège, 4020 Liège
Geinger, N., 19, Herrenrode Bosstraat, 3511 Kuringen
Herzeel, R., Rietstraat 53, 9440 Erenbodegen
Laey, J. de Witte Leertouwerstraat 17, B 8000
Leys, A., Universitaire Klinieken 'St. Rafaël', Capucijnenvoer 9, 3000 Leuven
Missotten, L., Leo Dartelaan 12, 3030 Leuven
Nieus, Chr., Josse Goffinlaan 118, Bruxelles
Poelman, A.H.M., Voskenslaan 99, 9000 Gent
Rousseau, A., Avenue Hippocrate 10, 1200 Bruxelles

Canada
Singh, O.S., Endeca Place Suite 3, 402-5 Avenue S.O., Lethbridge, Alberta

Denmark
Fledelius, H., Rigshospitalet, Eye Dept. 2061, DK—2100 Copenhagen
Møller, P.M., Hunderuovej 204B, 5230 Odense M.

Egypt
El Aswad, M.A., 44, El Khalifa El Mamounstreet, Helliopoli, Cairo
Mortada, A., 18A, 26 July Street, Cairo.

Fed. Rep. of Germany
Buschmann, H.W., Joseph Schneiderstrasse 11, 8700 Würzberg
Busse, H. Augenklinik der Westfälischen Wilhelms-Universität, Westring 15, Münster
Dormarus, H., Ratzeburger Allee 160, MHL, 2400 Lübeck
Fischedick, O., W. Kaiserweg 8, 46 Dortmund
Friederich, H., Neuhauserstrasse 14, D8000 München
Hida, T., Robert Kochstrasse 13, 4300 Essen 1.
Hollwich, F., Westring 15, Münster

Kirchner, Chr., Wandsbeker Ch. 12, 2000 Hamburg 76
Klehr, H.U., Venusberg, 53 Bonn 1
Kruse, H. Josef Stelzmannstrasse 9, 5000 Köln 41
Lange, S., Spandauer Damm 130, 1000 Berlin 19
Lemmingson, W., Diakonissenstrasse 28, 7500 Karlsruhe 51
Linnert, D., 2 Jozef Schneiderstrasse, Würzburg
Marx, K.U., Massenerstrasse 1, 4760 Unna
Mühlendyck, H., Am Zollstock 13, Giessen
Müller Jensen, K., Moltkestrasse 14, 75 Karlsruhe
Nover, A.H., Langenbeckstrasse 1, D 65 Mainz
Osmers, F., Augenklinik der Westfälischen Wilhelms-Universität, Westring
    15, Münster
Poeschel, W., Ratzeburger Allee 160, MHL, 2400 Lübeck
Raabe, M., Steinhauserstrasse 18, Karlsruhe
Roggenkämper, P., Hochkalter Strasse 12, 8 München 90
Schmidt, B., Hindenburgdamm 30, 1000 Berlin 45
Schmitt, E.J., Langenbeckstrasse 1, 63 Mainz
Schroeder, W., Martinistrasse 52, D–2000 Hamburg
Spalecck, C., Holbeingasse 2, 8833 Eichstätt
Stefani, F.H., Mathildenstrasse 8, D–8000 München 2
Waubke, Th.N., Universitäts-Augenklinik, Hufelandstrasse 55, Essen
Weigelin, E., Venusberg, 53 Bonn 1

Finland
Liesmaa, M., Väinämöisenkatu 9 B 19, 00100 Helsinki 10

France
Abitol, Y., 66 Avenue Victor Hugo, 75116 Paris
Aron-Rosa, D., Hopital Trousseau, 24 Av. du Docteur Arnold-Netter, Paris
    12
Barbier, A., 2 Place Saint Jacques, Besançon
Bonnin, P., 6, Rue des Peupliers, 02270 Bois Colombes
Bregeat, P., Rue Théodule-Ribot, Paris 17
Cabanis, E.A., 28 Rue de Charenton, 75571 Paris
Clay, C., 25 à 29 Rue Manin, 75019 Paris
Derremeaux, C., 25 à 29 Rue Manin, 75019 Paris
Diconstanzo, P., Fond. Rothschild, Manin 25, 75019 Paris
Iba-Zizen, M.Th., 28 Rue de Charenton, 75571 Cedex 12, Paris
Lasjaunias, P., 25 à 29 Rue Manin, 75019 Paris
Lebuisson, D.A., 24 Avenue du Docteur Arnold-Netter, Paris 12
Marchac, D., 24 Avenue du Docteur Arnold-Netter, Paris 12
Merlihot, M., 71 Boulevard Notre Dame, 13006 Marseille
Mouly, A.J., Les Borromees, Bat X 3 T. de la Fourragere, 13012 Marseille
Passot, M., Rue Damrémont 133, 75018 Paris
Poujol, J., 108 Avenue du Général Michel-Bizot, 75012 Paris

Ris, M., Chamonix
Rodallec, A., 24 Rue Edouard Nortier, 92000 Neuilly S/S
Toufic, N., 69 Rue Haxo, 75020 Paris
Vignaud, J., 25 à 29 Rue Manin, 75019 Paris

German Dem. Republic
Lommatzsch, P., Städtisches Klinikum Berlin-Buch, Karowerstrasse 11,
 1115 Berling-Buch

Italy
Bonavolontà, G., Seconda Clinica Oculistica, Policlinico Nuovo, Napoli
Cennamo, G., Seconda Clinica Oculistica, Policlinico Nuovo, Napoli
Gerosa, M., Via Giustiniani 5, Padova 351000
Gerosa-Tomazzoli, L., Instituto di Clinica Oculistica dell' Università di
 Padova, Padova 351000
Iraci, G., Università di Padova, Padova
Salvolini, U., Corso Stamira 49, Ancona 60100

Indonesia
Aswan-Gumansalangi, E., Jalan Kemjeran 6, Soerabaja
Bakri, A.B., Darmawangsa, Dalam Selapan 17, Soerabaja
Kadi, J., Jalan Tidar 17, Soerabaja
Sanjoto, H., Jakarta
Santoso, R., Medical Faculty of the University of Soerabaja, Soerabaja
Suwono, W., Jalan Diponegoro 213, Soerabaja
Tamin-Radjamin, R.K., Jalan Kalimantan 14, Soerabaja

Iran
Chams, H., Hafez Avenue, Teheran

Ireland
Dwyer Joyce, P., 11 Merrion Square, Dublin 2

Japan
Fujino, T., 35 Shinamomachi, Shinjuku-ku, Tokyo 160
Fukado, Y., 1-8-5 Nagasaki, Toshima-ku, Tokyo 171
Hamada, R., 6-7-1 Nishishinjuku, Shinjuku-ku, Tokyo
Imachi, J., 1652-Venoyama, Mikagecho, Kobe
Inoue, Y., Shibuya-ku jingumae 6-33-3, Tokyo
Kaneko, A., 5-1 Tsukiji Chuwo-ku, Tokyo 104
Kawai, K., 2-450 Tejin-cho, Kodaira-shi, Tokyo
Makita, T., 2-4-1 Tsukimi, Fukui City, 910
Matsuo, H., 6-7-1 Nishishinjuku, Shinjuku-ku, Tokyo

Okuzawa, L., Okamoto, Higashinada, Kobe

Ozawa, T., 7-3-1 Hongo, Bunkyo-Ku, Tokyo

Shimo-Oko, M., Akamatsu 2-2-16, Nada Kobe

The Netherlands

Abdelgawad, M.M., Wilhelmina Gasthuis, Dept. of Ophthalmology, Amsterdam

Akker, A., van den, Bachtstraat 2, Amsterdam

Baarsma, G.S., Schiedamse Vest 180, Rotterdam

Bazuin, M. Wilhelmina Gasthuis, Eerste Helmersstraat 104, Amsterdam

Bergen, M.P., Strandvliet 46, Amstelveen

Bertens, P., Milosdreef 13, Utrecht

Blaauw, G., Dijkzigt Ziekenhuis, Rotterdam

Bleeker, G.M., Muzenplein 1, Amsterdam

Boen-Tan, Y., Kathleen Ferrierlaan 34, Amstelveen

Brenkman, R.F., Vossenschwanslaan 142, Woerden

Buiter, C.T., Oostersingel 59, Groningen

Bijsterveld, O.P. van, Prinses Marijkeweg 4, Houten

Crone, R.A., De Custerstraat 19, Amsterdam

Dalen, J.Th.W. van, Wilhelmina Gasthuis, Dept. of Ophthalmology, Amsterdam

Dethmers, H.W., Staniastate 12, Almelo

Dorsman, H.W. Wilhelmina Gastduis, Eerste Helmersstraat 104, Amsterdam

Gelderman, P.W., Veer Allee 54, Zwolle

Gier, D.L. de, B.W. Laan 164, Amersfoort

Gillissen, J.P.A., Pekkendam 3, Amsterdam

Goettsch, F.J.B., Veer Allee 7, Zwolle

Gommers, P.A.M., A. v. 's-Gravesandestraat 82, Rotterdam

Gortzak-Moorstein, N., Muzenplein 7, Amsterdam

Haan, A.B. de, Valeriusstraat 163, Amsterdam

Henry, P., Stationsweg 23, Leiden

Hornstra, H., Academisch Ziekenhuis, Dept. of Ophthalmology, Rijnsburweg 10, Leiden

Horst-Breetvelt, H. van der, Corn. van der Lindenstraat 33, Amsterdam

Hoying, P.F.J., Houtrijk 21, Nieuw-Vennep

Jansen-Capriles, G.J.A., Zonneweilaan 7, Vught

Jong, B.D. de, Kerklaan 4, De Bilt

Jong, D.H. de, Leopoldlaan 37, Uithoorn

Keizer, R.J.W. de, Koopvaardijstraat 52, Zaandam

Kerlen, C.H., Alb. Perkstraat 50, Hilversum

Kok-van Alphen, C.C., Warmonderweg 12, Oegstgeest

Koornneef, L., Dorpsstraat 47, Zuiderwoude

Kuik, D.J. van, Händellaan 55, Enschede
Kuiper, J., Overspitting 30, Joure (Fr)
Kurstjens, J.H., Wassenaarse weg 29, Den Haag
Kusen, G.J., Wilhelmina Gasthuis, Eerste Helmersstraat 104, Amsterdam
Lefèbre, A., H. Swarthlaan 109, Groningen
Liem H.K., Elsbeek 33, Zwolle
Linden, H.J. van der, Waterhoenhof 7, Purmerend
Lindenburg, P.A.W., Prinses Marielaan 4, Amersfoort
Los, J.A., Janshof 21, Abcoude
Maren J.G. van, Abel Tasmanlaan 42, Gouda
Meer, J. van der, Wilhelmina Gasthuis, Dept. of Ophthalmology, Amsterdam
Mesker, R.P., Minervaplein 44, Amsterdam
Meulen, J.C.H. van der, Lambertweg 40, Rotterdam
Nijgaard, P., Prinsestraat 8, Cadzand
Oei, T.H. Koninginneweg 257, Amsterdam
Oosterhuis, J.A., Prinsenweg 57, Wassenaar
Oosterink, J.G., De Bosporus 45, Amstelveen
Oudhof, G., Ferd. Huycklaan 46, Baarn
Peeters, F., Wilhelmina Gasthuis, Dept. of Radiology, Amsterdam
Peeters, H.J.F., Ruimzicht 322, Amsterdam
Pol, B.A.E. van der, Hélène Swarthlaan 15, Groningen
Prick, L.J.J.M., St. Oolofspoort 5, Amsterdam
Renkema, H.F., Campersingel 61, Groningen
Ros, F.E., Max Havelaarlaan 329, Amstelveen
Rozemeyer, J.A., Roosendaalseweg 29, Etten-Leur
Scheffer, C.H., 2e Beukenlaan 8, Apeldoorn
Schepel, S.J., Mozartstraat 28, Nieuwerkerk a/d IJssel
Schipper, J., Academisch Ziekenhuis, Catharijnesingel 101, Utrecht
Schoeman, A.N., Wilhelmina Gasthuis, Dept. of Ophthalmology, Amster-
dam
Slooten, E.A. van, Prinsengracht 973, Amsterdam
Smith, G.M., Wulverderlaan 32, Santpoort
Snow, G.B., Vrije Universiteit, De Boelelaan 1117, Amsterdam
Stilma, J.S., Vrije Universiteit, De Boelelaan 1117, Amsterdam
Tan, A.S.T., Limburghof 15, Amsterdam
Tan, K.E.W.P., Jan Steenlaan 16, Bilthoven
Tjan, T.T. de Kempenaerstraat 88, Oegstgeest
Tjia, D.T.T., Vrije Universiteit, De Boelelaan 1117, Amsterdam
Touber, J.L., Borssenburg 42, Amstelveen
Valk, L.E.M., Rooseveltlaan 20, Helmond
Veld, M. in 't, Academisch Ziekenhuis, Rijnsburgerweg 10, Leiden
Velzeboer, C.M.J., Oranje Nassaulaan 18″, Amsterdam
Verbeek, A.M., De Weezenhof 66-43, Nijmegen
Verbeeten, B.W.J.M., Wilhelmina Gasthuis, Dept. of Radiology, Amsterdam

Vermey-Keers, Chr., Wassenaarseweg 62, Leiden
Versteeg, N.T., Wilhelmina Gasthuis, Dept. of Ophthalmology, Amsterdam
Versteege, C., Wilhelmina Gasthuis, Amsterdam
Vieluoye, G.J., Sweilandstraat 26, Warmond
Vrooland, J., Eastonstraat 87, Amsterdam
Wezer, J.E.C.M. van, Van Boerzelaerlaan 34, Den Haag
Wildervanck de Blécourt, P., Dijkzigt Ziekenhuis, Rotterdam
Witmer, J.P., Wilhelmina Gasthuis, Dept. of Ophthalmology, Amsterdam
Wijngaarde, R., Oogziekenhuis Rotterdam, Schiedamsevest 180, Rotterdam
Zeijntjes, G.A., Genistalaan 17, Apeldoorn

Norway
Bertelsen, T., Haukelandsbakken 26, 5000 Bergen
Borthne, O.A., Nordland Sentralsykehus, N-8000 Bod
Bynke, H., Väpplingvägen 17 C, Lund
Syversen, K., Solbakken 1, 3000 Drammen

Surinam
Themen, Chr.G.W., Prinsessestraat 39, Paramaribo

Sweden
Brismar, G., Persikev 17, S-22355 Lund
Brismar, J., Persikev 17, S-22355 Lund
Jerneld, B., Karolinska Sjuhuset, 104 01 Stockholm
Kock, E., Karolinska Sjukhuset, 104 01 Stockholm
Mertens, O., Röingegatan 33, S-281 00 Hässleholm
Prame, G., Slalomgatan 14, Västeras 72240
Singh, G., Karolinska Sjukhuset, 104 01 Stockholm
Tengroth, B., Karolinska Sjukhuset, 104 01 Stockholm
Wennhall, O., Jakobsberggatan 28, 722 13 Västerås

Switzerland
Bigar, F., Augenklinik Kantonspital, Raminstrasse 100, 8091 Zürich
Bosshard, C., Berghaldenstrasse 4, CH-9010, St. Gallen
Fabinyi, C.E., 1 Rue Achille Marguin, 2900 Porrentruy-Bern
Huber, A., Stadelhoferstrasse 42, Zürich
Spiess, H., Zürich
Wieser, D., Universität Augenklinik, Mittlerestrasse 91, CH-4056 Basel

United Kingdom
Bosanquet, R.C., Manchester Royal Eye Hospital, Oxford Road, Manchester
Chavis, R.M., Moorfields Eye Hospital, City Road, London EC1V 2PD
Coster, D., Moorfields Eye Hospital, City Road, London EC1V 2 PD
Gordon, D., 2 Gooden Court, Sudbury Hill, Harrow, Middlesex HAI 3 PZ

Lawton, N.F., Moorfields Eye Hospital, City Road, London EC1V 2 Pd
Levy, I., Moorfields Eye Hospital, City Road, London EC1V 2 PD
Lloyd, G.A.S., Dept. Radiology, Royal National Throat Nose and Ear Hospital, Gray's Inn Road, London WC1X8DA
MacFaul, P., Harley Street, London WIN IHH
Restori, M., Moorfields Eye Hospital, City Road, London EC1V 2 PD
Smith, V.H., Birmingham & Midland Eye Hospital, Church Street, Birmingham B3 2NS
Wright, J., Moorfields Eye Hospital, City Road, London EC1V 2 PD

U.S.A.
Blodi, F.C., University of Iowa, Iowa City, Ia 52240
Bullock, J.D., 60 Wyoming Street, Dayton, Ohio 45409
Callahan, A., 903 South 21st Street, Birmingham, Alabama 35205
Carrol, R.P., 1889 Summit Avenue, St. Paul, MN 55105
Grove, A.S., Dept. of Ophthalmology, Mass. Eye and Ear Infirmary, 243 Carles Street, Boston, Mass. 02114
Huang, T.T., University of Texas, Medical Branche, Galveston, Tex 77550
Jakobiec, F.A., 73 East 71st Street, New York N.Y. 10021
Kara, G.B., 654 Madison Avenue, New York N.Y. 10021
Kennedy, P.J., 32 Hampden Road, Upper Darby, Pa. 19082
Kronenberg, B., 605 Park Avenue, New York, N.Y. 10021
Menachof, I., 2634 Grand Avenue, Waukegan III 60085
Ossoinig, K.C., Dept. of Ophthalmology, University of Iowa, Hospitals and Clinics, Iowa City, Iowa
Sisler, H.A., 34 West 12th Street, New York, N.Y. 10011
Smith, B., 32 East 64th Street Suite One E., New York, N.Y. 10021
Snow Jones, I., 73 East 71st Street, New York, N.Y. 10021
Trokel, S.L., 635 West 165th Street, New York, N.Y. 10032
Walata, E.F., 563 Broadway, Everett 02149 Mass.
Weber, A.L., Mass. Eye and Ear Infirmary, Dept. of Radiology, 243 Charles Street Boston, Mass. 02114

OPENING SPEECH

G.M. BLEEKER

(Amsterdam, The Netherlands)

The organizers and sponsors of the 'Third International Symposium on Orbital Disorders', represented by
1. the Orbital Centre of the Eye Hospital of the University of Amsterdam,
2. the New York Eye and Ear Infirmary,
3. the Netherlands Ophthalmic Research Institute (I.O.I.), and
4. the Netherlands Ophthalmological Society, consider it a great privilege to receive so many guests, from so many countries, from so far away.

You wonder why it is, this world-wide interest in the orbit and its disorders, this tremendous attention to such a small geographical area of the body? The orbit is one of the vital parts of the head, surrounded by a number of structures of such importance that each one is covered by its own medical speciality. Neurologist, neurosurgeon, ophthalmologist, otorhino-laryngologist and maxillo-facial surgeon are all in touch with the orbit and its disorders. From this point of view it is more or less suprising to find the orbit without a patronage of its own. However, the number and variety of these disorders are impressive and the sophistication of the diagnostic and therapeutic armature is so extreme that it is impossible for one single person or discipline to handle orbital disorders at top grade level.

Interdisciplinary consultation and concentration of the material in a limited number of centres have considerably improved our technical skill and clinical experience during the last decade. It is because of the need for interdisciplinary consultation that an orbital symposium thrives.

It is true that nowadays ophthalmological meetings occasionally include orbital disorders in their program. It is also true that internal medicine devotes an occasional meeting to endocrine exophthalmos and that oto-rhino-laryngologists occasionally touch on the subject of orbital complications, but these meetings are always intended to inform the participants of the latest developments in orbitology as far as these are of interest for the members of the discipline concerned.

The gratifying response to this symposium on orbital disorders may serve to illustrate that a meeting where the orbital disorder is placed centrally, with' all the complications draped around it, is filling a clear gap in the system of medical information.

During the present meeting you will be confronted with a proposal to found an 'International Society for Orbital Disorders' in order to promote mutual contact and exchange of information at international and regional levels.

It was eight years ago that the First International Symposium on Orbital Fractures was held in Amsterdam. Although on a small scale, it was this symposium that started a lively interest in orbital disorder. The second symposium was held in 1973, and it culminated in a first class display of pathology, angioradiology and ultrasonography of the orbit.

You will see that the present symposium flies the flag of computerized tomography of which you will enjoy the latest developments. It will become clear that ultrasonography and angiography have hardly lost ground to this new radiological technique, and that it is precisely a combination of the three methods that is essential. Moreover, this meeting will bear evidence of reviving interest in orbital anatomy where new techniques have opened the gates to unexpected new fields.

Further news is coming of the diagnostic possibilities in endocrine exophthalmos where the Thyrotropin-releasing hormone and the T.S.H. test have added so much to the accuracy of defining the nature of exophthalmos.

I would like to conclude by expressing our gratitude to the University of Amsterdam that made the generous gesture of offering the dignified surroundings of the old University building as a stage for this symposium.

In addition, we have to acknowledge our debt to the Minister of Science and Education, together with the Minister of Health and the municipal authorities of Amsterdam for receiving the members of this symposium in the beautiful Van Gogh Museum tomorrow night.

The Third International Symposium on Orbital Disorders is opened.

SUMMARY OF THE THIRD INTERNATIONAL SYMPOSIUM
ON ORBITAL DISORDERS
September 5–7, 1977

BERNARD KRONENBERG
(USA)

It is my pleasant task to summarize the proceedings of the 3rd International Symposium. It has become tradition for me to do this, because I am doing it for the second time. Such is the manner in which Tradition is born.

The 3rd International Symposium on Orbital Disorders was convened at a very crucial period in the technology of the diagnosis of orbital disorders. Since the last meeting, four years ago, the management of orbital disorders has been revolutionized and a new dimension has been added. A 'Star was Born' — Computerized Axial Tomography — formerly known as CAT.

All of you are aware that a CAT has nine lives and thus this technique is assured of a long existence and will survive many modifications. This little CAT has grown into a roaring TIGER in only a few years. Enthusiasm at this Symposium for CAT was obvious, and many authors exchanged their experiences with CAT both axial and coronal, in a large series of presentations. There were several voices of caution, not in a negative fashion but to emphasize the need of combining it with older techniques, such as ultrasound, phlebography and arteriogaphy for the definitive localization of orbital lesions. Several papers compared the diagnostic value of these techniques.

The papers on the anatomy of the orbit added a great deal to our knowledge. There were a number of beautiful studies on the vasculature of the orbit, especially the veins, giving us a new insight into the blood circulation of the orbit. Orbital connective tissue was the subject of an exhibit as well as of a paper and made us understand the close relationships between the connective tissue septa and the vessels. These papers were of the highest scientific quality and perhaps explained some puzzling results in muscle surgery. The vascular supply of the extraocular muscles was beautifully demonstrated by radiographic techniques. One paper showed the ophthalmic artery can have various origins.

The optic nerve was the subject of several unusual papers. One paper described a very rare cyst of the optic nerve and the management of this case. Hypoplasia of the optic nerve and its differential diagnosis was discussed in great detail. The use of CAT to evaluate papilledema was

3

indeed challenging. These papers, among others, added to the spice of the meeting.

The medical aspect of dysthyroid disease was discussed. The superiority of TRH Test in comparison with T3 was demonstrated. It is most valuable in combination with the CAT in unilateral exophthalmos. A possible relationship between thyroid disease and myasthenia gravis was presented. The mortality rate of orbital infections was shown to be reduced to almost zero by the intensive use of anti-biotics, giving the patients a much better prognosis. An interesting paper on the poor prognosis of mucormycosis of the orbit was presented.

Several papers on painful ophthalmoplegia, known as Tolosa-Hunt Syndrome were presented. The diagnostic criteria and the value of corticosteroid therapy were demonstrated. The disease although rare must be managed properly.

Blow-out fractures, of course, received some attention. In particular the muscle problems associated with this injury were discussed. An experimental model demonstrated the force required to cause the blow-out fracture and concluded that less force was required to cause an intra-orbital fracture than was necessary to traumatize the eye-ball.

Ultra-sonography has not been abandoned by the rush for the CAT, but actually in many papers the combined use of ultrasonography and CAT was stressed. In addition an excellent paper on 'C' scan was presented. Ultra-sound is still very much alive.

No orbital meeting can be complete without a discussion of orbital surgery. Two aspects of decompression were presented — lateral and medial. A film demonstrating a rather heroic procedure for remodelling of a craniostenosis made the audience sit up and wonder. Facial anomalies and associated eye problems were the subject of several papers. Reconstructive surgery was shown.

There were very many fascinating papers on the management of orbital tumors, pseudo-tumors, neurofibromas, benign and malignant tumors. These papers should be read in the published form. One author called attention to the presence of germinal follicles on biopsy or pseudo-tumors. This was considered a good prognostic sign to determine whether the pseudo-tumors would recur. In addition there were several thought provoking papers on the causation of choroideal folds. The possibility of traction on the optic nerve causing these folds was expressed by one author.

Radio-active scanning techniques were presented and it was stressed that these techniques should be used in addition to ultrasonography and computerized axial tomography in the differential diagnosis of orbital disorders.

An excellent paper on ossifying fibroma was presented, calling attention to this frequently overlooked disease.

A new instrument for Ophthalmodynamometry was presented. A question was raised as to its accuracy in determining the true diastolic pressure of the ophthalmic artery.

4

In this brief presentation, I cannot mention all the subjects covered, but they were all of the highest quality.

The concept of an International Orbital Society, I believe, will come to fruition. Most of the participants of the Symposium were in favor of this Society and voted for its formation. I want to thank our hosts of the Orbital Centre and the Netherlands Ophthalmological Society for their very efficient organization and excellent program. We had a very instructive and enlightening meeting. I will look forward to the next Orbital Symposium.

Proc. 3rd Int. Symp. on Orbital Disorders, Amsterdam 1977

MODERN DIAGNOSTIC METHODS FOR ORBITAL LESIONS

F.C. BLODI

(Iowa City, Iowa, USA)

We have a number of valuable modern diagnostic methods available which make the detection and classification of an orbital lesion relatively easy and highly reliable. The diagnostic work-up of a patient with unilateral exophthalmus has to proceed logically and step-by step:

1. *History:* The main questions are whether the patient has any other signs or symptoms of Graves disease and what is the duration of the exophthalmus. The answers may give us a clue as to the underlying cause. The rapidly increasing proptosis due to an orbital rhabdomyosarcoma is a good example. A history of chronic periorbital sinus troubles would point toward a mucocele or a pyocele. The history of a systemic affection (leukemia, vasculitis, etc.) may indicate an orbital involvement by this disease.

2. *Physical examination:* The direction and extent of the exophthalmus may give us a clue as to the site of the lesion. Interference with ocular motility, pressure on the globe, damage to the optic nerve and other factors have to be evaluated.

Ausculation and palpation still remain an important aspect in the diagnostic work-up. The palpation should be done vigorously using the little finger. When a tumor can be palpated, its consistency and surface can be evaluated.

3. *Evaluation for Graves disease:* We always have to keep in mind that the most frequent cause for a unilateral exophthalmus is the orbitotopathy of Graves disease. The systemic manifestations may be minimal and even the most sophisticated laboratory tests may be inconclusive. The clinical picture (retraction of the lids, periorbital edema, etc.) is often indicative for this condition.

4. *Radiologic examinations:* Plain skull x-rays are indicated in every patient with an orbital lesion. The yield of positive findings is admittedly small, but important clues may be obtained.

Tomography will be necessary when a bony lesion is suspected.

Invasive radiodiagnostic methods used to be popular, but they have become obsolete and have been superseded by modern non-invasive methods, such as echography or computed tomography. Orbitography (injecting air or a radiopaque material into the muscle cone) had to be abandoned because of the rate of complications. This diagnostic method, as well as phlebography, is not only painful and unpleasant to the patient but also gives incomplete information to the examiner. While these methods may delineate

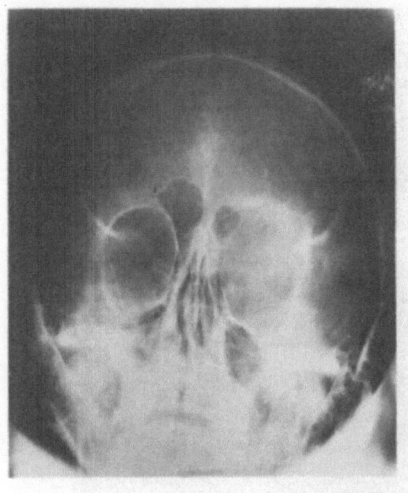
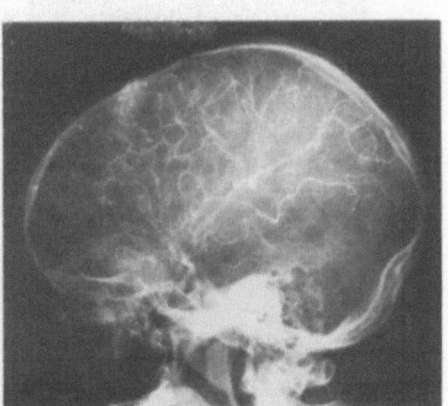
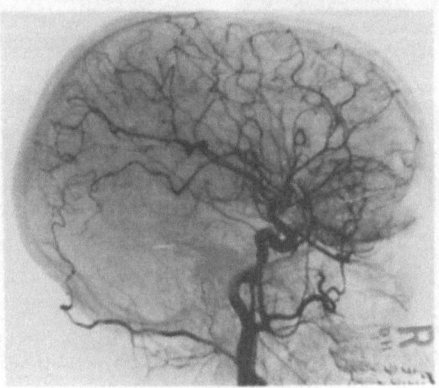

Fig. 1. A) Plain x-ray picture shows lesion of left orbital roof; B) Angiogram of the same patient: The displacement of the intracranial vessels around the frontal lesion is well visible; C) By the subtraction method the outlines of the orbital lesion are demarcated.

an orbital lesion as to its size and site, they can give little information on its nature.

Arteriography, on the other hand, is still occasionally indicated. It should be used in patients in whom a vascular anomaly is suspected or in whom the lesion may involve the intracranial cavity (Fig. 1).

5. *Echography* has become the most valuable diagnostic method for the detection of orbital mass lesions. The accuracy of this method exceeds 98% and in nearly 90% of the patients a correct tissue diagnosis can be made. The B-scan technique is used for better demonstration and documentation of the site and the shape of the lesion. The standardized A-scan is, however, necessary to establish a differential diagnosis and an experienced examiner can translate the tracings into a reliable histologic diagnosis (Fig. 2).

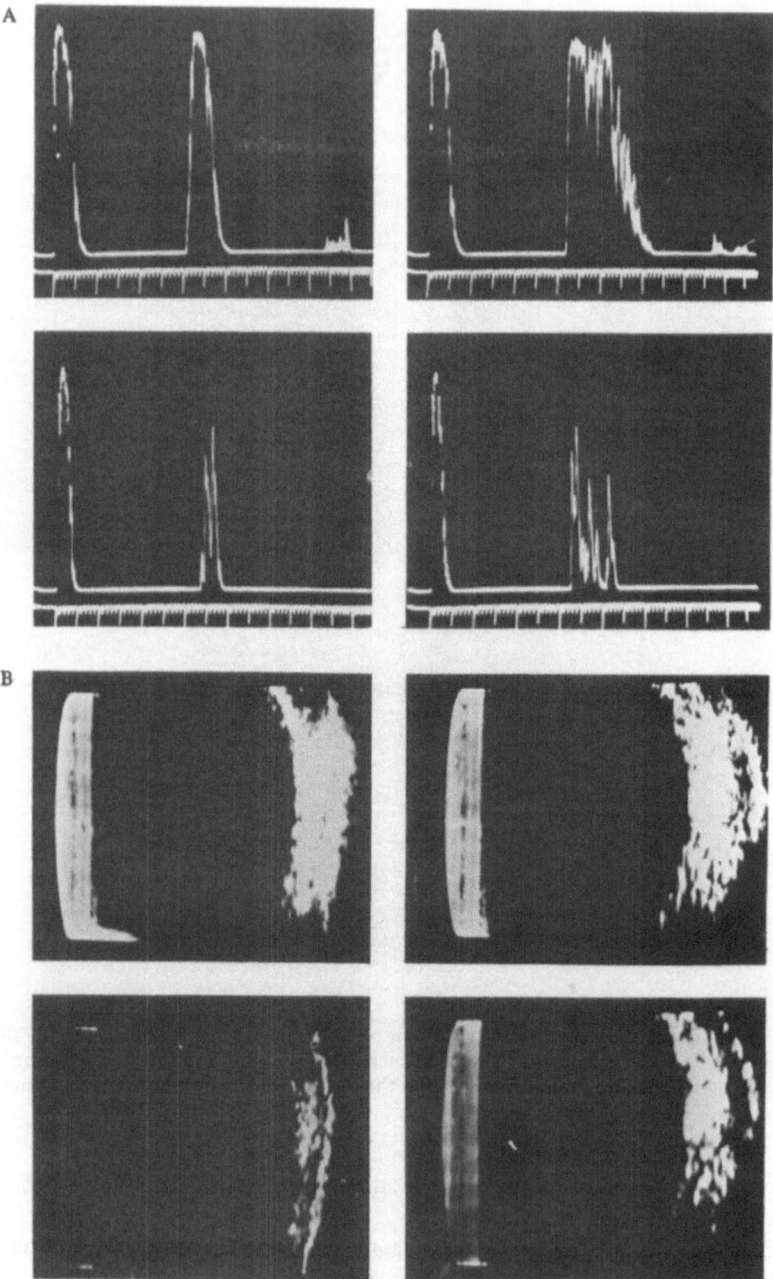

Fig. 2. A) Examples of an A-scan echogram in a patient with fibrous dysplasia of the orbital bones. The two pictures on the left side are from the affected side. The orbital echoes are nearly absent as the pathologic bone nearly touches the posterior ocular pole. The right pictures show normal orbital echoes. The lower pictures are obtained at reduced tissue sensitivity and the spike from the sclera and the orbital bone spike are now slightly separated.

B) A B-scan echogram for the same patient. The pictures on the left side are from the affected orbit and show the close proximity of bone to the eye. The pictures on the right show normal orbital echoes. The lower pictures are taken at reduced tissue sensitivity.

Ossoinig (1974) has proposed a differential diagnostic schema which also takes into account topographic and kinetic echography.

While this type of diagnostic examination has many advantages (reliability, non-invasive nature, relative low cost) a physician experienced in the methodology has to supervise the examination and evaluate the results.

6. The other great advance in the diagnosis of orbital lesions has been the introduction of *computerized axial tomography* (CAT). With appropriate positioning the orbits can be depicted and pathologic processes can be illustrated with an ease not matched by any other method (Fig. 3). Compared with echography computerized tomography has two disadvantages: 1) It is much more expensive. Not only is the equipment extremely expensive, the charges for an examination are several times that for an echographic examination. 2) The present methods give us a good clue as to the size and site of a lesion, but often cannot establish a differential diagnosis or a tissue diagnosis as we usually can obtain with the quantitative A-scan echography.

There is, however, no question that computerized tomography adds considerably to our diagnostic armamentarium for orbital lesions. If available, it should be obtained when other diagnostic methods give equivocal results.

Of great advantage has been in our hands the judicious combined use of echography and computed tomography.

The characteristic findings of these two diagnostic methods in the most important orbital lesions are:

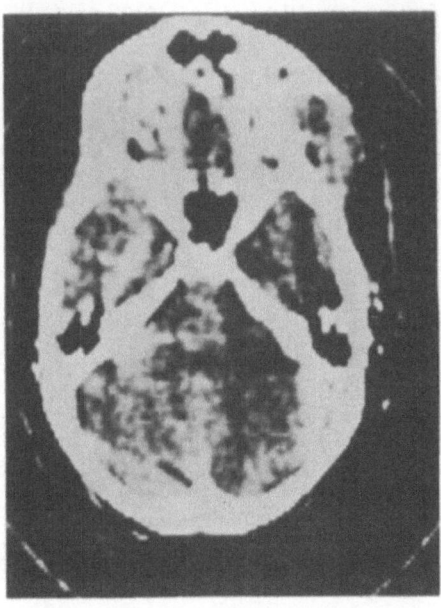

Fig. 3. EMI-scan of an orbital osteoclastoma on the right side. There is considerable destruction of the lateral orbital wall.

9

1) No orbital tumor present

This negative result is a most important and frequent one. Many patients are referred in whom the presence of an orbital tumor is suspected. These are patients with a vague unilateral exophthalmus, with Graves orbitopathy which is difficult to diagnose, with orbital edema, etc. In these patients an orbital tumor cannot be easily excluded. Before the two modern diagnostic methods were available it was often impossible to exclude the presence of an orbital lesion and an exploratory orbitotomy was often necessary. This is hardly ever the case any more. A quick echographic screening will establish the fact that no tumefaction is present in the orbit. The correct diagnosis can then be made and the appropriate treatment initiated.

2) Graves disease

The echographic characteristics consist of:
a) absence of circumscribed tumor mass in the orbit
b) increased bulk of the orbital tissues, especially of the orbital fat with increased acoustic reflectivity
c) thickening of the ectraocular muscles (Fig. 4)
   On EMI-scan the thickened muscles may be seen at the apex of the orbit. They should not be confused with an orbital neoplasm.

3) Cavernous hemangioma

The cavernous hemangioma is a benign lesion and probably the most frequent orbital tumefaction regardless of age of the patient.

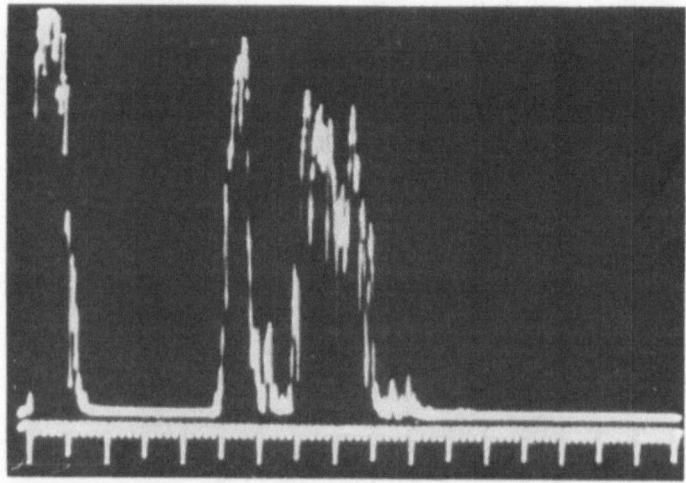

Fig. 4. Thickened medial rectus in a patient with Graves disease. There is a zone of low reflectivity between two high spikes, the first one of which presents the posterior ocular wall.

Echographically, it is characterized by a high acoustic reflectivity, strong sound attenuation, round shape and regular structure.

The EMI-scan will show the well-outlined, round tumor within the muscle cone.

The diagnosis of this benign lesion can now be made with such a high degree of reliability that an operation has become indicated only in those patients in whom the tumor produces a cosmetic blemish or causes a disturbance of visual function. The majority of patients with orbital hemangioma need only to be followed and observed.

4) Small cell tumors

This group comprises all lesions which consist of dense, homogenous infiltrations with relatively small cells. This includes lymphomas, inflammatory pseudotumors (benign lymphoid hyperplasia) and most sarcomas.

All these tumors have in common a low acoustic reflectivity which is due to the homogenous infiltration which produces no acoustic interfaces (Fig. 5). They usually show a hard consistency and have a slight sound attenuation.

Irregular soft tissue densities are seen on the CAT-scan. These densities may show considerable contrast enhancement (Fig. 6).

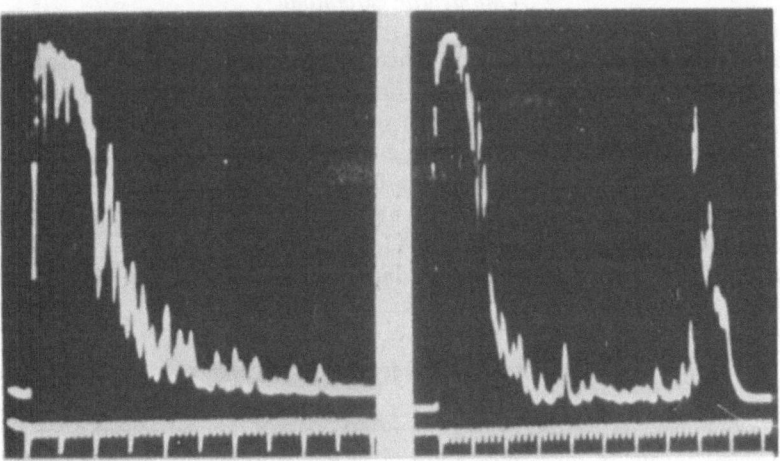

Fig. 5. A-scan picture of an inflammatory pseudotumor of the orbit characterized by low acoustic reflectivity. On the left is the picture of a diffuse infiltrative process without any sharp border. The right picture shows an encapsulated pseudotumor. The high spike on the right presents the posterior capsule.

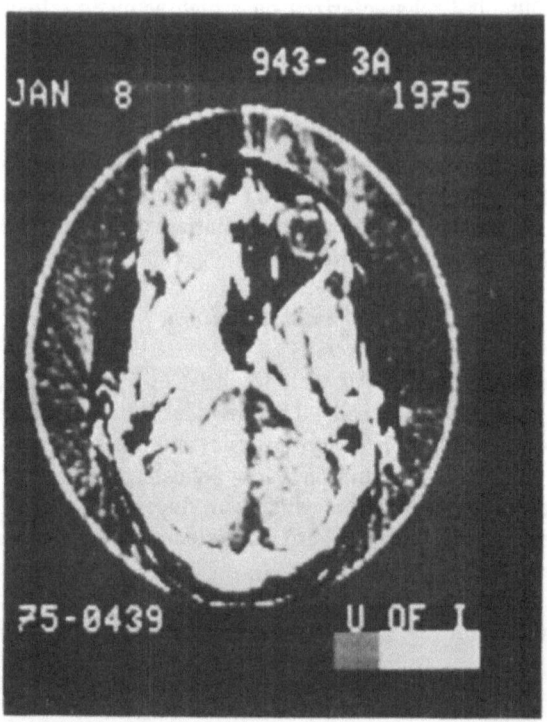

Fig. 6. EMI-scan of sarcoma on the left side. The tumor nearly fills the orbit.

5) Metastatic carcinoma

These lesions have a high acoustic reflectivity, as the strands and chords of neoplastic cells invading the orbital tissues produce numerous layers and membranes which strongly reflect the sound beam. The center of the metastatic tumor, however, shows homogeneity because of the dense cellular infiltration, producing a low acoustic reflectivity. The entire lesion produces the characteristic V-pattern with the high reflectivity in the periphery and the low reflectivity in the center of the lesion (Fig. 7).

On the CAT-scan these lesions produce irregular densities in the orbital tissues.

6) Optic nerve gliomas and meningiomas

These two lesions cannot easily be differentiated by echography or on CAT-scan, except in those meningiomas in which numerous calcified psammoma bodies produce increased reflectivity and shadows.

The lesions cause a widening of the optic nerve echo. They are of medium acoustic reflectivity, sharply outlined and of a typically elongated shape. The sound attentuation (angle kappa) is average, about 45 degrees (Fig. 8).

12

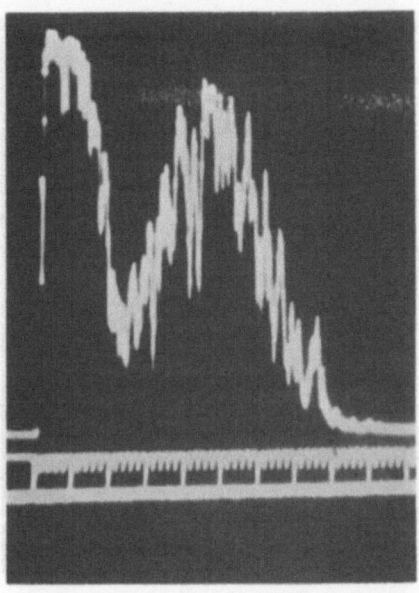

Fig. 7. The typical V-pattern of the A-scan echogram from a metastatic carcinoma in the orbit.

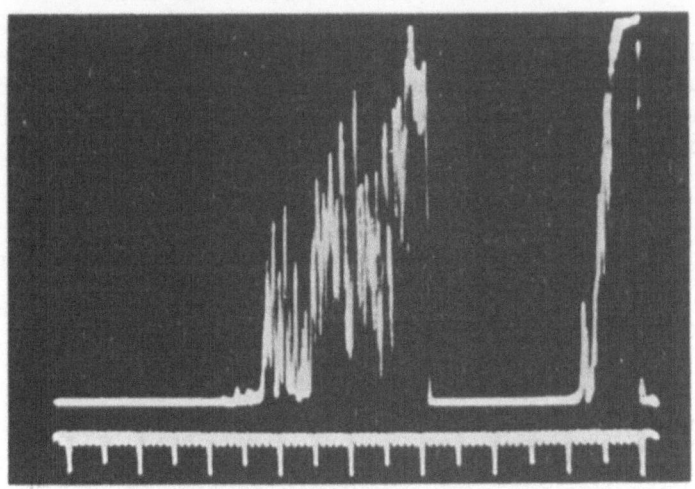

Fig. 8. Echogram from a meningioma of the orbital optic nerve.

On the EMI-scan the thickening of the optic nerve is usually well visible (Fig. 9).

7) Neurofibroma

The tumor signals show on echography high reflectivity and a strong sound attentuation.

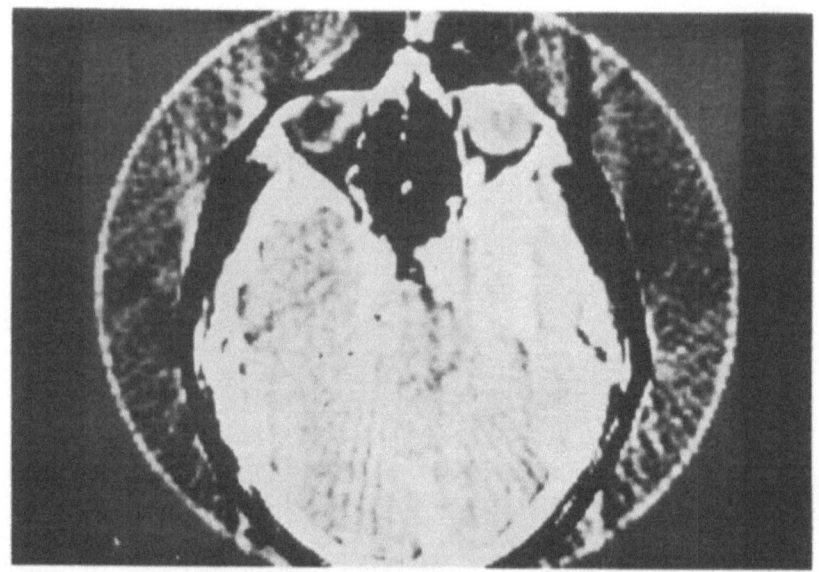

Fig. 9. The same tumor is seen at the apex of the right orbit.

8) Mucoceles and pyoceles of a periorbital sinus

Here, the defect in the orbital bones can usually be detected on plain x-rays, echography and on the CAT-scan. The lesion is well-outlined and round. It shows a low acoustic reflectivity. The bony defect is large, regular and confined to one area.

REFERENCES

Ossoinig, K.C. & F.C. Blodi. Diagnosis of orbital tumors. In: Current Concepts in Ophthalmology, IV (F.C. Blodi, ed.). C.V. Mosby Co., St Louis (1974).
Hodes, B.L. & P. Weinberg. A combined approach for the diagnosis of orbital disease. *Arch. Ophthal. 95: 781 (1977).*

Author's address:
Department of Ophthalmology
University of Iowa
Iowa City, Iowa 52242
USA

Proc. 3rd Int. Symp. on Orbital Disorders, Amsterdam 1977

COMBINED ULTRASONOGRAPHY, COMPUTERIZED TOMOGRAPHY, AND RADIOLOGY IN EVALUATION OF ORBITAL DISEASE

RICHARD L. DALLOW & ALFRED L. WEBER

(Boston, Massachesetts, USA)

INTRODUCTION

Several very effective non-invasive tests have become available for evaluation of orbital disorders in recent years, increasing diagnostic accuracy considerably. Ultrasonography and computerized tomography have each proven capable of demonstrating soft tissue abnormalities, including inflammatory changes as well as tumors, many of which could not be detected with other tests. Hypocycloidal polytomography has improved the evaluation of bony changes often associated with orbital tumors. Vascular contrast studies have a specific role in the diagnosis of arteriovenous malformations and shunts. We have analyzed the results of these tests in a series of 421 consecutive cases of exophthalmos to check their diagnostic accuracy for various orbital problems and to learn of specific sources of errors with them.

CLINICAL MATERIAL

Over a recent two year period we studied 421 patients with exophthalmos. For the cases of unilateral exophthalmos in this group, definitive diagnosis of the specific orbital disorder was established clinically or surgically in 342 patients with an adequate follow-up of at least six months in all cases.
The sources of referral of these patients was quite broad including general hospital populations and the speciality services of endocrine, neurology, neurosurgery, otolaryngology and ophthalmology from several institutions in our geographic area.
The orbital disorders represented in this series were documented by histopathologic study of surgical specimens for all tumors, by endocrine tests for all thyroid related cases, and by clinical behavior and therapeutic responses or surgical exploration in most others.
The distribution of diseases documented in this study is given in Table 1. Tumors of all types, primary and secondary, comprised 34%. Inflammatory disorders including thyroid conditions, cellulitis and pseudotumor, were 50%. Arteriovenous malformations, shunts and fistulas were 4%. Traumatic hemorrhage or foreign bodies were 5%. Bony abnormalities such as fibrous dysplasia, Paget's disease, etc. were 1%. Pseudoproptosis, usually a unilaterally large globe, a shallow bony orbital configuration, or simply a normal

Table 1. Causes of unilateral exophthalamos; 342 consecutive cases

Disease category	Cases	
Tumors	115	34%
Inflammatory conditions	170	50%
Vascular disorders	13	4%
Traumatic changes	16	5%
Bony abnormalities	3	1%
Pseudoproptosis	25	6%
	342	100%

orbital asymmetry, represented 6%. With the wide range of referral sources of patients in this series, we believe the orbital disease distribution found is representative of the general population rather than reflecting a skewed distribution usually seen within any one medical specialty.

TESTING TECHNIQUES

All tests were performed in the laboratories of the Massachusetts Eye and Ear Infirmary and the Massachusetts General Hospital, Boston, Massachusetts, U.S.A. Interpretations of tests were done by experienced physicians. Only tests from the 342 documented cases of unilateral exophthalmos are included in this analysis. Studies were ordered on a somewhat selective basis with consideration of expense, availability and patient tolerance.

Radiographic studies

Plain radiographs of the orbits were taken in 220 cases using the standard projections (Water's, Caldwell, lateral, base and optic foramen views). Hypocycloidal polytomography was done additionally in 170 cases. Major findings were bony and soft tissue abnormalities in the orbits and sinuses associated with tumors.

Computerized axial tomography

The EMI cranial computerized tomographic (CT) scanner was used for orbital and intracranial study in 145 cases. The fine matrix of 160 x 160 gave resolution of 1.5 mm. Variation of the window setting permitted differentiation of all major soft tissue components of the orbit — globe, fat, muscles, and optic nerve. The plane of sections was made parallel to the orbital floor and the width was 8 mm unless special 4 mm sections were needed. Intravenous infusion of iodinated contrast material was done routinely.

With CT scan, tumors were differentiated by density characteristics into cystic and solid types, with contrast uptake indicating a highly vascular lesion. Enlarged extraocular muscles and some diffusely increased density were seen with some inflammatory disorders. Dilated orbital veins may be seen with some arteriovenous shunts.

Ultrasonography

Combined A-scan and B-scan ultrasonography was performed on 297 patients using the water immersion technique and sophisticated electronics and diagnostic criteria described by Coleman and his associates. The ultrasound equipment was manufactured by Sonometrics Systems, Inc., of New York. Multiple horizontal and vertical sections were made on each orbit examined. Weakly focused transducers of both 5 mHz and 10 mHz were used to obtain a combination of good penetration (5 mHz) to the orbital apex, and reasonable resolution of 0.5 mm (10 mHz). The B-scan image demonstrated the two-dimensional morphology of orbital structures and tumors, while the simultaneous A-scan presentation provided the echo characteristics for differentiation of tissue types. The combination of A-scan and B-scan was more valuable than either one display alone.

With ultrasonography the globe, optic nerve, extraocular muscles, orbital fat, and lacrimal gland were all readily demonstrated. Tumors could be characterized into cystic, solid, angiomatous, or infiltrative. Inflammatory changes were recognized as exaggeration of normally occurring structures, i.e. enlarged extraocular muscles with thyroid disorder.

Venography and arteriography

Vascular contrast studies were performed only on patients with specific suspicion of arteriovenous malformations, venous malformations, and as an aid to neurosurgeons for intracranial tumor vascular supply. In general, these invasive studies with potential morbidity were avoided whenever possible in favor of the other tests described here.

RESULTS

Criteria for judging the accuracy of each diagnostic test were established as follows:

A test was considered *correct* if it demonstrated signs unequivocally diagnostic of the orbital disorder that was ultimately found.

Equivocal test results were those showing suspicious but not definitely diagnostic findings of the finally proven orbital disorder.

Incorrect results were test findings interpreted as one type of disease, whereas an entirely different disease was proven by other methods. With regard to tumors, for example, a false positivie incorrect result would be a test interpreted as demonstrating tumor when none was present, and a false negative incorrect result would be the interpretation of inflammation or other disorder when a tumor was, in fact, present.

Normal or non-contributory test findings were grouped separately, and not included in the false negative category.

Original test interpretations were used even though retrospective analysis might have led to a different interpretation in some cases. Similar criteria were applied to the diagnosis made on clinical examination prior to any laboratory testing.

17

For simplification of analysis, orbital disorders were divided into three categories: *tumors, inflammatory diseases,* and all *others.* The 'others' category is somewhat meaningless clinically, since it includes such disparate disorders as vascular malformations and pseudoproptosis, and it is statistically a minor category, although necessary for analysis of the total series.

The accuracy of clinical diagnosis is given in Table 2. Of 315 patients with unilateral exophthalmos examined prior · to any laboratory testing, the specific type of orbital disorder was diagnosed correctly in 39% of cases. This figure was remarkably similar for tumors, inflammatory disorders and other abnormalities. Cases of bilateral exophthalmos were much easier to diagnose clinically because of the prevalence of thyroid disorders, although no figures are given in this study. Clinical signs of specific orbital disorders are well known and will not be reviewed here. The incorrect diagnosis rate of 7% coupled with the equivocal findings in 54% indicates that 61% of unilateral orbital disorders could not be diagnosed on clinical examination alone. We are obviously dependent on laboratory tests to detect diseases in the majority of cases. Even when clinical diagnosis was accurate, the extent of disease, particularly with tumors, could be appreciated only with the tests.

Plain radiography (Table 3) and polytomography (Table 4) are best considered together for analysis. Of the cases in which orbital tumors were actually present, only 38% were diagnosed by plain radiography. With polytomography tumor diagnosis increased to 50% as the equivocal rate was reduced. There were no significant incorrect diagnoses of tumors with radiography; positive findings were, indeed, indicative of tumor. Inflammatory diseases showed essentially no positive radiographic findings except

Table 2. Clinical diagnosis. Accuracy for orbital diagnosis.

Cases	Tumors 124	Inflam. 148	Others 43	Totals 315
Correct	37%	40%	40%	39%
Equivocal	57%	54%	47%	54%
Incorrect	6%	6%	13%	7%
	100%	100%	100%	100%

Table 3. Plain radiography. Accuracy for orbital diagnosis.

Cases	Tumors 95	Inflam. 94	Others 31	Totals 220
Correct	38%	5%	3%	19%
Equivocal	12%	2%	3%	6%
Incorrect	–	–	3%	1%
Normal	50%	93%	91%	74%
	100%	100%	100%	100%

for cellulitis associated with sinusitis. This inflammatory disease category has a low diagnostic rate by radiography, since most appeared normal.

In this series 50% of the tumors were primary in the orbit and 50% secondary. Benign tumors represented 64%, mostly primary types, while the 36% malignant tumors were most commonly secondary. Secondary tumors invading the orbit from the surrounding sinuses, nasopharynx, intracranial tissues, or from metastatic sources characteristically show abnormalities with radiographic studies. Tumors are manifested either by osteolytic or hyperostotic changes. Mucoceles and other benign mass lesions may show smooth attenuation or erosion of bone. Primary orbital tumors, however, rarely show any positive signs except non-specific increased density of soft tissue. Childhood hemangioma producing generalized orbital enlargement is one unusual benign tumor causing bony abnormality.

Increased tissue density on radiography was not a helpful sign in differential diagnosis because it is seen with inflammatory disorders as well as with benign tumors. Opacification of the sinuses is an exception to this statement when it indicates a sinusitis associated with orbital cellulitis.

The overall positive yield of orbital diagnosis with radiography, combining the tumors, inflammatory diseases, and others, was 28% positive diagnostic results. However, radiographic tumor diagnosis was 50% with emphasis on the secondary orbital tumors.

Computerized tomography (CT) (Table 5) with its capacity for demonstrating variable soft tissue densities has a considerably higher accuracy in diagnosis of both tumors and inflammatory disorders. Tumor diagnostic accuracy was 86% correct, showing most primary as well as secondary types. Intravenous contrast infusion was helpful in confirming many suspected

Table 4. Radiographic polytomography. Accuracy for orbital diagnosis.

Cases	Tumors 84	Inflam. 61	Others 25	Totals 170
Correct	50%	8%	4%	28%
Equivocal	5%	3%	–	4%
Incorrect	–	–	–	–
Normal	45%	89%	96%	68%
	100%	100%	100%	100%

Table 5. Computerized tomography. Accuracy for orbital diagnosis.

Cases	Tumors 76	Inflam. 47	Others 22	Totals 145
Correct	86%	43%	23%	62%
Equivocal	11%	4%	9%	8%
Incorrect	1%	15%	9%	7%
Normal	2%	38%	59%	23%
	100%	100%	100%	100%

tumors, as the contrast uptake within a mass lesion corresponds to its degree of vascularity and distinguishes it more readily from surrounding soft tissues. Even in known tumor cases the full extent of most of them was appreciated only with computerized tomography and ultrasonography.

Equivocal findings with CT occurred in 11% of tumor cases, due largely to ambiguous soft tissue masses that could not be adequately characterized. Incorrect diagnosis rate was 1% and normal findings were found in 2% of actual tumor cases. False negative findings were seen with some cystic tumors, such as dermoids and mucoceles, because their density characteristics approximate fat instead of solid tumor.

With inflammatory conditions CT may show enlargement of the extra-ocular muscles, particularly associated with thyroid disease, and occasionally some diffuse increased orbital density with generalized inflammation. The correct diagnosis was made with CT in 43% of inflammatory conditions. A major source of CT error is the mistaking of enlarged muscles at the orbital apex for a tumor. When the vertical rectus muscles are cut obliquely by the scan plane, they appear as a circumscribed round mass in the orbital apex. Furthermore, this mass effect enhances with contrast infusion, thereby meeting all criteria for tumor. The false positive rate of CT for incorrect diagnosis of tumor was 15%, which is a rather significant error rate.

Computerized tomography was capable of detecting other orbital abnormalities, also. A large globe causing pseudoproptosis was evident if the size difference between the two eyes exceeded about 2 to 3 mm. Foreign bodies of all types from trauma were readily detected, regardless of size, because of the marked deflection artifacts created on the scan. Arteriovenous shunts may be suggested by a dilated superior ophthalmic vein coursing obliquely through the superior aspect of the orbit, although this diagnosis requires arteriography for confirmation.

The overall diagnostic accuracy of computerized tomography for all type types of orbital disorders was 62% correct, with 8% equivocal, 7% errors, and 23% normal findings. A striking difference exists between the 86% correct tumor diagnosis and the 43% correct inflammatory disease diagnosis. False negative and false positive tumor diagnoses were significant with CT.

Ultrasonography depicts soft tissues, also, but by an entirely different method. It detects reflections of sound from anatomical interfaces, thus making it particularly effective for graphically demonstrating tissue boundaries. Computerized tomography, on the other hand, works by detecting the photons transmitted through tissues and relating these absorption coefficients to actual tissue densities. Ultrasonography does not penetrate bone well, and therefore is limited to diagnosis within the bony orbit. Its resolution exceeds that of CT, making possible detection of smaller lesions down to 0.5 mm in the orbit.

Ultrasound diagnosis (Table 6) of tumors approximates that of CT with 80% correct, 17% equivocal, and 3% false negative errors. Differentiation of tumor type was somewhat more effective with ultrasonography. Cystic, solid, angiomatous and infiltrative tumors are distinguished with ultrasonography by their characteristics of shape on B-scan and by the sound trans-

Table 6. Ultrasonography. Accuracy for orbital diagnosis.

Cases	Tumors 112	Inflam. 142	Others 43	Totals 297
Correct	80%	87%	42%	78%
Equivocal	17%	6%	23%	13%
Incorrect	3%	1%	5%	2%
Normal	–	6%	30%	7%
	100%	100%	100%	100%

mission and internal tissue echo patterns seen on A-scan. Cystic masses are well seen with ultrasonography, but not with CT, whereas secondary infiltrating tumors are difficult diagnoses with ultrasound and readily apparent with CT.

Inflammatory disorders had characteristic findings with ultrasound in 87% of cases, far more effective than other tests. Enlargement of extraocular muscles, sub-Tenon's and optic nerve sheath edema, and diffuse inflammatory edema of the orbital fat are readily evident on ultrasonography with orbital inflammation. Scanning in the sagittal plane allows this test to identify the enlarged vertical muscles of thyroid disease, thus avoiding the false positive tumor diagnosis seen with CT scan in some of these cases. In only 1% of inflammatory disease cases was tumor diagnosed mistakenly with ultrasound.

In the category of other orbital abnormalities, the large globe of pseudo-proptosis is easily diagnosed with ultrasound even if minor in degree. Hemorrhage is usually apparent also. Orbital foreign bodies may be very difficult because of the high reflectivity of fat interferences. Arteriovenous malformations give no characteristic signs on ultrasonography, although general orbital congestion and occasionally a dilated superior ophthalmic vein may be seen with this test.

Overall orbital diagnostic accuracy with ultrasonography was 78% correct, 13% equivocal, 2% errors, and 7% normal. Ultrasonography appears to be the most versatile technique for soft tissue evaluation in general, but comparable to CT scan for tumor diagnosis. The two studies of ultrasomography and computerized tomography are quite complementary in their capabilities, each correcting for errors of the other. Together these two tests combined were correct in 98% of all cases.

Only a few patients in this series required vascular contrast studies for diagnosis. Venography was helpful in demonstrating venous malformations and arteriography for arteriovenous malformations and carotid-cavernous shunts. Tumors were not seen well or consistently with either test, and both were non-contributory in all inflammatory disorders. The number of cases having vascular contrast studies was too small to be statistically significant. Except for these specific vascular disorders, other tests were preferred for orbital diagnosis.

SUMMARY

We have compiled a series of over 300 consecutive cases of unilateral exophthalmos with definitive diagnosis of the causes of disease process and an adequate follow-up period. Orbital and periorbital tumors constitute 34% of this series, inflammatory diseases including thyroid disorders 50%, arteriovenous abnormalities 4%, and miscellaneous disorders 12%.

All patients were thoroughly evaluated clinically and with appropriate diagnostic tests, including ultrasonography (combined A-scan and B-scan), computerized axial tomography (EMI cranial scan), and radiographic techniques (plain films and hypocycloidal polytomography), orbital venography, and carotid arteriography. Each test was found to have diagnostic capabilities which complemented other studies, depending upon the specific disease process involved. No one test was entirely adequate without the others.

Radiographic studies demonstrated bony abnormality in 50% of tumor cases, but in only 28% of the entire series of exophthalmos cases. Primary orbital tumors had a lower hield with radiography than did secondary tumors. Computerized tomography demonstrated diagnostic soft tissue abnormality in 86% of tumors, 43% of inflammatory diseases, and an overall yield of 62% positive results. Ultrasonography proved the most versatile test for evaluation of orbital soft tissues, with 80% positive results for tumors, 87% for inflammatory disorders, and 78% overall acurate diagnosis. Usefulness of vascular contrast studies was limited to definition of arteriovenous malformations, being somewhat unreliable for tumor diagnosis. Erroneous tumor diagnosis of 7% with computerized tomography and 3% with ultrasonography was corrected by combining these two studies, because they tend to err in opposite directions – computerized tomography showing some abnormal densities that were not tumor, and ultrasonography mistaking some tumors as inflammatory lesions. Combination of these two soft tissue diagnostic tests resulted in 98% correct diagnosis of orbital diseases of all types.

REFERENCES

Ambrose, J., G.A.S. Lloyd & J.E. Wright. A preliminary evaluation of fine matrix computerized axial tomography in diagnosis of orbital space-occupying lesions. *Br. J. Radiol.* 47: *747* (1974).

Baker, H.L., T.P. Kearns, J.K. Campbell & J.W. Henderson. Computerized transaxial tomography in neuroopthalmology. *Am. J. Ophthal.* 78: *285* (1974).

Bilaniuk, L.T. & R.L. Dallow. Diagnostic techniques in orbital surgery. p. 17, in: Complications of Ophthalmic Plastic Surgery (D.B. Soll, ed.). Aesculapius, Birmingham, Alabama (1976).

Brismar, J., K.R. Davis, R.L. Dallow & G. Brismar. Unilateral endocrine exophthalmos: Diagnostic problems in association with computerized tomography. *Neuroradiol.* 12: *21* (1976).

Coleman, D.J. Reliability of ocular and orbital diagnosis with B-scan ultrasonography. Part II: Orbital diagnosis. *Am. J. Ophthal.* 74: *704* (1972).

Dallow, R.L. Evaluation of unilateral exophthalmos with ultrasonography. *Laryngoscope* 85: *1905* (1975).

Dallow, R.L., K.J. Momose, A.L. Weber & S.H. Wray. Comparison of ultrasonography, computerized tomography, and radiography techniques in evaluation of exophthalmos. *Trans. Am. Acad. Ophthal. Otolaryngol.* 81: *305* (1976).

Hanafee, W.N. Plain views of the orbit. *Rad. Clin. of N.A.* 10: *167* (1972).
Lombardi, G. Orbital pathology and contrast media. *Rad Clin. of N.A.* 10: *115* (1972).
Ossoinig, K.C. Clinical echo-ophthalmology. p. 101, in: Current Concepts in Ophthalmology, Vol. 3 (F.C. Blodi, ed.). C.V. Mosvy Co., St Louis (1972).
Purnell, E.W. Ultrasonic interpretation of orbital diseases. p. 249, in: Ophthalmic Ultrasonography (K.A. Gitter, A.H. Keeney & L.K. Sarin, eds.). C.V. Mosby Co., St Louis (1969).
Zizmor, J. & G. Lombardi. Atlas of Orbital Radiography. Aesculapius, Birmingham, Alabama (1973).

Authors' address:
Departments of Ophthalmology and Radiology
Harvard Medical School
Massachusetts Eye & Ear Infirmary
243 Charles Street
Boston, Mass. 02114
USA

Proc. 3rd Int. Symp. on Orbital Disorders, Amsterdam 1977

A SCAN ULTRASONOGRAPHY AND DIAGNOSIS
OF UNILATERAL EXOPHTHALMOS

J. FRANÇOIS & F. GOES

(Ghent, Belgium)

We have analyzed the diagnostic results in 129 cases of unilateral exophthalmos of at least 2 mm. All cases were examined with A scan ultrasonography. Besides, other technical investigations such as X-rays and tomography, angiography of the ophthalmic artery, gammagraphy of the orbit, and orbital phlebography, were also carried out. The computerized axial tomography introduced in ophthalmology by Lloyd & Wright in 1974 (Wright et al., 1975) could only be used in a limited number of patients.

All associated clinical signs, which could be helpful for the etiological diagnosis, were recorded and discussed: onset; degree and reducibleness of the exophthalmos; retraction of the upper eyelid; signs of congestion of the anterior segment; limitation of the external eye motility; changes of the retina and the optic nerve.

DIAGNOSIS OF EXOPHTHALMOS

The mean exophthalmos of the normal eye is 15 to 17 mm. An exophthalmos exceeding 22 mm is pathological (Rundle, 1964; François & Goes, 1977).

Lavergne & Winand (1973) reported that successive measurements made by the same examiner with the Hertel exophthalmometer are only significantly different when the difference exceeds at least 2 mm. When the measurements are made by different examiners only a difference of at least 3 mm is statistically significant (Tengroth et al., 1964).

On the other hand, the maximal difference between the exophthalmos of both eyes in normal conditions is 3 mm. There is no difference between both sides in 44% of cases and there is a difference between 1.5 and 3 mm in only 3,5% of normal subjects (Knudtzon, 1949). Moreover, the exophthalmos does not change with age.

Therefore, an exophthalmos can be considered as pathologic when:

1. The value exceeds the limits of the normal distribution (> 22 mm).

2. There is a difference of 3 mm or more between both eyes.

3. There is a change in the exophthalmos reading of more than 2 mm, when the measurement is made by the same examiner, and of more than 3 mm, when the measurement is made by different examiners.

We must keep in mind that a change in the position of the corneal apex in relation to the temporal orbital wall can also be caused by a change in the form of the eye (myopia, hyperopia, atrophy of the globe) as well as by the presence of an infiltrative process in the orbit. Especially in the presence of opaque ocular media, the diagnosis of pseudo-exophthalmos can be made by measuring the position of the eye apex in relation to the temporal orbital wall. This position is given by the formula $E - \dfrac{A}{2}$, where E represents the exophthalmometric value (mm) and A the axial eyelength (mm). Buschmann & Schwaar (1967) have calculated a mean value of 2.90 (± 0.28) in emmetropic eyes, with a maximum difference between both eyes of 1 mm. In anisometropic eyes the maximum difference between the position of the centre of both eyes was always less than 2 mm.

METHOD OF EXAMINATION

All our orbital examinations were made with A-scan ultrasonography. Our survey covers a period from 1969 to 1976. Up to 1971 we used the 7000 Kretz apparatus which had a very strong amplification, but a too small dynamic range (26 db), so that a differential diagnosis was very difficult. Since 1971 we have been using the 7200 MA standardized Kretz apparatus with a good dynamic range (36 db), a strong amplification and a built-in calibration scale.

We used the standard amplification for tumour diagnosis, which is calculated according to the technique of Ossoinig (1971). For the differential diagnosis this setting was usually diminished by two to four decibels.

A possible change in width of the orbital echogram was studied after compression of the eyeball-orbit complex by the transducer.

A frequency of 8 MMZ was used. This allows a sufficient resolution and penetration, so that the normal orbit can be explored to a depth of 15 mm behind the eye. In the case of tumour a distance of 35 mm behind the eye may be demonstrated on the screen because of less attenuation. The normal human orbit changes according to the position of the transducer, and the absorption of ultrasound varies according to the composition and the hydration of the fat tissue, which is variable from one eye to another. For these reasons the examination has to be transbulbar and parabulbar in symmetrical positions for both eyes, the transducer being in a limbal, paralimbal or equatorial position.

ULTRASOUND DIAGNOSIS OF ORBITAL DISORDERS

Ultrasonography was introduced in ophthalmology in 1956 (Mundt & Hughes, 1956) and in orbital diagnosis in 1960 (B-scan, Baum & Greenwood). A-scan was first considered to be less appropriate than B-scan, but since 1963 Ossoinig and co-workers stressed the high reliability and accuracy of A-scan ultrasound in detecting orbital disorders.

A-scan ultrasonography can demonstrate a circumscribed tumour of the anterior orbital part, which has a diameter of at least 3 mm. When the lesion is situated in the apical region the diameter has to be at least 5 mm to be detected. Moreover, A-Scan may give information on the solid, vascular or cystic structure of the lesion. It allows the correct measurement of the diameter as well as the localisation of the tumour. These data are very helpful for the follow-up of a possible space-occupying process.

The orbital echogram is characterised by:

1. *Echo-height.* The normal orbital echogram shows a dense uninterrupted chain of high (100% for maximal amplitude) to medium amplitude mobile spikes with rapidly decreasing amplitude from left to right (Fig. 1). This high reflectivity is caused by the heterogeneity of the normal orbital structure, which includes fat, muscle and fibrous tissue. All orbital solid tumours show usually a more irregular and always a lower amplitude echogram because of their more homogeneous structure (Fig. 2). A cystic tumour shows no echos or only low-amplitude echos because of its inner structure (Fig. 3).

2. *Kappa angle.* This angle, formed by the baseline and a line traced through the peaks of the tumour spikes, represents the decline of the echo amplitudes and is normally high because of the strong sound attenuation in the normal orbit. As this sound attenuation is always less pronounced in tumour cases, the kappa angle is decreased in these cases.

3. *Width of the echogram.* The diameter of the orbital echogram depends on the available retro-orbital space. It shows individual variations and changes according to the localisation in the orbit. The normal echogram is limited at the right side by a high amplitude orbital wall echo when the ultrasonic beam is directed perpendicular to the bony orbital wall. The orbital echogram becomes broader in the case of a space-occupying lesion,

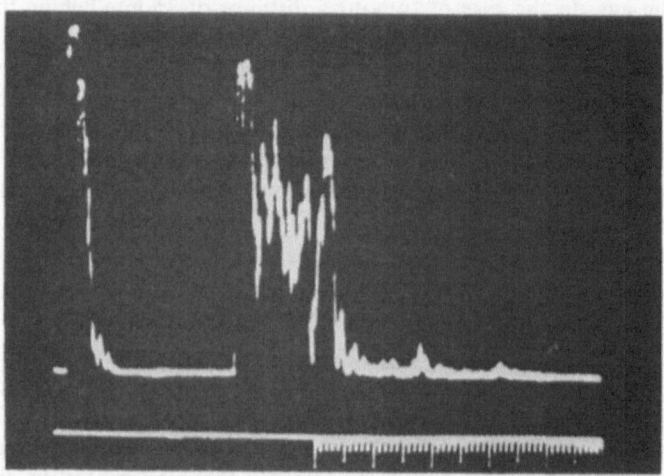

Fig. 1. Normal orbital transbulbar echogram.

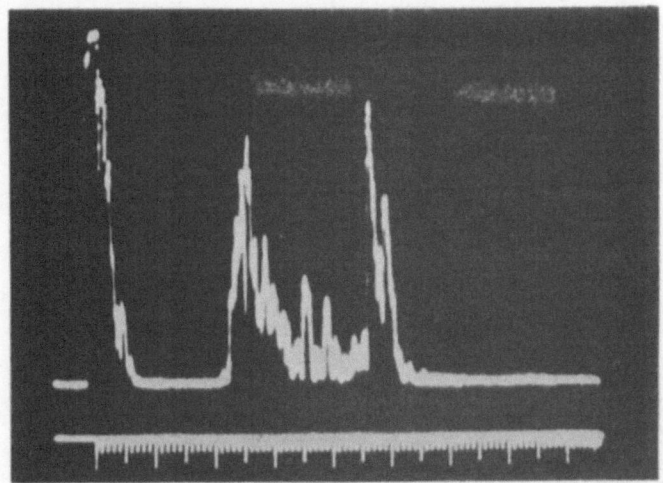

Fig. 2. Echogram of a solid orbital tumour, with lower amplitude echos.

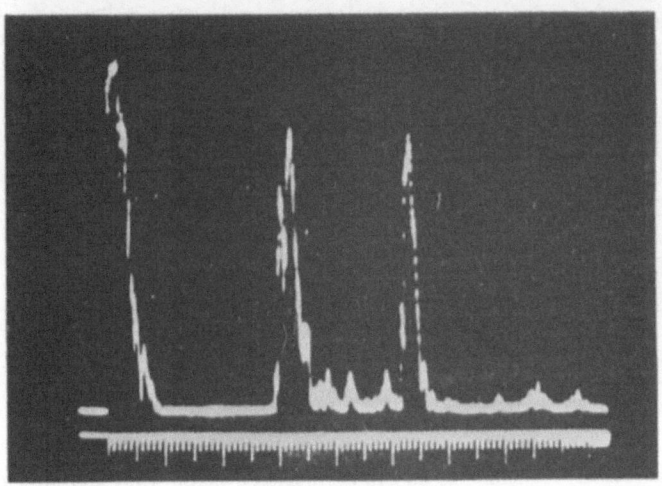

Fig. 3. Echogram of an orbital cyst (mucocele) with very low amplitude echos between the walls of the tumour.

while a terminal echo corresponding to the posterior tumoral surface may become visible.

4. *Compression of the echogram.* The normal echogram becomes narrower after compression of the orbit content, because the normal orbital structure is more easily deformed than the eyeball itself. In the case of a solid orbital tumour the width of the echogram does not decrease after compression of the orbital tissue, because the consistency of the tumour is harder than that of the eyeball. On the contraru, in the case of an orbital cyst the echogram is more easily deformed than the eye itself (Fig. 4).

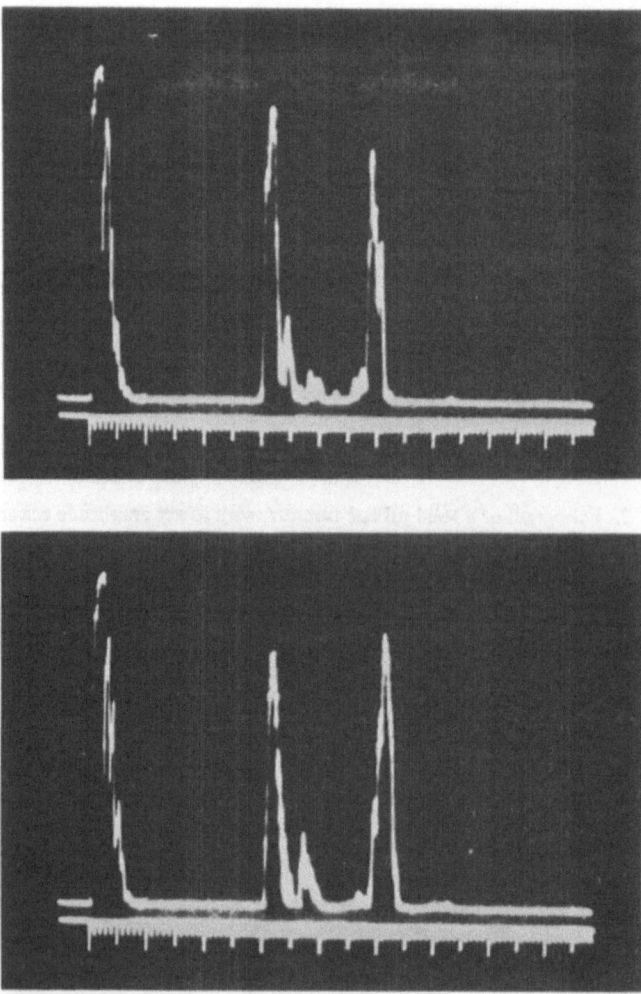

Fig. 4. Transbulbar echogram of an orbital mucocele before (up) and after (down) compression, with resulting shortening of the echogram.

5. *Spontaneous movement.* The normal orbital echogram shows a continuous spontaneous movement caused by the vascular pulsations. In tumour cases (with the exception of vascular tumours) this spontaneous movement is absent, the echogram remaining rigid on the screen. It is, however, not always easy to observe this spontaneous movement of the orbital echogram.

MATERIAL

The diagnostic results of A-scan orbital examinations are dicussed in comparison with those of other technical examination in 129 cases of unilateral exophthalmos of at least 2 mm. Thirteen cases were not verified, because the patients refused surgery or because the follow-up was incomplete. Ultrasound was positive in 8 of these cases, while X-ray examination was positive in only 4 of them. In 116 cases we made an etiological diagnosis, which could be verified by histological examination in the case of tumour or pseudo-tumour, by X-rays in the case of non-tumoral vascular disorder, by laboratory examinations in the case of thyroid dysfunction, and by the reaction to systemic antibiotic treatment in the case of orbital inflammation.

Endocrine exophthalmos

We made the diagnosis of unilateral endocrine exophthalmos in 21 cases (18%): hyperthyroidism in 20 cases and hypothyroidism in 1 case (Table 1). In 14 of these 21 cases (67%) the unilateral exophthalmos was the first clinical sign of the endocrine dysfunction. Other authors found for unilateral endocrine exophthalmos a percentage of 16% (McMillan-Moss, 1962; Pohjola, 1964), 12% (Kuchle & Guizzetti, 1966), or 8% (Lazorthes et al., 1969).

The mean age of the patients was 52 years, 12 being women and 9 men. The mean value of the exophthalmos was 3 mm. It never exceeded 5 mm. This corresponds to the conclusion of Rundle & Wilson (1965), who stated that an exophthalmos of 6 mm or more is a positive sign for an orbital tumour.

The maximal value of the exophthalmos was 32 mm. It exceeded 24 mm in three other cases. In nearly 50% of the cases there was also a high exophthalmometric reading for the fellow eye: in 8 cases the exophthalmos was of 18 mm and in 2 cases even more than 20 mm. This asymmetry of the exophthalmometric readings in endocrine exophthalmos has been observed by other authors in 10 to 26% of the cases (MacMillan-Moss, 1962; Kuchle & Guizzetti, 1966; Pohjola, 1964).

As far as the associated clinical signs are concerned, we found that the onset of the exophthalmos was rather sudden (less than one month) in only 3 cases (15%) and that important symptoms of the anterior eye segment (chemosis, redness) were present in 10 cases (45%). A limitation of the ocular motility was present in 9 cases (42%), the upwards eye-movement

Table 1. Unilateral endocrine exophthalmos

Frequency (21 cases)	18% of cases
Mean age	52 years
Sex	12 women, 9 men
Exophthalmos	mean 3 mm, always $\leqslant$ 5 mm
Onset	fast in 15% of cases
Associated signs, of the anterior segment	in 45% of cases
of the motility	in 42% of cases
Reducibleness	in 75% of cases
Retraction upper lid	in 76% of cases

being limited in 7 of these cases. Papilloedema (1 case) or retinal folds (2 cases) were seen in 3 cases (14%).

In 75% of the cases the exophthalmos was reducible.

The most characteristic clinical sign was the retraction of the upper eye lid (François, 1951), which existed in 16 of our cases (76%). This high percentage is confirmed by other authors (Kuchle & Guizzetti, 1966, 36%; Brihaye et al., 1968, 75%; Samaran, 1971, 84%).

A-scan ultrasonography provided us with little specific information as far as the etiologic diagnosis was concerned. In about 30% of the cases a significant enlargement of the orbital echogram could be demonstrated. Moreover, the amplitude of the orbital echos was usually higher than normal because of the diffuse oedematous infiltration and the higher reflectivity of the orbital tissue. Ultrasonography could in any case exclude the presence of an orbital tumour, at least after repeated examinations.

Orbital tumours

In 70 cases (61%) the exophthalmos was caused by an orbital tumour (Table 2). In 37 cases (53%) we were dealing with a malignant tumour and in 33 cases (47%) with a benign one. The mean value of the exophthalmos was 5,3 mm, and the extreme values were situated between 2 and 15 mm. In 7 cases (10%) the exophthalmos exceeded 10 mm, but there was no significant difference between the mean value for malignant tumours (5.4 mm) and that for benign tumours (6.0 mm).

In 18 cases a metastasis was responsible: tumour of the breast (6 cases), of the lung (4 cases), melanoma (2 cases), prostate carcinoma (2 cases), sympathicoblastoma (1 case), unknown primary tumour (3 cases) (Table 3).

In 10 cases there was an orbital sarcoma: rhabdomyosarcoma (4 cases), lymphosarcoma (4 cases). In 9 cases there was a mucocele. A carcinoma of the peri-orbital sinuses was responsible for 7 cases, and a meningioma for 6 other cases.

We observed 5 cases of cavernous hemangioma, 4 cases of lacrimal gland tumour, 4 cases of orbital cyst, 2 cases of neurinoma, 1 case each of multiple myeloma, of fibrous bone dysplasia, of benign lymphoma, of fibrolipoma and of lacrimal sac carcinoma.

In this series of 70 orbital tumours the A-scan ultrasonography gave a positive diagnosis in 66 cases (94%). There were only 4 erroneously negative echograms (6%) (Table 4). In these 4 cases the exophthalmos was respectively 1, 4, 7 and 8 mm, and the responsible tumour was twice a metastasis,

Table 2. Etiology of unilateral exophthalmos
(≥ 2 mm): 116 cases

	No	%
Endocrine exophthalmos	21	18
Orbital tumour	70	61
malignant	37	53
benign	33	47
Non tumoral affection	25	21

Table 3. Nature of the orbital tumours (70)

Nature	No
Metastasis	18
Sarcoma	10
Mucocele	9
Carcinoma of the sinus	7
Meningioma	6
Cavernous hemangioma	5
Tumour of the lacrimal gland	4
Cyst	4
Neurinoma	2
Myeloma	1
Bone dysplasia	1
Lymphoma	1
Fibrolipoma	1
Cancer of the lacrimal sac	1

Table 4. Percentage of positive diagnosis with various examination techniques in unilateral exophthalmos.

Methods of examination	% of positive diagnosis
Ultrasonography	94
Angiography	70
Gammagraphy	65
Phlebography	45
Radiology	30

once a sinus carcinoma and once a meningioma. In this ultrasound-negative orbital tumour group gammagraphy was 3 times positive, X-rays and arteriography 2 times positive.

When we compare the diagnostic value of other technical examinations, we see that arteriography of the ophthalmic artery was positive in 18 cases out of 26 (70%). In 8 cases where ultrasonography could demonstrate the presence of a tumour, the arteriography remained negative (2 mucoceles, 2 sarcomas, 2 sinus carcinomas, 1 metastasis, 1 lymphoma) and the orbital phlebography in 4 cases out of 5.

Orbital gammagraphy with technetium 99 m was positive in 33 cases out of 51 (65%). The examination was negative in 4 of the 5 orbital mucocele cases, but it was positive in all the meningioma cases. In about 50% of the cases with negative gammagraphy the carotid arteriography was positive.

Orbital phlebography was positive in 9 cases out of 20 (45%).

In the tumour series X-rays gave positive pathological results in 21 cases out of 70 (30%). This percentage increased to 80% for the meningioma-group.

In 3 cases where all technical investigations were negative, only ultrasonography could demonstrate the presence of an orbital tumour (sinus carcinoma, sarcoma, mucocele).

Table 5. Etiology of the noñ-tumoral orbital affections (25)

Pseudo-exophthalmos	1
Vascular affection	13
orbital hematoma	4
carotid-cavernous fistula	4
thrombosis of the ophthalmic vein	3
orbital varices	1
carotid artery aneurysm	1
Pseudotumour	9
Cellulitis	2

Non-tumoral unilateral exophthalmos

In 25 cases out of 116 (21%) the exophthalmos was caused by a non-tumoral disorder (Table 5). A myopic pseudoexophthalmos was responsible for 1 case. A vascular lesion was involved in 13 cases (4 cases of orbital hematoma and carotid-cavernous fistula, 3 cases of thrombosis of the ophthalmic vein, 1 case of orbital varices and 1 case of aneurysm of the carotid artery). A. pseudotumour existed in 9 cases and an orbital cellulitis in 2 cases.

In this group ultrasonography remained negative in 7 cases out of 25 (28%): 2 cases of pseudo-tumour, 2 cases of thrombosis of the ophthalmic vein, 1 case of diffuse orbital hematoma, 1 case of orbital cellulitis and 1 case of carotid-cavernous fistula. In this ultrasound-negative series the mean exophthalmos value was 4 mm, and the other technical examinations were negative in 3 of the 7 cases.

In the pseudotumour series ultrasonography showed a sarcoma-like echogram with low reflectivity (15 to 20%) and narrow kappa angle. In more than 75% of these echograms there was no change after compression of the orbit content (Fig. 5). A-Scan ultrasonography could not differentiate a

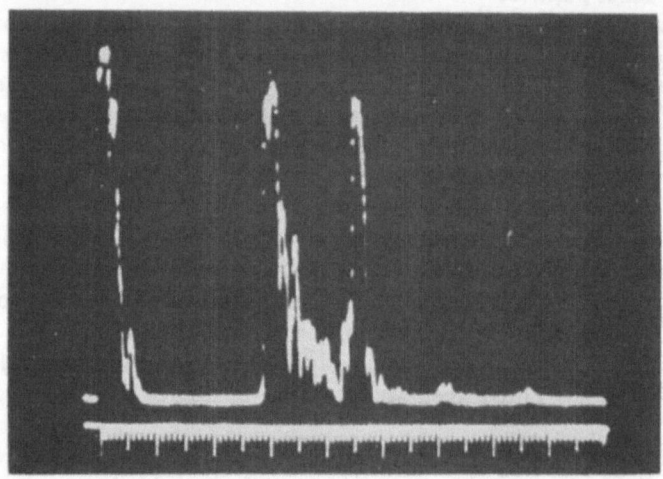

Fig. 5. Orbital pseudotumour with very low amplitude echos.

sarcoma from a pseudotumour because of the similar histological structure of both disorders.

In some vascular non-tumoral disorders ultrasonography could demonstrate a typical echogram.

An orbital hematoma produces echos of very low amplitude, well defined border echos, and a shortening of the echogram after compression (Fig. 6). In a case of carotid-cavernous fistula we observed a typical fast spontaneous movement with rapidly moving mobile echos due to the blood circulation between the walls. The amplitude of the echos was very low (10%).

In this group X-ray examination was positive in 40% of the cases, but it

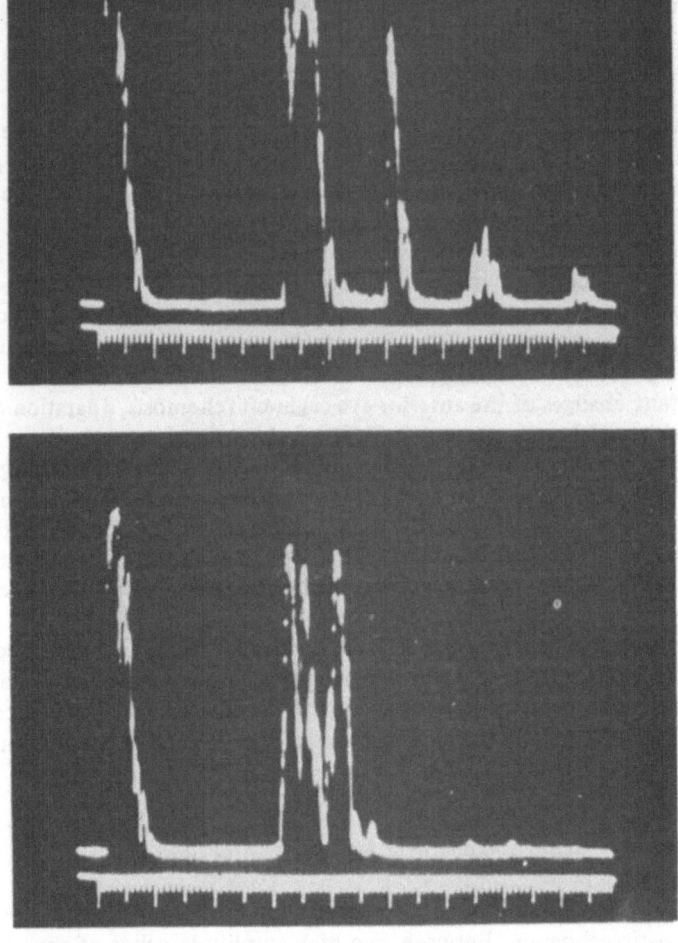

Fig. 6. Orbital hematoma (posttraumatic) immediately after (up) and six months after (down) the traumatism.

Table 6. Percentage of positive diagnosis in cases of non tumoral orbital affections causing exophthalmos.

Examination technique	% of positive diagnosis
Ultrasonography	72
Radiology	40
Gammagraphy	37
Angiography	33

was always negative in pseudo-tumour cases (Table 6). Gammagraphy was positive in 37% of the 11 examined cases. In 4 pseudo-tumour cases, where a gammagraphy was made, the examination was only once slightly positive. Carotid angiography was positive in 3 cases out of 10 (1 case of thrombosis of the ophthalmic vein, 1 case of carotid aneurysm and 1 case of carotid-cavernous fistula).

Associated clinical signs

When we consider the onset of the unilateral exophthalmos in the non-endocrine group, this onset was usually rather slow in the benign group (more than one year in 4 out of 9 mucoceles and in 3 out of 9 meningiomas). It was usually rather fast (less than one month) in 7 out of 18 metastatic tumours and in 6 out of 10 sarcomas. It was, of course, also fast in the vascular non-tumoral group (fistulas, thrombosis).

The exophthalmos was accompanied by a pain sensation in 32% of the malignant orbital tumours. This percentage was lower in the benign tumour series, or in the non-tumoral group.

Important changes of the anterior eye-segment (chemosis, dilatation of the episcleral vessels) were present in 35% of the orbital tumour group. This percentage was the same in the benign as well as in the malignant group.

A limitation of the ocular motility was observed in 70% of the orbital tumours and in only 45% of the nontumoral disorders. The motility disturbances were nearly as frequent in the benign as in the malignant tumour group, although the percentage was higher in cases of orbital metastasis (85%).

In 19 cases the visual functions were disturbed because of papilloedema, retinal folds or optic atrophy. In the malignant tumour series the percentage was 30%, in the benighn tumour group 13% (hemangioma, syst, mucocele, neurilemnoma), and in the non-tumoral group 18% (3 pseudotumours, 1 carotid-cavernous fistula).

Echogram characteristics of orbital tumours

Among the orbital tumours it is the orbital mucocele which gives the most characteristic echogram. Between two high-amplitude echos of the anterior and of the posterior cyst wall, the inner part of the cyst produces only low-amplitude echos with a spike height varying from 0 to 15% at tissue sensitivity. As the tumour causes only a minimum attenuation of the ultra-sounds, the kappa angle is very small. This cystic echogram pattern is usually deformed when the transducer is pressed on the eye (Fig. 7). We found a shortening of the echogram after compression in 7 of the 9 muco-celes. In other cases a typical zig-zag movement of the posterior wall echo can be observed, when the beam strikes the bony orbital defect, which is demonstrated by the sudden displacement of the posterior wall echo to the right side of the screen.

A cavernous hemangioma of the orbit produces also a pathognomonic echogram. In our series this tumour has the highest reflectivity with an

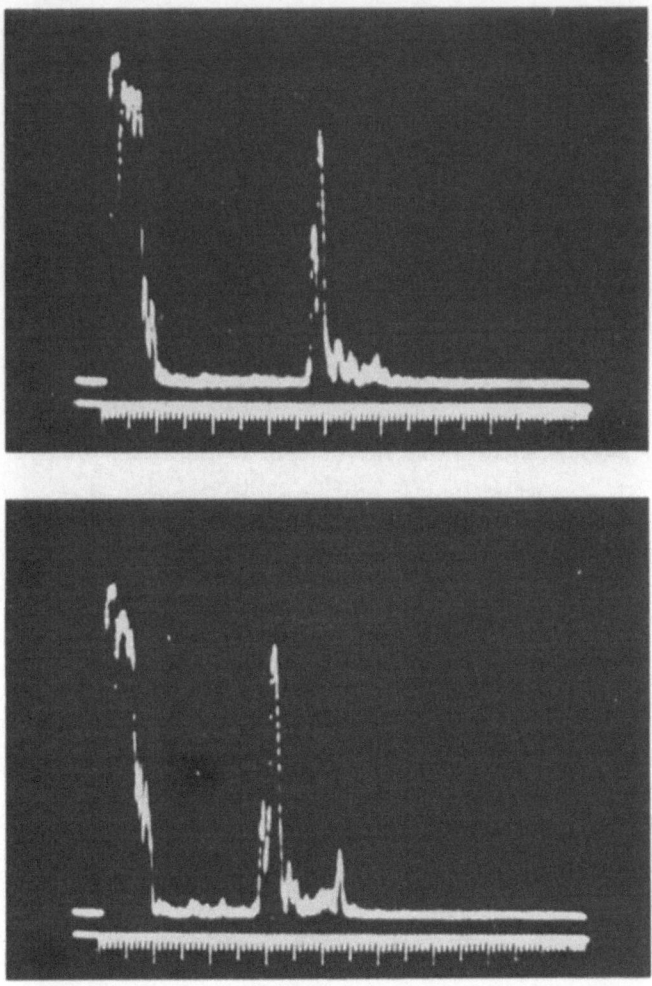

Fig. 7. Parabulbar echogram of an orbital mucocele, before (up) and after (down) compression.

echo-height of 35 to 60% at tissue sensitivity (Fig. 8). The typical echo-pattern is explained by the histological structure which shows highly reflective, large and regular surfaces. Because of the strong sound attenuation, there is a large kappa angle and in most cases the tumour wall echos are sharp.

A mixed tumour of the lacrimal gland may give an echogram similar to that of a hemangioma, but some iso-electric zones are generally seen because of large echo-free cystic areas inside the tumour. The typical localization in the upper temporal quadrant of the orbit facilitates the differential diagnosis, since a cavernous hemangioma is situated in the muscles.

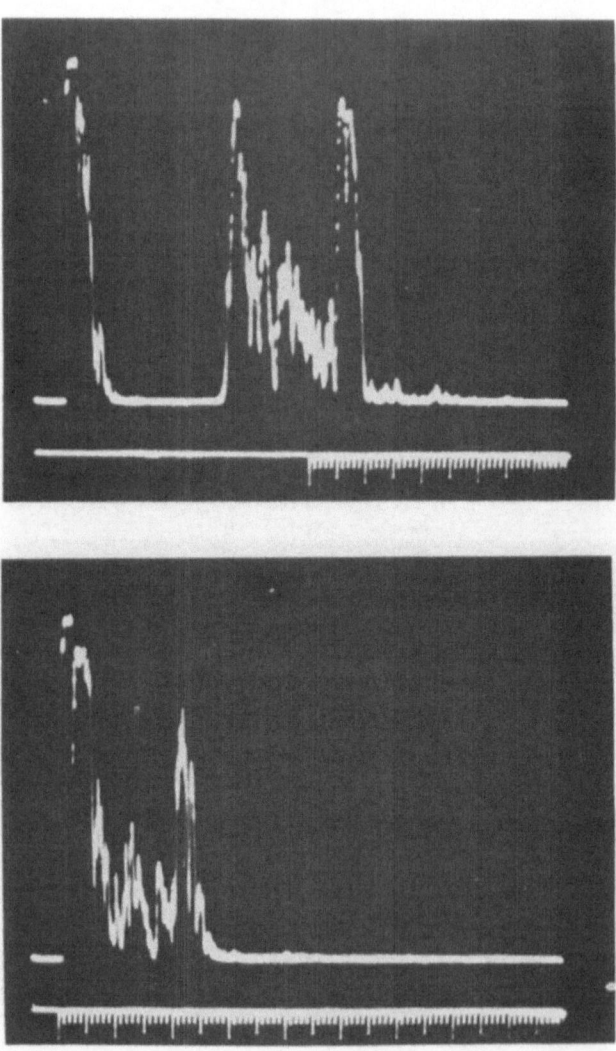

Fig. 8. Orbital hemangioma; parabulbar (up) and transbulbar (down) echogram.

The echogram of a sarcoma is also typical. The reflectivity of this tumour is low (10 to 20%) because of the absence of large interfaces. The kappa angle is small because of the minimal sound attenuation (Fig. 9). The tumour surfaces are usually well demonstrated on the screen. In our series the sarcomas had the lowest reflectivity of all the solid tumours.

In the case of a pseudotumour we mostly obtain the same echo-pattern as in the case of sarcoma. Ultrasonography is unable to make a differential diagnosis between both disorders. The sarcoma and the pseudotumour echograms do not change after compression.

An orbital metastasis shows a rather irregular echo-pattern with a low reflectivity (10 to 20%). The echogram length does not change, when the transducer is pressed on the eye (Fig. 10).

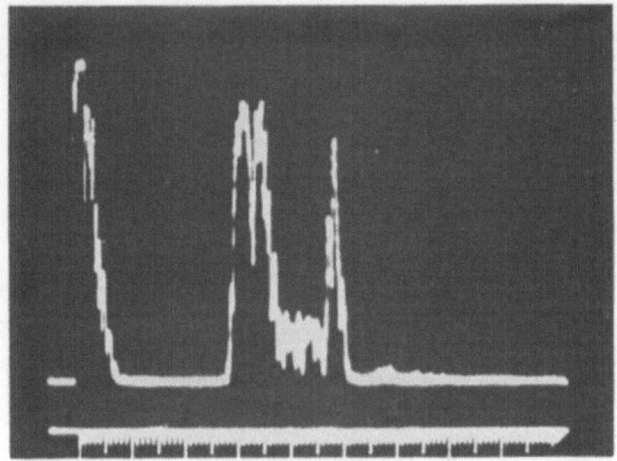

Fig. 9. Orbital sarcoma.

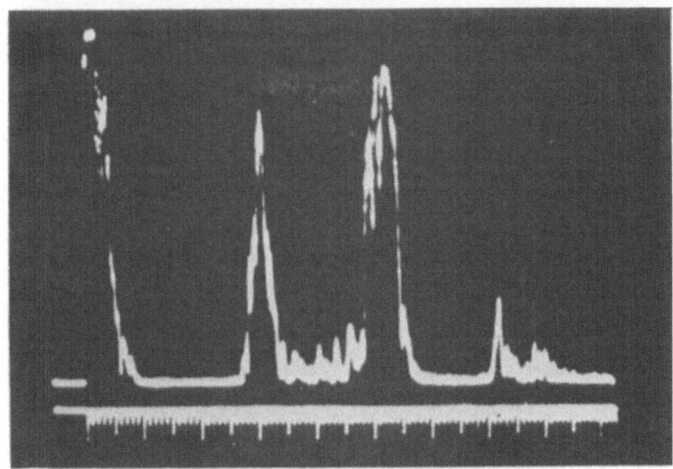

Fig. 10. Orbital metastasis from Oat cell carcinoma.

Meningiomas produce usually a rather irregular echo-pattern because of the presence of homogeneous zones, as well as of zones with high reflectivity (calcifications), so that high spikes alternate with low echos and echo-free zones (Fig. 11). In our series the reflectivity of these tumours varied from 15 to 60%, and the echogram could not be deformed after compression.

Malignant tumours of the peri-orbital sinuses present an irregular echogram with high and low spikes alternating with short base line homogeneous zones, due to the irregular acoustic structure of the tumour. The reflectivity of the echogram is larger than normally (15 to 75%). The kappa angle is narrow (Fig. 12).

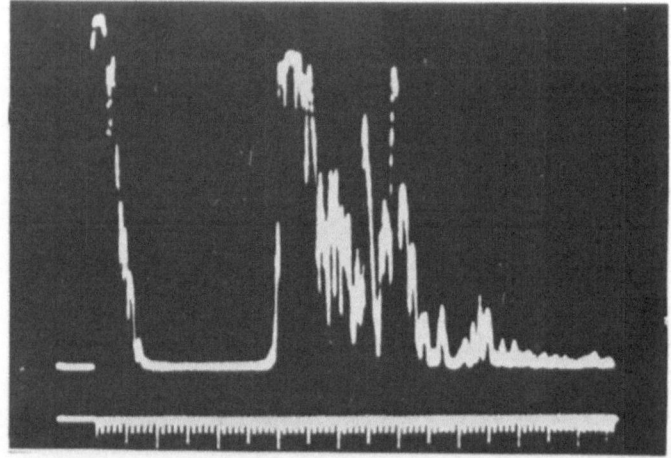

Fig. 11. Orbital meningioma.

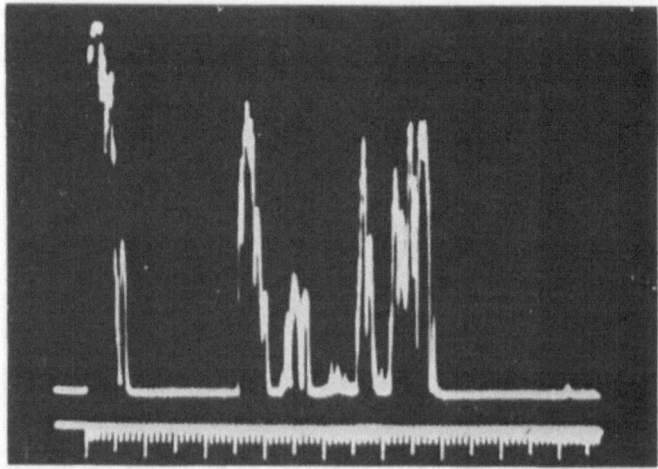

Fig. 12. Liposarcoma: high amplitude echos areas alternating with low amplitude echos and echo-free zones.

In our fibrolipoma case we found a very irregular echogram, the spikes having an amplitude from 10 to 70% at tissue sensitivity. This was explained by the typical histological structure of the tumour. The echogram showed the characteristics of solid tissue and remained unchanged after compression of the eye by the transducer.

DISCUSSION

Among our 116 cases of unilateral exophthalmos we found an endocrine etiology in 18%, a tumoral etiology in 61% (47% benign, 53% malignant) and non-tumoral etiology in 21% of the cases. In many of these non-tumoral cases the history and the clinical signs were sufficiently typical to make a correct diagnosis (hematoma, carotido-cavernous fistula, cellulitis).

A retraction of the upper eye-lid, seen in 76% of the endocrine exophthalmos cases, was nearly pathognomonic for this etiology. In this group the exophthalmos never exceeded 5 mm, and there was frequently a high exophthalmos reading in the fellow eye. Ultrasonography showed specific patterns in 1/3 of these endocrine cases, but never gave a tumour positive diagnosis.

In the tumour group the fast onset of the exophthalmos and the existence of pain were in favour of malignancy. We were surprised by the high number of metastasis cases in this group.

Ultrasonography gave a positive diagnosis in 94% of the tumour cases, which was a much higher percentage than could be obtained with other techniques. The tissue differentiation was possible in about 50% of the cases, especially in the cases of mucocele, sarcoma, lacrrimal gland tumour and hemangioma.

When a shortening of the orbital echogram could be obtained after compression of the globe by the transducer, this sign was strongly in favour of a benign etiology. It was positive in 60% of our cases. All mucocele echograms (except 2), all non-tumoral vascular disorders echograms, and 5 out of the 9 pseudotumour echograms could be deformed.

In the non-tumoral group the diagnosis of the etiology of the exophthalmos was made in 72% of the cases by ultrasonography only.

Using A-Scan ultrasonography, Ossoinig & Seher (1967) could diagnose an orbital tumour in 97% of 153 clinically suspected cases. Gitter et al. (1968) could demonstrate an orbital tumour in 60% of their 20 cases. Five of the 8 tumours, which were not diagnosed by ultrasonography, were situated in the apex of the orbit. Valençak (1969) could localize an orbital tumour in 96% of his 152 cases. Psilas et al. (1970) made a correct ultrasound diagnosis in 12 of 13 examined exophthalmos cases. Poujol (1973) diagnosed a tumour in 95.4% of 112 verified unilateral exophthalmos cases, and made a differential diagnosis between solid, vascular and cystic tumours in 81.8% of the cases. Söllner et al. (1975) found a tumoral etiology in 45 out of 78 unilateral exophthalmos cases. In more than 90% of these cases the tissue diagnosis was proved to be exact. Ossoinig & Till (1975) made a correct

39

diagnosis in 98% of 767 verified cases with suspected orbital lesion, and between 1971 and 1973 they obtained a correct differential diagnosis in 87% of 73 verified cases. Schwab & Nover (1975) examined 119 unilateral exophthalmos cases and obtained a tumour positive echogram in 67 of the cases (56%). In 40% of these cases the tissue differentiation was possible. In 10 of 13 operated cases the nature of the tumour was confirmed.

Wright et al. (1975) examined 41 unilateral exophthalmos cases by the E.M.I. scan technique and obtained a tumour positive result in 84% of 25 orbital tumours. The B-Scan ultrasonography was positive in 76%, and the orbital phlebography in 84% of the cases. After having modified the examination technique and improved the equipment, better results could be obtained and a positive tumour diagnosis was made in 93% of the cases.

We think that the B-Scan technique may give supplementary information in demonstrating the shape and sometimes the localization of the lesion. It may also allow a better tissue differentiation.

CONCLUSION

In 116 controlled unilateral exophthalmos cases ultrasonography could make a correct tumour diagnosis in 94% of the cases, while angiography of the ophthalmic artery gave a positive result only in 70%, orbital gammagraphy only in 65%, orbital phlebography only in 45%, and X-rays only in 30% of the cases. In most of the cases an information on the solid, cystic or vascular structure of the orbital lesion could be obtained.

REFERENCES

Baum, G. & I. Greenwood. Ultrasonography – an aid in orbital tumour diagnosis. *Arch. Ophthal.* (Chicago) 64: *180–194* (1960).

Bertelson, T.I. Diagnostische Methoden bei einseitigen Exophthalmos. *Ophthalmologica* 151: *309–330* (1966).

Brihaye, J., G.R. Hoffmann, J. François & M. Brihaye-Van Geertruyden. Les exophtalmies neurochirurgicales. *Neurochirurgie* 14: *185–487* (1968).

Buschmann, W. Die Ultraschall Exophthalmometrie. pp. 303–306 in: Diagnostica Ultrasonica in Ophthalmologia (J. Böck & K. Ossoinig, eds.). Wiener Med. Akademie (1973).

Buschmann, W. & D. Linnert. Visualisation of orbital tissues using various echographic techniques. *Ultrasound in Med. Biol.* 2: *295–300* (1977).

Buschmann, W. & R. Schwaar. Zur Exophthalmometrie. Die Lagebeziehungen zwischen Bulbusmitte und Orbitarand bei Emmetropen. *Graefe's Arch. Ophthal.* 173: *261–268* (1967).

Danis, P. & J. Mahaux. Les exophtalmies simples et oedémateuses d'origine endocrinienne. *Bull. Soc. belge Ophtal.* 97: *1–108* (1951).

Fledelius, H. Ultrasound oculometry in high myopia with reference to the occurrence of retinal detachment. *Acta Ophthal., Kbh.* 49: *707–714* (1971).

François, J. L'hypertonie unilatérale du releveur de la paupière supérieure dans le syndrome de Basedow. *Bull. Soc. belge Ophtal.* 97: *138–160* (1951).

François, J. & F. Goes. Echographie A et exophtalmies unilatérales. *Bull. Soc. belge Ophtal.* 155: *475–486* (1970).

François, J. & F. Goes. Kyste dermoïde de l'orbite. *Bull. Soc. belge Ophtal.* 161: *738–747* (1972).

François, J. & F. Goes. L'ultrasonographie dans l'exophtalmie unilatérale. In press (1977).

François, J., F. Goes & P. Yobbagyu. L'échographic ultrasonique en ophthalmologie. *Ann. Oculistique* 201: *609–405* (1968).
Gitter, K., D. Meyer, R. Goldberg & L.K. Sarin. Role of ultrasound in diagnosis of unilateral proptosis. pp. 327–331 in: Diagnostica Ultrasonica in Ophthalmologia. Universita J.E. Purkinje, Brno (1968).
Hildebrandt, I. Die Lagebeziehungen zwischen Bulbusmittelpunkt und temporalem Orbitarand bei Exophthalmos. *Wiss. Z. Humboldt Univ.*, Berlin 14: *213–216* (1965).
Knudtzon, K. On exophthalmometry. *Acta Psych. Neurol., Kbh.* 24: *523–537* (1949).
Küchle, H.J. & K. Gyuzetti Zum Tumor bedingte einseitigen Exophthalmos. Acta II. Congr. Soc. Europ. Ophtal. 1964. pp. 780-783, Karger, Basel (1966).
Lavergne, G. & R. Winand. L'exophtalmie endocrinienne. *Bull. Soc. belge Ophtal.* 163: *15–23* (1973).
Lazorthes, G., J. Espagno, L. Arbus, J. Zadeh & Y. Lazorthes. Exophtalmie unilatérale par atteinte des parois orbitaires. *Rev. Oto., Neuro., Ophtal.* 41: *93–94* (1969).
Lloyd, G.A.S. & J.E. Wright. Computerized axial tomography. *Br. Med. J.* 3: *114* (1974).
MacMillan Moss, H. Expanding lesions of the orbit. A clinical study of 230 consecutive cases. *Am. J. Ophthal.* 54: *761–770* (1962).
Mundt, G.H. & W.E. Highes. Ultrasonics in ocular diagnosis. *Am. J. Ophthal.* 42: 488–498 (1956).
Ossoinig, K. Zum Problem der akustischen Tumordiagnostik von Auge und Orbita. *Wiss. Z. Humboldt Univ.*, Berlin 14: *185–191* (1965).
Ossoinig, K. Die Ultraschalldiagnostik der Orbita. *Klin. Mbl. Augenheilk.* 149: *817–839* (1966).
Ossoinig, K. Grundlagen der klinische Echo-Ophthalmographie. Wiener Med. Akademie, Wien (1971).
Ossoinig, K. & K. Seher. Ergebnisse der Ultraschalldiagnostik orbitaler tumoren. *Klin. Mbl. Augenheilk.* 151: *519–524* (1967).
Ossoinig, K. & P. Till. Ten year study on clinical echography in orbital diseases. pp. 200–216 in: Ultrasonography in Ophthalmology (J. François & F. Goes). Bibl. Ophthal., Basel 83 (1975).
Ossoinig, K. & E. Valençak. Ultrasonography and other diagnostic methods. Importance in orbital tumors. pp. 301–305 in: Ophthalmic Ultrasound (K. Gitter, A. Keeney, L.K. Sarin & D. Meyer). C.V. Mosby Co., St Louis (1969).
Pohjola, S. Unilateral exophthalmos with special reference to endocrine exophthalmos and pseudp-tumor. *Acta Ophthal., Kbh.* 42: *456–464* (1964).
Poujol, J. pp. 107–113 in: Echographie de l'oeil et de l'orbite (H. Hamard, M. Massin & J. Poujol, eds.). Bull. Soc. Ophtal. France 73 (1973).
Psilas, K., J.P. Houber & H. Soriano. Le diagnostic par l'échographie A d'exophthalmie unilatérale vérifiée histologiquement. *Bull. Soc. Franç. Ophtal.* 83: *434–439* (1970).
Rundle, F.F. Some observations on exophthalmos. *West J. Surg.* 55: *578–583* (1947).
Rundle, F.F. Eye signs of Graefe's disease. p. 172 in: The thyroid gland (B. Pittrivers & W.R. Trotter eds.), Vol. 2. Butterworth, London (1964).
Rundle, F.F. & Wilson. Cited by Danis & Mahaux (1951).
Samaran, M. Les exophtalmies endocriniennes. Thesis, Toulouse (1971).
Schwab, B. & A. Nover. Ergebnisse der Orbita-echographie im A Bildverfahren. *Klin. Mbl. Augenheilk.* 166. *758–766* (1975).
Söllner, F., L. Wüstenberg & R. Kohlhase. Echografische Differentialdiagnostik der einseitigen Exophthalmus. *Klin. Mbl. Augenheilk.* 164: *114–117* (1975).
Tengroth, B., H. Bogren & V. Zackrisson. Human exophthalmometry. *Acta Ophthal., Kbh.* 42: *864–874* (1964).
Wright, J.E., G.A.S. Lloyd & J. Ambrose. Computerized axial tomography in the detection of orbital space occupying lesions. *Am. J. Ophthal.* 80: *78–84* (1975).

Authors' address:
University Eye Clinic
135 De Pintelaan
B-9000 Ghent
Belgium

Proc. 3rd Int. Symp. on Orbital Disorders, Amsterdam 1977

THE ROLE OF CLINICAL ECHOGRAPHY IN MODERN DIAGNOSIS OF ORBITAL AND PERIORBITAL LESIONS

KARL C. OSSOINIG

(Iowa City, Iowa, USA)

ABSTRACT

Following a brief review of currently useful A-scan, B-scan, and Doppler techniques, the role of diagnostic ultrasound in the management of the following objectives will be covered:
1. screening of the orbit and periorbit for lesions;
2. differentiation of lesions;
3. indication for specific diagnostic tests, such as carotid arteriography;
4. localization and measurement of lesions for optimal surgery or radiotherapy, and for follow-up evaluations;
5. measurement of the thickness of optic nerve and extraocular muscles.

The results of clinical echography and its relationship to other major diagnostic tests, such as plain x-rays, x-ray tomography and CT-scanning will be discussed.

Author's address:
Department of Ophthalmology
University of Iowa
Iowa City, Iowa 52242
USA

The complete article is to be found on page 495.

B-SCAN AND C-SCAN IMAGING IN THE ORBIT

MARIE RESTORI, JOHN E. WRIGHT & DAVID McLEOD

(London, England)

Many authors (Coleman et al., 1972; Ossoinig & Till, 1975) have reported the use of A-scan and B-scan techniques in orbital diagnosis.

METHOD

The B-scan facility has been described in a previous publication (McLeod et al., 1977), and only salient features are given here. A 10 MHz focused transducer is coupled to the eye by means of a bath containing warmed saline. The transducer is scanned mechanically to cover a 4 cm square aperture in which the eye is centralised. Each 4 cm sweep of the transducer takes 140 milliseconds to complete and comprises a linear B-scan section B-scans are taken at one millimetre intervals. The B-scan level is adjusted remotely and its position indicated on a millimetre scale. B-scans may be taken in the horizontal, saggital or oblique planes.

The coronal plane of the orbit may be displayed using C-scan imaging (Fig. 1). This technique is described fully in a forthcoming publication

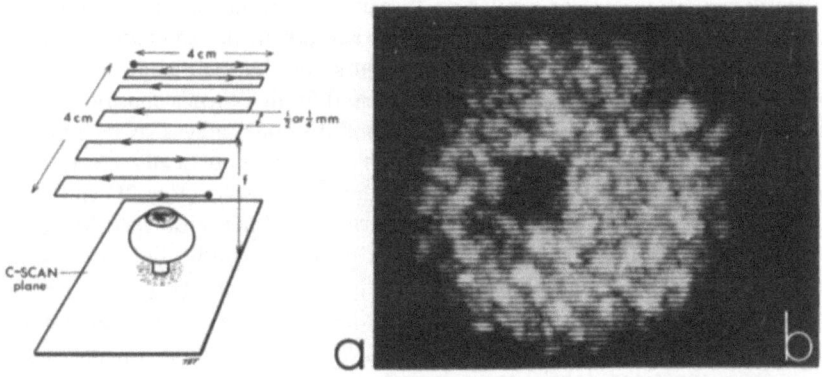

Fig. 1. a. C-scan imaging of orbital structures. b. C-scan section through a normal fat pad and optic nerve.

(Restori & Wright, 1977). To construct a C-scan a strongly focused 10 MHz transducer scans mechanically the 4 cm square aperture in which the eye is centralised. The C-scans require either 80 or 160 transducer sweeps and take 11 or 23 seconds to complete respectively. The focal plane of the transducer is arranged to lie at the plane of interest, and echoes from this plane only are recorded. These echoes are plotted as intensity registrations on a cathode ray tube. This focal plane imaging permits good resolution and sensitivity to be attained.

RESULTS

Orbital lesions can be localised to one of the following six regions: optic nerve, intraconal, orbital apex, extraocular muscles, lacrimal gland or paraorbital encroaching onto the orbital contents. Such lesions may be differentiated by a variety of features including shape, sound attenuating properties together with the number and amplitudes of echoes arising from acoustic interfaces within the lesion.

Optic nerve tumours

These masses are demonstrated as an increase in the optic nerve diameter. Often they appear acoustically homogenous (Figs. 2a, 3a) although they may give rise to medium amplitude echoes as illustrated in teh optic nerve meningioma of Fig. 3b. Optic nerve gliomas and meningiomas cannot be differentiated on an ultrasonic basis alone.

Intraconal masses

Many intraconal masses have been seen. Cavernous haemangiomas and neurilemmomas often appear similar on B-scan section, having regular borders, only modest sound attenuating properties and giving rise to medium amplitude echoes (Figs. 2b and c). Pseudotumours may be seen as discrete mass lesions (Fig. 2d), but inflammatory signs e.g. fluid in Tenon's capsule and/or around the optic nerve indicative of a pseudotumour, may also be demonstrated (Fig. 2e). Lymphomas have been seen as acoustically clear mass lesions producing modest attenuation of the sound beam (Fig. 2f) and may be lobulated. Metastases appear as infiltrative lesions with very irregular borders. These tumours give rise to scattered low amplitude echoes and attenuate the sound beam more strongly than lymphomas (Fig. 4a). Orbital metastases are often difficult to differentiate from discrete pseudotumour masses. Cystic lesions are usually acoustically homogenous (echoes may arise from contained debris) and attenuate the sound beam poorly (Fig. 4b). Varices may be differentiated from other orbital cystic lesions by their increase in size on jugular vein compression (Figs. 4c and d).

44

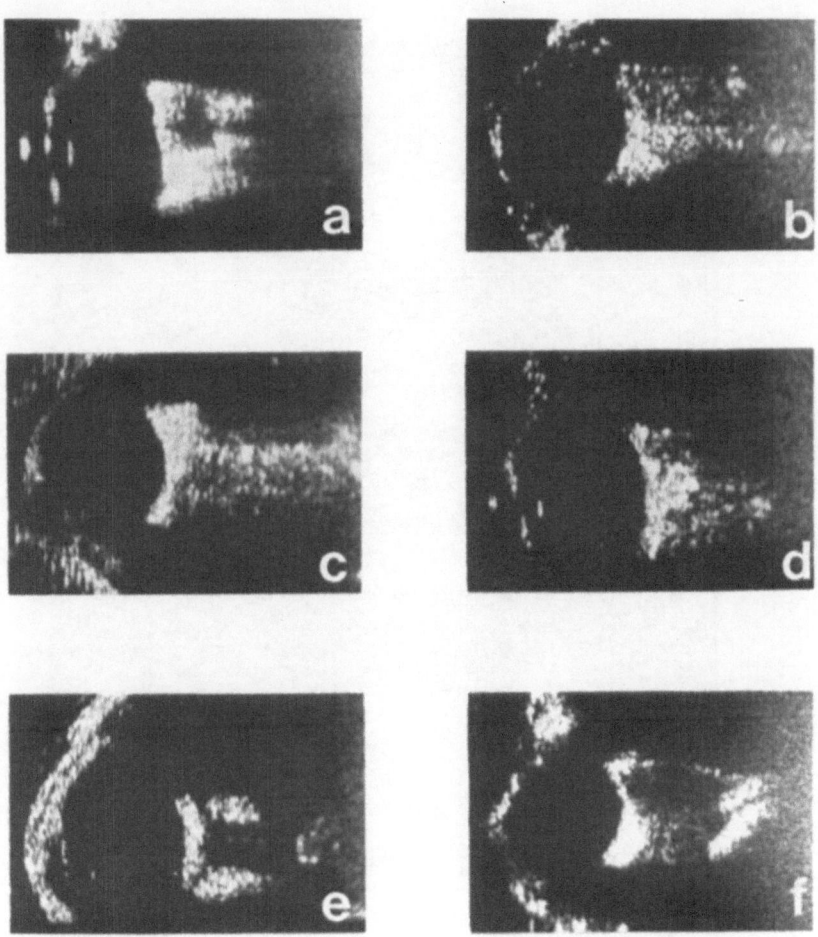

Fig. 2. Horizontal B-scan sections. a. Optic nerve glioma. b. Cavernous haemangioma. c. Neurilemmoma. d. Discrete pseudotumour mass with irregular anterior border; posterior border not outlined. e. Fluid in Tenon's space and around optic nerve – inflammatory signs of pseudotumour. f. Large lymphoma.

Orbital apex, extraocular muscle, lacrimal gland and paraorbital lesions

Tumours at the orbital apex are not demonstrated unless so large as to affect more anterior structures. Extraocular muscle disorders, for example, enlargement in dysthyroid disease may be demonstrated. Lacrimal gland tumours may be differentiated by many of the features mentioned in the section headed intraconal lesions. Paraorbital lesions, e.g. mucoceles of the paranasal sinuses may be demonstrated when encroaching onto the orbital contents. Mucoceles have clearly cystic features.

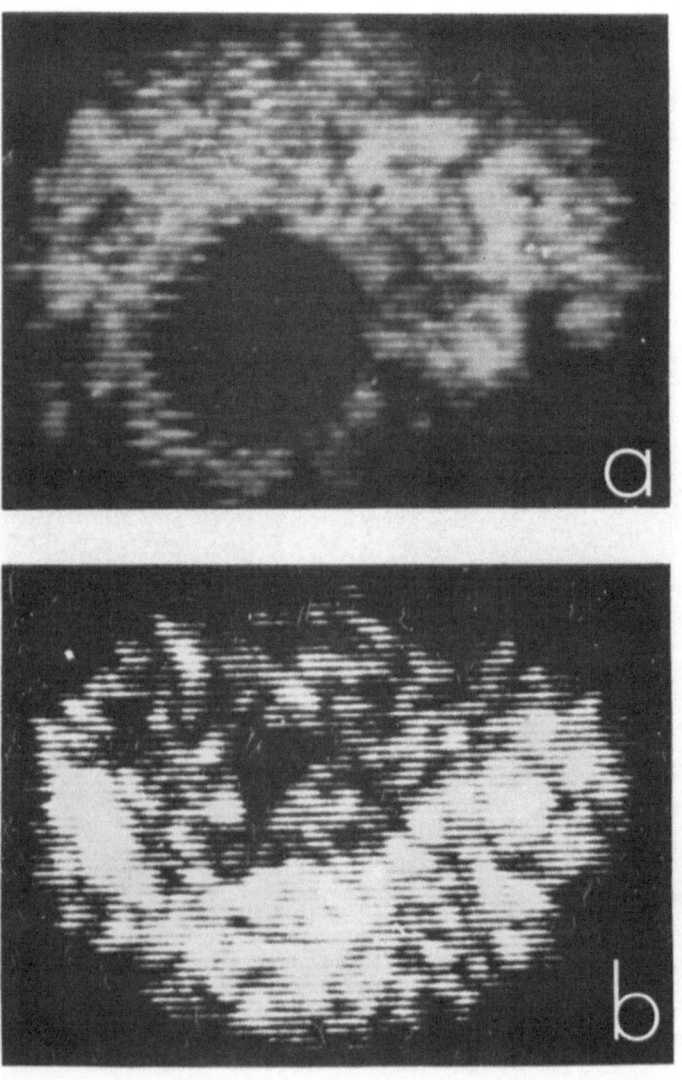

Fig. 3. a. Optic nerve glioma of Fig. 2a – C-scan section. b. Optic nerve meningioma C-scan section – atrophic nerve.

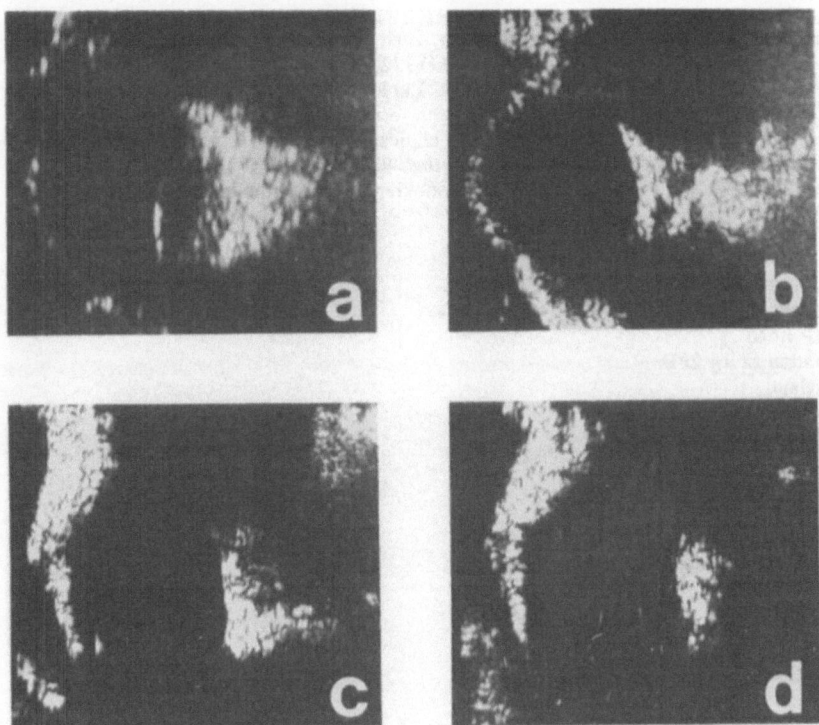

Fig. 4. a. A secondary intraocular carcinoma extending posteriorly; irregular posterior border (horizontal B-scan section). b. Orbital blood cyst (horizontal B-scan section). c. Orbital varix (saggital B-scan section). d. Varix of Fig. 4c following jugular compression; increase in size of varix.

CONCLUSION

B-scan imaging permits localisation of orbital lesions. The good resolution and tonal quality of the Moorfields B-scan system allows demonstration of acoustic interfaces and their relative echo amplitudes. The rapid B-scanning facility enables studies in motion to be undertaken. The coronal plane of the orbit may be displayed using the C-scan modality. High resolution and sensitivity allow accurate optic nerve measurement and good presentation of orbital lesions.

ACKNOWLEDGEMENTS

The authors wish to thank Terry Tarrant for the illustrations shown, and Sarah Cole for her secretarial assistance.

REFERENCES

Coleman, D.J., R.L. Jack & L.A. Franxen. High resolution on B-scan ultrasonography of the orbit. *Arch. Ophthal.* 8: 000–000 (1972).

McLeod, D., M. Restori & J.E. Wright. Rapid B-scanning of the vitreous. *Br. J. Ophthal.* 61: *437* (1977).

Ossoinig, K. & P. Till. Ten-year study on clinical echography in orbital disease: ultrasonography in ophthalmology. *Bibl. Ophthal.* 83: *200–216* (1975).

Restori, M. & J.E. Wright. C-scan ultrasonography in ophthalmic diagnosis. In press (1977).

Authors' address:
Moorfields Eye Hospital
City Road
London EC14 2PD
England

ULTRASOUND EXOPHTHALMOMETRY, ORBITAL ECHOGRAPHY AND CAT IN DIAGNOSIS OF ORBITAL DISORDERS*

H.W. BUSCHMAN & D. LINNERT

(Würzburg, W. Germany).

We are using the Kretztechnik 7100 MA With time-gain compensation and a flat-stalked 8 MHz transducer for A-scan ultrasonography. Echo amplitudes and echo distances can be evaluated accurately. This is especially useful for tissue differentiation. Position movements become visible as well as ultrasound attenuation. However, to determine the localisation to adjacent structures is often difficult. Anatomic schemes of corresponding size proved to be helpful for echo identification.

B-scans have been taken with Coleman's 'Ophthalmoscan' (Sonometrix), using focused 5 and 10 MHz probes in a waterbath coupling technique. Differentiation and contour enhancement were applied. Parallel, horizontal and vertical scans have been preferred since the scanning device is circumstantial to adjust for meridional scans. The unfavourable angle of beam incidence results in poor presentation of the orbital walls and the equatorial parts of the sclera. However, the localisation to adjacent structures can be shown much better than in A-scan technique. The lateral resolution is 1.0 mm and the depth resolution 0.3 mm for 6 dB amplitude decrease within the 30 μsec focal zone (10 MHz probe).

The Departments of Neuroradiology at Mainz and at Würzburg use the EMI-scanner with 160 by 160 matrix for computerized X-ray tomography. One absorption figure corresponds to a tissue volume of about 1.5 by 1.5 by 8 mm. Scanning is restricted to planes parallel to the orbital floor. This restricts the vertical resolution. Orientation of flat structures to the scan plane is decisive. Therefore, the medial and lateral rectus muscles are well presented, but the others are not. Flat horizontal tumour parts may be missed. Tumours penetrating into the orbit from neighbouring cavities, however, can be shown clearly.

Hertel's optic exophthalmometry can be supported by ultrasonic A-scan measurements of the axial length of both eyes. We called this technique 'ultrasound exophthalmometry' and first apply it after clinical examination. As an example a patient is shown with a growing unilateral exophthalmos that raised tumour suspicion, but it was only a pseudoprotrusion due to an increasing posterior staphyloma. The corneal vertex of the left eye was

---

* The full text of this paper, including figures and references, will be published in 'Klinische Monatsblätter für Augenheilkunde' (1978).

displaced anteriorly. But the rear wall of the eye was displaced backwards, and to an even greater extent. Therefore, the bulbus center (which stands for the position of the whole eye) was also displaced backwards, as compared with the other eye. Such findings exclude any suspicion of a retrobulbar space-occupying lesion. No further examinations are needed.

Contrary to this, in case of a retrobulbar tumour cornea, rear wall and bulbus center are all displaced anteriorly. This proves the existence of a retrobulbar mass. Then, A- and B-system ultrasonography of the orbital tissues as well as computerized tomography would be indicated to clarify the location and nature of this lesion.

Some results may demonstrate the use of both methods in a combined approach.

In a patient with unilateral exophthalmos, tumour suspicious A-scan echograms were recorded from the lower temporal part of this orbit, and compared with the corresponding echograms from the healthy right orbit. Computerized tomography was done at Würzburg. The tumour was also foudnd, but said to be in the upper temporal region. The patient was operated in another clinic. No tumour was found in the upper parts of the orbit. After that, B-scan ultrasonography stated the presence of the tumour in the lower part of this orbit. Exenteration was done and a large melanoblastoma was found in this area.

In a patient with intermittent exophthalmos the change of bulbus position with and without compression of the jugular veins could be measured by ultrasound exophthalmometry. B-scans 8 mm above the optical axis, taken after compression of the jugular vein demonstrated multiple large echo-free areas in the orbital fat which collapsed after release of the vein compression within some minutes. Venography confirmid the diagnosis of orbital varicosis which was treated via a Krönlein operation.

A boy, aged 9, developed 9 mm protrusion of the left eye. Ultrasonography as well as computerized tomography could be done successfully. Ultrasonography demonstrated defects in the orbital fat pattern. The orbital walls could only partially be shown with the present technique. Computerized tomography, performed at Mainz by Prof. Wende, revealed intact orbital walls and a retrobulbar mass extending into the tip of the orbit. A Krönlein-Berke operation was done; the clinical diagnosis of neurofibromatosis was stated, tumours were removed from the medial and lateral rectus muscles and the lacrimal gland.

In another patient, B-scan ultrasonography revealed a parabulbar lesion with echo-free areas. This was shown even better in the computerized tomogram, taken at the Würzburg Neuroradiology Department by Prof. Nadjmi. The absorption figures suggested fat. However. A-scan ultrasonography had demonstrated that the tumour contained no fatty tissue but waterlike fluid, and extended further backwards than B-scans and computerized tomography had shown. Both findings were confirmed by operation. The lymphangioma contained entrapped lymph and could be removed only after enlarging the lateral anterior orbitotomy to a Krönlein-Berke operation.

The clinical diagnosis of acute inflammatory proptosis was confirmed in a patient by A- and B-scan ultrasonography. A large, echo-free abscess cavity was visible in the depth of the upper half of the orbit. X-ray examination revealed frontal sinuitis. The diagnosis was confirmed during operation at the ENT-clinic at Würzburg.

Insufficient sensitivity adjustment may cause misleading abscess-like A-scan echograms in a tumour. In such a patient the B-scan appeared tumour-suspicious but was difficult to interpret due to massive intraocular and orbital pathology. The computerized tomography, performed at Würzburg, demonstrated a large tumour in the left eye and orbit with intact orbital walls. A melanoblastoma with extensive necrosis was found during exenteration.

Muscle swellings due to Grave's disease can be diagnosed by A- and B-scan ultrasonography. The orbital fat echoes become displaced. Computerized tomography yields positive findings especially when fibrosis has developed.

Ultrasound exophthalmometry, ultrasonic A- and B-scans of orbital tissues and computerized X-ray tomography have considerably improved the pre-operative diagnoses in patients with space-occupying orbital lesions. The combined evaluation of the results proved to be much more informative than the use of only one of the methods.

Ultrasonic B-scanning technique and frequency analyses should be further promoted. In computerized X-ray tomography other scan planes and a better resolution could yield further improvement.

Authors' address:
University Eye-Hospital
Josef-Schneider-Straße 11
D-8700 Würzburg
W. Germany

Proc. 3rd Int. Symp. on Orbital Disorders, Amsterdam 1977

B-SCAN ULTRASONOGRAPHY OF RHINOGENIC EXOPHTHALMOS

AKIHIRO KANEKO

(Tokyo, Japan)

Mucoceles and pyoceles are the most frequent cause of unilateral exophthalmos in Japan. They can be diagnosed usually with X-ray examinations. However, disorders of the orbital contents cannot possibly be visualized with these methods. They do not reveal the cystic characteristics of mucopyoceles.

Ultrasonography is a safe, noninvasive and economic procedure. Till (1975) reported A-scan ultrasonography concerning rhinogenic exophthalmos. But A-scan ultrasonography cannot visualize the localization and extent of orbital invasion from paranasal sinuses. Coleman (1972) reported B-scan ultrasonography of orbital mucoceles. However, his ultrasonic apparatus was not so sensitive as to disclose abnormality in paranasal sinuses.

The author (1977) has developed a high quality ultrasonic apparatus and investigated rhinogenic exophthalmos.

MATERIALS AND METHOD

Thirty cases of rhinogenic exophthalmos were examined with a high quality ultrasonic apparatus for the ophthalmological diagnosis using manual compound scanning (Aloka SSD-65). Special features of this apparatus are high sensitivity and resolution and a wide range of manual compound scanning. The wide range of scanning enables us to disclose abnormalities in the paranasal sinuses and to compare bilateral orbits. Sagittal sections were used to examine the frontal and maxillary sinus. Horizontal sections were used to assess the ethmoid sinus. The actual technique has been described in detail elsewhere (Kaneko et al., 1977).

The ultrasonic findings were confirmed by operation or X-ray examinations including computerized tomography. Causes of rhinogenic exophthalmos are shown in Table 1.

RESULTS

All cases of rhinogenic exophthalmos were shown to have an abnormality in the orbit and paranasal cavity except a case of mucocele of the posterior ethmoid sinus and several cases of neoplastic orbital invasion. Muco-pyo-

Table 1. Cases of rhinogenic exophthalmos

Mucocele or pyocele	18	
Ethmoid sinus		8
Frontal sinus		5
Both sinuses		5
Postoperative cyst of the maxillary sinus	5	
Neoplasm	7	
Epiparynx cancer		2
Hard palate cancer		2
Malignant lymphoma of the maxillary sinus		1
Benign lymphoma of the maxillary sinus		1
Rhabdomyosarcoma of the ethmoid sinus		1
Total	30	

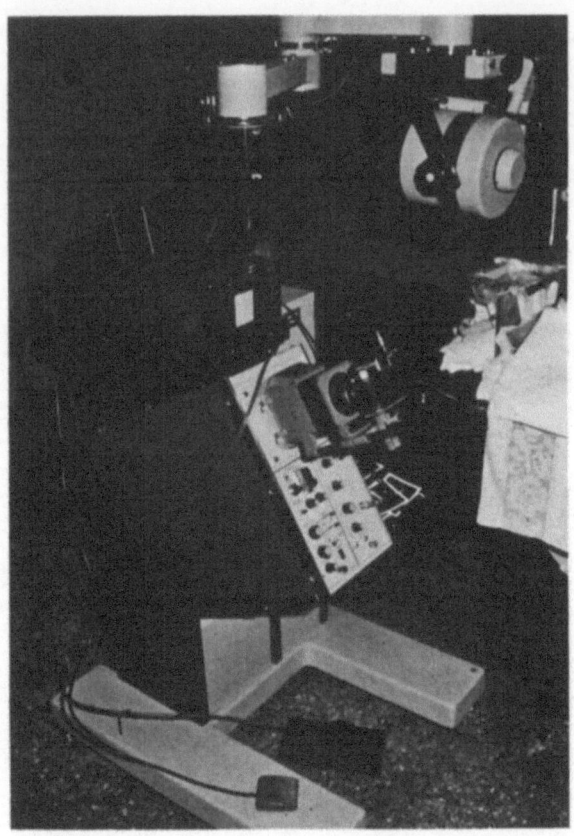

Fig. 1. The ultrasonic apparatus used in this investigation. Aloka SSD-65 (Aloka Co. Ltd., Japan).

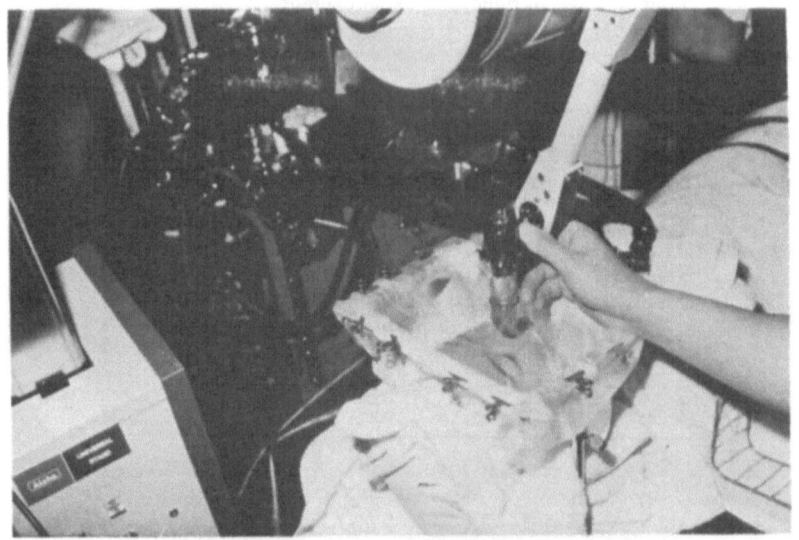

Fig. 2. Manual compound scanning is being done in the water bath.

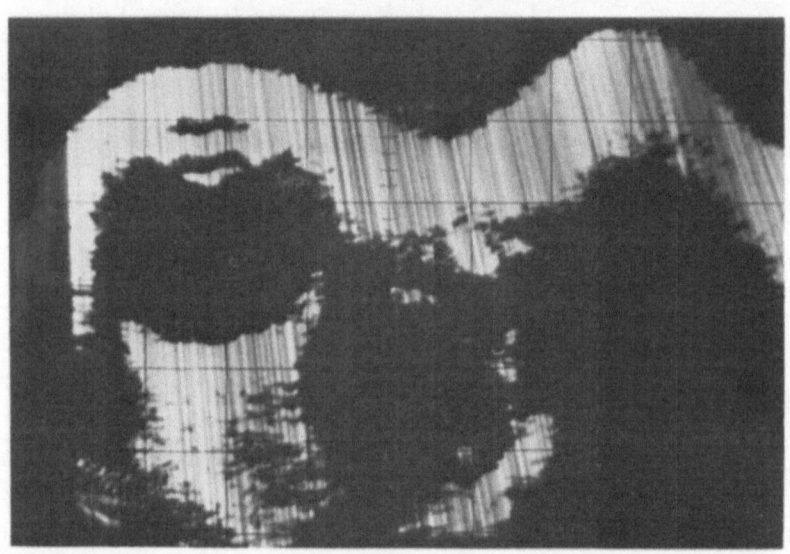

Fig. 3. Echogram of mucocele of the ethmoid sinus.

celes showed an acoustic hollowness between the orbit and the paranasal sinus. This finding corresponded to the cystic protrusion into the orbit from the sinus. Postoperative cysts of the maxillary sinus gave the same finding as muco-pyoceles. On the other hand, neoplastic invasion from the sinus did not show the cystic pattern. A portion of the retrobulbar tissue weakened reflectivity of ultrasound due to neoplastic invasion. The sinus was shown to be occupied with neoplasm. In some cases, only the abnormality of the orbit was demonstrated. Muco-pyoceles of the ethmoid and frontal sinuses were shown with B-scan ultrasonography as cystic protrusions from both sinuses.

Several cases were also examined with computerized tomography. Computerized tomography could reveal normal and abnormal conditions of bone, or a normal air-filled paranasal cavity. However, ultrasonography could reveal only abnormal bone and water-filled paranasal cavity. So, anatomical relations were more understandable with the computerized tomography than ultrasonography. But the cystic features of muco-pyoceles were more obviously disclosed with ultrasonography.

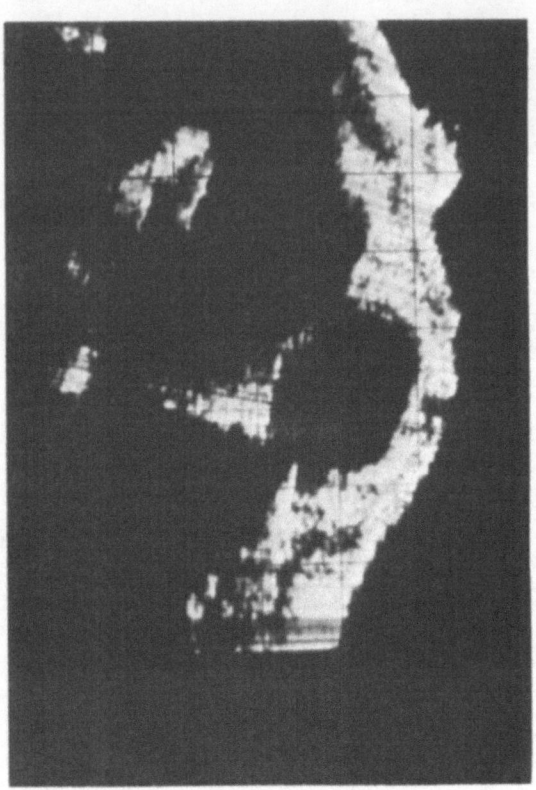

Fig. 4. Echogram of mucocele of the frontal sinus (sagittal section).

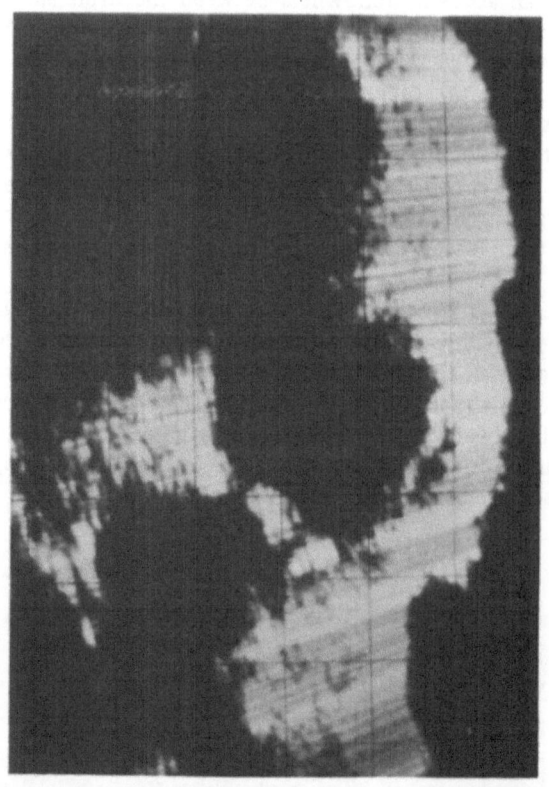

Fig. 5. Echogram of postoperative cyst of the maxillary sinus (sagittal section).

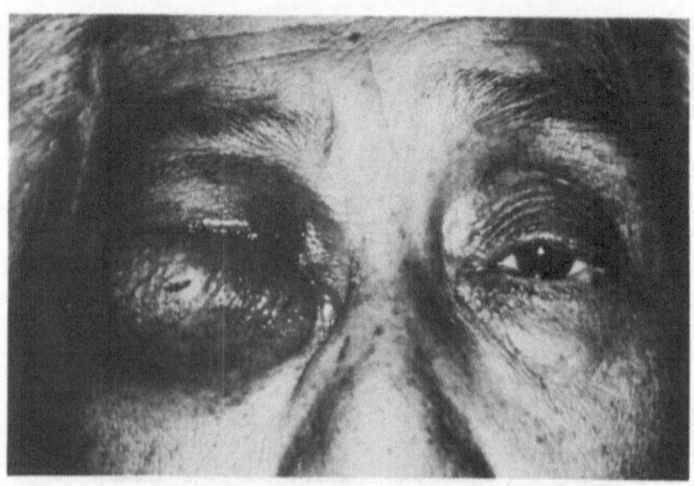

Fig. 6. Malignant lymphoma of the maxillary sinus invading the right orbit of an old woman.

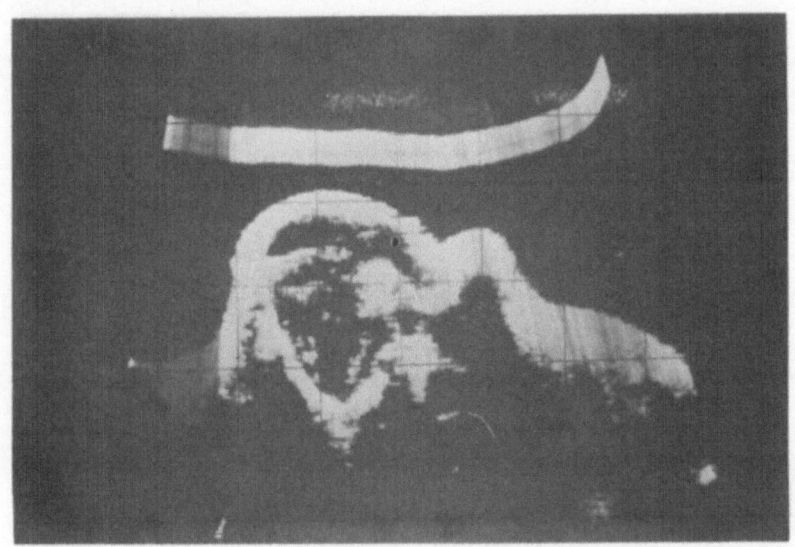

Fig. 7. Echogram of malignant lymphoma of the maxillary sinus. (horizontal section).

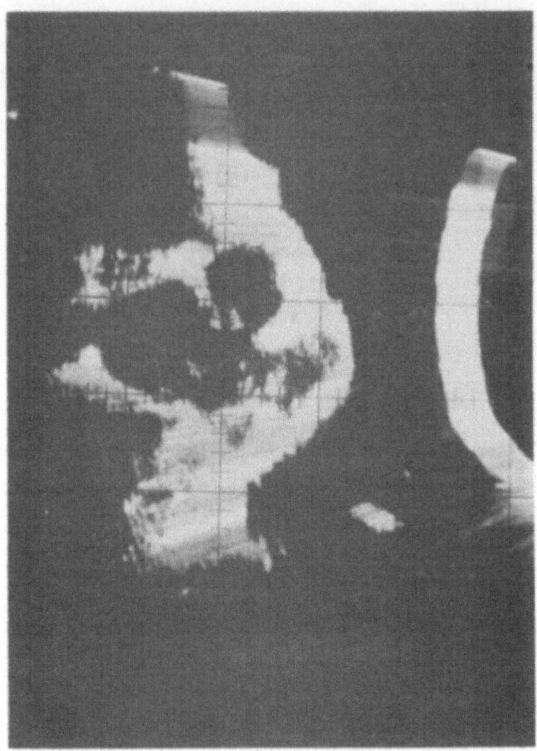

Fig. 8. Echogram of malignant lymphoma of the **maxillary** sinus (sagittal section).

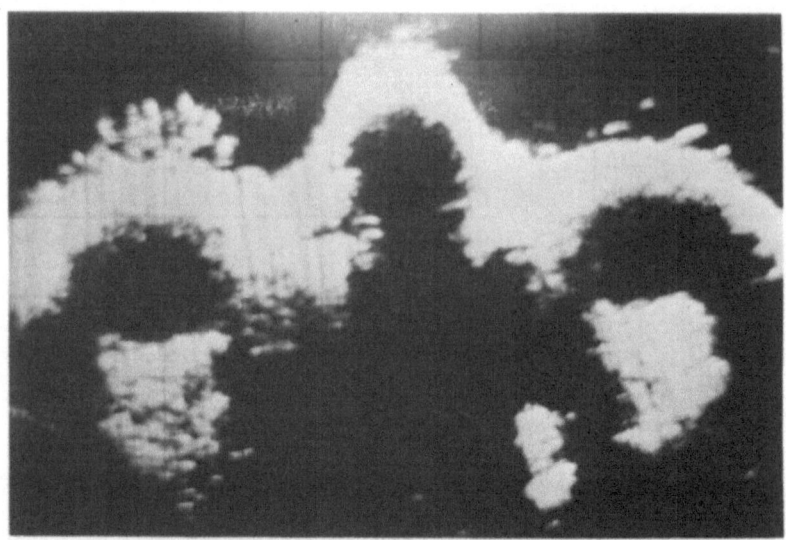

Fig. 9. Echogram of epipharynx cancer invasion of the left orbit. A solid mass in the ethmoid sinus was disclosed.

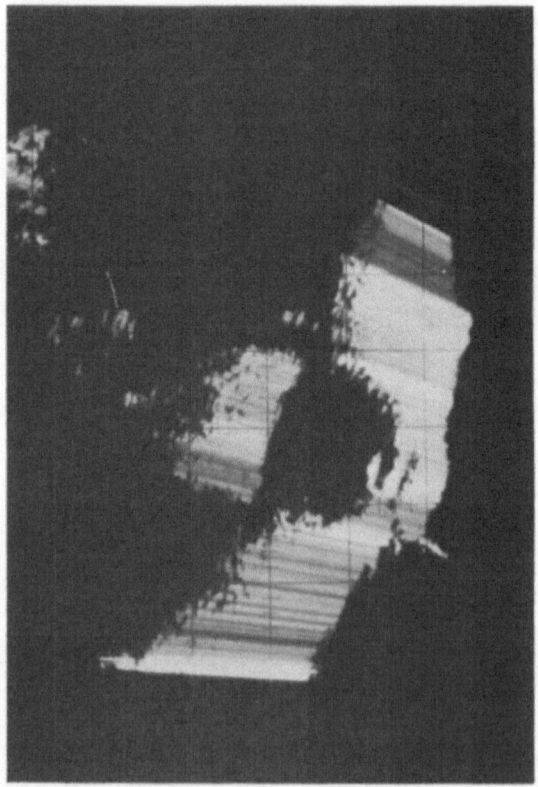

Fig. 10. Echogram of orbital invasion of rhabdomyosarcoma of the ethmoid sinus (sagittal section). No abnormality of the sinus was disclosed.

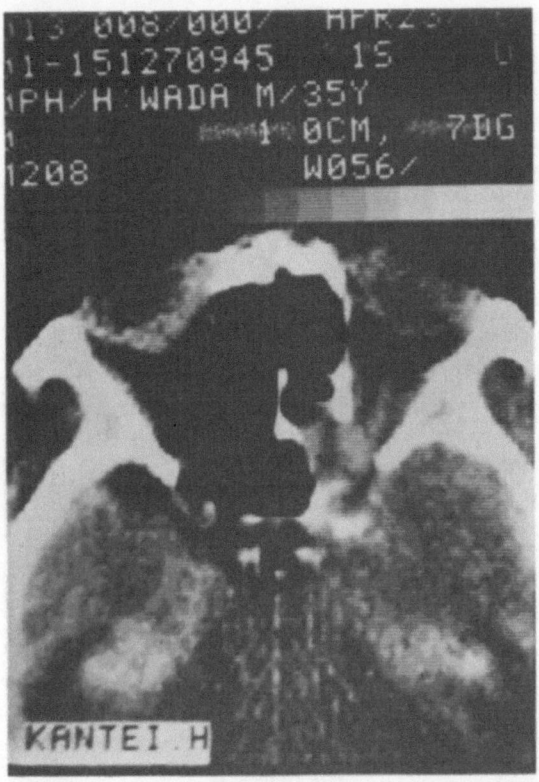

Fig. 11. Computerized tomogram of mucocele of the posterior ethmoid sinus. A well demarcated solid mass protruded into the orbit from a bony defect of the medial posterior wall. It extended very close to the optic nerve.

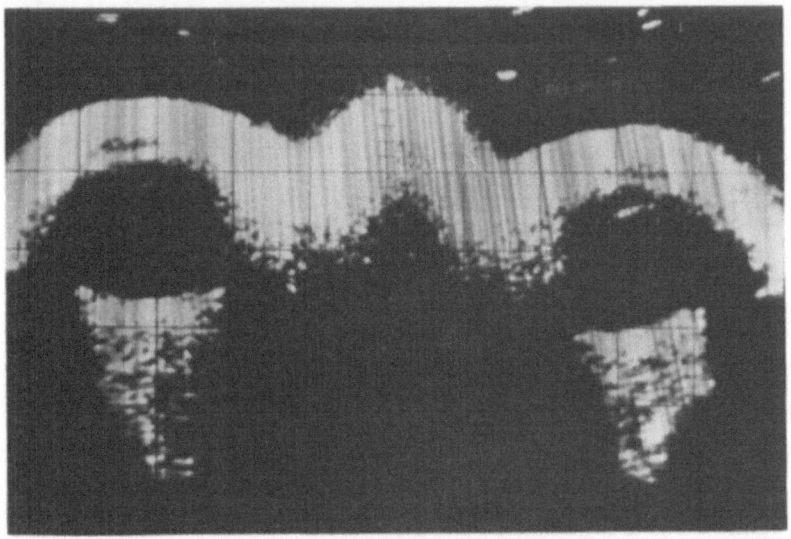

Fig. 12. Echogram of the same case as Fig. 11. The orbita fat in the nasal portion showed weak reflectivity, reflecting protrusion of mucocele from the posterior ethmoid sinus. No abnormality of the sinus was disclosed.

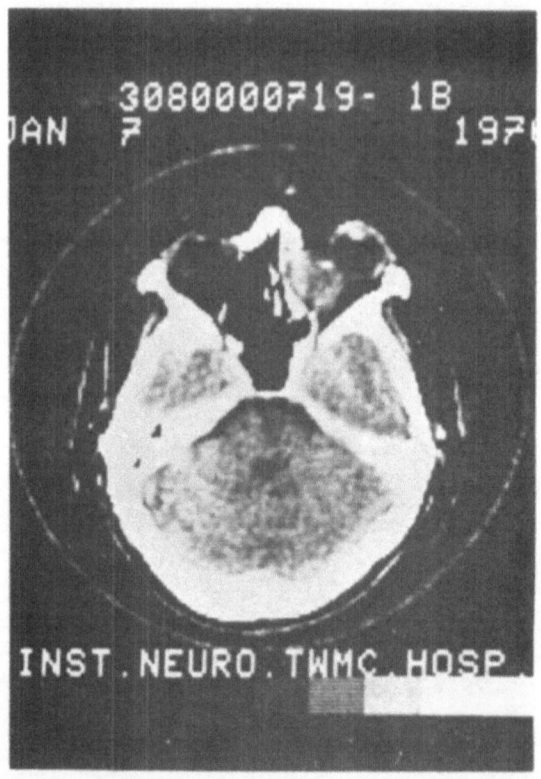

Fig. 13. Computerized tomogram of mucocele of the ethmoid sinus. A well demarcated mass exists between the ethmoid sinus and the eyeball.

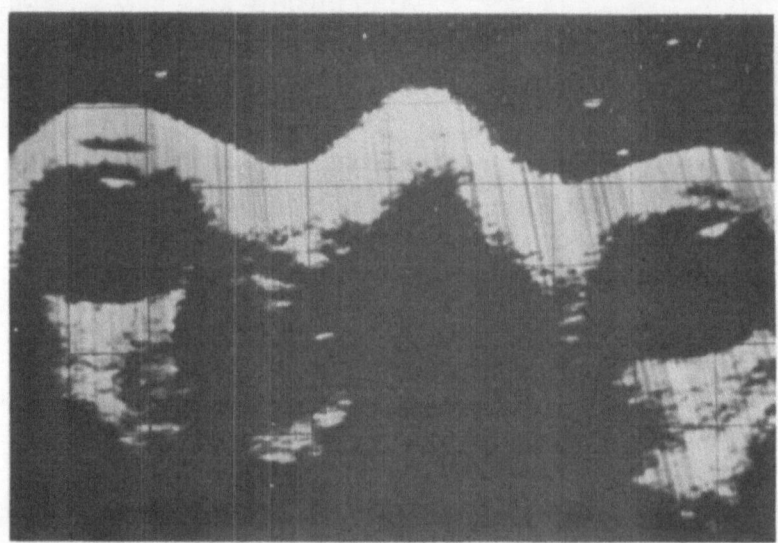

Fig. 14. Echogram of the same case as Fig. 13. Cystic characteristic of the mass was strikingly disclosed.

CONCLUSION

Using the high quality ultrasonic apparatur (Aloka SSD-65), B-scan ultrasonography was useful to visualize abnormality of the orbit and paranasal sinuses. The cystic feature of muco-pyoceles was more clearly demonstrated with ultrasonography than computerized tomography. Neoplastic invasion of the orbit can be differentiated from muco-pyocele with ultrasonography.

ACKNOWLEDGEMENT

This work was supported in part by a Grant-in-Aid for Cancer Research from the Ministry of Health and Welfare of Japan.

REFERENCES

Coleman, D.J., R.L. Jack & L.A. Franzen. B-scan ultrasonography of orbital muco-celes. *Eye, Ear, Nose, Throat Monthly* 51: *207–211* (1972).

Kaneko, A., S. Shigeyama & R. Uchida. A new ultrasonic apparatus for ophthalmology using manual compound scanning. *Doc. Ophthal.* 43: *137–146* (1977).

Till, P. Echography in rhinogenic orbital conditions. pp. 273–277, in: Proc. 2nd Int. Symp. on Orbital Disorders, Amsterdam 1973. Mod. Probl. in Ophthal. Vol. 14. Karger, Basel (1975).

Author's address:
Ophthalmologist-in-chief
National Cancer Center Hospital
5-1-1, Tsukiji, Chuwo-ku
Tokyo 104
Japan

Proc. 3rd Int. Symp. on Orbital Disorders, Amsterdam 1977

COMBINED A- AND CONTACT B-SCAN ULTRASONOGRAPHY OF ORBITAL DISEASE

J. POUJOL & N. TOUFIC

(Paris, France)

Having used the immersion B-scan method for examining the orbit at the beginning of our experience in echography (Massin & Poujol, 1968), we abandoned it in 1968 for the A-mode (Ossoing, et a., 1969; Poujol, 1970). Since 1974, we have been using A-mode combined with contact B-scan as a routine examination. In this paper we have tried to define the respective qualities of each method and the advantages to be gained from their combined use.

MATERIAL AND METHODS

This report concerns the conclusions obtained from 337 echographic examinations of the orbit made over the past three years using the combined A-mode and contact B-scan method. These cases are taken from the 560 orbit examinations carried out in our hospital over the past 13 years. Examinations of the orbit represent about 5% of all our echographic examinations, and 7% in the past three years.

Most of these cases (60%) were referred for examination because they presented a unilateral exophthalmos; 14% because they presented an obvious swelling, 11% a problem of ocular motility, 5% an oedema or an atrophy of the optic disc. Other reasons were retinal folds in the fundus (2.5%), blepharal oedema, loss of vision without any apparent reason, arterial or venous retinal thrombosis, progressive hypermetropia and orbital pains.

In A-mode we used the KRETZTECHNIK 7100, the FERLUX EO1 and the FERLUX EO2, the latter with a logarithmic amplification of 40 dB (Dory et al., 1972). For all the instruments, the probes were nond-focalised, 5 mm in diameter and with a frequency of 7 and 8 mHz. In contact B-scan, we used the BRONSON-TURNER apparatus (Bronson, 1972; Poujol, 1975) and the FERLUX EO2. All examinations were performed first in A-mode, then in B-scan.

DIAGNOSTIC ADVANTAGES OF EACH METHOD

The respective value of A-mode and B-scan according to the criteria required is presented in a schematic manner in Table 1, which may be summarized as follows:

Table 1. Reliability of A- and contact B-scan with regard to some characteristics of pathological orbital structures

Characteristics of structures		A-scan	B-scan
Detection	pathological orbits	+++	++
Topography in terms of the anatomical elements of the orbit	bony wall	++	++
	eyeball	++	++
	optic nerve	+	+++
	extraocular muscles	+	++
Dimensions and limits	measurements	+++	+
	general shape	+	+++
	boundaries	+	++
Content	mobility	++	++
	compressibility	+++	++
	homogeneity	++	+++
	reflectivity level	+++	+
	attenuation	++	+

— A-mode is preferable for measuring the dimensions of normal and pathological structures, which enables the ophthalmologist to follow their development and, more especially, gives precise information on the level of reflectivity of pathological structures, which is essential in differential diagnosis (Ossoinig, 1975). Logarithmic amplification, which eliminates echo saturation, helps the recognition of orbital, endocrinal or inflammatory hyper-reflectivity.

— B-scan gives more information on the exact location of a pathological, orbital structure in terms of the optic nerve, on its general shape and on the homogeneity of its structure (Fig. 1).

Two new criteria have been introduced by the contact B-scan method due to its real-time image which provides instantaneous topographic and kinetic data. These criteria are (a) the existence of horizontal, moving interfaces inside certain pathological structures (Fig. 2), (b) the existence of floating deposits whose echoes fill the whole of the pathological structure when the patient moves, then sediment when the patient is still, in a few seconds, in the lower part of the structure, being separated by a more or less horizontal line from the upper part which is not normally echogeneous.

DIAGNOSTIC RESULTS

Our results were verified mainly on the basis of anatomo-pathological examinations and on cases where an endocrinological examination had shown up sure signs of Grave's disease. Much less frequently, we took into account results of angiography, computerised tomography or extended follow-up. In this manner, out of 337 echographic examinations made with routine A- and contact B-scan, we were able to prove the exactitude

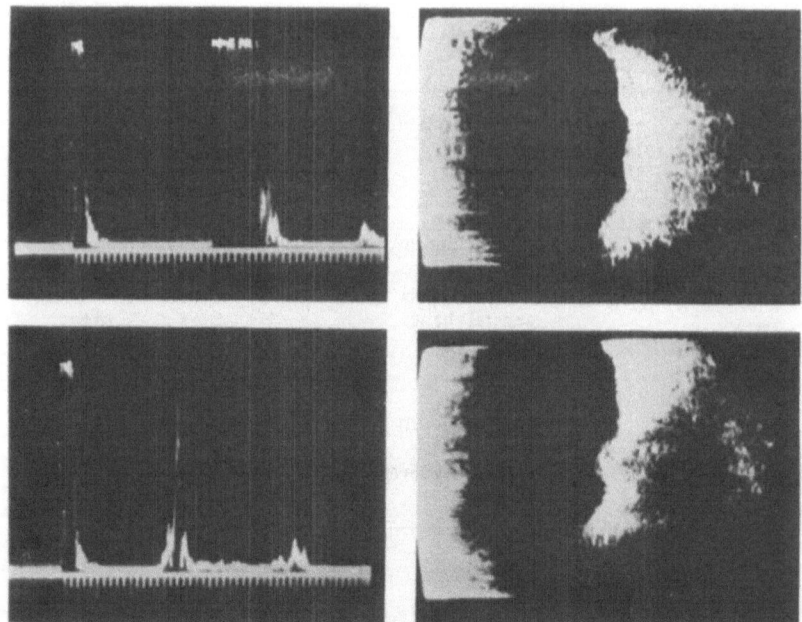

Fig. 1. Glioma of the optic nerve with papillary oedema. A six year old girl in whom a unilateral papillary oedema without exopthalmos had been discovered by chance. Top: normal globe and orbit. Bottom: pathological side. On the A-mode echogram, a shortening of the globe due to pressure from the tumour can be noted, and in the orbit a gap of 18 mm from front to back, the contents of which are only slightly reflective, of the dense type. The B-scan image shows the oedematous papilla and, behind it, on the right of the picture, a gap with ill-defined outer limits in the path of the optic nerve. The first diagnosis which comes to mind is that of a glioma of the optic nerve and this was confirmed by the anatomo-pathological examination.

of the echographic diagnosis of the presence or absence of intraorbital pathological structures in 234 cases.

Table 2 gives the possibility of comparing the exactitude of A-mode and B-scan separately and of the two methods combined in the detection of pathological intra-orbital structures. These figures do not include bony meningiomas of the orbit, which, even though they often provoke uni-lateral exophthalmos, do not actually form intra-orbital tumors. For this reason they are not very often detected by echographic methods but they can very easily be identified using simple radiological methods. A-mode and B-scan would seem to be of more or less the same value in the detection of pathological structures, although in our opinion A-mode is slightly superior, but this is possibly only a result of personal experience.

For differentiating by echographic methods between actual disease of the orbit, we have simply divided them into three categories: (a) heterogeneous structures (mainly cavernous angiomas) (Fig. 3), (b) dense structures (primary and secondary tumors and inflammatory pseudo-tumors) (Fig. 4), (c) liquid structures (mucoceles), cysts, cascular dilatation) (Fig. 5).This

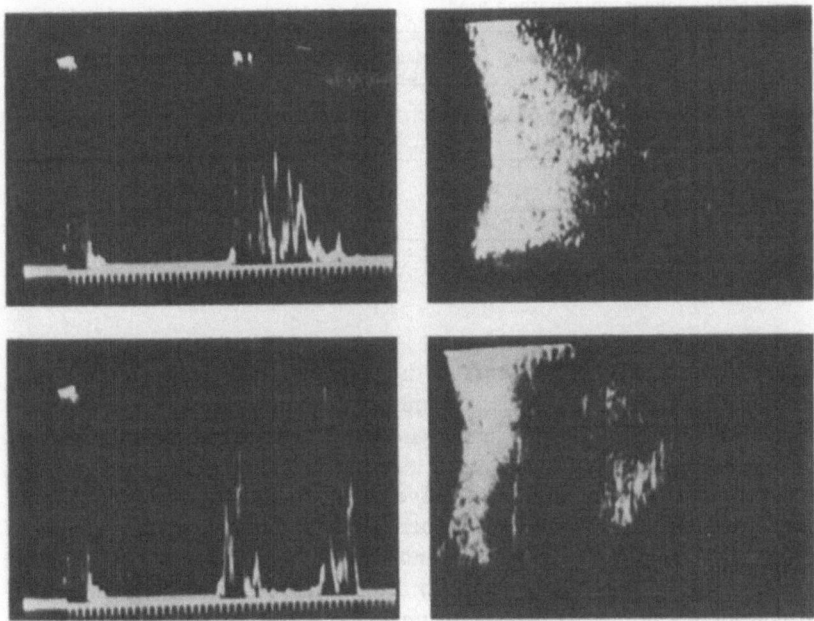

Fig. 2. Cystic hematoma associated with a small cavernous hemangioma. A twenty-eight year old man, who had been suffering from a sudden unilateral exophthalmos. Top: normal globe and orbit. Bottom: the presence can be noted of a gap in the pathological orbit. In A-mode the contents seemed mobile. The B-scan image shows that it is a well-defined bilobate structure with a horizontal interface (vertical on the photo), which looks like a membrane in the middle of a liquid, and in the posterior-upper part, a heterogeneous structure which corresponds to a small cavernous hemangioma.

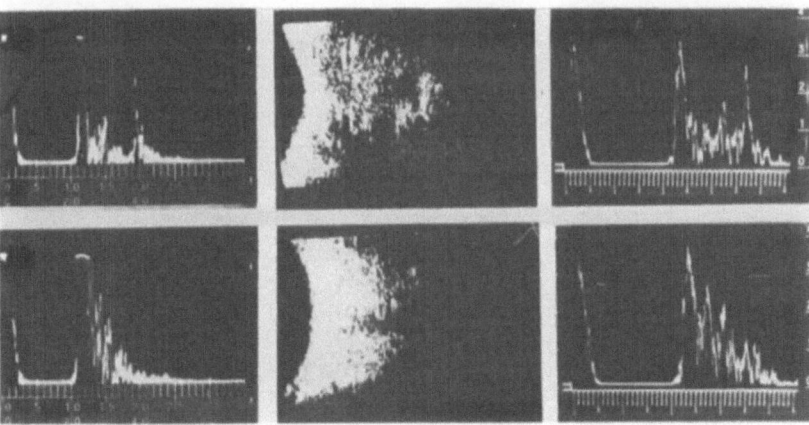

Fig. 3. Cavernous hemangioma of the orbit. A forty-eight year old man who had been suffering from an irregularly progressive unilateral exophthalamos for one year. Top: on the left, A-mode echogram obtained with a very simple and compact apparatus with linear amplification; it was sufficient for correct detection and differentiation. In the middle, B-scan, and on the right, A-mode echogram with logarithmic amplification.

Table 2. Accuracy of *detection* of orbital pathological structures in 234 verified cases, in terms of the echographic method used

Ultrasonic	Diagnosis	A-scan	B-scan	A- & B-scan	%
Correct: 225	positive negative			80 145	96.2
Incorrect: 9	positive negative	1 0	1 5	1 1	3.8

classification considerably orientates the diagnosis. Generally speaking, it is our opinion that a more precise differentiation cannot be obtained without the help of non-echographic clinical and paraclinical criteria. In the numerous cases where an echographic examination has allowed us to eliminate the diagnosis of an orbital tumor, we have often obtained purely echographic arguments pointing towards an endocrinal or inflammatory exophthalmos (mainly thickening of the muscles and orbital hyperreflectivity). We have not taken these case into account in the results presented here since they are considered simply as cases with no pathological intra-orbital structure.

From Table 4, we can conclude that combined A- and B-scan diagnosis is slightly more precise than A-mode for the differentiation between orbital pathological structures, with respect to our previous results (Poujol, 1975).

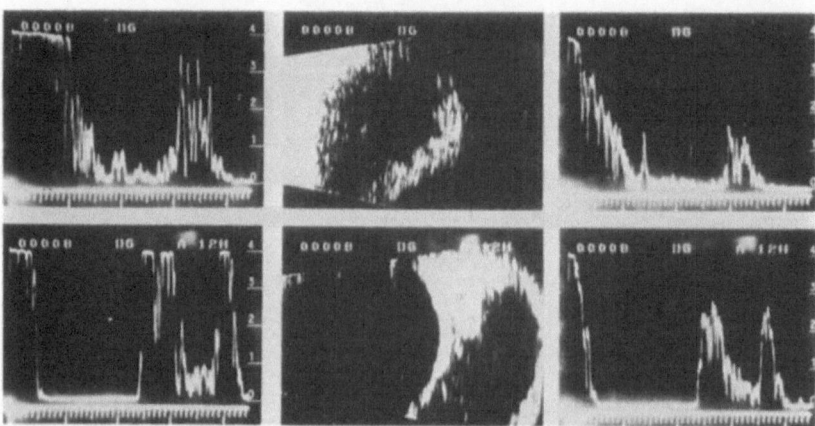

Fig. 4. Primary malignant tumor of the orbit. An eighty-one year old woman who had been suffering for two years from a progressive unilateral exophthalmos. Top: the para-ocular images: on the left, A-mode picture with linear amplification; in the center, contact B-scan and on the right, A-mode with logarithmic amplification. Bottom: the trans-ocular images, in the same order.

Table 3. Distribution of verified cases with regard to the acoustic appearance

I. Acoustically pathological orbits

Acoustic appearance	Diagnosis	Number of cases
(a) Heterogeneous		
	cavernous angiomas	7
	lymphangiomas	2
	hemolymphangioma	1
	infiltrative hematomas	5
	orbital emphysema	1
(b) Dense		
− Primary malignant or benign tumors:		
	lymphosarcomas	7
	reticulosarcomas	2
	lymphoma	1
	gliomas of the optic nerve	2
	neurofibromas	3
	neurinoma	2
	untypical malignant tumors	5
	myoblastomas	2
	cylindroma	1
	rhabdomyosarcoma	1
	plasmocytosis	1
	Waldenström's disease	1
	sarcoidosis	1
	lacrymal adenocarcinoma	1
	chronic dacryoadenitis	1
	fibrolipoma	1
	intra-orbital meningioma	1
	untypical chalazion	1
− Orbital extension of other tumors:		
	ethmoidal tumor	1
	maxillary sinus tumor	1
	choroidal melanoma	1
− Metastatic tumors originating from:		
	lung carcinoma	1
	opposite side choroidal melanoma	1
− Inflammatory pseudo-tumors		14
(c) Liquid		
	orbital mucoceles	5
	muco-pyocele	1
	dermoid	3
	abcess	1
	liquid hematomas	2
	orbital varices	1
	chronic dacryocystis	1

II. Acoustically normal orbits

endocrine diseases	27
diffuse inflammation	17
meningiomas (see text)	8
myopic pseudo-exophthalmos	19
extraocular muscle paralysis	18
disease of the optic nerve	14
arterial and venous retinal thrombosis	4
retinal folds	1
intracranial disorders	6
infraclinoid carotid aneurysms	2
trigeminal neuralgia	1
congenital appearance	4
negative long-term follow-up	30

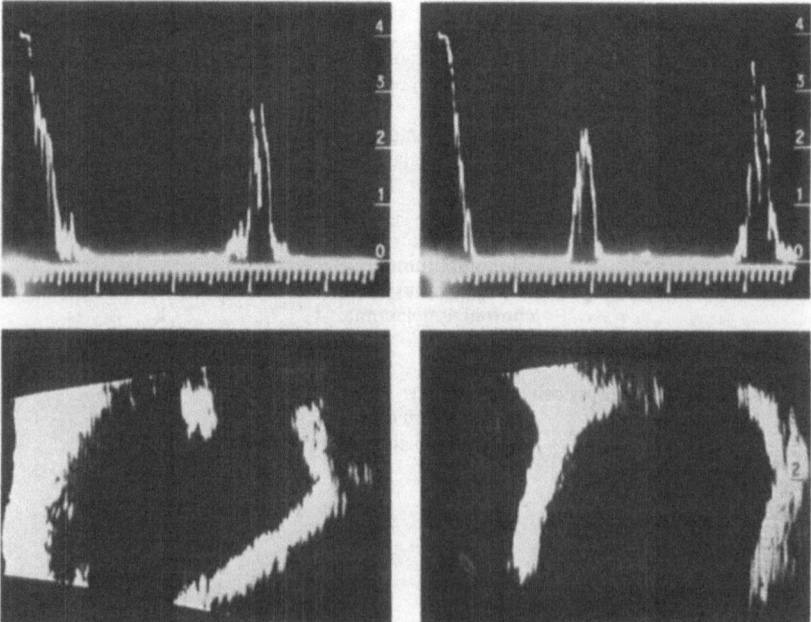

Fig. 5. Fronto-orbital mucocele. A forty-five year old woman who had been suffering for two years from an exophthalmos and a hard mass at the upper inner angle of one orbit. On the left, para-ocular images: the A-mode echogram shows a complete lack of reflectivity of the contents. The B-scan echogram shows the upper edge of the bony gap between the orbit and the frontal sinus, and also the bottom of the sinus. On the right, trans-ocular images: the roof of the frontal sinus is visible.

Table 4. Accuracy of *differentiation* between orbital pathological structures in 80 correctly detected cases

A- and B-scan diagnosis Number of cases	Heterogeneous 15	Dense 52	Liquid 13	Total %
Correct: 71	93.5%	91.5%	87.0%	88.7%
Incorrect: 9	6.5%	9.5%	23.0%	11.3%

CONCLUSION

The convenience and speed of contact B-scan have made it possible to use this method for routine examinations of the orbit (and of the globe), along with A-mode. It only takes a minute with either method to verify or eliminate the presence of a pathological orbital structure. It obviously takes longer to determine the nature of the pathological structure once it has been located but the examination remains easy to perform.

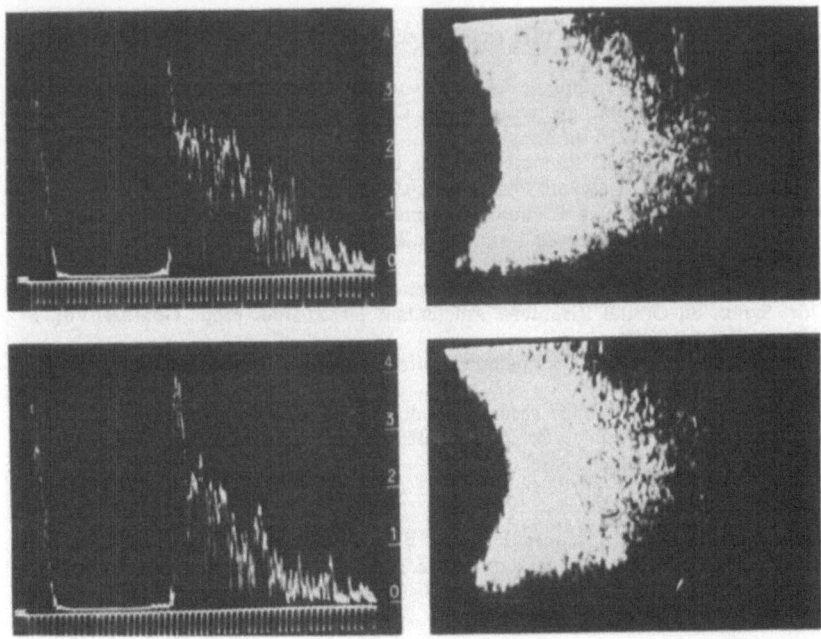

Fig. 6. Endocrine unilateral exophthalmos. A forty-three year old man who had been suffering from a rapidly progressive unilateral exophthalmos for eight months. Angiography and computerized tomography were highly evocative of a big retrobulbar tumor, whereas echography indicated only an enlargement of the retro-bulbar tissue and a higher reflectivity with regard to the opposite side. Top: pathological side. Logarithmic A-mode echogram on the left: the reflectivity level is about 5 dB higher than on the normal side below. This cannot be observed on the B-scan echograms on the right.

Each method provides information for the differential diagnosis of orbital diseases. The biometric and quantitative data provided by A-mode are associated with the topographical and kinetic data furnished by B-scan for a clearer picture of the structure being examined.

One major question may be asked: how does echography compare with other complementary examinations, especially the more recent ones? We felt that echography has a very important part to play since it provides completely different information from that provided by radiology. Echography gives information of the reflection and absorption of ultrasound by the tissues whereas radiology, no matter what method is used, only gives information on the extent to which the tissues are permeated by X-rays (Fig. 6). Radiology and echography are obviously complementary. The examination protocol followed at the Quinze-Vingts Hospital is in fact as follows: clinical examination, followed by simple X-rays and an echographic examination. If the latter is positive, computerised tomography is carried out, followed by angiography if the preceding examinations have not provided enough information to make the decision to operate or not.

REFERENCES

Bronson, N.R. Development of a simple B-scan ultrasonoscope. *Trans. Am. Ophthal. Soc.* 70: *365–408* (1972).

Dory, J., M. Massin & J. Poujol. A new instrument using logarithmic amplification for ophthalmic echographic diagnosis. World Congress on Ultrasonics in Medicine, San Francisco, August 1976 (in press).

Massin, M. & J. Poujol. Rapport d'un cas de tumeur orbitaire examinée par échographie 'B'. *Bull. Soc. Ophtal. France* 68: *303–33* (1968).

Ossoinig, K., M. Massin & J. Poujol. L'ultrasonographie, méthode de routine pour le diagnostic des affections de l'orbite. *Bull. Soc. Ophtal. France* 72: *1051–1058* (1969).

Ossoinig, K.C. A-scan echography and orbital disease. pp. 203–235, in: Proc. 2nd. Int. Symp. on Orbital Disorders, Amsterdam 1973. Mod. Probl. Ophthal. Vol. 14. Karger, Basel (1975).

Poujol, J. Introduction à l'échographie ultrasonique en ophtalmologie. Conf. lyon. Ophtal. No. 103 (1970).

Poujol, J. A-scan ultrasound: accuracy of diagnosis in orbital diseases. pp. 250–253, in: Proc. 2nd Int. Symp. on Orbital Disorders, Amsterdam 1973. Mod. Probl. Ophthal. Vol. 14. Karger, Basel (1975).

Poujol, J. Perspectives de l'échographie B de contact en ophtalmologie. *Bull. Soc. Ophtal. France* 2: *185–191* (1975).

Toufic, N. & J. Poujol. L'échotomographie B de contact en temps réel dans la pratique ophtalmologique. 3me Colloque de la Soc. franç. pour l'application des ultrasons à la Médicine et à la Biologie. Strasbourg, 28–29 juin 1976 E dit. Soc. Franç. Utrasons (1977).

Authors' address:
Centre National d'Ophtalmologie des Quinze-Vingts
28 rue de Charenton
75012 Paris
France

Proc. 3rd Int. Symp. on Orbital Disorders, Amsterdam 1977

ULTRASONOGRAPHY OF THE OPTIC NERVE

W. SCHROEDER

(Hamburg, W. Germany)

INTRODUCTION

In 1972 and 1973 the first papers regarding ultrasonography of the optic nerve were presented by Coleman & Abramson. During a discussion at the 2nd Symposium on Orbital Disorders in Amsterdam in 1973, Ossoinig mentioned that exact measurements of the optic nerve diameter were possible. Since then we have routinely performed examinations of the optic nerve. In the following an attempt is made to present a survey of our experience in this field.

METHODS

We use A-scan ultrasonography (Kretz 7200 MA) to measure the thickness of the optic nerve and its sheath. Figure 1 shows the various directions from

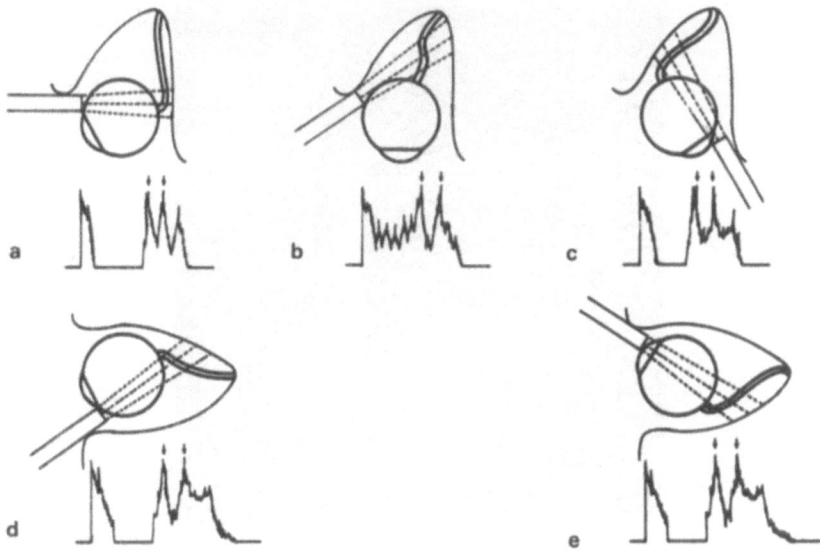

Fig. 1, a—e. Methods to measure the thickness of the distal part of the optic nerve and its sheath. a—c, horizontal; d,e, vertical plane. Arrows: patterns of the optic nerve.

71

which the sound beam can be projected to the distal part of the nerve. We prefer the first method (Fig. 1a) because in this way the nerve can be encountered perpendicularly. The globe is abducted and the transducer is placed on the temporal corneal limbus so that the sound beam is directed to the posterior pole. Beyond this it meets the optic nerve and the rectus internus muscle, which both lie there parallel to the medial orbital wall. The distance between the last spike of the 2nd and the first spike of the 3rd group of high echospikes indicates the double running time of ultrasound within the cross section of the distal part of the optic nerve (Fig. 2). We do not convert the running time into millimeters as this leads to inaccuracies because different optic nerve lesions may cause an unknown range of sound velocities.

With contact B-scan ultrasonography (Bronson-Turner unit) the position of the optic nerve is determined especially in its relationship to space occupying orbital lesions. Figure 3 shows some methods of examination. The optic nerve can be scanned longitudinally or in cross section. By alternating the direction of the scanplane vertically three-dimensional information is obtained, which naturally cannot be documented.

RESULTS AND COMMENTS

Under normal conditions cross-sectional measurements of the distal portion of the optic nerve give double running time of ultrasound between 4 and 6

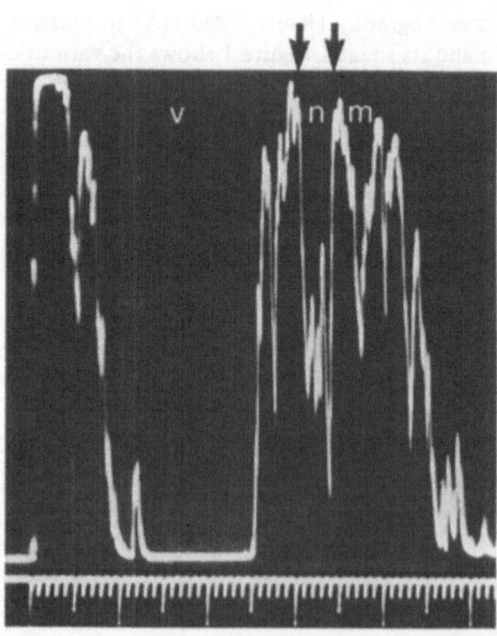

Fig. 2. Cross sectional A-scan ultrasonogram of the distal part of the optic nerve obtained by the method demonstrated in Fig. 1a. v, vitreous; n, optic nerve; m, medial rectus muscle. Arrows: echospikes used for measurement.

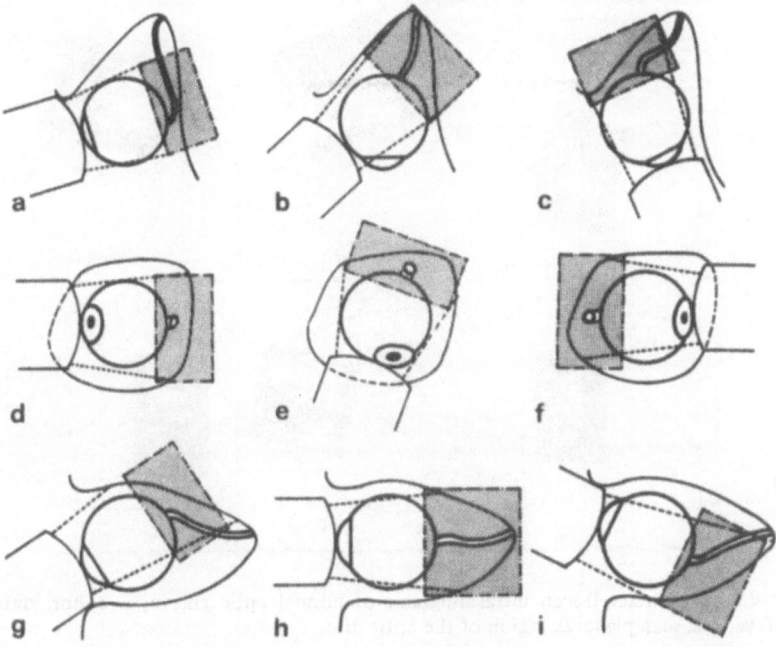

Fig. 3. Methods to examine the optic nerve with contact B-scan ultrasonography. a–c, horizontal; d,f,g–i, vertical and oblique; e, scan plane.

µsec (Table 1), which corresponds to an anatomical diameter of 3 to 4 mm. The patterns of the optic nerve in the contact B-scan ultrasonogram are shown in Figure 4. In the primary position of the eye the undulation of the optic nerve is seen (Fig. 4b,e). Vertical or oblique scanplanes show its cross section. Measurements of the diameter however appear more exact with A-scan.

Under pathological conditions thickening of the optic nerve is a constant finding in the fol owing lesions: intraorbital compression, papilloedema due to increased intracranial pressure, tumour, neuritis, injury (Table 2). Thus in orbital lesions which compress the nerve but do not dislocate its distal part ot a great extent – for instance in tumours of the orbital apex and the optic canal – the thickening correlates initially to the papilloedema. It persists even if the disc becomes pale provided the compression lasts. After a decom-

Table 1. The double running time of ultrasound within the cross section of the optic nerve.

x	4,7	µsec
s_x	0,9	µsec
n	160	

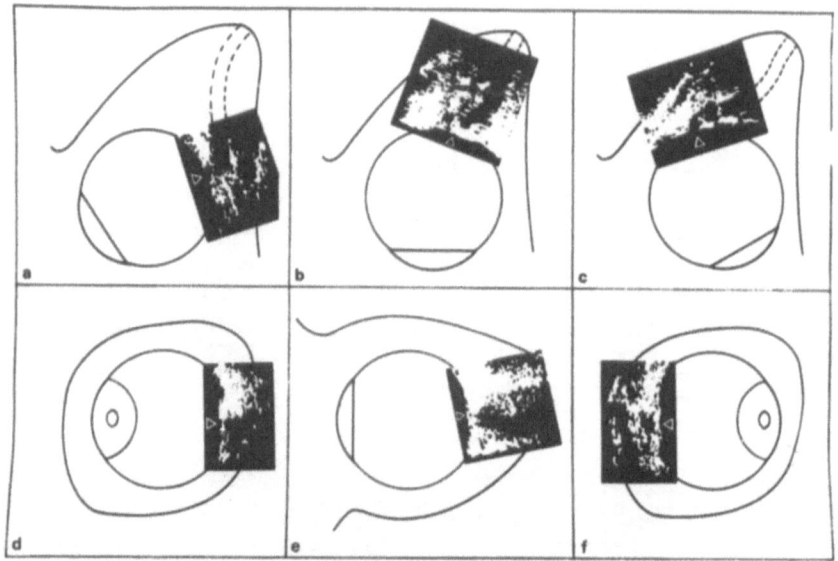

Fig. 4, a–f. Contact B-scan ultrasonograms of normal optic enerve; a–c, horizontal; d–f, vertical scan plane; △, region of the optic disc.

Table 2. Conditions causing optic nerve thickening

Compression, orbital and intracanalicular Papilloedema due to
    increased intracranial pressure ('Stauungspapille')
Tumours of the optic nerve and its sheath
Neuritis
Injury

---

pression is performed the diameter becomes normal immediately. We have seen similar patterns in cases of bilateral papilloedema and secondary optic atrophy due to raised intracranial pressure. Meningiomas of the optic nerve sheath are generally first suspected, if unilateral thickening of the optic nerve persists although the initial papilloedema has turned to disc atrophy and when visual loss continues. Glial hamartomas in neurofibromatosis produce a moderate permanent thickening of the optic nerve accompanied by a more or less pale disc. The three gliomas we have seen were so big that only echographic tumour patterns could be found, which could be hardly identified as a result of the optic nerve thickening. In neuritis with papilloedema the thickening of the optic nerve structures lasts several weeks in all cases, approximately up to the time when the disc becomes pale or vision improves. In contrast to this, thickening could be demonstrated in only about two-thirds of our cases with retrobulbar neuritis up to an average of 8 days after onset of the illness. Traumatic optic nerve lesions were found only in one-third to cause an increase of optic nerve diameter. This indicated a hematoma within the optic nerve sheath, which therefore disappeared a few weeks after injury.

We have never seen thickening of the optic nerve echographically in the following conditions: ischemic neuropathy, drusen of the disc, optic pits, atrophy due to ischemic neuropathy, neuritis, injury, prechiasmal or chiasmal lesions (Table 3). This is of interest especially in anterior ischaemic neuropathy and drusen of the disc to differentiate these relatively frequent conditions from the other lesions causing papilloedema. Optic atrophy secondary to ischaemic disease, neuritis, injury, prechiasmal or chiasmal lesions shows normal or diminished optic nerve thickness and is therefore easily distinguished from tumours and other causes of orbital optic nerve

Table 3. Conditions with normal or decreased optic nerve thickness.

Ischaemic neuropathy
Drusen of the disc
Optic pits
Atrophy due to ischaemic neuropathy,
    neuritis, injury, (pre) chiasmal
    intracranial lesions

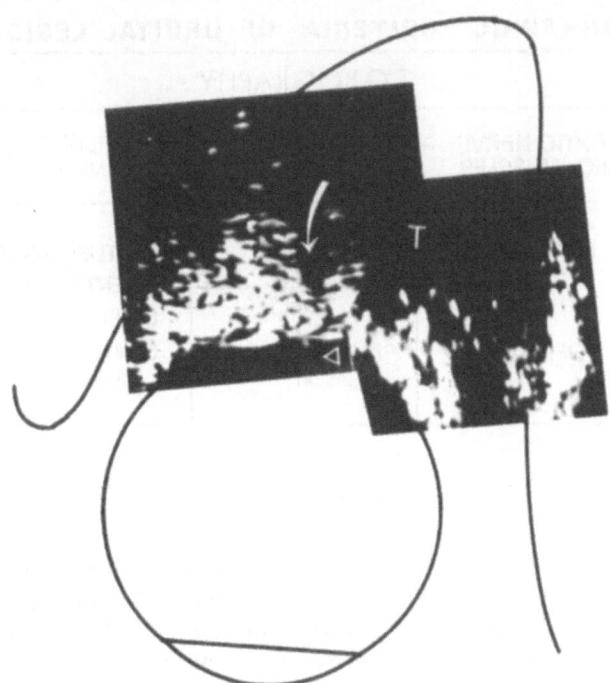

Fig. 5. Lateral dislocation of the optic nerve (arrow). Neurinoma (T) in the medial part of the inner orbital space. Δ, region of the optic disc

compression. It should be mentioned that we have never found patterns which allowed us to differentiate between neural and perineural affection of the optic nerve as Ossoinig (1977) had demonstrated.

Deficiencies of ocular motility, enophthalmus and non-co-operation of the patient are problems in the measurement of optic nerve thickness. Tumours of the inner orbital space frequently dislocate the nerve so that measurement of its diameter is not possible too. In these last cases the dislocation of the nerve demonstrated by contact B-scan ultrasonography indicates the expanding character of the tumour (Fig. 5). Till now we have seen cavernous hemangiomas, neurinomas, malignant melanomas and an abscess in this position. Infiltrating lesions are not expected to dislocate the optic nerve.

Finally it should be mentioned, that in drusen of the optic disc points of increased reflectivity are found with B-scan ultrasonography as described by Fisher & Henkind (1976). Cohen & Stone (1976) have also demonstrated extreme cupping of the disc by the B-scan method.

To conclude, we feel the value of ultrasonography in the diagnoses of orbital lesions is enhanced if examination of the optic nerve is included (Table 4). Firstly, information regarding its diameter is helpful in determining the part of the nerve affected. Secondly, a space-occupying orbital lesion when present can be further characterized by its spatial relationship to the optic nerve.

Table 4

ECHOGRAPHIC CRITERIA OF ORBITAL LESIONS

	TOPOGRAPHY		
REFLECTIVITY	OPTIC NERVE EO. MUSCLES	ORBITAL SPACES	ORBITAL WALL
	DIAMETER	EXPANDING	PROTUBERANCE INDENTATION DEFECT
	POSITION	INFILTRATING lesion	CONTINUATION into sinuses

SUMMARY

A survey of the results of echographic examination of the optic nerve is given. The clinical diagnoses include a great number of primary and secondary lesions of the optic disc as well as the orbital, intracanalicular and intracranial portions of the optic nerve. A-scan ultrasonography is used for measurement of the optic nerve diameter, whereas contact B-scan is especially helpful to determine the spatial relationship of an orbital lesion to the optic nerve. We conclude that examination of the optic nerve plays a vital role in the ultrasonographical diagnosis of orbital lesions.

REFERENCES

Abramson, D.H., D.J. Coleman & L.A. Franzen. Ultrasonography of optic nerve lesions. *Bibl. Ophthal.* 83: *131* (1975)

Cohen, J.S., R.D. Stone, J. Hetherington, Jr. & J. Bullock. Glaucomatous cupping of the disc by ultrasonography. *Am. J. Ophthal.* 82: *24* (1976).

Coleman, D.J. Evaluation of optic neuropathy with B-scan ultrasonography. *Am. J. Ophthal.* 74: *915* (1972).

Fisher, Y.L. Ultrasonic determination of optic nerve head drusen. First Meeting World Fed. for Ultrasound in Medicine (1976).

Henkind, P., H. Friedman & S. Gartner. Drusenpapille. *Klin. Mbl. Augenheilk.* 168: *164* (1976).

Ossoinig, K.C. The role of clinical echography in modern diagnosis of orbital and peri-orbital lesions. In: Proc. 2nd. Symp. on Orbital Disorders, Amsterdam 1973. Mod. Probl. Ophthal. Vol. 14. Karger, Basel (1975).

Ossoinig, K.C., S.L. Kaefring, L. McNutt & S.J. Weinstock. Echographic measurement of the optic nerve. First Meeting World Fed. for Ultrasound in Medicine (1976).

Schroeder, W. Ergebnisse der A-Bildechographie bei einseitigen Sehnerverkrankungen. *Klin. Mbl. Augenheilk.* 169: *30* (1976).

Schroeder, W. Schallaufzeitmessung im distalen Sehnervquerschnitt. *Klin. Mbl. Augenheilk.* 169: *743* (1976).

Schroeder, W. Topographische Orbitadiagnostik mit der Kontakt-B-Bildechographie. *Klin. Mbl. Augenheilk.* (In press.)

Stone, R.D. Ultrasonographic demonstration of glaucomatous cupping of the optic disc. First Meeting World Fed. for Ultrasound in Medicine (1976).

Author's address:
Universitäts Augenklinik
52 Martinistrasse
D-2000 Hamburg 20
W. Germany

Proc. 3rd Int. Symp. on Orbital Disorders, Amsterdam 1977

UNILATERAL HIGH MYOPIA:
COMPARISON OF ULTRASONOGRAPHY AND CT-SCANNING

P.A. GOMMERS, G. BLAAUW & R. WIJNGAARDE

(Rotterdam, The Netherlands)

The presence of high axial myopia can be deceptive in unilateral proptosis. The failure to recognize this condition may cause unnecessary trouble to the patient from redundant technical investigations.

Axial myopia can be demonstrated by streak retinoscopy and ultrasonographic oculometry. These methods are compared with computerized tomographic scanning (CT-scan) in this paper.

ILLUSTRATIVE CASES AND METHODS

Six patients with unilateral proptosis stated, when asked, that they had long standing low vision in one eye. Visual acuity, streak retinoscopy, ultrasonography, and CT-scanning were performed in all the cases.

Streak retinoscopy is a well-established method and we do not need to go into this further.

Oculometry is performed utilizing the ultrasonographic method. When maximal echos of the cornea, the anterior and posterior part of the lens, and of the retina are obtained, the axial length is measured. The apparatus used gives the exact values using an electronic system. A correction for the lens and the retina of 0.6 mm is necessary.

The registration is made by a polaroid camera. Figure 1 depicts the ultrasonographic measurements in a patient with a unilateral proptosis. The upper image represents the right eye, the lower part the left eye. The axial length is 30.3 and 24.3 mm respectively.

· For the measurement of the axis of the eye CT-scans are required visualizing both optic nerves. One tomographic section represents eight mm tissue, so a pure axial measurement is not possible. Only large differences between the two eyes are clearly visible (Fig. 2).

· Table 1 gives the results. Retrobulbar abnormalities could not be detected in any of the patients by both CT-scanning and ultrasonographic examination.

DISCUSSION

It appears that streak retinoscopy is not always possible in an advanced cataract or corneal dystrophy. Furthermore, its results represent the myopia

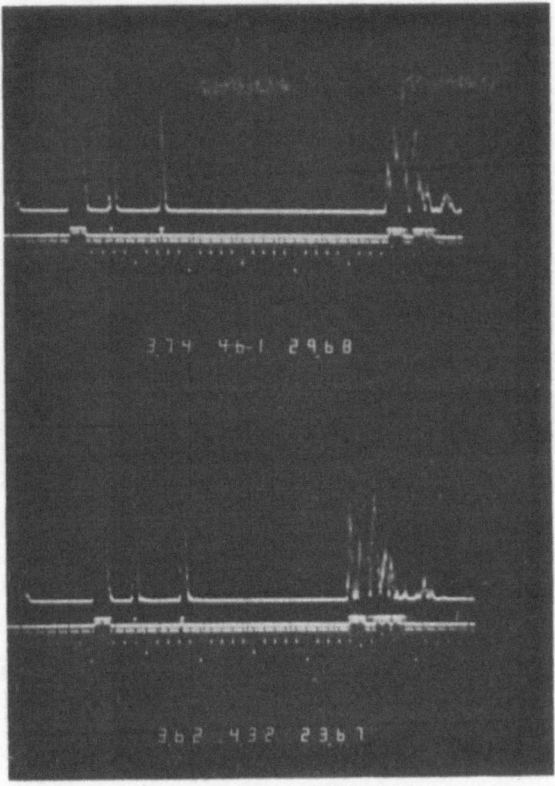

Fig. 1. Ultrasonographic measurements of the axial length in a patient with unilateral high axial myopia. Upper image is from the right eye, the lower image from the left. The last figure underneath the diagrams represents the axial length to which a correction of 0.6 mm must be added for the lens and retina.

as a whole and not the axial myopia which we want to know. Oculometry gives results with an accuracy of plus or minus 0.1–0.3 mm (François & Goes, 1969).

CT-scanning is less exact due to the methods employed. The inexactitude of CT-scanning for the measurement of the axis of the eye in comparison with ultrasonography makes the first method unsuitable for accurate axial measurements, although a rough estimate may be sufficient in these instances.

As the lens dose during CT-scanning of the orbit is 3–6 rad (Wende et al., 1977), routine CT-scanning in patients with unilateral proptosis should be avoided, unless the diagnosis cannot be made by conventional unharmful technical aids.

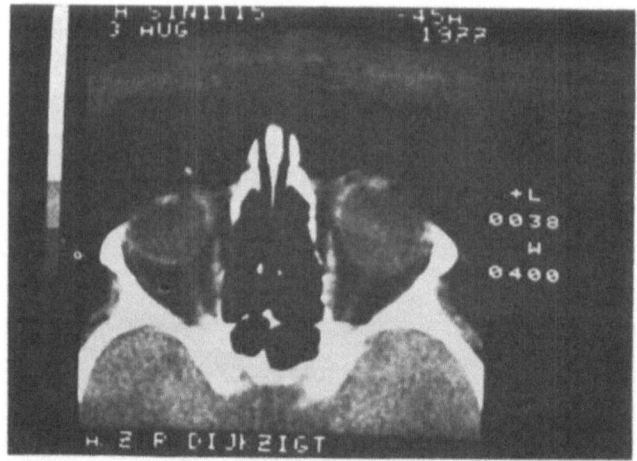

Fig. 2. CT-scans of a patient with unilateral high axial myopia. The greater length of the right eye is clearly visible.

CONCLUSION

Ultrasonographic oculometry and CT-scanning were compared in six patients with unilateral high axial myopia. Oculometry appeared to be more exact, is not harmful, easier to perform and cheaper. Oculometry is to be preferred in these instances to CT-scanning.

Table 1. Results of streak retinoscopy, visual acuity (V.A.), ultrasonographic oculometry, and CT-scanning in six patients with unilateral high axial myopia.

Patient	Age	Streak retinoscopy	V.A.	Oculometry mm	Δ OD/OS	C.T. Scan mm	Δ OD/OS
S.K. ♀	54	OD S − 5 = c − 0.5 x 150	1.0	27.3		28	
		OS S − 15	0.01	30.6	3.3	32	4
Y.O. ♀	77	OD S − 6	1.0	25.7		not to fix	
		OS S − 18 = c − 1 x 80	0.2	30.2	4.5		
S.B. ♀	63	OD S − 16	0.02	33.4		32	
		OS S + 2.25	1.0	23.7	9.7	24	8
H.L. ♀	66	OD S − 8	0.01	25.3		32	
		OS S + 4 = c − 1 x 105	1.0	22.1	3.2	28	4
K.V. ♀	59	OD S − 0.5 = c − 0.5 x 45	0.8	23.7		28	
		OS S − 14 = c − 2 x 160	0.5	30.1	6.4	32	4
L.M. ♀	67	OS S + 2 = c + 0.5 x 180	0.8	24.6		26	
		OS cataract	perc.	31.6	7.0	32	6

REFERENCES

François, J. & F. Goes. Comparative study of ultrasonic biometry of emmetropes and myopes with special regard to the heredity of myopia. pp. 165–180, in: Ophthal. Ultrasound Proc. 4th Int. Congress on Ultrasonics in Ophthalmology, Philadelphia. Mosby, St. Louis (1969).

Wende, S., A. Aulich, A. Nover, W. Lankich, E. Kazner, H. Steinhoff, W. Meese, S. Lange & T. Grumme. Computed tomography of orbital lesions. *Neuroradiology* 13: *123–134* (1977).

Authors' address:
Eye Hospital and Departments of
Neurosurgery and Ophthalmology
Erasmus University
Rotterdam
The Netherlands

Proc. 3rd Int. Symp. on Orbital Disorders, Amsterdam 1977

RADIOLOGICAL DIAGNOSIS OF ORBITAL FRACTURES
IN OPHTHALMOLOGY

E.A. CABANIS, M.T. IBA-ZIZEN, V. DANICEL & A. LOPEZ

(Paris, France)

The radiological diagnosis of orbital fractures in ophthalmological practice is different from the current traumatic maxillo-facial procedure. There are two types of patient. First, a patient who consults an ophthalmologist for a recent orbital trauma in most cases he has had a light trauma and presently suffers a more important maxillo-facial traumatism (with or without poly-traumatism): he is brought to an Emergency Unit (reanimation, neurosurgery . . .) because prognosis is above all vital.

We are primarily concerned with a patient of the first category. Radiologic exploration is altogether possible (therefore obligatory), immediate and complete in its findings. More often that not the bony lesion is difficult to find.

MATERIAL

Six hundred and thirty-five (635) patients with orbital concussions have been X-rayed during the last three years (1974-1976), in the X-ray Department of C.N.O. 15/20. Two hundred and twenty-nine (229) (36%) fractures have been diagnosed. Only twenty-two (22) surgical interventions have had to be done. The traumas were mostly recent ones, seen at the Emergency Unit of the Hospital. In thirty-four (34) cases, radiological investigation had been initiated for a different reason (diplopia, lagophthalmia); in these cases the initial traumatism had either been ignored or forgotten.

In each case, the radiological technique first takes a standard examination and in many cases it is followed by a tomographic study.

Standard X-ray

The 'orbital' P.A. view (projection of the superior edge of the petrous bone at the middle of the maxillary sinus) is fundamentally useful. The other views (P.A., Fronto-nasal, Waters, Optic canal, Axial, Lateral) are well known. They are a completion of the exam. Direct magnification is applied for orbital view.

Tomography

It is performed with Polytome ° (Hypocycloidal movement, constant magnification, cuts of 1 mm thickness). The cuts are repeated at 2.5 mm intervals for orbital walls and 1 mm for the optic canals. Two orthogonal planes are used: frontal and sagittal (superior and inferior walls), frontal and axial (lateral walls), unilateral and axial (optic canal). The frontal view is always taken in A.P. to prevent movement on the part of the patient.

DISCUSSION

We have adopted the P. Serres' clinical and anatomical classification (1975), which divides orbital fractures into six types.

Type I: orbital walls;

Type II: orbital walls and margins (with naso-orbital dislocation and zygomatic bone lesion);

Type III: orbital disjunction along the three lines of weakness (zygomatic bone, Lefort's types II and III, complete disjunction);

Type IV: extensive fracture of the skull (from the vault or the base, multiple fractures;

Type V: crushing (combination of types II and III, comminuted fractures);

Type VI: apex (superior orbital fissure, optic canal, sphenoid);

Other clinical aspects are concerned with ballistics, children and sequels.

The cases most frequently encountered were of type I, less frequently II and III, and still less frequently type VI; others were only exceptional occurences.

These results reflect that the traumas were light enough in severity to bring the patient to ophthalmology first. In fact, etiologies encountered are the following: scuffle (39%), road accident in second place only (23%), fall (13%) and unspecified injuries. The scuffles most frequently concerned males, 30–35 years old, having suffered a closed fist impact and the fracture is at the lower or medial wall (the most fragile). The floor is very rarely destroyed; the classical 'blow-out' fractures (CONVERSE) with incarceration are relatively rare. Tomography sometimes makes it possible to distinguish between submucous hematoma and preexisting sinusitis. The walls of the intraorbital groove must be analysed in tomographies: so that lateral microfractures may be detected.

Ethmoidal fracture (planum) often provoke 'pneumo-orbit'; the little air bubble is seen as a clear round area close to the roof: it must be distinguished from the normal palpebral lines. The second sign of planum fractures is the opacity of the homolateral ethmoidal cells. Tomography in frontal and axial views gives the exact extent of the fracture and the surrounding hematoma (Fig. 1).

In a similar manner, suspicion of a roof lesion demands a tomographic exploration. In fact, the danger has become threefold: direct cranio-cerebral injury, fracture of the frontal sinus walls, and to a lesser degree lesion of the trochlear fovea (superior oblique trochlea). For that reason, a millimetric tomographic examination is called for.

Type II corresponds to a more violent impact (small surface). The nasal pyramid and the naso-lacrimal duct are often affected in internal trauma-

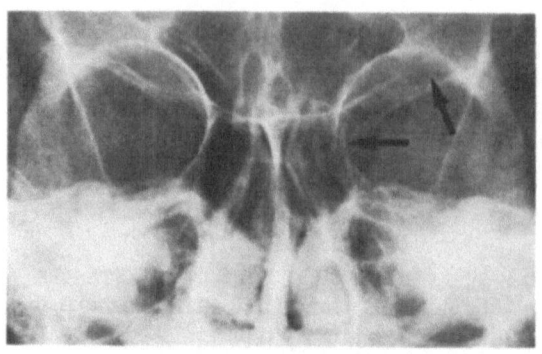

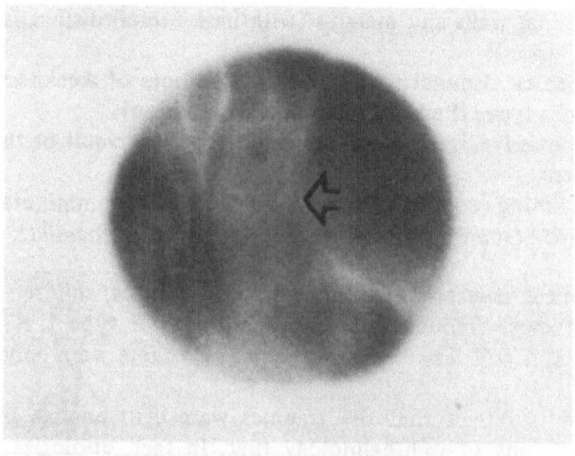

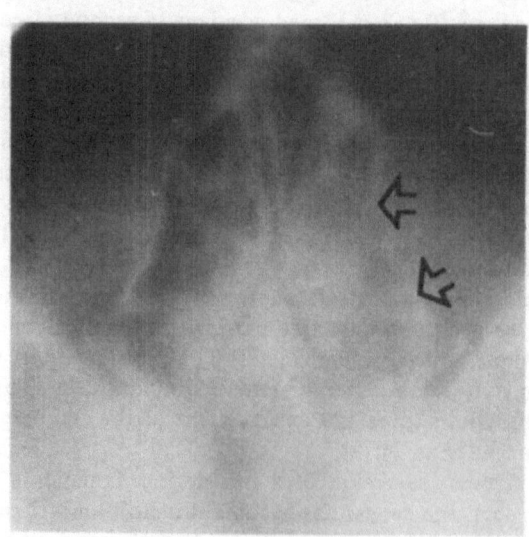

Fig. 1. Fracture of the left lamina papyracea. G. Henri, 54, closed first (left).
1a. Standard X-ray (P-A). Small/pneumo-orbit (superior) and opacity of left ethmoidal cells (↗).
1b. Tomography (A-P). Opacity of ethmoidal cells, planum discontinuity (↑).
1c. Tomography (Axial). Antero-posterior extension of the opacity, planum deformation (↑).

tisms. Millimetric cuts are again necessary. Furthermore dacryocystography may be necessary.

Type III (disjunction) is found at the three lines of weakness which converge at the orbital apex at the middle of the planum, along the infraorbital groove and the external wall.

Type IV and V escape any radiological description: prognosis is vital.

Type VI (apex fractures). A fracture of the optic canal must be immediately suspected in cases of post-traumatic amaurosis. In standard X-ray, we must check the integrity of jugo-optico-clinoidal line. Millimetric tomographies are in Hartmann-Gilles (unilateral) and axial (comparative) views.

Clinical aspects

Foreign bodies visible close to the roof demand tomographies (craniocerebral injury). A child with an even small superior palpebral wound must be immediately suspected of cranio-cerebral injury; the child frequently

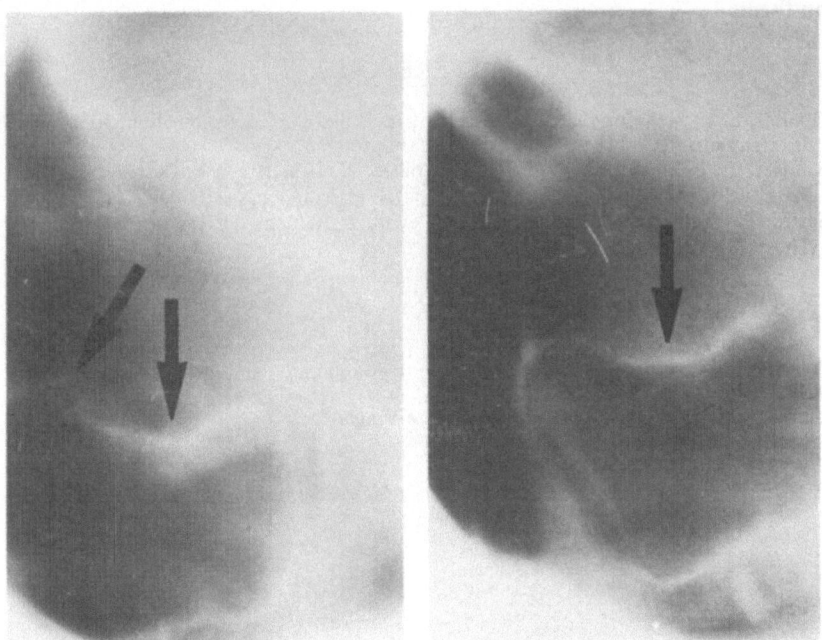

Fig. 2. Fracture of the orbital floor = spontaneous reconstruction. C. Brev, 41, closed fist.

2a. Post-traumatic lateral tomography (immediate). Discontinuity of the floor, inferior displacement and angulation of the fragments, mucosal thickening (hematoma?) (↗).

2b. Control lateral tomography, 7 weeks later. Spontaneous reconstruction in vicious position, with secondary enlargement of the vertical orbital diameter; disparition of the mucosal thickening (↗).

does not admit the circumstances of the trauma (e.g. foreing body having entered?) Orbital roof tomographies are imperative.

The radiological aspect of sequels must be emphasized. In case of fractures of the internal or lower walls with minimal displacement, a control examination made a few weeks after the initial traumatism may show the disappearance of sub-periostal reconstruction.

These findings must be compared with similar findings in patients examined for diplopia: the initial traumas in these cases had been forgotten or ignored. The secondary enlargement of the orbital diameters may result in oculomotor disfunction. A secondary diplopia could then be explained by a prolonged hematoma resorption or a secondary fibrosis.

A post-traumatic exophthalmos may appear in two circumstances: carotido-cavernous fistula and retrobulbar hematoma. The latter demands a complete neuroradiological examination (standard, tomographies, CT and angiography) to look for a preexisting vascular malformation.

In conclusion, we may assert that the orbital 'concussion' is suspect of fracture (floor of planum). Standard X-ray and complex tomography beyond the slightest doubt must all be performed with particular attention. Therapeutic and medico-legal consequences (secondary diplopias) depend on them.

REFERENCES

Canabis, E.A., M.T. Iba-Zizen, R. Cavezian, A. Kujas & U. Salvolini. Radio-diagnostic des traumatismes orbitaires. Masson, Paris (in press).
Rougier, T., P. Tessier, F. Hervouet, M. Woillez, M. Lekièffre & P. Derome. Chirurgie plastique orbito-palpébrale. Soc. franç. Ophtal. Masson, Paris (1977).
Serres, P. Etat actuel de la classification et du traitement des fractures de l'orbite. Thèse, Médicine. Paris (1975).

(In collaboration with G.R.E.N.R.O.)

Authors' address:
X-Ray Dept.
Centre National d'Ophtalmologie des Quinze-Vingts
28 rue de Charenton
Paris 75571
France

Proc. 3rd Int. Symp. on Orbital Disorders, Amsterdam 1977

THEORETICAL OPHTHALMOLOGIC RISK OF EMBOLIZATION

C. CLAY, P. LASJAUNIAS, J. MORET & J. VIGNAUD
(Paris, France)

Selective angiography of the external carotid artery has led us to evaluate the possibilities of treatment by embolization, and, at the same time, the theoretical risks of such treatment in relation to anastosmoses between the external and the internal carotid arteries.

Radio-anatomical studies show that the anastomotic vessels between these two arteries concern (Fig. 1):

1. The sensorial territory (second cranial nerve) through ophthalmo-meningeal channels.

2. The territory of the orbital motor nerves (third, fourth and sixth cranial nerves), through anastomotic branches between the accessory meningeal artery and the infero-lateral trunk of the internal carotid siphon: this occurs in 78% of the cases. In 22% there is no anastomosis. The orbital motor nerves are then exclusively vascularized by the external carotid artery (i.e. the accessory meningeal artery).

3. The sensitive territory (fifth cranial nerve, trigeminal ganglion): through anastomotic branches between the middle meningeal artery and the infero--lateral trunk of the carotid siphon.

4. The territory of the internal carotid artery (fronto-parietal cortex) through anastomotic branches with different arteries from the carotid siphon (infero-lateral branch and ophthalmic artery).

Keeping in mind these anatomical data, we may evaluate the theoretical risks incurred by the embolization of the branches of the external carotid artery. These risks may be:

the migration of the embolism in the 'wrong' arterial branch;

– the migration of the embolism beyond its aim ('overshooting');

the complete occlusion by the embolism of an arterial pedicle which is the only vascular source of a major organ.

These risks incite caution, and make it necessary to discuss in each case

1. *The type of treatment* - embolization or therapeutic occlusion. The choice depends on the pathological lesion and on the distribution of the arteries in the anatomical region to be treated.

2. *The choice of material* to be used, in case of embolization.

3. *The technique of embolization.*

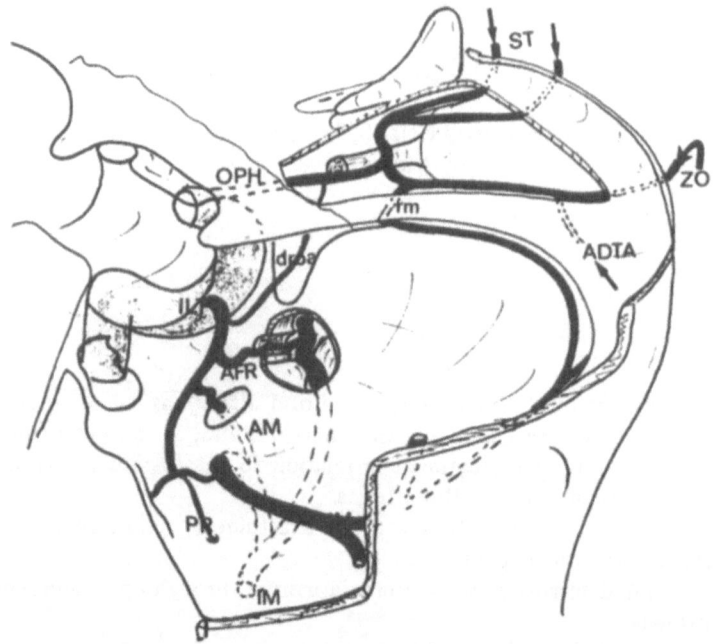

Fig. 1. Supra-lateral view of the base of the skull. Schematic drawing to indicate the anastomotic channels between the internal maxillary stem and the ophthalmic stem.

Explanation of symbols: ILT — infero-lateral trunk; ST — superficial temporal artery; AFR — artery of the rotund foramen; IM — internal maxillary artery; AM — accessory meningeal artery; PR — petrous ramus; ZO — zygomatico-orbital artery; ADTA — anterior deep temporal artery; rm — recurrent meningeal artery; droa — deep recurrent ophthalmic artery.

CHOICE OF TREATMENT

The choice of the type of treatment is based on the following conditions:
   the pathological zone is hypervascularized;
– there is no dangerous anatomical variation in the arterial distribution;
   selective or supraselective, catheterism is possible.

CHOICE OF MATERIAL

The materials which may be used are:
1. *Fluid* at thetime of injection, but undergoing polymerization when in contact with the circulating blood. This material may even reach the tiniest branches and determine a durable obstruction. The major risk involved is overshooting; for this reason such materials are rarely used.
2. *Solid and resorbable* (sponge). This is injected alone or with hyperthrombotic drugs. The size of the embolism may be adapted to the size of the vessel to be embolized. The risks are slight, since these materials are tran-

sient. This treatment is, however, never permanent as there is a repermeation of the embolized vessels in the first days following treatment.

3. *Solid and non-resorbable* (e.g. lyophilized duramater). The advantages are easy handling, readier appreciation of the size of the embolism and the permanency of obstruction in cases where the lesion receives only one arterial pedicle, or in cases where all pedicles have been embolized. The risk is the migration of the embolism into the wrong arterial branch and overshooting the embolism into the internal carotid system.

TECHNIQUE OF EMBOLIZATION

Whenever possible, the catheter is to be positioned as distally as possible, and beyond the anastomosis between the external and the internal carotid arteries. Embolization is only performed when the catheter is fixed in order to avoid reflux of the material.

The course of the material must be carefully observed by a preliminary injection of a small quantity of contrast medium before embolization. This helps to ascertain that the contrast medium is really directed towards the right arterial branch and that there is no reflux. The size of the emoblism used should not be greater than the size of the embolized vessel. These sizes are difficult to appreciate accurately.

Cases of arterial spasm should be treated by slow local perfusion of vascodilators.

CONCLUSIONS

In practice, we may evaluate the theoretical risks after an exact study of the anatomy and of the permeability of the arterial anastomoses.

There should be no anastomotic channel beyond the catheter, if correctly placed between the vessel to be embolized and the various territories mentioned above. It is then possible to embolize the vessel completely, using any material, fluid or solid. However, the embolized territory should receive more than one arterial pedicle, or else complete embolization would determine a necrosis of this territory.

If there is a tiny anastomosis, embolization is, theoretically, possible without risk if the embolism is of resorbable or non-resorbable material and of a size greater than that of the anastomosis. Fluid materials are absolutely contra-indicated in such cases.

If there is an important anastomosis, two situations may occur:

1. Selective embolization is possible. The catheter is fixed beyond the anastomosis in such a way as to avoid reflux. Radioscopic control is done by injection of contrast medium. Technical problems are considerable in such cases, and require a highly trained team for this treatment. In this particular case, fluid material is absolutely contra-indicated.

2. Selective embolization is not possible and consequently the risk is enormous. The functional disorders must then be re-evaluated and the risks of surgical treatment should be weighed against those of the spontaneous course of the affection.

What are the clinical consequences of embolization? In our cases we observed:
— no neurological complications;
— no sensorial complications;
— no orbital motor nerve paralysis;
— very constant but transient trigeminal neuralgia (twelve hours) after internal maxillary artery embolization.

In the literature, trigeminal neuralgia is reported as being frequent, but only two cases of facial paralysis were published.

In summary, it seemed important to underline the theoretical risks of arterial embolization and to stress the necessity of precise studies of angiographies by a highly trained team, familiar with radio-anatomy.

Authors' address:
C. Clay
Service de Radiologie
25 à 29 rue Manin
75019 Paris
France

THE VALUE OF COMPUTER TOMOGRAPHY (CT-SCANNING), ORBITAL VENOGRAPHY AND CAROTID ANGIOGRAPHY IN THE DIAGNOSIS OF EXOPHTHALMOS

F. PEETERS, R. KRÖGER, B. VERBEETEN Jr. & C. VERSTEEGE

(Amsterdam, The Netherlands)

INTRODUCTION

The results obtained by computer tomography (CT-scanning) in the diagnosis of exophthalmos have been so favourable that this new method of investigation should be regarded as the radiological aid of choice in the diagnosis of this condition. The literature reports a diagnostic efficacy of over 90%. Table 1 lists the values reported by a number of authors who compared the CT-scan with conventional radiological methods of investigation. The so-called efficacy concerns only the demonstration or exclusion of pathological tissue as a cause of exophthalmos. In the differential diagnosis of the pathological tissue, CT-scanning is often not more effective than conventional methods. The possibilities of differential diagnosis can be somewhat extended by contrast intensification. Moreover, optimally accurate determination of the localization and extent of the process can also be helpful in differential diagnosis. For this purpose, Hilal et al. (1977) make use of very thin sections (4 mm).

Despite all these measures, even experienced authors point out that in many cases it is impossible to determine the nature of an intra-orbital process (Hilal et al., 1977; Salvolini et al., 1977; Wende et al., 1977).

The question arises whether, beside CT-scanning, there is still any use for the conventional radiological methods of investigation. This contribution attempts to answer this question on the basis of data from the literature and personal observations. We also attempt to establish whether, if there is still any use for these conventional methods, there are cases in which they are to be preferred to CT-scanning; and, if so, in which cases.

MATERIAL AND METHODS

Orbital CT-scans in our patients were obtained with an E.M.I. Mark I brain scanner with 160x160 matrix, using 8 mm sections, 140 kV$_p$ 28 mA. The patient's head was so positioned that the sections lay in a plane at an angle of $10-15°$ with the orbitomeatal line.

The total group of patients to be discussed consisted of 42 patients in whom orbital venography (and sometimes carotid angiography) was carried out as well as CT-scanning.

91

In the entire series, we determined to which extent the diagnosis based on the CT-scan was less accurate than that based on orbital venogram and carotid angiogram. This was found to be the case in two patients with carotid/cavernous sinus fistulae and in three patients with a venous malformation, in whom the nature of the process was diagnosed on the basis of the orbital venogram.

One of the last mentioned patients was a 13-year-old boy with a haemangioma of the chest and a varix in the left superficial jugular vein. This boy showed intermittent exophthalmos which increased upon blowing or stooping. The orbital CT-scan showed tissue of increased density in the left retrobulbar region, immediately above the vascular nerve strand (Fig. 1). The orbital venogram revealed a direct anastomosis between the superior orbital vein and a venous plexus, characteristic of a venous malformation (Fig. 2). The carotid angiogram failed to reveal this malformation.

Orbital venography proved to be superior in the diagnosis of varices and venous malformations, whereas carotid angiography was superior in the diagnosis of cavernous sinus fistulae and carotid aneurysms. These results are listed in Table 1, which compares them with corresponding findings (so far as discovered) in the literature. The series in which this information could be found were small, and did not include some syndromes in which exophthalmos is likewise prominent. Apart from the indications for orbital venography which can be deduced from the data in Table 1, some authors have mentioned a number of syndromes in which orbital venography supplies more diagnostic information than CT-scanning. These instances involved differential diagnosis between infalmmation and tumour (Lloyd et

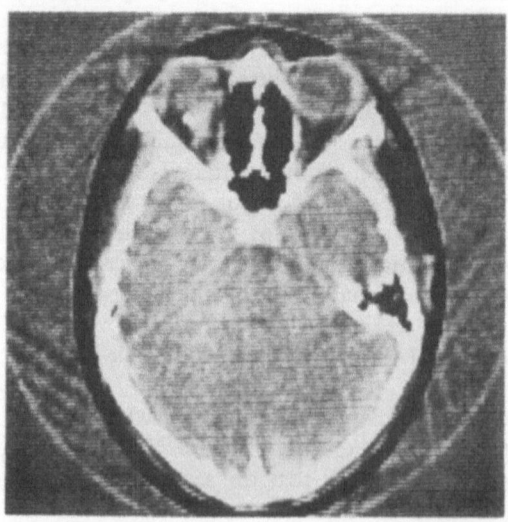

Fig. 1. CT-scan of the orbits in a patient with venous malformation of the left superior ophthalmic vein. Pathological tissue of increased density is visible in the retrobulbar space.

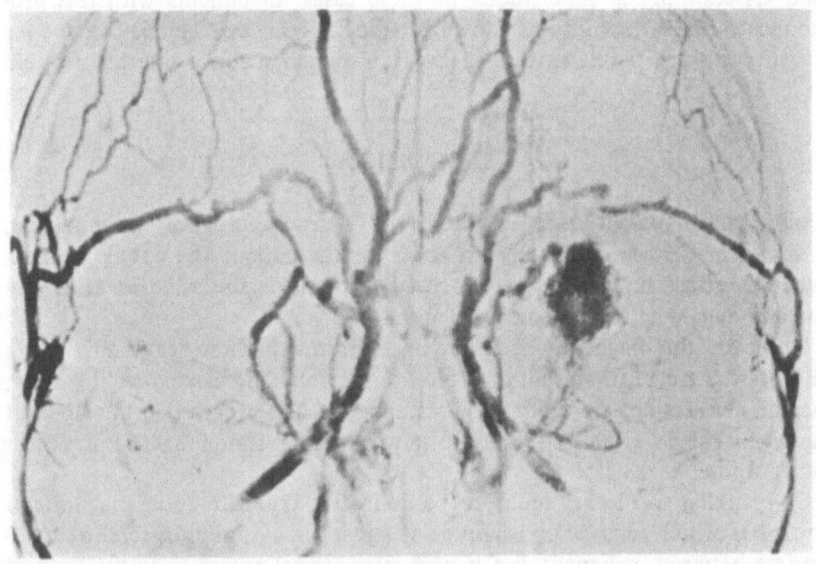

Fig. 2. Orbital venography in the same patient as fig. 1. Unlike the CT-scan, the venogram reveals the venous malformation as such.

al., 1977), small tumours in the apex which would be overlooked at CT-scanning (Moseley et al., 1975), differential diagnosis between endocrine exophthalmos and tumour (Brismar et al., 1976), and the diagnosis of thrombosis of orbital veins (Brismar et al. 1977).

To summarize: it can be maintained that orbital venography is indicated in exophthalmos when the CT-scan reveals no pathological tissue within the orbit, the ocular muscles show normal features, and the clinical picture can be consistent with venous malformation or venous thrombosis. Careful determination of the indication for orbital venography is imperative because recent publications have indicated that this examination is not entirely without risks (Safer & Guibor, 1975; Brismar et al., 1976). In a few patients, bleeding from the congested orbital veins has been observed, probably as a result of the sudden rise in pressure in these veins upon injection of the contrast medium. In the case of cavernous sinus fistulae the clinical features are often sufficiently characteristic to warrant diagnosis,

Table 1. Diagnostic efficacy of CT-scanning and conventional methods of investigation.

Author	CT-scan	Orbital venogram	Carotid angiogram
Wright et al. (1975)	84%	84%	
Lloyd et al. (1977)	91%	91%	
Gyldensted et al. (1977)	97%		65%

and CT-scanning is superfluous in these cases. In patients with less pronounced clinical symptoms, however, the CT-scan can be indicative of a cavernous sinus fistula in that it reveals a dilated superior ophthalmic vein (Fig. 3).

DISCUSSION

Unlike the conventional methods of neuroradiological examination, CT-scanning involves virtually no stress for the patient and entails no risk. When contrast intensification is used, the risk is the same as after any intravenous injection of contrast medium.

Moreover, the diagnostic accuracy in diagnosing pathological tissue within the orbit is greater than that of orbital venography and carotid angiography. As thinner sections are used in CT-scanning, smaller processes in the apex of the orbit can be visualized, and orbital venography is no longer required for this purpose.

CT-scanning still leaves much to be desired in the differential diagnosis of processes which cause exophthalmos. In most cases it is impossible to differentiate between malignant and benign intra-orbital processes on the basis of the CT-scan (Wackenheim et al., 1977).

Orbital venography is superior to CT-scanning in the diagnosis of venous malformations. In case of sinus cavernosus fistula angiography is imperative. In these cases the vertebral artery and the internal and external carotid artery should be separately examined.

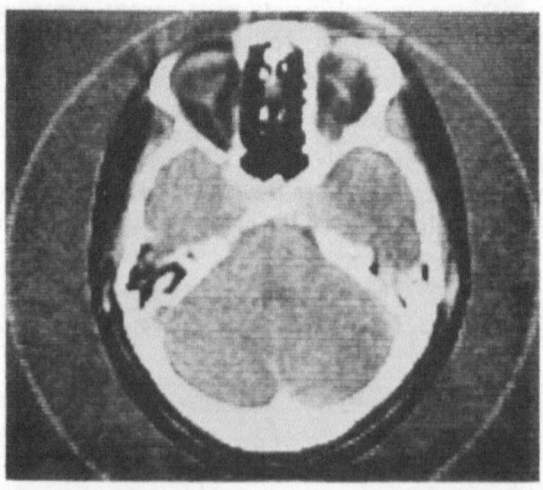

Fig. 3. CT-scan of the orbits in a female patient with a right sided carotid/ cavernous sinus fistula. The dilatated superior ophthalmic vein is recognizable.

SUMMARY

On the basis of 25 patients examined by orbital venography, CT-scanning and sometimes carotid angiography, the diagnostic value of each of these methods is evaluated. The data obtained are compared with the corresponding information from the literature. In view of the findings it can be stated that CT-scanning can be regarded as the primary neuroradiological examination in cases of exophthalmos. Orbital venography gives supplementary information in cases of varices and venous malformations. Angiography is the method which supplies the maximum of information when cavernous sinus fistulae are clinically suspected, in such cases selective angiography of the internal and external carotid and the vertebral artery is indicated.

Authors' address:
Central Department of Radiology
Wilhelmina Gasthuis
University of Amsterdam
104, 1e Helmerstraat
Amsterdam

Proc. 3rd Int. Symp. on Orbital Disorders, Amsterdam 1977

VARYING ORIGIN OF THE OPHTHALMIC ARTERY

P. LASJAUNIAS & J. MORET

(Bicètre/Paris, France)

INTRODUCTION

Since the basic work of Padget (1948) the embryological development of the arterial stem of the human orbit is well known. With very few modifications (Lasjaunias, 1975; Lasjaunias et al., in press) one can understand and memorise all the anatomical varieties of arterial supply to the orbit.

We have chosen to limit our development scheme to the key stages (five stages). None of the other stages in which secondary collaterals are concerned will be presented here.

EMBRYOLOGY

Stage 0

Two arteries arising from the internal carotid stem supply the orbit:
— ventral ophthalmic artery originating from the anterior cerebral artery joining the orbit via the future optic canal;
— dorsal ophthalmic artery arising from the internal carotid syphon and coursing through the future superior orbital fissure.

Stages 1 and 2

Intra-orbital anastomosis of these two main pedicles from which arise: the two posterior ciliary arteries and the hyaloid artery. Simultaneously the ventral ophthalmic artery migrates posteriorly to originate finally from the carotid syphon (future C2 portion).

Stage 3

Incomplete regression of the dorsal ophthalmic artery, remnant of which will be the deep recurrent ophthalmic artery in the usual adult arrangement (Lasjaunias et al., in press).

The main trunk is, at this time the ventral ophthalmic artery, or primitive ophthalmic artery. Its territory includes only the sensorial structures of the orbit (optic nerve, "eye ball").

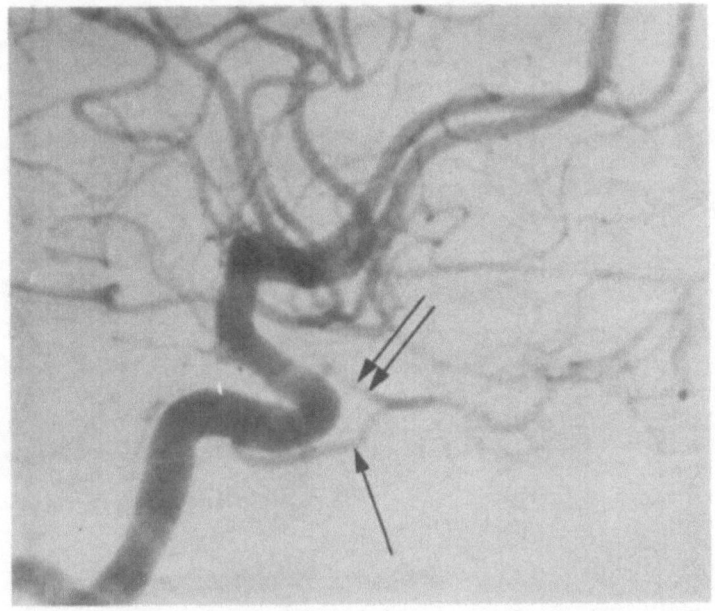

Fig. 1. Lateral view of internal carotidogram (by courtesy of Dr. T. Hasso). **Double arrow** = ventral ophthalmic artery; single arrow = dorsal ophthalmic artery.

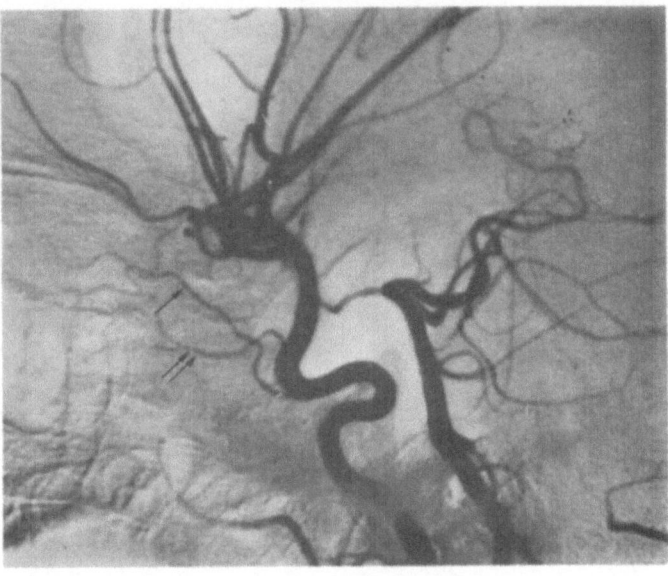

Fig. 2. Lateral view of humeral angiogram (by courtesy of Dr. Ernest). Double rooted non-anastomosed ophthalmic artery. Same legend as Fig. 1.

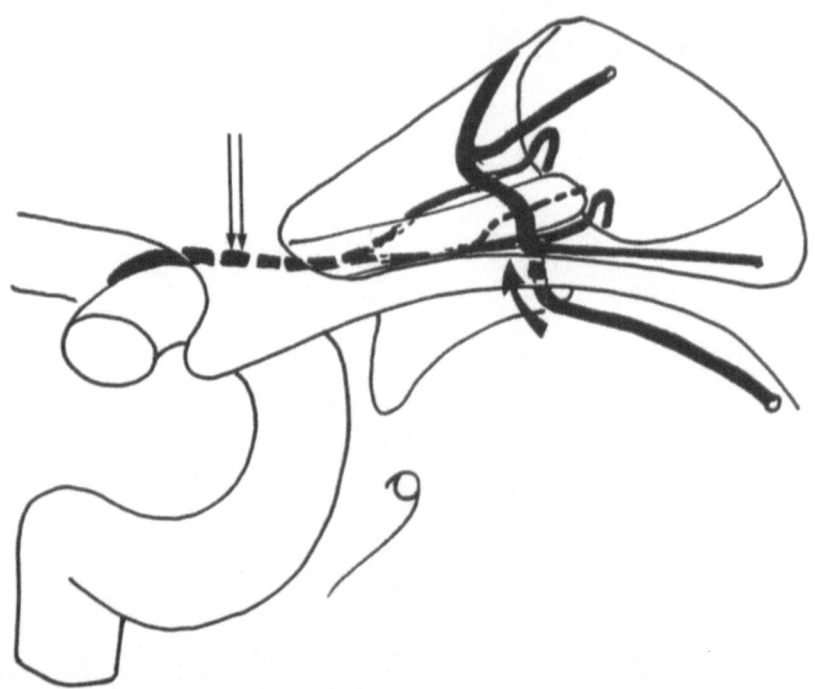

Fig. 3. Chanmugan's case. Postero-lateral view of the cavernous area after removal of the orbital roof. Schematic drawing. Double arrow = primitive ophthalmic artery; curved arrow = orbital artery (from the middle meningeal artery).

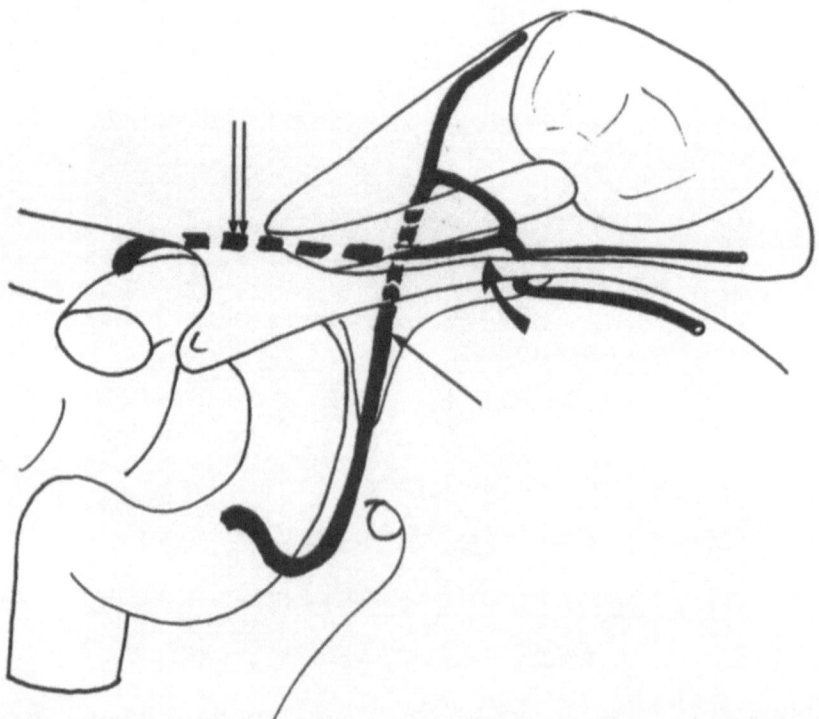

Fig. 4. Poirier's case. Same schematic drawing. Double arrow = ventral ophthalmic artery; single arrow = dorsal ophthalmic artery; curved arrow = middle meningeal contribution.

Table 1.

Varieties of origin from	Migration of the OPH_v	Orbital anastomose of the OPH_v-OPH_D	Regression of the OPH_D	Orbital anastomose of the stapedial branch	Regression of the proximal orbital artery
C2 portion of the internal carotid	+	+	+	+	+
Anterior cerebral artery	−	+	+	+	+
Double root non-anastomosed	+	−	−	+ with the OPH_d	+
Double root anastomosed	+	+	−	+	+
Intracavernous	+	+	wrongly on the OPH_v	+	+
Chanumgam's case	+	+	+	−	−
Poirier's case	+	−	−	double	−
Middle meningeal	+	+	+	+	wrongly on the primitive ophthalmic

Stage 4

Development of the orbital branch of the stapedial artery which enters the orbit through the superior orbital fissure and branches in two:
– the lacrymal artery, laterally;
– the naso ciliary artery medially (it becomes later the distal portion of the ophthalmic artery with its collaterals: supraorbital and ethmoidal).

The later branch of the orbital stapedial collateral will anastomose with the primitive ophthalmic stem; this anastomosis (future second portion of the ophthalmic) takes place medial or lateral to the optic nerve.

Stage 5

Incomplete regression of the juxta foraminal portion of the orbital artery, and annexion of its intra-orbital collateral by the primitive ophthalmic stem. As a remnant, a small artery persists in the adult arrangement, known as the recurrent meningeal artery anastomosing the lacrymal artery with the middle meningeal artery.

ANATOMICAL VARIETIES

If this program is not followed precisely or if these key stages are not executed, or on a wrong site, an anomalous origin of the definitive ophthalmic artery will occur. (Table 1).

To our knowledge only these varieties have been described:
– anterior cerebral origin;
– double rooted from the internal carotid syphon (second and fourth portion) with or without intra-orbital anastomosis (Fig. 1 and 2);
– double rooted origin from the internal carotid syphon and the middle meningeal artery non-anastomosed (Chanmugan, 1936) (Fig. 3);
– Triple rooted origin from the syphon (C2 + C4) and the middle meningeal with arterial anastomotic ring round the optic nerve (Poirier, 1896) (Fig. 4);
– middle meningeal origin.

CONCLUSION

To our knowledge no other variety is described in the literature. Personally, we have seen all these varieties angiographically except the anterior cerebral origin. The sylvian origin of the ophthalmic artery cannot be retained because of the absence of internal carotid artery.

REFERENCES

Chanmugan, P.K. Case report. *J. Anat.* 70: *580* (1936).
Lasjaunias, P. L'artère méningée moyenne. Thèse en médicine. Paris (1975).
Lasjaunias, P. et al. The recurrent branches of the ophthalmic artery. Accepted for publ. in *Acta Radiol.*

Moret, J., P. Lasjaunias, J. Theron & J.J. Merland. The middle meningeal artery to the
  orbit. To be publ. in *J. franç. de Neuro-Radiol.*
Padget, D.H. The development of the cranial arteries in the human embryo. *Contr.
  Embryol.* 32: *207, 205–261* (1948).
Poirier, P. Traité d'anatomie humaine, Tome II. Masson Ed., Paris (1896).

Authors' addresses:
P. Lasjaunias
Radiological Department
Bicètre Hospital
Le Kremlin Bicètre 94270
France

J. Moret
Radiological Department
Fondation Ophtalmolgique A. de Rothschild
25 rue Manin
Paris 75019
France

Proc. 3rd Int. Symp. on Orbital Disorders, Amsterdam 1977

RADIOGRAPHICAL ANATOMY
OF THE MUSCULOSENSORIAL VESSELS

C. DERREMEAUX, C. CLAY, P. LASJAUNIAS & J. VIGNAUD

(Paris, France)

ABSTRACT

This work is based on microradiographs of injected specimens correlated to normal magnified arteriographics.

Comparison of similar projections permits one to define criteria for the identification of the different muscular and sensorial arteries.

Authors' address:
Service de Radiologie
25 à 29 rue Manin
75019 Paris
France

Proc. 3rd. Int. Symp. on Orbital Disorders, Amsterdam 1977

DYNAMIC ANGIOGRAPHY OF THE ORBIT

M.T. IBA-ZIZEN, E.A. CABANIS, P. BONNIN & G. PORRET

(Paris, France)

The vascular anatomy of the orbit is well known and yet it is subject to a great number of variations. These have become the source of many investigations in pathological cases.

In one and the same patient one cannot avoid being surprised by the variance between the right and the left angiograms resulting from the external or internal curve of the ophthalmic artery surrounding the optic nerve.

The choroid blush is irrigated by the internal carotid in the majority of cases. It may also have a preferential vascular passage from the external carotid by means of meningo-lacrimal anastomosis. Here is an example. In the case of a eighteen months old child stricken by a palpebral angioma, the opacification of the choroid is kept to a minimum by the internal carotid. On the contrary, it remains well visible starting from the external carotid.

But, let us remember, the eye is a moving organ. The amplitude of these movements is of great importance. This can be seen on X-Ray. We can observe a metallic foreign body on the disc. The displacement is ten millimeters on the vertical and nine millimeters on the horizontal. The movement of the globe is made possible by the flexibility and curvature of the optic nerve, which is tightly wound around and attached to the ophthalmic artery.

One might ask, why is it not possible to consider angiography from a dynamic point of view rather than taking it as a fixed entity? This can be achieved under the following two conditions. One must have:
1. a non-anaesthetised patient;
2. the head is to be placed in a fixed position.

With pathological cases we insist on the fact that vascular examination must be subtracted. In spite of this, the contribution of phlebography to diagnosis has until now been of limited consequence.

Before approaching the indication of this arteriographic dynamic model, let us first consider cases in which it does not need to be used. First, there is the case of atrophy of the eyeball six months after a hunting accident. Then we have the case of a widespread tumor, a melanoma's metastasis. Further, there are some negative cases in which there is simply an element of doubt where only computerized tomography will bring a tumor into evidence.

On the other hand, the movements of the eyeball will permit us to set the limits of the tumor into better perspective. It will become possible to deter-

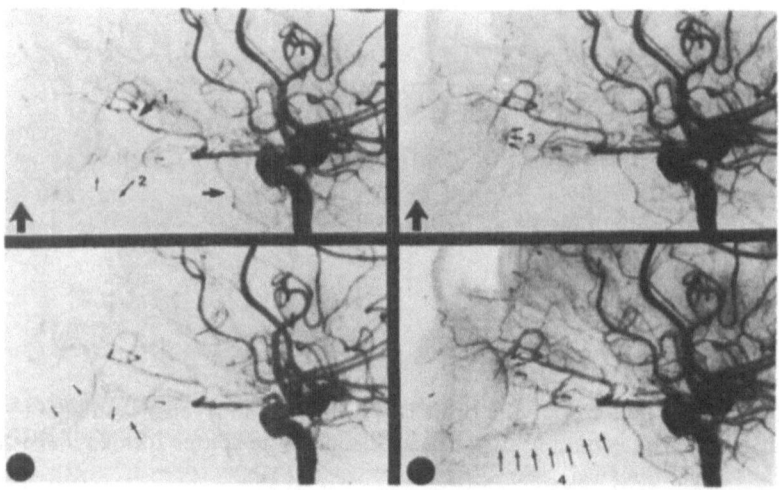

Fig. 1. Internal carotid arteriography: indifferent and upward (↑) positions. (1) Displacement of the second segment of the ophthalmic artery. (2) Displacement of an inferior muscular artery. (3) Enhancement of the papilla. (4) Inferior rectus physiological 'blush'.

mine the exact interrelations of the pathological process with ophthalmic vessels, and the globe.

Furthermore some indirect signs come into evidence where a retro-ocular tumor produces folds on the posterior portion of the eye.

Finally, we can make a contrast between two types of intra-ocular tumors: choroid melanomas and angiomas. Melanomas are not greatly vascularized and hence badly visible. Without angiography, however, it is true that, whatever their volume, they may be detected by computerized tomography.

In contrast, the choroid angiomas present one of the best opportunities for the use of this dynamic proof. At the capillary stage the choroidal blush is nearly always visible. The disc is of a greater density. The position of the visual axis is easily determined. At the arterial stage the position of the trunk of the ophthalmic artery varies in its second segment. The intracanalicular and terminal portions are stationary. The flattening out of the latero-optic curve takes place at the same time as at the opening of the anterior bow. The movement of the eyeball also permits one to see the ciliary artery's plexus. The course of the branches going from the artery move also. This can be easily observed at the inferior muscular arteries when the visual axis rises. When this happens the disc and the ciliary plexus can also be seen more clearly. Let it be noticed that at the capillary stage the vortical vein also becomes visible.

With the superimposition of the traced pattern one can measure the degree of displacement of the ophthalmic artery and its branches. One can take still another criterion. This is determined by the cooperation on the part of the patient. A muscular blush appears in the muscle which is most active at any given position. Here we can see the contraction of the superior rectus during

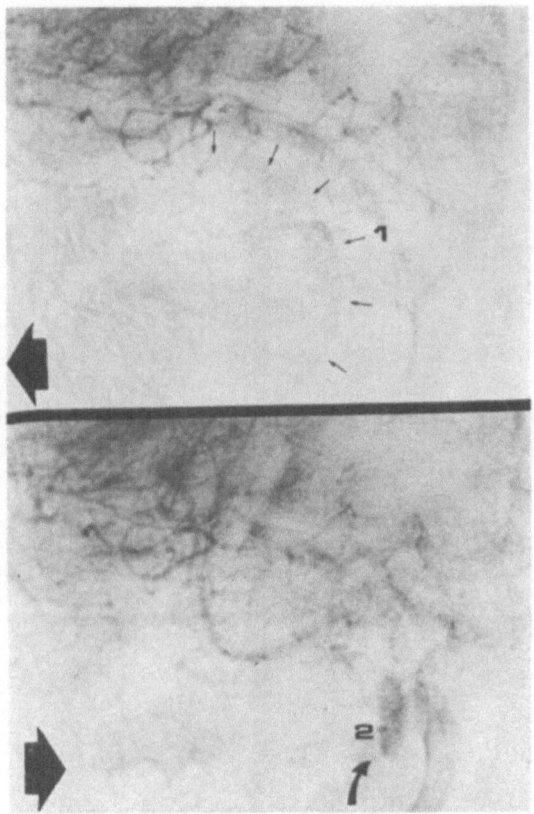

Fig. 2. Right internal carotid arteriography: choroïd melanoma. (1) Choroïd crescent visible on A.P. view; absence of tumoral blush. (2) Blush during contraction of the medial rectus muscle (lateral gaze).

an upward glance, the inferior rectus during a downward glance, and the medial rectus during a lateral position, toward the left.

The hypervascularization can be explained by the existence of a great number of intramuscular vessels. The anatomical cuts, give, in this slide, an impression of the minute displacement of the vessels by estimating their distance from the eyeball and the optic nerve. In normal cases the inferior ophthalmic vein is displaced to a far greater degree than the superior ophthalmic vein. This fact is made apparent by means of tracing patterns.

In conclusion:
1) The eye is the only nervous organ which has movements of such an amplitude that dynamic observations are made possible. The vascular anatomy cannot be studied unless it is studied on a functional basis.
2) Dynamic observations should be made as often as possible. They support the diagnosis of space occupying lesions and vascular lesions next to and within the globe.

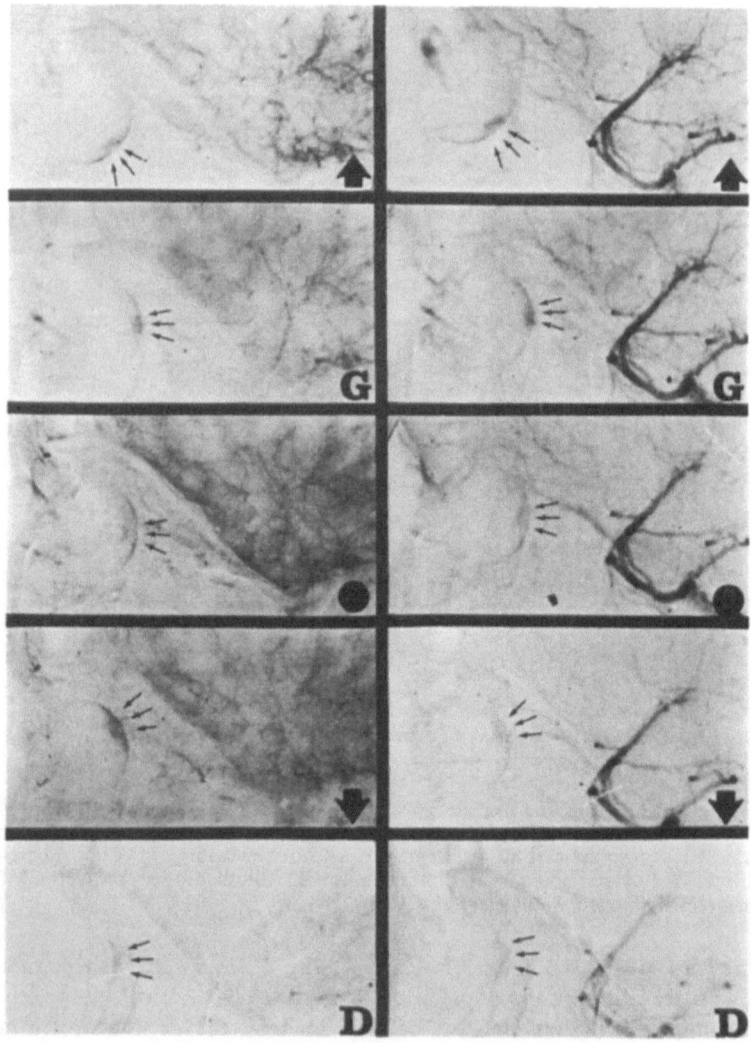

Fig. 3. Carotid arteriography: capillary stage; indifferent, upward, downward, lateral gazes. Enhancement of choroïd angioma.

Authors' address:
Service de Neuroradiologie
Centre National d'Ophtalmologie des Quinze-Vingts
28 rue de Charenton
75571 Paris Cedex 12
France
(with the collaboration of G.R.E.N.R.O.)

Proc. 3rd Int. Symp. on Orbital Disorders, Amsterdam 1977

THIN SECTION COMPUTERIZED TOMOGRAPHY: ANALYSIS OF 600 ORBIT STUDIES

STEPHEN L. TROKEL & SADEK K. HILAL

(New York, N.Y.)

Diagnosis of orbital lesions has traditionally been difficult when the orbital walls are not involved. Pathologic processes involving the orbit walls have been accurately analyzed by plain films and tomograms which can detali bone changes. Contrast angiography is useful when orbit tumors are large or have a significant blood supply. However, small avascular tumors in the orbit have been difficult to detect, define, and localize by these techniques (Trokel, 1976). Confusion also arises because swollen extraocular muscles may become large enough to mimic a neoplasm using these angiographic techniques.

This clinical problem has made the advent of computerized tomography particularly welcome since it directly visualizes the orbital soft tissue structures. In the four years that computerized tomography has been generally available it has become the preferred diagnostic technique for clinical investigation of orbital disease (Wright et al., 1975; Dallow et al., 1976; Hilal et al., 1976, 1977). This is because its tomographic image has unusual soft tissue discrimination and shows subtle differences among orbital structures. Fat is distinguished from water which in turn is distinguished from solid tissues. Soft tissue contours are imaged simultaneously with bony structures and their relationship determined. The sclera, vitreous, crystalline lens, optic nerve, extraocular muscles, and orbital fat are reliably seen in relationship to the adjacent bone. Intracranially it is routinely possible to demonstrate the cerebral ventricles, subarachnoid spaces, the cerebral sulci, and grey and white matter. Small amounts of calcium not visible on plain x-rays are shown. Similarly, a wide range of foreign material of low radiographic density is readily detected.

Many commercial machines have been developed but the first available and most widely distributed is the EMI scanner produced by the EMI corporation in England. This machine, designed for analysis of intracranial disease, is well suited for modification for orbital study. A newer machine, the AS&E-CT scanner has recently become available (Hilal et al., 1977, in press) and significantly increases the resolution of orbital detail. We are reporting the results of thin section CT scanning of 603 patients of whom 5 were studied with the AS&E scanner.

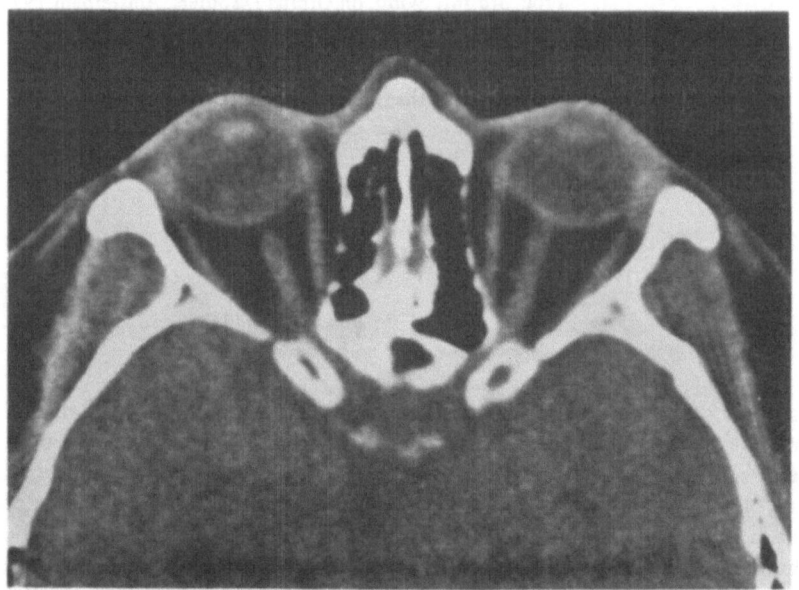

Fig. 1. Normal orbit prepared with AS&E CT scanner. The resolution of the bone detail approaches conventional pleuridirectional tomography. Soft tissue structures are detailed into the orbit apex in this 2 mm section.

METHODS

Thin section tomography

High resolution in the EMI machine is achieved by decreasing the thickness of the slices from the standard (Hilal & Trokel, 1977) 10 mm to 3.5 mm. It is only with these thin sections that details of the orbit apex are resolved sufficiently to be used clinically. Briefly, necessary modifications for orbital CT scanning include proper skull positioning with rigid stabilization. Maximal extension of the head is required to include the entire orbital volume within the scanning area of the machine. The narrow x-ray beam width is necessary for scanning because of the small sizes of orbital structures. The wide scan beam does not resolve the extraocular muscles and the optic nerve at the apex of the orbit.

The AS&E machine is based on a 512 matrix and produces sections of two mm thickness. This capability is supplemented by a zoom magnification which provides exquisite details of orbital structures. Figure 1 is a CT scan of a normal orbit prepared with the AS&E scanner. The horizontal recti can be followed to their origins in the orbit apex and the normal variation in thickness and anatomic contour appreciated. The resolution of the bone detail approaches that which is obtained with conventional pleuridirectional tomography. We show both oblique muscles in scans with the AS&E machine. The obliques have not been demonstrable in the EMI scanner even with collimation.

Contrast enhancement

All patients studied for orbital lesions have had contrast enhancement. An intravenous injection of 100 ml 75% Conray is administered over three to four minutes and the CT scan is repeated. Both the vascularity of the tumor and its absorbance of organic iodine are factors involved in improving the visibility of lesions. The bulk of the enhancement is due to breakdown of the blood tissue barrier by the pathologic process.

RESULTS OF SCANNING

In Table 1 is an overall summary of the broad classification of the results of scan studies. The total is greater than six hundred three patients because a few patients had lesions which required placement in two categories, i.e. one young child with a proven retinoblastoma developed a glioma of the contralateral optic nerve. An impressive two hundred thirty-seven patients or 39.5% of the total number of studies had scans which were normal in all respects. Table 2 shows the reason for the study in these patients. The majority had vascular or demyelinating disease. Three were test controls to determine normal anatomy. Ninety patients had vision loss ultimatley ex-

Table 1. Thin section CT of the orbit.

Normal orbits	236
Graves (abnormal EMI)	76
Pseudotumor	40
Granulomas	4
Vascular lesions	17
Thick optic nerve	20
Neoplasms	171
Ocular lesions	25
Retinoblastoma	10
Miscellaneous	17
No diagnosis	3
619	619

Table 2. Thin section CT of the orbits. Normal orbits.

Vision loss	90
Motility disturbance	35
Papilledema	5
Pain, headaches	19
Pseudoproptosis	9
Controls	3
Graves (grade 2 or less)	16
Orbital varix	1
Basal cell Ca lid	1
Sella, sinus lesion	57

plained as optic neuritis, retrobulbar neuritis, ischemic optic neuropathy, congeintal optic atrophy, amaurosis fugax, central retinal vein occlusion, low tension glaucoma, or optic nerve injury. Most of these examinations were ordered by neurologists and reflect the strong desire to rule out an unsuspected mass lesion with a markedly atypical presentation. Usually, the accurate diagnosis was known at the time of the study. A similar large group of thirty-five patients with disturbances of extraocular motility were studied with negative results. Most of these patients turned out to have a vascular cause (usually diabetic) for the ocular paresis. No single underlying diagnosis was present in patients with headaches and pain in the orbits. Three of the patients with papilledema had benign central retinal vein occlusions and two optic neuritis. Sixteen patients with thyroid disease had non-toxic nodular goiter or Grade 1 to 2 Graves' disease with no exophthalmos present. In the absence of exophthalmos, we have not been able to show abnormalities of the extraocular muscles.

In sixty patients with normal orbits, an adjacent sinus or brain lesion was suspect or present. In these patients, most of whom had sella or parasella lesions, the orbits were all normal.

NON-NEOPLASTIC CAUSES OF EXOPHTHALMOS

1. Graves' disease

Seventy-six patients of three hundred thirty-two with exophthalmos were ultimately determined to have Graves' disease. Serologic testing included routine circulating T3 and T4 (RIA); T3 suppression test, and a TRH test. In only two of these patients was it impossible to obtain evidence of abnormal pituitary-thyroid function.

The CT findings in seventy-six patients which correspond to the American Thyroid Association classification of Graves' disease is summarized in Table 3. Patients with Graves' disease Grade 3 to 6 show findings similar to those in Figure 2. The medial and lateral recti are swollen with prolapse or the orbital fat and the anterior displacement of the septum. It is probable that

Table 3. High resolution CT scans in Graves' disease

Class	Patients	Findings
0	2	Normal orbit
1	4	Normal orbit
2	10	Normal orbit
3	21	Proptosis, large muscles, mild lid swelling
4	48	Proptosis, larger muscles, lid swelling
5	2	Proptosis, large muscles, lid swelling, variable optic nerve enlargement
6	5	Proptosis, large muscles, lid swelling, large optic nerve

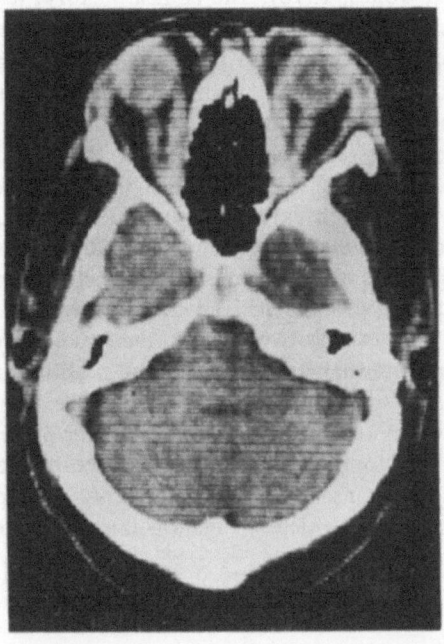

Fig. 2. CT scan of an eighty-five year old woman with exophthalmos and vision loss. The medial and lateral recti are swollen as is the optic nerve. Ultrasonography in this patient usggested that a metastatic tumor was present.

the swollen recti produce a mass effect where it converges in the orbit apex to compress the optic nerve and cause vision loss. The swollen optic nerve, seen in the CT scan are present only in patients with Grade 5 and 6 Graves' disease. The origin of the inferior recti, the entire length of the medial and lateral recti and the full length of the superior group of muscles are seen when enlarged. It has not been possible to distinguish among the levator, superior rectus and superior oblique as they run in a contiguous mass. The obliques have not been identified on this scan. No patients with Graves' disease have been studied with the AS&E scanner.

It is *extremely* important to distinguish the swollen inferior recti and superior muscles from tumor masses which may be mimicked when the swollen recti are obliquely sectioned. The presence of the fading edge suggests that the muscle is moving out of the scan plane while a tumor shows a sharp edge. A CT scan made with a wide window is necessary to demonstrate this fading edge. In addition, several extraocular muscles are almost always noted to be enlarged in patients with Graves' disease.

2. 'Orbital pseudotumor'

Forty patients in this series were ultimately diagnosed as having orbital pseudotumor. The clinical criteria for this diagnosis have recently been reviewed (Jakobiec & Jones, 1976). The clinical history, response to steroid therapy, and biopsies when done all contributed to the diagnosis.

When the inflammatory condition produces a focal mass a focal radiodensity was found. Diffuse orbital inflammation in patients who respond to steroid therapy show varying enhancement of the sclera and optic nerve. Ultrasonic abnormalities were usually present in this group of cases. In fact this conjunction of findings was specific in this series for pseudotumor.

Some patients with swollen extraocular muscles are diagnosed as having 'pseudotumor' because their exophthalmos rapidly regresses with steroid treatment. These patients also show motility disturbance and local pain and injection. The muscle swelling was shown to regress after treatment. In Figure 3 are scans of a twenty-two year old man taken seven months apart. Initially, there was exophthalmos, chemosis, and motility disturbance which regressed entirely after treatment with corticosteroids. The massive swelling of the lateral rectus in the initial scan is no longer present seven months later. Seven of the forty patients had similar findings of enlarged extraocular muscles with rapid response to anti-inflammatory therapy. We classified these as orbital myostitis, which we believe may be distinguishable from other forms of pseudotumor.

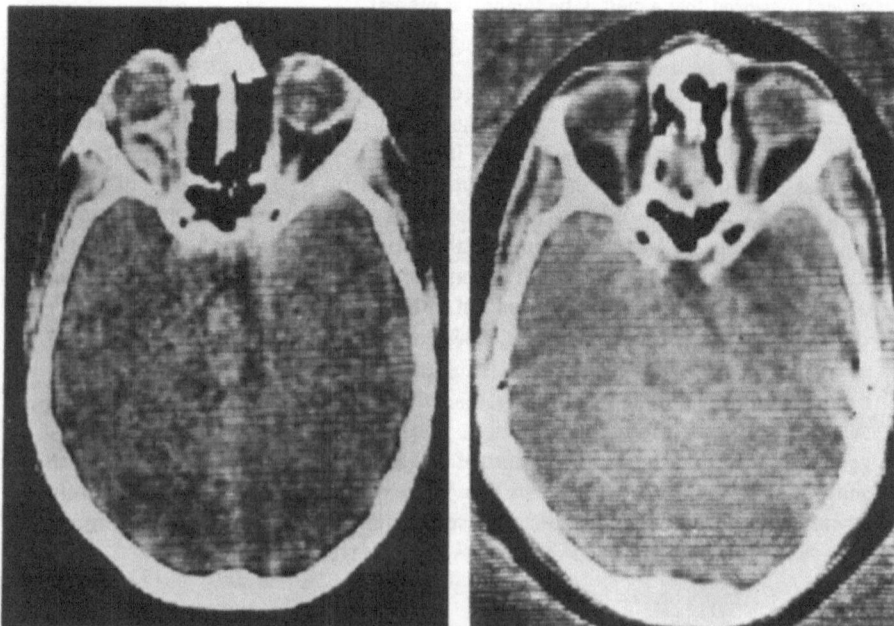

Fig. 3. Pre and post treatment scans of orbits of a twenty-two year old man with acute exophthalmos, injection and chemosis. The massively enlarged lateral rectus muscle disappears after coritcosteroid therapy.

3. Other inflammatory conditions

Five patients had specific orbital granulomas recognized after biopsy while four patients had an orbital cellulitis and one had inflammation following a dislodged acrylic implant.

Specific granulomas were foreign body granuloma, xanthogranuloma, Wegner's, and two patients with tuberculous granulomas. It is believed that the orbital cellulitis was pyogenic in origin.

4. Vascular lesions causing exophthalmos

Seventeen patients with exophthalmos were ultimately found to have a vascular lesion. Table 4 summarizes the distribution and findings in this group. In only one patient was the EMI scan normal. This one had an orbital varix which collapsed entirely with the patient positioned for scanning. The findings in the eight patients with carotid cavernous fistulae and four patients with arteriovenous malformation were similar. In eight of these twelve patients, diagnosis was initially made on the basis of the CT scan. It had been suspected in six of the twelve patients although some degree of episcleral venous congestion was present in all. Other clinical findings in this group include glaucoma (4 of 12), bruit (3 of 12), central retinal vein enlargement (6 of 12). In six patients only exophthalmos and vascular injection was present. The EMI findings showed diffuse uniform enlargement of the medial rectus and lateral rectus muscles. There was no anterior fat prolapse as seen in thyroid disease. The optic nerve contour was normal. In all patients, an *enlarged superior ophthalmic* vein was demonstrable. In one patient, Figure 4, the massively enlarged superior ophthalmic vein could be traced easily to the cavernous sinus.

5. Bone dysplasias

Six patients with exophthalmos had fibrous dysplasia which was visible on the CT scan although conventional radiographic methods led to the proper diagnosis. Three of thirteen patients with neurofibromatosis had dysplastic sphenoid wings with associated exophthalmos.

Table 4. Vascular lesions.

Carotid-cavernous fistula	
(large muscles)	
(superior ophthalmic vein)	8
Arterio-venous malformation	
(large muscles)	
(superior opththalmic vein)	4
Orbit varix (1 negative)	2
Aneurysm	
(Apical enhancing mass)	2
Hemangiomatosis	
(diffuse vascular structures)	1

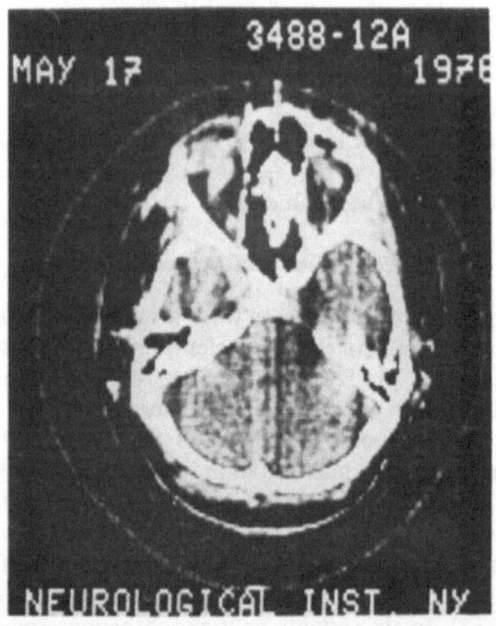

Fig. 4. Massively enlarged superior ophthalmic vein seen entering cavernous sinus. This was due to a traumatic carotid cavernous fistula following an automobile accident.

NEOPLASTIC CAUSES OF EXOPHTHALMOS

1. One hundred ninety-eight patients had orbit tumors causing exophthalmos. Ultrasonography can produce false-positive echo patterns in patients with orbital inflammation and false-negative studies when orbit tumors are subperiostal or do not touch the globe. For example, a patient with exophthalmos and vision loss had a normal ultrasonic study. The CT scan shows a hemangioma (Figure 5) in the retroocular space. The tumor is separate from the optic nerve and displaces it medially. The distribution of these tumors (Table 5) reflects the wide variety of orbit diseases. Eleven hemangiomas had a benign, encapsulated appearance. The six lymphangiomas were less regular. Tumor localization is extremely precise vis-a-vis the optic nerve and orbit walls. This gives planning of orbit surgery an accuracy that has not been heretofore possible. In two patients with enlargement of the optic nerve and progressive vision loss, the resolution was not adequate nor was the enhancement sufficient to determine with certitude if this optic nerve enlargement was a meningioma. The angiomatous lesions are perhaps the most dramatic for precise visualization and localization of orbit tumors. Other lesions include four osteomas, five mucoceles, three orbital dermoids and one focal orbital abcess.

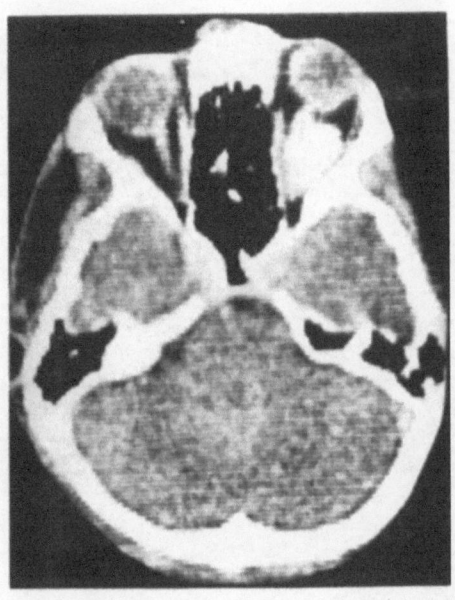

Fig. 5. Hemangioma in the orbit apex. This lesion had reduced the visual acuity to 6/60 and was not identified with the ultrasonogram.

Table 5. Orbital neoplasms

Optic nerve gliomas	41
Orbit meningioma	27
Optic nerve meningiomas	7
Hemangiomas	11
Lymphangiomas	6
Hemangiopericytomas	3
Lymphomas	5
Neurilemmoma	3
Neurofibroma	13
Lacrimal gland	5
Sarcoma	4
Sinus neoplasms	15
Metastatic (breast, kidney, melanoma, neuroblastoma, lung)	13
Retinoblastoma	10
Miscellaneous (osteoma, dermoid, bone cyst, mucocele)	18

2. Malignant tumors

The entire spectrum of malignant tumors is represented in Table 5 in the ninety-two lesions studied. Only two lymphomas and one neurilemmoma of relative benign cytology had an appearance that suggested confusion with

115

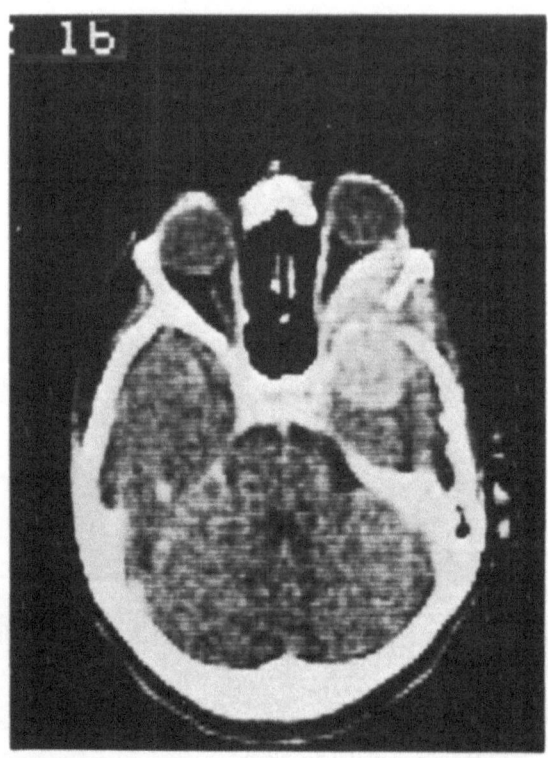

Fig. 6. Metastatic breast cancer producing orbit apex syndrome. The tumor had destroyed much of the sphenoid wing.

an angiomatous mass lesion. The hemangiompericytomas, sarcomas, and metastatic tumors all had irregular contours with bone destruction. Figure 6 is a CT scan of a metastatic breast cancer to the orbit apex with extensive destruction. Seven optic nerve meningiomas were diagnosed although two other patients had thick optic nerves in whom the diagnosis could not be made with certainty. Twenty-seven patients had meningiomas involving other portions of the orbit including the classical sphenoid meningiomas.

Because the CT scan records a wide range of radiodensities, abnormal bone structures of paranasal sinuses are seen as well as soft tissue abnormalities. The bone destruction caused by these tumors can be outlined by conventional radiographic methods but the extent of the soft tissue tumor is demonstrable on the CT image. This has been a great assistance in planning biopsy and radiotherapy. Carcinomas arising within the sinuses as well as mucoceles can be detected and distinguished from other causes of exophthalmos.

116

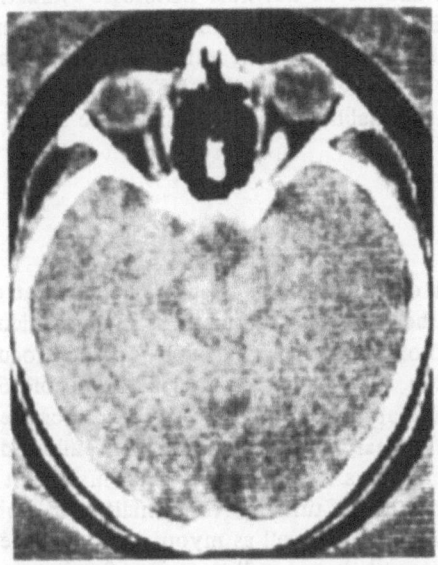

Fig. 7. Irregular enhancing optic nerve lesion in a forty-two year old woman with vision loss progressing to count fingers acuity. We believe this appearance is typical of meningioma of the optic nerve sheath.

3. Optic nerve tumors

A small amount of exophthalmos associated with vision loss suggests that the orbital portion of the optic nerve is involved with a mass lesion. This orbital portion of the optic nerve has been most difficult to anlyze since no bone change is caused by these tumors and they may cause significant vision loss when quite small. Vascular displacement is unreliable. The CT scan of a patient (Figure 7) with progressive vision loss of four years duration and two mm exophthalmos shows a tumor covering the optic nerve. This proved to be a miningioma and was removed through a transfrontal craniotomy.

Forty-one patients with gliomas of the optic nerve have been studied. In no patient was a glioma of the orbital portion of the optic nerve not diagnosed on a CT scan and found on either subsequent testing or by another diagnostic method.

4. Retinoblastoma

Eleven patients were studied with retinoblastoma within the eye or suspect orbital recurrence. In seven of these eleven patients an ocular retinoblastoma was known to be present. Six of the seven patients had calcification visible within the mass. The seventh patient had a small lesion less than one disc diopter in size immediately adjacent to the optic nerve. This eye had not been removed and we do not have histologic evaluation of this tumor mass. In two patients, the presence of the retinoblastoma was only suspected as the patient presented with retinal detachment and no history of tumor. In these two patients only the CT scan showed the calcification within a tumor mass enabling the diagnosis to be made with confidence.

OCULAR LESIONS

A varying amount of ocular detail is shown dependent on the degree of movement during the scanning examination. In one patient the eye was immobilized by retro-orbital xylocaine which increased ocular of detail and allowed visualization of a malignant melanoma. Table 6 summarizes the intraocular lesions that we studied. The diffuse increased density of the vitreous cavity in primary hyperplastic vitreous allowed it to be distinguished from other causes of leucocoria. Two malignant melanomas were seen out of four intraocular tumors. Abnormalities in globe size allow congenital buphthalmic globes as well as myopic globes to be recognized. It is possible to recognize aphakia as well as various foreign materials within and adjacent to the eye. Intraocular foreign bodies, silicone bands, silicone sponges, as well as silicone explants can easily be shown. Figure 8 is a scan of a young woman with congenital glaucoma who recieved trauma to the globe. She has a choroidal effusion and deep choroidal hemorrhage. The effusions as well as the hemorrhage can be recognized and distinguished from each other because of the greater radiodensity of the blood.

LARGE OPTIC NERVES

In twenty patients (excluding Graves' disease and tumors) enlargement of the optic nerve was noted. Table 7 summarizes the apparent cause of these. Most commonly, intracranial hypertension with resulting papilledema produces a large irregular optic nerve. Other causes of a prominent nerve have been acute optic neuritis and acute central retinal vein occlusion.

We look forward to studying optic nerve pathology with machines of greater resolution.

Table 6. Ocular lesions

Tumors	5
Abnormal size	4
Congenital abnormalities	4
Trauma	5
Foreign bodies	3
Miscallaneous	4

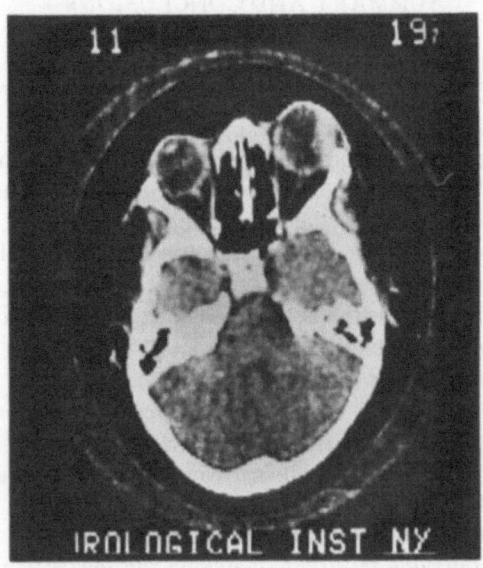

Fig. 8. Scan shows the buphthalmic globe with both choroidal effusion and hemorrhage visible. Note the difference in radiodensity between the effusion and the darker blood.

Table 7. Large optic nerve. More than 6 mm corrected (window width 200) (window level 30).

Papilledema	9
Optic neuritis	5
Intracranial hypertension	3
Trauma	1
Vein thrombosis	2

TRAUMA

Seven patients were studied with recent trauma to the orbit. Increased density was noted associated with orbital hematoma and fibrosis following its resolution. The extensive fracture of the orbit apex associated with blindness in an automobile accident is demonstrated as well as a traumatic encepholocele and porencephalic cyst associated with cranial trauma. One patient had segmental atrophy of the optic nerve noted following trauma and vision loss. The method is widely used to detect subdural hematoma associated with trauma and avoids angiography.

119

SUMMARY AND CONCLUSIONS

The six hundred and three patients who were studied with this technique represent a wide range of pathologic problems. CT scanning is dramatically effective in analyzing patients with exophthalmos with only one orbit varix completely missed by the method. In no patient did subsequent follow-up and repeat examination indicate that an exophthalmos producing neoplasm had been missed at the time of the initial study.

This precision of detection and localization has considerably altered our surgical approaches. No longer is it necessary to have an exploratory orbitotomy to achieve a diagnosis. The number of lateral orbitotomies has been considerably diminished as many tumors can be approached from an anterior route because the tumor location is known.

More important, medially located tumors can be approached without traversing the optic nerve with the attendant risks.

It appears that the machine is being overused in analyzing patients with problems of vision loss. However, there is no overutilization by the orbital surgeon as the diagnostic value in orbital disease is high.

In fact, the encouraging results in analyzing the few patients with trauma and ocular lesions, suggest that as the resolution of the machine increases, we may well find increadsing uses for it in analyzing patients with trauma to the eye and orbit as well as the wide variety of intraocular lesions.

REFERENCES

Dallow, R.L., K.J. Momose, A.L. Weber & S.H. Wray. Comparison of ultrasonography, computerized tomography and radiographic techniques in evaluation of exophthalmos. *Trans. Am. Acad. Ophthal. Otolaryng.* 81: *323–333* (1976).

Hilal, S.K., P.M. Joseph, F. Kelcz & W.B. Seaman. Development of a new computed tomography scanner with stationary detectors. Part II: Initial experimental and clinical evaluation. *Radiology* (in press).

Hilal, S.K., P.M. Joseph, J.A. Stein & L.A. Shepp. Development of a new computed tomography scanner with stationary detectors. Part I: Design considerations. *Radiology* (in press).

Hilal, S.K., L. Shepp, P.M. Joseph & J. Stein. Desirable features for advanced computerized tomography scanners. pp. 541–549, in: Reconstruction Tomography in Diagnostic Radiology and Nuclear Medicine (Workshop on Reconstruction Tomography, San Juan, Puerto Rico, April, 1975) (P.M. Ter-Pogossian et al., eds.) (1977).

Hilal, S.K. & S.L. Trokel. Computerized tomography of the orbit using thin sections. pp. 137–147, in: Seminars in Roentgenology, Vol. XII, No. 2 (April 1977).

Hilal, S.K., S.L. Trokel & D.J. Coleman. High resolution computerized tomography and B-scan ultrasonography of the orbits. *Trans. Am. Acad Ophthal. Otolaryng.* 81: *607–617* (1976).

Hilal, S.K., S.L. Trokel & S.M. Kreps. Diseases of the orbit: computerized tomography. Chapter 23, in: Clinical Ophthalmology (T.D. Duane, ed.), Vol. 2 (1976).

Jakobiec, F.A. & I.S. Jones. Orbital inflammations. Chapter 35, in: Clinical Ophthalmology (T.D. Duane, ed.), Vol. 2 (1976).

Trokel, S.L. Radiology of the orbit. Chapter 22, in: Clinical Ophthalmology (T.D. Duane, ed.), Vol. 2 (1976).

Wright, J.E., G.A.S. Lloyd & J. Ambrose. Computerized axial tomography in the detection of orbital space-occupying lesions. *Am. J. Ophthal.* 80: *78–84* (1975).

Authors' addresses:

S.L. Trokel
Asst Professor of Clinical Ophthalmology
College of Physicians and Surgeons
Columbia University
New York, N.Y.
USA

S.K. Hilal
Professor of Radiology
Director of Neuro-radiology
Neurological Institute
New York, N.Y.
USA

Proc. 3rd Int. Symp. on Orbital Disorders, Amsterdam 1977

A COMPARATIVE EVALUATION OF COMPUTERIZED TOMOGRAPHY IN ORBITAL DIAGNOSIS

GLYN LLOYD & JAMES AMBROSE

(London, England)

For the past four years we have been sending patients from the Orbital Clinic for CT examination at Atkinson Morleys Hospital. Initially the prototype 80 x 80 scanner was used. Then in January 1974 a 160 x 160 matrix was fitted and more recently the CT 1010 scanner, incorporating a 320 x 320 matrix has been employed. We have now examined nearly 250 patients with histological verification of the pathology found in the orbit in 100 of them. These patients form the case material for this paper; only lesions arising primarily within the orbit were included (see Table 1).

The series of patients was examined by four techniques listed in Table 2 and a direct comparison made between the various methods of examination. Diagnostic accuracy was assessed as a simple positive/negative response; that is whether there was or was not a mass lesion present in the orbit. Although there is little to choose between the first three techniques listed in Table 2 in numerical terms, in practice we have found CT scan to be by far the most emphatic method of demonstrating the presence of a space-occupying lesion. Small lesions in the forward part of the muscle cone may be missed entirely on venography; and in our experience Ultrasonography produces a

Table 1. Primary orbital mass lesions

Pseudotumour (granuloma)	23
Lacrimal gland tumour	17
Meningioma	17
Lymphoma	10
Haemangioma	10
Optic nerve glioma	4
Neurilemmoma	3
Venous malformation	2
Haemangiopericytoma	2
Malignant melanoma	2
Blood cysts	2
Metastasis	2
Dermoid	2
Arterio-venous malformation	1
Cystic Hygroma of optic nerve	1
Leimyoma	1
Fibroxanthoma	1
Total	100

122

high number of false positive scans in the orbit, a fact not reflected in the simple percentages listed in Table 2. However, it is not enough to leave the diagnosis at this first stage of demonstrating whether there is a mass lesion present. If possible some idea of the aetiology should be given. This is because the treatment varies according to the pathology. For example, a venous malformation in the orbit is ofter best treated by excision of superficial varices only. Deep surgical intervention is usually contraindicated. On the other hand benign tumours should be excised preferably by lateral orbitotomy; malignancies require radiotherapy, and granulomata steroid therapy.

Table 2. Diagnostic accuracy

100 proven primary orbital space occupying lesions	
C.T. scan	90%
Venography	88%
Ultrasound	87%
Axial hypocycloidal tomography	74%

The diagnostic accuracy was assessed as a simple positive/negative rsponse

There are three ways in which CT scanning may further the diagnosis and indicate the likely aetiology of a space-occupying lesion in the orbit:
a) By identifying the site of origin of the mass, for example, the lacrymal gland or optic nerve.
b) By its shape and density.
c) By consideration of the absorption values before and after intravenous contrast injection.

The optic nerve tumours, both gliomata and meningiomata were clearly identified as arising from the optic nerve with scans made on the 160 x 160 matrix or 320 x 320 matrix scanner, and could be differentiated from other encapsulated tumours in the muscle cone such as haemangiomata. The latter tumours are also readily diagnosed on their typical morphology as depicted on the CT scan. They give a clear-cut image, usually rounded, with well defined edges and even density values. Another tumour arising within the muscle cone which may give similar appearances is a neurilemmoma. In our experience these are usually larger than the haemangiomata, and the size of the mass may suggest the diagnosis. However, this differentiation is of little practical significance since the treatment is the same for both tumours; namely, excision by lateral orbitotomy.

The benign encapsulated tumours referred to above could be clearly differentiated by their clear-cut margins from infiltrative lesions in the muscle cone, such as granulomate, lymphomata or secondary tumours. These latter space-occupying lesions typically showed an ill-defined mass of irregular outline and uneven density. The commonest lesion to present these features is the pseudotumour in the orbit. Sometimes these masses may involve the lacrimal gland, extending both intraconally and extraconally, and the inflammatory process may involve a rectus muscle, causing local enlargement. This is, however, a non-specific sign. It was recorded 14 times in the series, and in addition to its association with pseudotumour, was also observed in dysthyroid exophthalmos, and in 3 examples of lacrimal gland tumours in which the mass had extended into the lateral rectus muscle; it also occurred in one patient with an orbital varix in the muscle cone.

It was not found possible to differentiate the lymphomata occurring in the orbit from pseudotumours by the morphology of the lesion as depicted on CT. Differentiation of inflammatory processes from true tumours in the orbit is particularly idfficult when they occur in the orbital apex where all mass lesions have a very similar appearance on CT scans.

ABSORPTION VALUES

The findings in this series have been recorded previously (Lloyd & Ambrose, 1977). No evidence of tissue recognition could be obtained from the absorption values, pre or post contrast injection. The mean values, derived from 7 menigiomata enhanced after contrast approximately 18% more than other tumours evaluated, but this was insufficient to make an differentiation in individual cases. The finding of negative EMI values in some pseudotumours, was regarded as indicative of their infiltrative nature rather than being tissue specific.

THE ROLE OF OTHER TECHNIQUES

The various techniques now available for orbital investigation are listed in Table 3 along with their suggested order of employment. Bone imaging by plain X-ray aided, where necessary by conventional tomography in the axial plane, should never be neglected. In a series of 1070 patients examined for unilateral exopthalmos, it was found that 33% showed abnormality on plain X-ray and, more important, in 21% there were totally diagnostic features present.

With regard to the other method of soft tissue imaging — ultrasonography: we have found this most useful in demonstrating pathological changes in the optic nerve, sometimes with tissue recognition. It has, for example, been possible to recognise an optic nerve meningioma on C scan ultrasonography by the high reflectivity produced by the presence of psammoma bodies in the tumour. For these purposes C mode imaging of ultrasound has proved more effective than A or B scan ultrasonography.

ANGIOGRAPHIC TECHNIQUES

There are several reasons for performing orbital venography in the investi-

Table 3. The three stages in the radiological investigation of unilateral exophthalmos

I	Bone structure	Plain X-ray	Conventional tomography
II	Soft tissue imaging	CT scanning	Ultrasonography
III	Vasculature	Venography	Carotid angiography

gation of orbital disease. It is essential for the demonstration of venous malformations in the orbit; this is important because this type of vascular anomaly was found in our series to form over 20% of all intraconal space occupying lesions. Venous malformations can be missed entirely on CT scan scan, and when suspected still require venography for diagnostic confirmation and to show their extent. A second important function of orbital venography lies in the diagnosis of inflammatory lesions in the orbit. Listed in Table 4 are 48 consecutive patients showing intraconal obstruction of the venous system on venography, i.e. obstruction in the second or third parts of the superior ophthalmic vein. It can be seen that in over two thirds of

Table 4. The aetiology of 48 consecutive lesions showing intraconal venous obstruction on frontal venography

Inflammatory lesion (granuloma	33
Miningiomata (four secondary)	7
Metastases	4
Neurilemmoma	2
Dysthyroid	1
Lymphoma	1
Total	48

these patients the cause of the obstruction was inflammatory. Furthermore, if secondary neoplasia can be excluded either clinically or by plain X-ray, and the CT scan shows an infiltration in the muscle cone, there is an over 90% probability of an inflammatory process. It should be remembered that in the Tolosa Hunt syndrome, the cause of which is generally regarded as inflammatory, the veins are often obstructed in the posterior orbit or in the cavernous sinus.

Orbital venography may also be useful in the differential diagnosis of dysthyroid exophthalmos, and the exclusion of spurious mass lesions on CT scan which may occur as the result of rectus muscle enlargement in this condition (Brismar et al., 1976).

The introduction of the non-invasive technique of CT scanning and ultrasound have made carotid arteriography less necessary for the routine investigatigation of proptosis. CT scanning has largely taken over the role of carotid angiography in the exclusion of intracranial lesions causing proptosis, and these techniques have made intraorbital diagnosis far more exact pre-operatively, so that in most patients the appropriate surgical approach is clearly indicated and can be safely undertaken without the risk of the morbidity which attends carotid puncture. The investigation should therefore, only be carried out on selected patient, principally those who are clinically suspected of having an arteriovenous malformation in the orbit or a caroticocavernous fistula or other vascular anomaly intracranially. Another category of patient requiring carotid angiography includes those with a very vascular tumour in the orbit, in which it is important to identify the feeding vessels prior to surgery.

REFERENCES

Brismar, J., K.R. Davis, R.L. Dallos & G. Brismar. Unilateral endocrine exophthalmos. Diagnostic problems in association with computed tomography. *Neuroradiology* 12: *21–24* (1976).

Lloyd, G.A.S. & J.A.E. Ambrose. An evaluation of C.A.T. in the diagnosis of orbital space occupying lesions. pp. 154–160, in: Computerised Axial Tomography in Clinical Practice. Springer-Verlag, Berlin (1977).

Authors' address:
Moorfield Eye Hospital
City Road
London EC14 2PD

126

Proc. 3rd Int. Symp. on Orbital Disorders, Amsterdam 1977

CORONAL SECTIONS IN C.T. OF THE ORBIT

J. VIGNAUD & M.L. AUBIN

(Paris, France)

Out of more than 50 cases of orbital disease 34 were selected for coronal sections of computerized tomography. In 16 cases this examination was not possible because of old age or because of the presence of too many metallic fillings in the dentures.

TECHNIQUE

The sections were performed in general in the prone position. Only children under anesthesia were examined in supine position. In cases of severe cervical arthrosis, basilar insufficiency or of posterior fossa tumor with papilledema the method is contra-indicated.

The plane of the section must be perpendicular to Virchow's plane in order to cut perpendicularly to the optic nerve. Corrections have to be made as regards teeth and head deflection. Metallic prothetic teeth induce artifacts which completely blur the image. This can be avoided by tilting the plane of section. If too many of such teeth are present or if they are located too far superiorly and posteriorly, coronal sections are impossible.

With our ACTA 200 FS, the thickness of the sections for the orbit is five 5 mm. Sections were made at every 5 mm. In our cases, coronal sections, if necessary, were always made after the axial sections and, consequently, they are generally done after contrast perfusion.

RESULTS

Normal radio anatomy

When compared to anatomical sections, the main components of the orbit can be identified easily. The optic nerve, the eye ball and the lens, the muscle cone (muscles and aponeurosis), the oblique muscles, the superior ophthalmic vein and its roots, the eyelids, the lacrimal gland, and sometimes even the ophthalmic artery (Fig. 1).

Orbital tumors

In orbital tumors, coronal sections were decisive in defining the exact location of superior and inferior extraconal tumors. In axial CT it is sometimes

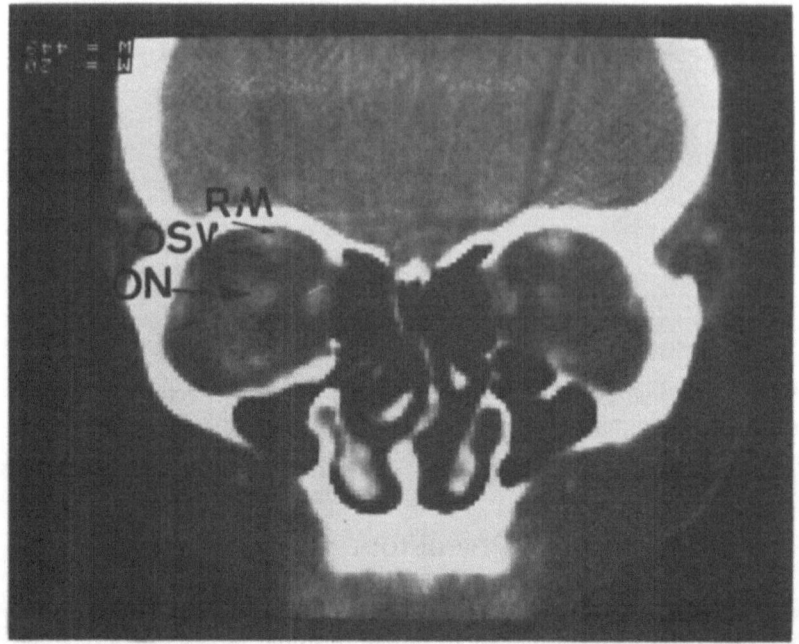

Fig. 1. Coronal sections - normal case. RM = Rectus muscle; OSV = Ophthalmic sup. vein; ON = Optic nerve.

difficult to differentiate a tumor from the superior or inferior rectus muscle, in particular if the tumor is small, e.g. lymphoid tumors and lacrimal tumors (Fig. 2).

It is sometimes very difficult to locate the optic nerve in cases of intraconal tumor on axial sections. This is particularly true when the optic tract is close to the tumor when it is hard to say whether the optic nerve is involved or not. Coronal sections demonstrate without any doubt the location of the optic nerve with regards to the tumor. If it is included in the tumor, the diagnosis of glioma or meningioma is the more probable. The coronal sections give the surgeon a more acurate diagnosis and a more precise location of the tumor than the axial CT.

Venous malformations

These malformations may be filled incompletely with phlebographic technique. With axial and coronal sections of computerized tomography the entiremalformations may be delineated.

Eye ball tumors

The importance of coronal CT depends on the location of the tumor. If it is at the posterior part of the eye ball, axial tomography is sufficient. On

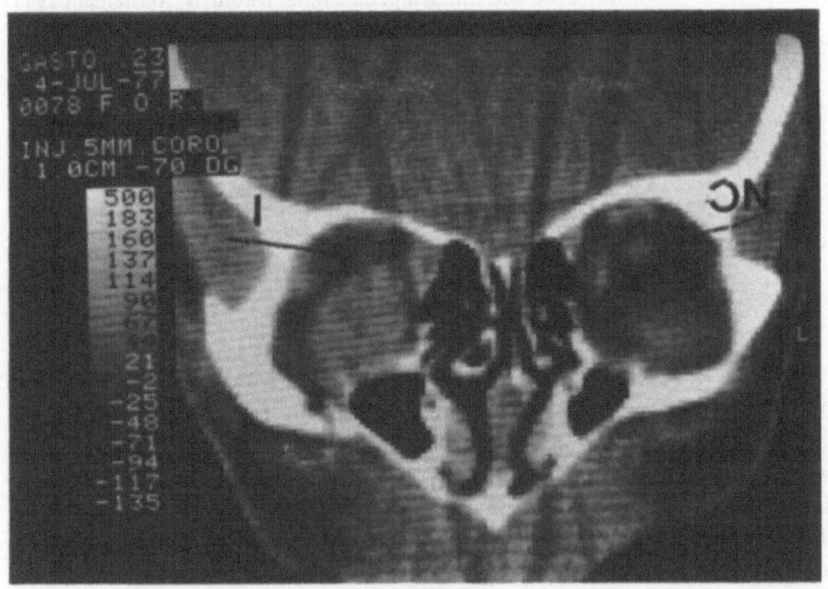

Fig. 2. Coronal section - Hodgkin disease (T). ON = Optic nerve.

the other hand, when it is located more anteriorly, coronal sections will be of much help. For a positive diagnosis of a tumor, the possibility of an artifact should be excluded.

Foreign bodies

For the exact localisation of foreign bodies, coronal sections may be helpful. Five millimeter thick sections may include at the same time different components of the orbit. Consequently, the accuracy will never be less than 5 mm. Coronal sections in an orthogonal plane might provide better localisation of the foreign body.

Papilledema and degenerative disease represent the most difficult and the most interesting problem. In such cases coronal sections seem to be of great importance. The optic nerve is tortuous to allow easy motion of the eye ball. It makes such a downward loop that one axial section cannot contain the entire optic nerve but encloses at the same time a part of the adjacent fat. For these reasons measurement of diameter and density in axial projections is very inaccurate. Coronal sections raised high expectation. However, the sections are oblique and include so much fat that only the density measurements of the central part of the nerve are dependable.

Authors' address:
Department of Radiology
Fondation Ophtalmologique A. de Rothschild
25 rue Manin
75019 Paris
France

Proc. 3rd Int. Symp. on Orbital Disorders, Amsterdam 1977

COMPUTERIZED TOMOGRAPHY FOR EVALUATION OF FRACTURES AND FOREIGN BODIES OF THE ORBIT

ARTHUR S. GROVE, Jr., RINA TADMOR,
K. JACK MOMOSE, & PAUL F.J. NEW

(Boston, Massachusetts, USA)

Orbital trauma may injure soft tissues, damage the facial bones, and imbed foreign bodies. Injury may also occur to structures adjacent to the orbits, leading to cerebrospinal fluid leaks, carotid-cavernous sinus fistulas, and damage to the brain, nasolacrimal pathways, or paranasal sinuses (Smith et al., 1976; Grove, 1977). Because of the difficulty in determining the extent of soft tissue injuries in patients with orbital fractures, and in localizing intraorbital foreign bodies, computerized tomography has been used to aid in the management of patients with mid-facial injuries (Grove, 1977; Grove et al., 1974, 1977; Momose et al., 1975; Kollarits et al., 1977).

Patients at the Massachusetts Eye and Ear Infirmary who have suffered serious orbital trauma are first examined to determine the extent of injury to the eyes, optic nerves, and intracranial structures (Grove, 1974). Conventional orbital x-rays are usually supplemented by hypocycloidal tomograms. Selected patients who are found to have orbital fractures or who are suspected of having intraorbital foreign bodies are studied by computerized axial tomography (CAT) or by computerized coronal tomography (CCT).

TECHNIQUE

Computerized axial tomography can be performed with either a head or total body scanner. Axial scans visualize cross-sections of the orbits in the same plane as Reid's baseline, which nearly parallels the course of the optic nerves and horizontal rectus muscles (Grove et al., 1974; Momose et al., 1975). However, details near the orbital floor and maxillary sinuses are difficult to distinguish on axial scans (Grove, 1977).

Computerized coronal tomography is performed using a total body scanner with the patient in either a 'hanging head' or 'elevated chin' position. Coronal scans visualize cross-sections of the orbits in a plane which is analogous to Caldwell view x-rays. The plane of coronal scans is perpendicular to Reid's baseline, with scans spaced at 5 mm intervals. Images are viewed as direct enlargements of quadrants of a scan, so that bones and soft tissue structures can be examined in detail (Grove et al., 1977).

Examples of computerized tomograms of patients with orbital floor fractures and intraorbital foreign bodies will be presented to demonstrate the usefulness of this technique for evaluating orbital trauma.

ORBITAL FRACTURES

Linear fracture of orbital floor with entrapment of
inferior rectus muscle

This woman was struck over the right orbit, after which vertical movements

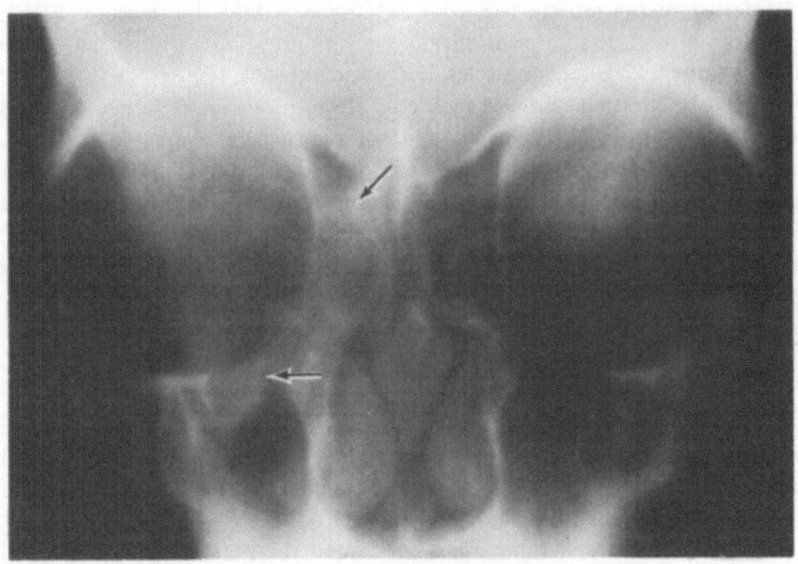

Fig. 1A. X-ray shows densities (arrows) in right maxillary and ethmoid sinuses.

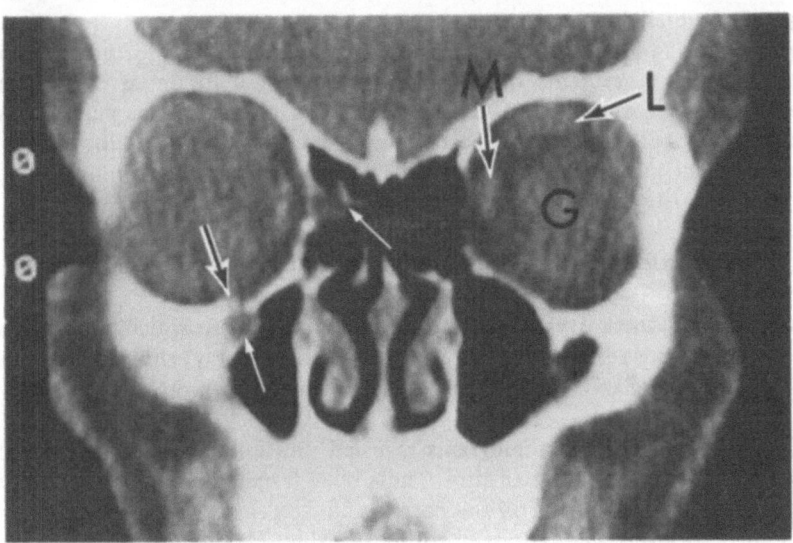

Fig. 1B. Corresponding CCT scan shows small fracture (black arrow) in right orbital floor and soft tissues (white arrows) in right maxillary and ethmoid sinuses. Normal tissues in left orbit include globe (G), medial rectus (M), and levator (L).

131

of that eye were restricted. On x-rays a linear fracture could be seen in the right orbital floor and soft tissue densities were visible in the right maxillary and ethmoid sinuses (Figures 1A and 2A).

Computerized coronal tomograms revealed similar densities in the paranasal sinuses (Figures 1B and 2B). The linear fracture was seen more clearly than on the corresponding x-rays. In sections through the posterior orbits, the inferior rectus muscle was seen entrapped within the fracture (Figure 2B). Normal soft tissues seen within the uninjured left orbit included the globe, levator, extraocular muscles, and optic nerve.

A forced traction test showed restricted elevation of the right eye. Limited movements of the right eye persisted for two weeks, and the patient suffered diplopia in primary gaze. Because of these findings, the orbital floor was explored and the right inferior rectus muscle was found entrapped within the fracture in the position seen on the computerized tomograms. Postoperatively, vertical movements of the right eye were normal except for slightly restricted downgaze.

Depressed fracture of orbital floor with entrapment of inferior rectus muscle

This man was struck over the right orbit, with resulting limitation of vertical movements of that eye. X-rays showed a fragment of the right orbital floor depressed into the maxillary antrum (Figure 3A).

Computerized coronal tomograms confirmed the presence of a depressed bone fragment. On these scans, the inferior rectus muscle was seen entrapped between the displaced bone and the lateral portion of the orbital floor (Figure 3B). Dental fillings caused radiating linear artifacts which are typical of metallic foreign bodies.

Elevation of the right eye was found to be restricted by a forced traction test. Limited movements of the right eye persisted for more than three weeks and the orbital floor was explored. The inferior rectus muscle was found entrapped as seen on the computerized tomograms. Following surgery, vertical movements of the right eye were improved, although some diplopia persisted.

Comminuted fracture of orbital floor withouth muscle entrapment

This man was struck over the left orbit, immediately after which movements of that eye were restricted in all positions of gaze. X-rays showed densities within the paranasal sinuses and bone fragments within the maxillary antrum (Figure 4A).

Computerized coronal tomograms revealed multiple pieces of the orbital floor within the maxillary antrum. These bone fragments were more clearly defined on the scans than on the corresponding x-rays. Soft-tissue densities and air-fluid levels were also seen within this sinus (Figure 4B). No evidence of muscle entrapment was found on these scans.

Diplopia rapidly disappeared in primary gaze, and movements of the eye improved. No restriction of eye movements was evident by a forced traction

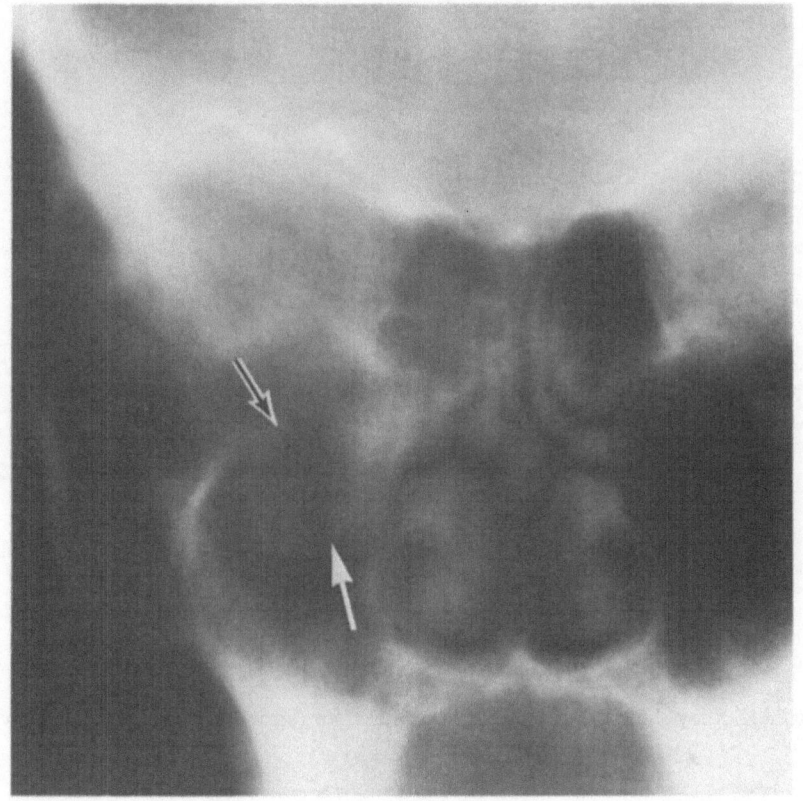

Fig. 2A. X-ray of posterior orbit shows linear fracture (black arrow) and teardrop-shaped density (white arrow) in right maxillary sinus.

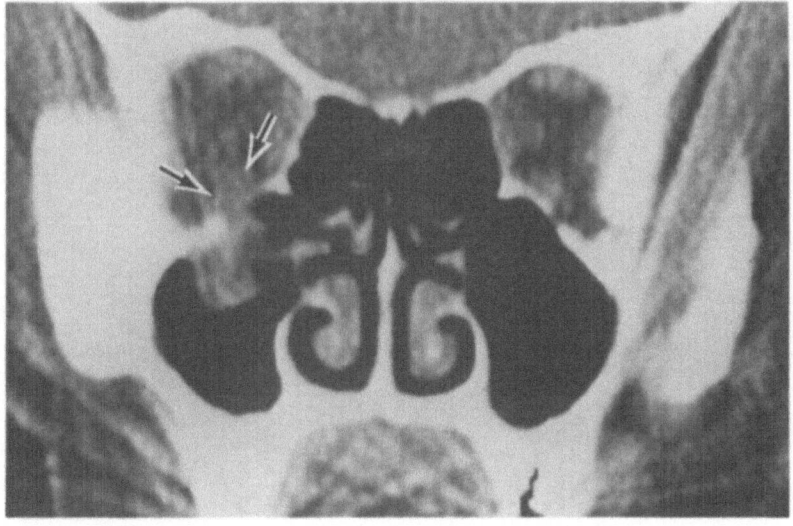

Fig. 2B. Corresponding CCT scan shows right orbital floor fracture and soft tissue density in sinus. Entrapped inferior rectus muscle (arrows) is visible adjacent to fracture.

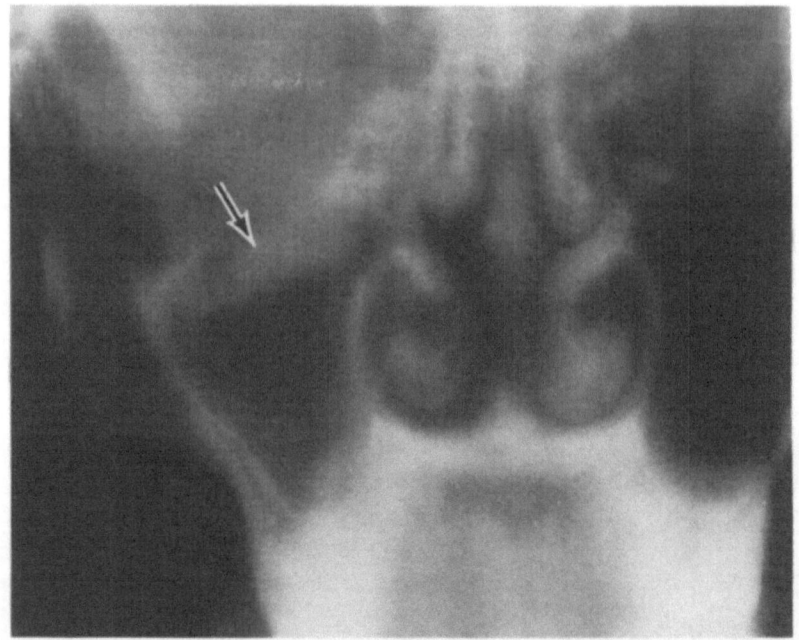

Fig. 3A. X-ray shows fragment of right orbital floor (arrow) depressed into maxillary sinus.

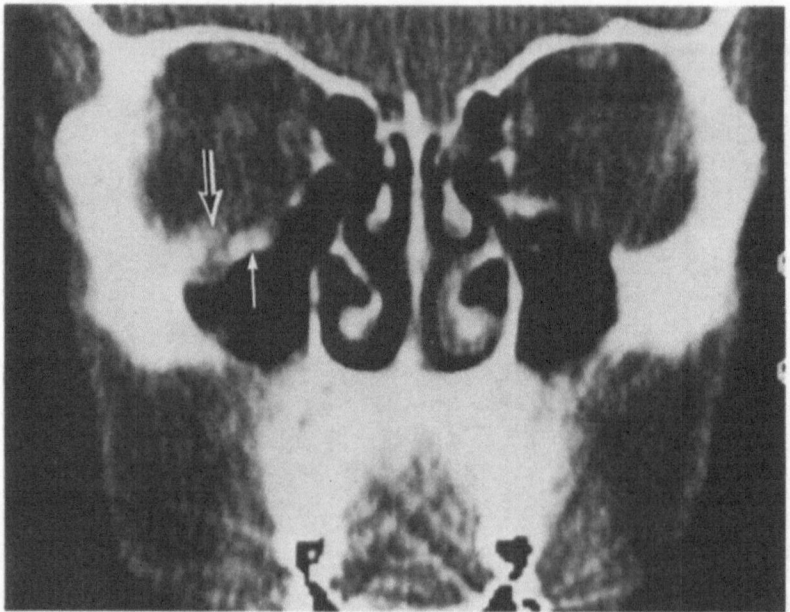

Fig. 3B. Corresponding CCT scan shows entrapped inferior rectus muscle (black arrow) adjacent to depressed bone fragment (white arrow). Dental fillings with radiating artifacts are visible in maxilla.

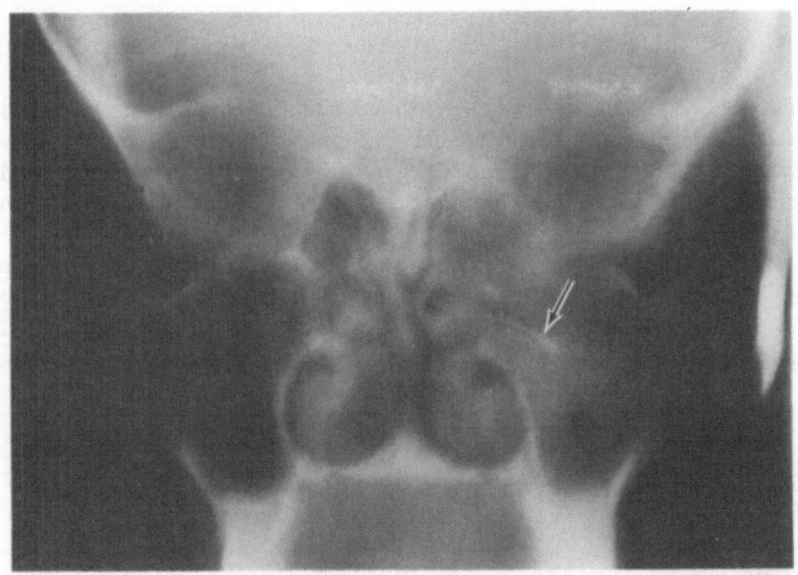

Fig. 4A. X-ray shows opacification of left paranasal sinuses and bone fragment (arrow) displaced into maxillary antrum.

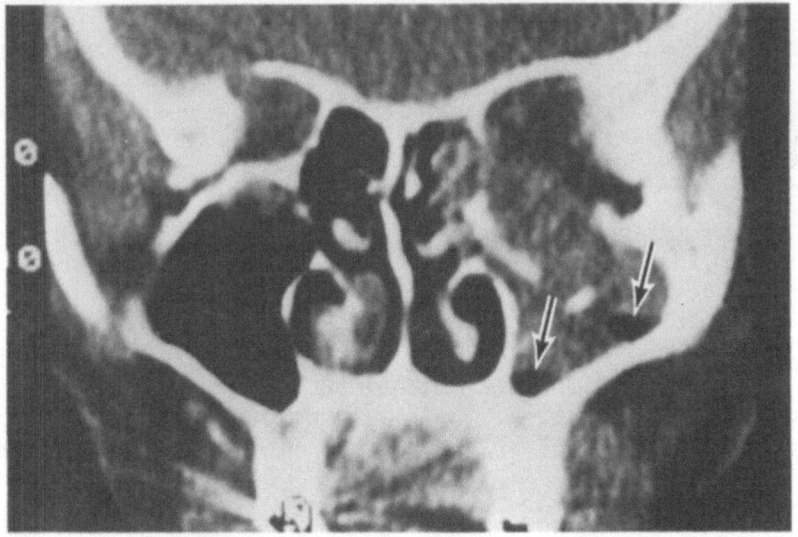

Fig. 4B. Corresponding CCT scan shows comminuted fragments and air fluid levels (arrows) which are not apparent on x-ray.

test. No surgical repair of this fracture was performed, although the patient continues to be followed to determine whether enophthalmos may develop in the future.

135

INTRAORBITAL FOREIGN BODIES ·

Metal pellet

This boy was struck by a copper-covered air-gun pellet which penetrated the conjunctiva near his right medial canthus. X-rays revealed an oval opacity behind the right eye (Figure 5). Even by using ultrasound B-scans and radiographic localization techniques, the position of the pellet relative to the globe and the optic nerve could not be accurately determined.

Computerized coronal tomograms showed the foreign body, directly above which a small air pocket was seen which was not visible on x-rays (Figure 6A). By using different density settings to eliminate the surrounding soft tissues, the foreign body could be more clearly distinguished (Figure 6B).

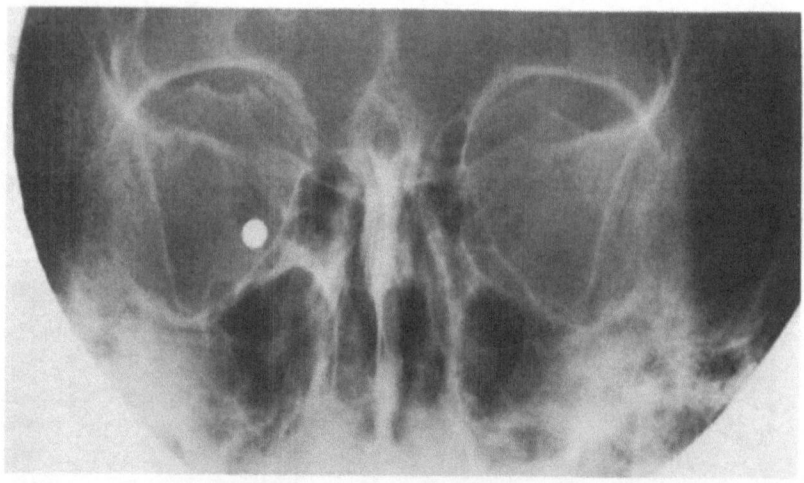

Fig. 5. Metallic foreign body in right orbit is visible on x-ray.

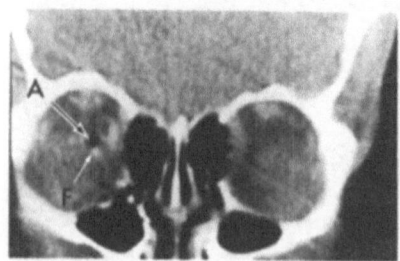 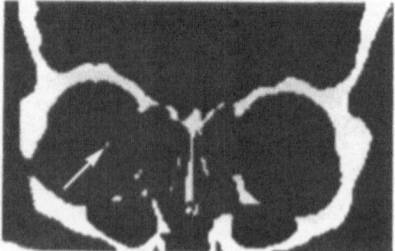

Fig. 6A. CCT scan of patient with metallic foreign body (F) in right orbit. Air pocket (A) located directly above foreign body was not seen on corresponding x-ray (Figure 5).

Fig. 6B. CCT scan of same orbital section using density setting which only visualizes bones and metallic foreign body (arrow).

Computerized axial tomograms of the same patient demonstrated the foreign body in the middle of the right orbit directly behind the globe (Figure 7A). Linear artifacts could be seen radiating from the metallic object. In the section above the foreign body, the air pocket which had been found on coronal tomograms was seen between the medial rectus and the optic nerve (Figure 7B). Since the foreign body was located near the optic nerve, no surgery was performed and the patient uneventfully recovered from the injury.

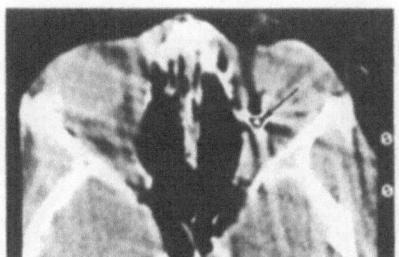 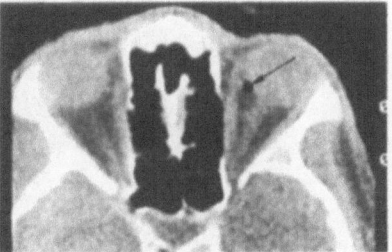

Fig. 7A. CAT scan of same patient in previous two Figures. Metallic foreign body (arrow) produces radiating artifacts which obscure soft tissue details.

Fig. 7B. CAT scan in section above foreign body shows air pocket (arrow) between medial rectus and optic nerve.

Glass fragment

This boy's right upper eyelid was lacerated by a broken piece of a glass door. Computerized axial tomograms localized a small foreign body in the posterior orbit adjacent to the globe (Figures 8A and 8B). A residual glass fragment was removed through an incision near the orbital roof.

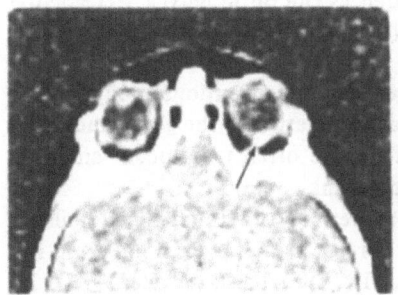 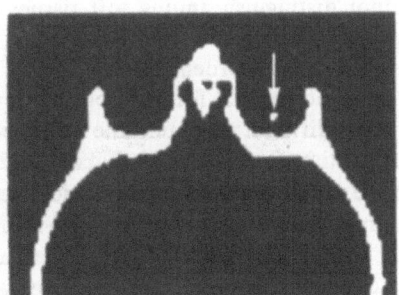

Fig. 8A. CAT scan of patient after right upper lid was cut by glass. Foreign body (arrow) not clearly seen because both high and low density tissues are visualized.

Fig. 8B. CAT scan of same orbital section using density setting which only visualizes bones and glass foreign body (arrow).

Wooden stick

This boy was struck by a piece of wood which penetrated the right lateral conjunctiva. The right upper lid was ptotic after the injury but x-rays revealed no abnormality within the orbit. Computerized axial tomograms showed a linear foreign body between the eye and the lateral surface of the orbit (Figures 9A and 9B). A wooden stick was removed through an incision beside the lateral rectus muscle.

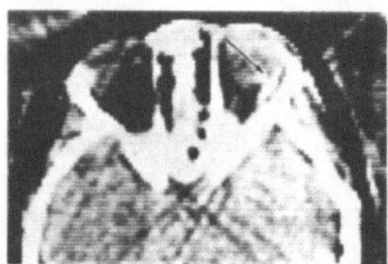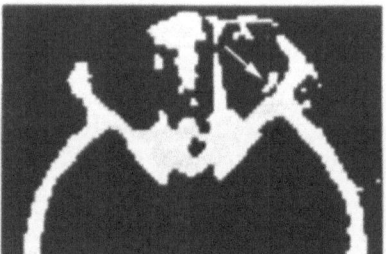

Fig. 9A. CAT scan of patient with ptosis after stick penetrated right lateral conjunctiva. Foreign body (arrow) seen along lateral orbital wall.

Fig. 9B. CAT scan of same orbital section using density setting which eliminates most soft tissues, clearly demonstrating bones and wooden foreign body (arrow).

COMMENT

Most fractures of the orbital floor can be seen on conventional Caldwell or Walters view x-rays. Radiographic tomography will almost always demonstrate fractures which are not apparent on plane films. However, x-rays cannot distinguish among soft tissues such as the optic nerves, extraocular muscles, orbital fat, and hematomas (Grove, 1977; Grove et al., 1977; Emery & von Noorden, 1975).

Many intraorbital foreign bodies can be seen on conventional x-rays, but it is often difficult to determine their location relative to the globe and other normal tissues. Wooden and glass fragments are often radiolucent and may not be visible even on hypocycloidal tomograms.

Computerized tomography provides a method of visualizing details of soft tissues and facial bones, as well as foreign bodies even if they are not radiopaque (Grove, 1977; Grove et al., 1974; Kollarits et al., 1977). By utilizing both axial and coronal plane scans, the orbits can be evaluated in three dimensions. Entrapped extraocular muscles may sometimes be seen adjacent to orbital floor fractures. Bone fragments can often be seen more discretely on scans than on conventional x-rays. Air-fluid levels and intraorbital air pockets may sometimes be seen on computerized tomograms

(Figures 4B, 6A, and 7B) when they are not visible on x-rays. By using computerized tomography, foreign bodies may be accurately localized relative to normal orbital soft tissues, scars, and blood clots. These examinations may help to determine if a traumatized orbit should be explored, and to plan the surgical approach when necessary.

SUMMARY

Computerized axial tomography (CAT) and computerized coronal tomography (CCT) can be used to aid in the evaluation of orbital fractures and the localization of intraorbital foreign bodies. Entrapped extraocular muscles and other soft tissues may be visualized and anatomically identified. Bone fragments, foreign bodies, and air shadows may sometimes be distinguished more clearly than on x-rays. Computerized tomograms may help to determine when it is necessary to surgically explore a traumatized orbit.

REFERENCES

Emery, J.M. & G.K. von Noorden. Traumatic 'pseudoprolapse' of orbital tissues into the maxillary antrum: a diagnostic pitfall. *Trans. Am. Acad. Ophthal. Otolaryng.* 79: *893–896* (1975).

Grove, A.S., Jr. Legal aspects of ocular trauma. *Int. Ophthal. Clin.* 14: *193–203* (1974).

Grove, A.S., Jr. New Diagnostic techniques for the evaluation of orbital trauma. *Trans. Am. Acad. Ophthal. Otolaryng.* In press (1977).

Grove, A.S., Jr., P.F.J. New & K.J. Momose. Computerized tomographic (CT) scanning for orbital evaluation. *Trans. Am. Acad. Ophthal. Otolaryng.* 79: *137–149* (1974).

Grove, A.S., Jr., R. Tadmor, P.F.J. New & K.J. Momose. Orbital fracture evaluation by coronal plane computed tomography (CCT). *Am. J. Ophthal.* (in press, 1977).

Kollarits, C.R., G. Di Chiro, J. Christiansen, J.B. Herdt, P. Whitmore, M. Vermess & R.G. Michels. Detection of orbital and intraocular foreign bodies by computerized tomography. *Ophthal. Surg.* 8: *45–53* (1977).

Momose, K.J., P.F.J. New, A.S. Grove Jr. & W.R. Scott. The use of computed tomography in ophthalmology. *Radiology* 115: *361–368* (1975).

Smith, B., A.S. Grove Jr. & P. Guibor. Fractures of the orbit. Chapter 48, pp. 1–10, in: Clinical Ophthalmology (T. Duane, ed.), Vol. 2. Harper & Row, Hagerstown, Md (1976).

Authors' addresses:
Department of Ophthalmology
Harvard Medical School

and

Ophthalmic Plastic Surgery Service
Massachusetts Eye and Ear Infirmary
Boston, Mass.
USA

Reprint requests to:
Dr A.S. Grove
Massachusetts Eye and Ear Infirmary
243 Charles Street
Boston, Mass. 02114
USA

140

Proc. 3rd Int. Symp. on Orbital Disorders, Amsterdam 1977

STANDARDIZED A-SCAN ECHOGRAPHY AND COMPUTERIZED TOMOGRAPHY FOR EVALUATION OF ORBITAL DISEASE

FRANCIS BIGAR, HANS SPIESS & CHRISTIAN BOSSHARD

(Zürich/St. Gallen, Switzerland)

Since the introduction of computerized tomography (Ambrose, 1973), many reports on the use of this newer examination technique for evaluation of orbital disorders have been published (Lloyd & Wright, 1974; Baker et al., 1974; Gawler et al., 1974; Wright et al., 1975; Grove et al., 1975; Nover et al., 1976; Wollensak et al., 1976; Bronner et al., 1976). Neuroradiologists easily overlook the fact that since the early sixties ophthalmologists have used high-frequency ultrasonography for demonstrating orbital soft tissue abnormalities. Baum & Greenwood (1960), Purnell (1969), and Coleman (1972) mainly advocated the use of immersion B-scan methods, whereas Ossoinig (1975) introduced standardized A-scan echography.

A combined approach of standardized A-scan echography and computerized tomography was used in a series of 37 consecutive patients. This study analyses the results of 18 of these patients with surgical and histological proof of the location and type of lesion present in the orbit.

INSTRUMENTATION AND EXAMINATION TECHNIQUE

Computer Tomography (CT)

All CT scans included in this report were performed with the SIRETOM unit, utilizing the 128 x 128 matrix, except one case examined with the 160 x 160 matrix EMI-scanner. The sections were taken parallel to the infraorbitomeatal plane with the 5 or 10 mm collimator. In routine examinations three to five overlapping sections were obtained with and without intravenous contrast enhancement (1 mg/kg of a 38% iodinated contrast material). Additional scans of the intracranial structures were taken in most patients.

Echography

Standardized high-frequency A-scan echography with a KRETZ-unit 7200 MA was used for the echographic examination of the orbit. In rare instances, the contact Bronson-Turner B-scanner was used in addition to A-scan echography for better documentation of changes op the optic nerve or other lesions within the muscle cone. An attempt to differentiate the lesion

141

was made with the help of quantitative, topographic and kinetic echography after detection of a lesion during the basic examination. The examination technique is best demonstrated by video-tape or 16 mm film with split frame showing simultaneously the guiding of the 8 MHz pencil-shaped probe in the transocular and paraocular approach, and the resulting A-scan echogram on the oscilloscope.

RESULTS

One of the 18 patients with histologically verified space-occupying orbital masses showed a lesion with secondary extension to the orbit from adjacent structures. 11 patients had primary tumors, and 7 had secondary lesions (Table 1).

Computerized tomography and standardized A-scan echography clearly detected and demonstrated the expanding process within the orbit in all 18 cases. A preoperative tissue diagnosis using computerized tomography was performed in 9 cases (50%) (Table 2). This diagnosis proved to be correct in 4 cases, and incorrect in 5. Computerized tomography made a correct diagnosis of an optic nerve glioma, an expanding malignant process of the orbit with partial destruction of the sphenoid wing and infiltration of the middle fossa, a mucocele and a hematoma of the optic nerve. Incorrect diagnoses were: 2 supposed meningiomas of the sphenoid wing. One proved to be a malignant lymphoma adjacent ot the sphenoid, and one a large rhabdo-

		Tissue diagnosis				
	computer tomography			A-scan echography		
Primary orbital tumors	none	correct	incorrect	none	correct	incorrect
4 malignant lymphomas	3	–	1	–	4	–
1 rhabdomyosarcoma	–	–	1	–	1	–
2 mixed tumors lacrimal gld.	2	–	–	–	2	–
2 optic nerve gliomas	–	1	1	1	1	–
1 meningioma	–	–	1	1	–	–
1 malignant tumor	–	–	1	1	–	–
Secondary orbital lesions						
3 metastatic carcinomas	3	–	–	–	3	–
1 plasma cell myeloma	–	1	–	–	1	–
1 mucocele	–	1	–	–	–	1
1 abscess	1	–	–	–	–	1
1 hematoma optic nerve	–	1	–	–	1	–
18 orbital lesions	9	4	5	3	13	2

Table 1. Results of preoperative evaluation of 18 orbital lesions by computerized tomography and standardized A-scan echography.

Pre-operative evaluation of tissue type.

	not made	made correct false
computer tomography	9	9	4	5
A-scan echography	3	15	13	2

Table 2. Summary of results of preoperative tissue type evaluation.

myosarcoma. One supposed glioma of the optic nerve was found to be a malignant tumor of the optic nerve, and one was a meningioma of the optic nerve. The elongated configuration of the latter tumor and little enhancement after contrast material was more suggestive of a glioma 9 (Fig. 1). One diagnosed meningioma of the optic nerve was histologically a glioma (Table 1).

With standardized A-scan echography the enlargement of the optic nerve was correctly detected and measured in three cases, but no differential diagnosis was attempted (Table 1). In 15 patients (83%), an acoustic preoperative tissue evaluation was made. This was correct in 13 cases (85%) and incorrect in 2 cases.

The incorrect diagnoses were one lesion thought to belong to the entity of the lymphoma/sarcoma/pseudotumor group which was found to be a clinically unsuspected abscess. A dermoid cyst was found to be a small mucocele. No bone defect was detected by plain X-ray examination nor by echography. Computerized tomography, however, suspected a mucocele, on the basis of the density values and the location of the lesion.

The classification of orbital disorders with the help of Ossoinig's standardized A-scan echography is based mainly on quantitative echography. Different groups of lesion can be distinguished, based on the height and arrangement of the spikes in abnormal echograms. The echographic tracings can be correlated with the coarse low power microscopic appearance of the lesions in relation to the used wavelength of 0.2 mm at 8 MHz. Further information with regard to location and size, shape and borders, consistency and vascularity of lesions can be gained with additional criterias.

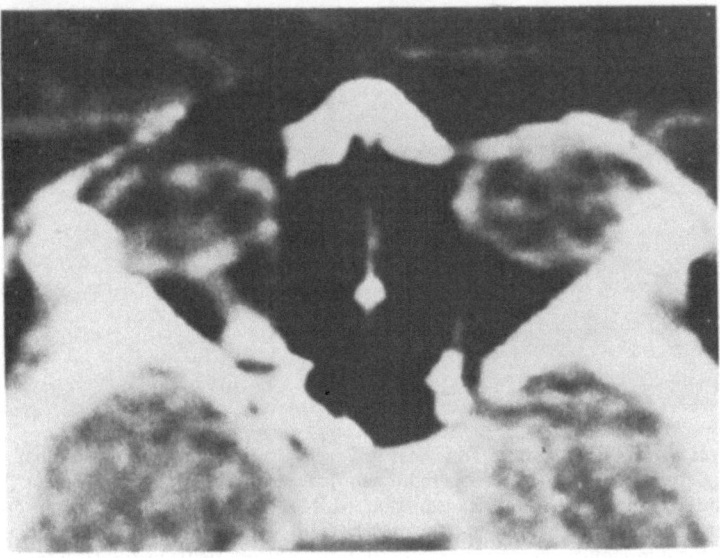

Fig. 1. Meningioma of the optic nerve. The lesion was diagnosed as a glioma on the basis of its shape and little enhancement.

In the following, an example of the 4 most frequent mass lesions of this series is presented together with a CT scan, the echograms and the histology.

Malignant lymphoma (Fig. 2)

A 71 year old woman had a rapid onset of a left-sided proptosis. Tomograms showed an osteolytic process of the orbital roof and the small sphenoid wing. CT demonstrated a large, well delineated elongated mass in the upper parocular and retrobulbar space reaching back to the apex. No contrast enhancement was found. A-scan showed the mass to be well-outlined and low-reflective, typical of a lesion of the lymphoma/sarcoma/pseudotumor group. None of these densely packed cellular lesions can be further differentiated with ultrasound. On the parocular approach, the maximal extension of depth was found to be 25 mm. An anterior biopsy was recommended, but a fronto-temporal craniotomy was performed showing a tumor reaching from the anterior part of the orbit back to the apex. A complete extirpation of the mass was not possible. The diagnosis of malignant lymphoma was made.

The echographic tracing of the tumor is explained on the basis of the homogenous histologic appearance with absence of large interfaces. The

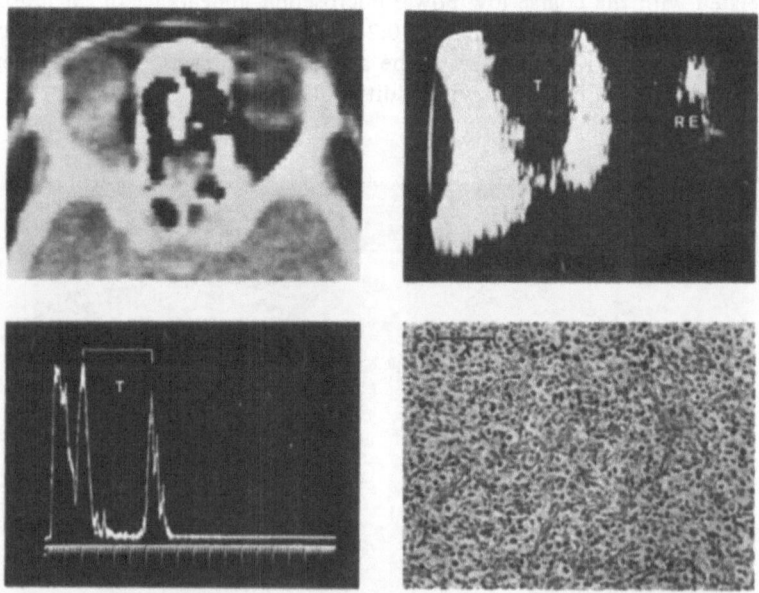

Fig. 2. Malignant lymphoma. Top left: CT scan with elongated retrobulbar mass reaching the left orbital apex. Top right: contact B-scan echogram with defect (T) in the orbital tissue; good sound transmission with low-reflective echoes (RE) in double distance. Bottom left: parocular A-scan echogram with lof-reflective echospikes (T) typical for lymphoma, sarcoma or pseudotumors. Bottom right: histological section of the tumor with regular distribution of small densely packed cells producing weak echoes. The magnification is indicated by a mark corresponding to one wavelength (0.2 mm).

144

regularly distributed densely packed small cells and scarce fibers replace the normal irregular, acoustically high-reflective orbital tissue with large interfaces.

Optic nerve glioma (Fig. 3)

A 20 year old woman was seen with a proptosis of 4 mm of her right eye and a vision of 20/25. On ophthalmoscopy retinal striae and papilloedema were present. The optic canal appeared somewhat distorted on X-ray, but not enlarged. A CT scan showed an elongated enlargement of the optic nerve with the largest diameter in the posterior third of the orbit. Only slight enhancement after contrast material suggested a glioma of the optic nerve. A-scan echography demonstrated a sharply outlined space-occupying lesion within the muscle cone of medium reflectivity (40—60% of the display height) with regular shorter and longer spikes typical for a glioma. The diagnosis was confirmed after a fronto-temporal craniotomy and excision of the tumor. It reached from the apex to the immediate retrobulbar area of the optic nerve.

The acoustic texture of this tumour with regular content of fibrous connective tissue and cells arranged in bands is coarser, and the homogeneity is

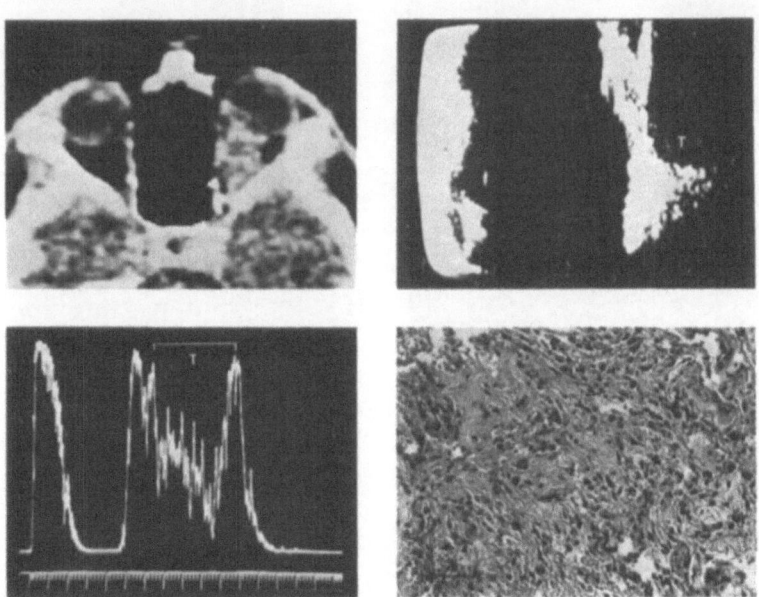

Fig. 3. Glioma of the optic nerve. Top left: CT scan with elongated tumor of the right optic nerve, 5 minutes after contrast material, only slight enhancement. Top right: contact B-scan with indentation in the retrobulbar fat due to the optic nerve tumor. Bottom left: transocular echogram with medium-reflective lesion with longer and shorter spikes. The tumor surface signals are sharply rising and consist of 2—3 peaks. Bottom right: histological section of the tumor with fibrous connective tissue and cells arranged in bands.

145

looser compared to the cellular lesion of the presented malignant lymphoma. This produces the medium reflectivity of this lesion.

Benign mixed tumor of lacrimal gland (Fig. 4)

A 25 year old man presented an exophthalmos and a downward displacement of the right eye as well as diplopia. Superior and lateral orbital bone erosions were found in polytomograms. CT scan showed a tumor with increased density in the upper temporal, anterior and middle orbit, adjacent to the lateral orbital wall. No enhancement was seen after intravenous contrast material. The optic nerve was found to be displaced nasally and the extraocular muscles were considered normal. No specific tissue diagnosis was given. A-scan echography indicated a large solid tumor within the upper temporal parocular space with some retrobulbar extension above the optic nerve. The oval lesion was well delineated and of a high reflectivity (60–95%), typical for a mixed tumor of the lacrimal gland or a cavernous hemangioma. The location within the fossa lacrimalis was in favor of a mixed tumor. This diagnosis was confirmed histologically when the tumor was removed by a lateral orbitotomy.

Histology shows a picture with a distinct regular change of the tissue

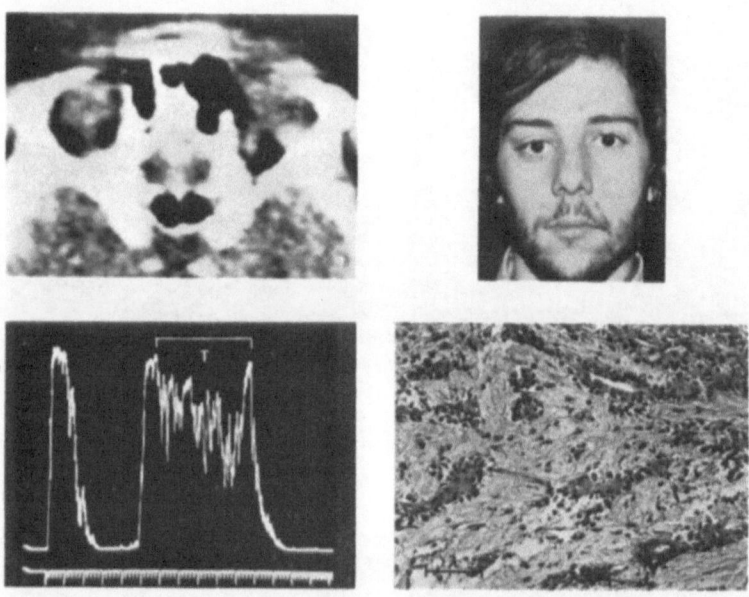

Fig. 4. Benign pleomorphic adenoma of lacrimal gland. Top left: CT scan with large tumor in anterior and middle third of the right orbit adjacent to the lateral orbital wall. No significant enhancement after contrast material. Bottom left: transocular A-scan echogram: high reflective tumor (T) with long regular spikes. The spike height decreases from left to right due to the sound attenuation (medium angle kappa) and are bordered by high surface spikes. Bottom right: the echogram is best explained by the regular change of epithelial cells arranged in bands layed in areas with mesenchymal myxomatous cells.

146

structure. Areas with an accumulation of epithelial cells arranged in bands are layered in areas with mesenchymal myxomatous cells. These changes of large interfaces are responsible for the high-reflectivity of the inner tissue texture.

Carcinoma (Fig. 5)

A progressive proptosis with downward displacement of the left eye and diplopia was found in a 77 year old man. Plain X-ray showed a sclerosis of the upper orbital roof with suspicion of an osteoplastic metastasis. CT scan indicated erosions of the orbital bones on the integral picture and a tumor in the superior orbit possibly starting from the superior rectus muscle. A slight enhancement appeared after contrast material. A-scan echography: a high reflective incompressible lesion with V-shaped pattern and poor outlines above the superior rectus muscle and bone defects of the orbital roof was detected. Surgery confirmed the tumor above the rectus muscle and a softened orbital roof. Histology showed a metastasis of a poorly differentiated adenocarcinoma.

The large interfaces between sheets of carcinoma cells, the eroded bone tissue and the remnants of normal orbital tissue are the source of the echographic high reflectivity.

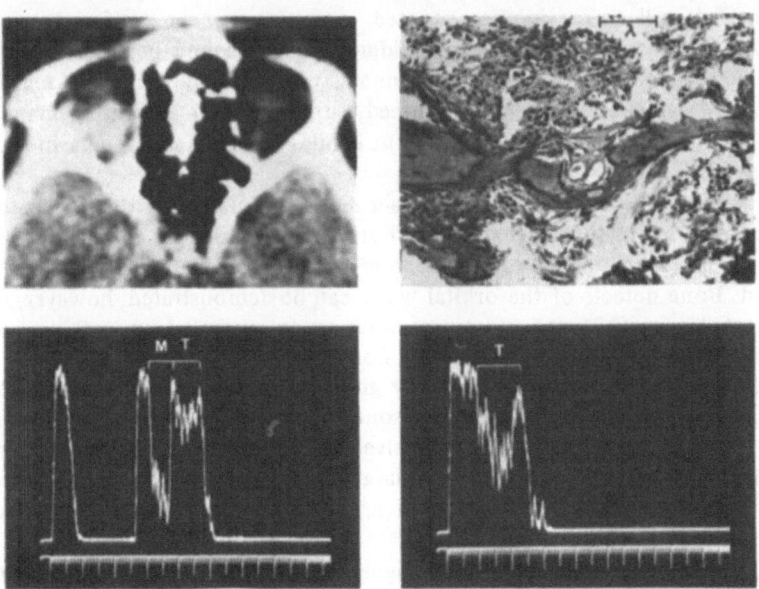

Fig. 5. Carcinoma. Top left: CT scan with tumor in the upper anterior orbit. Bottom right: parocular A-scan echogram with high reflective and poor outlined tumor pattern (T). Bottom left: transocular A-scan echogram with low-reflective pattern of enlarged superior rectus muscle (M) followed by high-reflective tumor spikes (T). Top right: histological section of this tumor with large interfaces compared to the wavelength of 0.2 mm (λ).

COMMENTS

This study shows that computerized tomography and standardized A-scan echography detected all surgically and histologically verified space-occupying lesions of the orbit in this series. A preoperative tissue diagnosis was attempted in half of the 18 patients with computerized tomography. It was correct in 4 out of 9 cases. The relative density and location of mass lesions give some suggestion of their actual nature. Additional information can be gained by enhancement studies after the injection of radioopaque dyes. But reliable differential tissue diagnosis with computerized tomography is not yet possible today. This is in contrast to standardized A-scan echography which defined the nature of the disorder in over 80% of the cases with a diagnostic accuracy of over 80% (Table 2). These data confirm previously published results of other investigators (Ossoinig & Till; Söllner et al., 1974) and of our laboratory (Bigar et al., 1976). Further evaluation of the tissue type of detected lesions is based on their reflectivity, location, extension, shape, borders, consistency and vascularity. As demonstrated with the presented cases, the echographic pattern depends on the coarse tissue structure of the lesion at low power magnification in relation to the acoustic wavelength.

The possibility of reliable classification of lesions is of help in chosing the appropriate treatment. A low reflective lesion of the lymphoma/sarcoma/pseudotumor group is a contraindication for a transfrontal approach. These lesions as well as carcinomas situated anteriorly can be verified by fine needle puncture under the exact guidance of the sound beam. The echographic diagnosis of the cavernous hemangioma is highly reliable. If regular follow-up examinations are guaranteed, surgery is not absolutely mandatory. That is why this rather frequent orbital tumor is not represented in this series.

An important advantage of the contact method as used over the immersion ultrasound techniques is that anterior structures hidden by the orbital rim can be easily evaluated. Normal bone is a barrier for high frequency ultrasound. Bone defects of the orbital walls, can be demonstrated, however, by contact A-scan (17) and the extraorbital space evaluated when the sound beam is directed through the detected bony hole.

Computerized tomography generally gives better topographic information on the involved structures than ultrasound. In most cases CT can tell more easily whether the optic nerve is involved in a lesion of the muscle cone or whether the nerve is displaced by a large expanding process. Furthermore, only CT recognizes the extension of an orbital process of the optic nerve within the intracranial space.

As demonstrated in the case of malignant lymphoma, it can be difficult to indicate by echography the correct maximal depth extension of a lesion situated in the upper orbit with the parocular approach. This is due to the smallness of the parocular space and the concave shape of the orbital roof. Here again, the topographic information of the computerized tomography is of great help.

Computerized tomography and standardized A-scan echography comple-

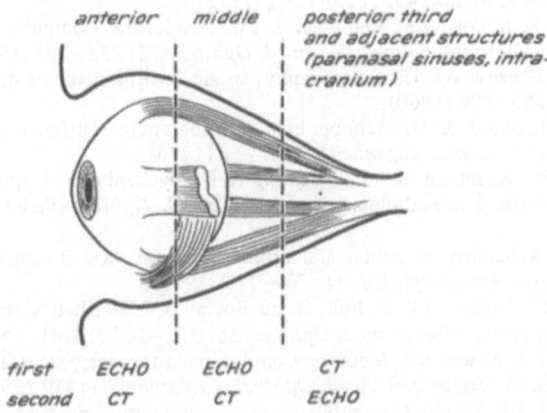

Table 3. Evaluation of exophthalmos with computerized tomography and echography.

ment each other for the evaluation of orbital disorders. We advocate first echography in conjunction with conventional radiology. If this shows and differentiates a lesion within the antereior third of the orbit, an additional examination by computerized tomography is not necessary. If the lesion reaches the middle third of the orbit or originates in this area standardized A-scan echography and computerized tomography are equally desired. The advantage of echography is the better and more accurate tissue differentiation. If however, a lesion is situated within the apex of the orbit or is in connection with adjacent structures, as the intracranial space, computerized tomography is superior and of greater help (Table 3).

SUMMARY

Computerized tomography (CT) and standardized A-scan echography detected all space-occupying lesions of the orbit in a series of 18 patients with surgical and histological proof of the location and type of the lesion. A-scan echography allowed a more reliable preoperative differentiation whereas CT gave more accurate topographic information. This is particularly true if the lesion is situated within the orbital apex.

ACKNOWLEDGEMENTS

The histological examinations were performed in the Pathological Laboratory of the University Eye Clinic of Zurich (Prof. E. Landolt), the University Neuropathological Institute of Zurich (Prof. Friede) and the Pathological Institute of St. Gallen (Prof. Gloor).

149

REFERENCES

Ambrose, J. Computerized transverse and axial scanning (tomography). Part 2: Clinical applications. *Br. J. Radiol.* 46: *1023–1047* (1973).

Baker, H.L., T.P. Kearns, J.K. Campbell & I.W. Henderson. Computerized transaxial tomography in neuroophthalmology. *Am. J. Ophthal.* 78: *285–294* (1974).

Baum, G. & I. Greenwood. Ultrasonography, an aid in orbital tumor diagnosis. *Arch. Ophthal.* 64: *180–194* (1960).

Bigar, F., C. Bosshard & H. Tschopp. Echo-Orbitographie: Differentialdiagnose des Exophthalmus. *Klin. Mbl. Augenheilk.* 168: *151* (1976).

Bronner, A., Ph. Kosmann, W. van Damme & C. Wackenheim. L'application de la tomodensitométrie à la pathologie des orbites. *Arch. Ophtal.* (Paris) 36: *789–796* (1976).

Coleman, D.J. Reliability of ocular and orbital diagnosis with B-scan ultrasound. II. Orbital diagnosis. *Am. J. Ophthal.* 74: *704–719* (1972).

Gawler, G., M.D. Sanders, I.W.D. Bull, G. du Boulay & J. Marshall. Computer assisted tomography in orbital disease. *Br. J. Ophthal.* 58: *571–187* (1974).

Grove, A.S., P.F.J. New & K.J. Momose. Computerized tomographic (CT) scanning fo: orbital evaluation. *Trans. Am. Acad. Ophthal. Otolaryng.* 79: OP *137–149* (1975).

Lloyd, G.A.S. & J.E. Wright. Computerized axial tomography. *Br. Med. J.* 3: *114–115* (1974).

Nover, A., J. Schmitt, S. Wende & A. Aulich. Computertomographie in der Ophthalmologie. *Klin. Mbl. Augenheilk.* 168: 461–467 *(1976).*

Ossoinig, K.C. A-scan echography and orbital disease. pp. 203–239 in: Proc. 2nd Symp. on Orbital Disorders, Amsterdam 1973. Mod. Probl. Ophthal, Vol. 14. Karger, Basel (1975).

Ossoinig, K.C. & P. Till. A ten year study of clinical echography in orbital disease. pp. 200–216 in: Ultrasonography in ophthalmology (J. François & F. Goes, eds). Bibl. Ophthal. Vol. 83. Karger, Basel (1975).

Purnell, E. Ultrasonic interpretation of orbital diseases. pp. 249–255 in: Ophthalmic ultrasound (Gitter et al., eds.). Mosby, St Louis (1969).

Söllner, F., L. Wüstenberg & R. Kohlhase. Echographische Diagnostik des einseitigen Exophthalmus. *Klin. Mbl. Augenheilk.* 164: *117–124* (1974).

Till, P. Echography in rhinogenic orbital conditions. pp. 273–277 in: Proc. 2nd Symp. on Orbital Disorders, Amsterdam 1973. Mod. Probl. Ophthal., Vol. 14. Karger, Basel (1975).

Wollensak, J., H. Bleckmann, S. Lange & T. Grumme. Computertomographie des Auges und der Orbita. *Klin. Mbl. Augenheilk.* 168: *467–475* (1976).

Wright, J.E., G.A.S. Lloyd & J. Ambrose. Computerized axial tomography in the detection of orbital space-occupying lesions. *Am. J. Ophthal.* 80: *78–84* (1975).

Authors' addresses:
F. Bigar
University Eye Clinic
Kantonsspital
Rämstrasse 100
CH-8091 Zürich
Switzerland

H. Spiess
Neuroradiologisches Institut
Talstrasse 65
CH-8001 Zürich
Switzerland

C. Bosshard
Augenklinik
Kantonsspital
CH-9007 St. Gallen
Switzerland

MISLEADING FINDINGS OBTAINED BY
ULTRASONOGRAPHY AND COMPUTERIZED TOMOGRAPHY

A. NOVER & J. SCHMITT

(Mainz, W. Germany)

Our diagnostic possibilities in examination of orbital lesions have been considerably enlarged by ultrasonography and computerized tomography. In a high percentage of those of our patients who have been examined with both methods, retrobulbar lesions could be verified. In a number of cases, however, we have been misled by the outcome of one of these methods. This may be illustrated by the following clinical examples.

CASE REPORTS

First case

G.A., a 79 year old woman, had had an excision of a malignant lymphoma from the right groin. Now a bilateral exophthalmus had developed one month earlier. Ultrasonography repeatedly revealed bilaterally a free retrobulbar space. Because of the anamnestic data metastasis into both orbita was likely. Therefore a CT was done as a result of which areas with greater density and tuberous appearance could be seen. Since a tumor could also be detected in the right abdominal area and edemas were present in both legs, the cause of the protrusion was presumably a metastasis of the malignant lymphoma. This, however, could not be proved because the patient was not operated on but exposed to cobalt-60 radiation.

Second case

W.Cl., a 13 year old girl, was seen with a progressive protrusio bulbi of the right eye of 2 years' duration, together with decreasing visual acuity. The difference in exophthalmometry finally was 13 mm, the right optic nerve was pale. Ultrasonography and CT both showed a bulb-like swelling of the right optic nerve and dilatation of the right optic foramen. The girl was operated on because of a glioma of the right optic nerve in the Neurosurgical Department of the University Hospital of Mainz; the optic nerve was removed.

The result of a CT done six months after the operation was very surprising because it clearly showed optic nerves in otherwise almost empty retrobulbar spaces. This was also the case on the side where the optic nerve had been removed during the operation.

We have been unable to find an explanation – and neither can our neuro-radiologists – for this whitish cord that apparently corresponds to the optic nerve and extends from the posterior pole of the bulbus to the orbital tip.

Third case

P.P. This 29 year old man had had a blow on the left eye during a row, and immediately thereafter lost the sight in that eye. He showed a massive retro-bulbar hematoma together with the pertinent protrusion; the visual acuity was light perception; the upper lid had a cut.

Ultrasonography showed a moderate widening of the para- and retrobulbar space but no foreign body echos. CT then, besides a spot-like density within the whole retrobulbar space which was interpreted as a hematoma, showed two sharply demarcated foreign bodies, one located nasally, having displaced the nervus opticus laterally. According to density they might have been glass pieces. During the subsequent operation an overall number of five glass fragments was removed; some of them were relatively large.

Fourth case

B.H. This 47 year old man had noticed a transient slight deterioration of visual acuity during the last five months, accompanied by a simultaneous transient swelling of the lids and progressive protrusion and dislocation of the left eye. Ultrasonography – in correspondence with the clinical picture – revealed a solid process, 30 mm in depth with a clear terminal spike in the upper nasal quadrant. A mucocele could be excluded. The CT picture did not reveal a solid process but only a well demarcated area of soft tissue density at the nasal wall of the orbita. The neuroradiologists interpreted these findings as a thickening of the internus rectus muscle and also saw the superior rectus thickened. Therefore, they assumed a unilateral endocrine ophthalmopathy. Despite this, subsequent surgical intervention in the superior nasal quadrant revealed an encapsulated tumor macroscopically resembling a lipoma. In the subsequent discussion with the neuroradiologists it was said that the structures in the pictures revealed by CT could also be interpreted as being a lipoma. What was at first taken for thickened eye muscles, could also have been the denser border of a lipoma and the dark and apparently unsuspicious tissue in between would have been the centre of the tumor.

Despite the fact that the diagnostic value of both procedures together with the approved methods is uncontested, the analysis of the results demands great experience and even then – as documented by our cases – it still leaves considerable scope for misdiagnoses. Therefore, one should always take also into account the individual history and the clinical picture as well as the other methods of examination available.

Authors' address:
Universitäts-Augenklinik
Langenbeckstrasse 1
6500 Mainz
W. Germany

Proc. 3rd Int. Symp on Orbital Disorders, Amsterdam 1977

COMPUTERIZED TOMOGRAPHY IN ORBITAL DISEASES

S. LANGE, Th. GRUMME, S. WENDE, K. KRETZSCHMAR,
E. KAZNER & H. STEINHOFF

(Berlin, W. Germany)

Computer tomography is an important new non-invasive radiological method which has been used for the exploration of the orbit for 4 years (Ambrose et al., 19   ; Gawler et al., 1974; Momose et al., 1975). Today it may undoubtedly be considered the most advanced radiographic representation of soft tissue orbital structures.

In a cooperative study of the clinics in Berlin, Mainz and Munich we have studied 210 cases of orbital lesions including 25 vascular malformations, 50 meningiomas, 8 diseases of the optic nerve, 24 benign space occupying processes, 5 pseudotumors, 10 malformations, 53 malignant tumors, 22 endocrine exophthalmus, 9 traumas and 39 lesions not yet histologically verified. The computer tomograms were obtained using an EMI-machine (Mark I) with a matrix of 160 x 160 pixels. The sections were positioned parallel to Reid's base line. Each slice has a thickness of 8 mm and usually 4 slices are sufficient to cover the whole orbital space.

The orbit and its contents form an ideal situation for computer tomography because of the low density fat surrounding the anatomic or pathological structures. In general, the eyelids, the globe with its sclera, the optic nerve, the extra-ocular muscles namely the external rectus and the bony walls of the orbit may be discerned.

In Grave's disease proptosis and the thickening of the extra-ocular muscles – namely the internal rectus and the posterior cone of the ocular muscles – are characteristic computer-tomographic features. However, in myositis extra-ocular muscles may also be thickened and the differential diagnosis between the two diseases cannot be made on computer tomographic grounds. Also, a congestion of the orbit due to a carotid-cavernous fistula may present a similar picture.

The main indication for computer tomography in ophthalmology is the confirmation or exclusion of a space occupying lesion suspected on clinical grounds. An orbital tumor whose diameter is smaller than 4 mm cannot be detected by the machines now in use, and the resolution of the method may even be much worse if the lesion is adjacent to bony structures (Fig. 2).

For clinical purpose, however, the determination of the lesion's size is – apart from exceptions – accurate. Also the location of a lesion and its invasion of bony structures can be identified. The confidence level of the computer tomographic localisation permits one to decide on the surgical

153

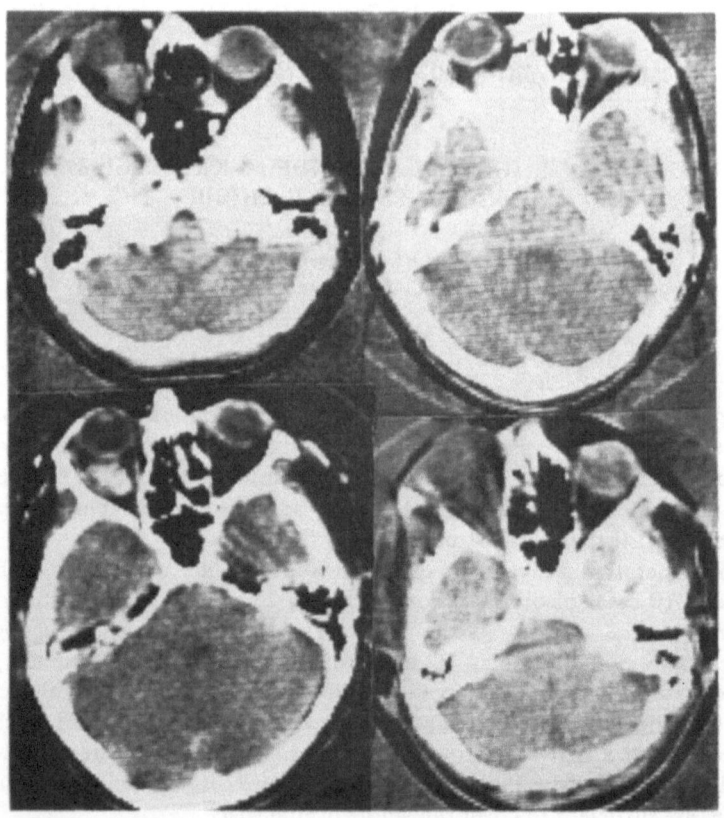

Fig. 1. a) Meningioma. b) Carcinoma of epipharynx invading orbit. c) Cavernous hemangioma. d) Congesion of orbit due to carotid-cavernous fistula.

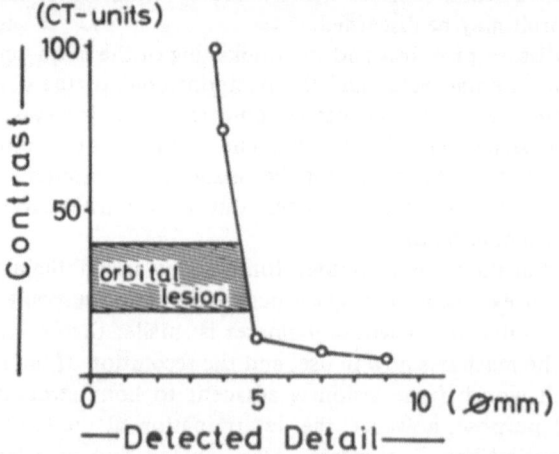

Fig. 2. In phantom studies, balls of increasing diameter and density were scanned. The smaller the diameter of a ball the larger its density difference with the surroundings (= contrast) has to be in order to permit detection.

technique, namely on the anterior, lateral or transcranial approach.

It has been claimed that by relying on computer tomographic criteria (density of lesion, its affinity to contrast medium, its size and its shape) some information may be gained concerning the etiology and histologic nature of a lesion (Lloyd & Ambrose, 1977). To our knowledge and experience this is, however, not possible. Comparing various orbital lesions it was found that the difference of both the plain density values and the density values of the contrast enhancement was too small to permit a reliable diagnosis as to the etiology. Also, the position of a lesion, namely its connection to intraorbital structures, was of little diagnostic value as we have found a wide variety of lesions connected to the optic nerve, such as a reticulosarcoma, meningoma, glioma or cavernous hemangioma. Also, tumors connected to the lacrimal glands may be of quite different origin. A destruction of the orbital wall may be found in malignant tumors as well as in benign lesions such as mucoceles or pyoceles. Therefore, he who interprets computer tomograms of the orbits should avoid a diagnosis concerning the etiology of a lesion.

Computerized tomography is easily performed, and may readily be repeated in a patient. The examination is of little discomfort, there is no risk, and radiation dose is relatively low. Conventional radiographic methods are only in a few cases superior, namely arteriography for carotic-cavernous fistula, venography for venous malformations and lesions within the superior fissure of the orbit, a region which is relatively inaccessible to computerized tomography.

The destruction of the orbital walls may be seen on computer tomograms but due to its better resolution conventional tomograms may yield more detailed information. Because of its easy performance and high diagnostic accuracy computerized tomography should always be used as the first radiological method in suspected orbital disease.

REFERENCES

Ambrose, J.A.E., et al. A preliminary evaluation of fine matrix computerized axial tomography (Emiscan) in the diagnosis of orbital space-occupying lesions. *Br. J. Radiol* 47: *747–751* (1974).

Gawler, J., et al. Computer assisted tomography in orbital disease. *Br. J. Radiol.* 58: *571* (1974).

Lloyd, G.A.S. & J.A.E. Ambrose. An evaluation of C.A.T. in the diagnosis of orbital space-occupying lesions. Proc. ESCAT Seminar, London 1976. Springer, Berlin (1977).

Momose, K.J., et al. The use of computer tomography in ophthalmology. *Radiology* 115: *361* (1975).

Wende, S., et al. Computed tomography or orbital lesions. *Neuroradiol.* 13: *123* (1977).

Authors' address:
Stralenklinik
Universitätsklinikum Charlottenburg
130 Spandauer Damm
1000 Berlin 19
W. Germany

Proc. 3rd Int. Symp. on Orbital Disorders, Amsterdam 1977

C.T. OF THE OPTIC NERVE IN PAPILLEDEMA

U. SALVOLINI, F. MENICHELLI, U. PASQUINI,

(Ancona, Italy)

A. RODALLEC, E.A. CABANIS & P. BONNIN

(Paris, France)

In the Ospedale 'Umberto 1°' (Ancona, Italy) we noticed that in certain patients C.T. showed abnormally thick optic nerves. Most of them were known to have papilledema. Ambrose & Mosely had already noticed an increase in the size and shape of optic nerves with irregular thickness. Enlarged optic nerves were seen with or without any intra-cranial lesion (Fig. 1).

CRITERIA

Certain criteria must be followed in optic nerve examinations:
1. position and immobility;
2. incidence and thickness;
3. overlapping;
4. diagnostic display console;
5. partial volume effect.

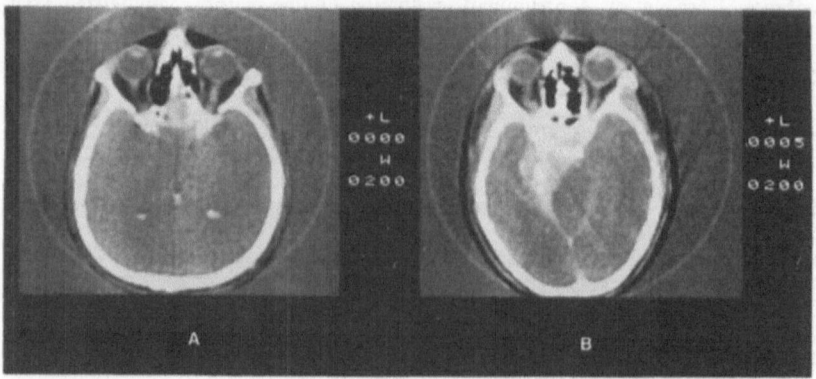

Fig. 1. C.T. in two cases of papilledema with enlarged and deviated optic nerves. A. Benign cranial hypertension. Bilateral augmentation of O.N. caliber. B. Sphenoidotentorial meningioma. Predominance of the caliber augmentation homolateral to the tumor.

Position and immobility

It is important to make sure that the eyeball does not move during the examination because of inaccurate measurements which may result from movement. The optic nerves move with the eyeball movements. Under general anesthesia, the eyes are in Charles Bell's position, i.e., rotated up and outwards.

Incidence and thickness; neuro-ocular plane

Fig. 2 shows the C.T. exploration of normal orbits (Fig. 2B). Sequence of vertical scans, 8 mm thick, with a 5 mm overlap. The optic nerve visible in 2 and 3 may only be studied on scan 3, as it is the only one conforming to the Lens-Optic disc-Optic canal alignment criteria. It is what we call the 'neuro-ocular plane' in which we are interested.

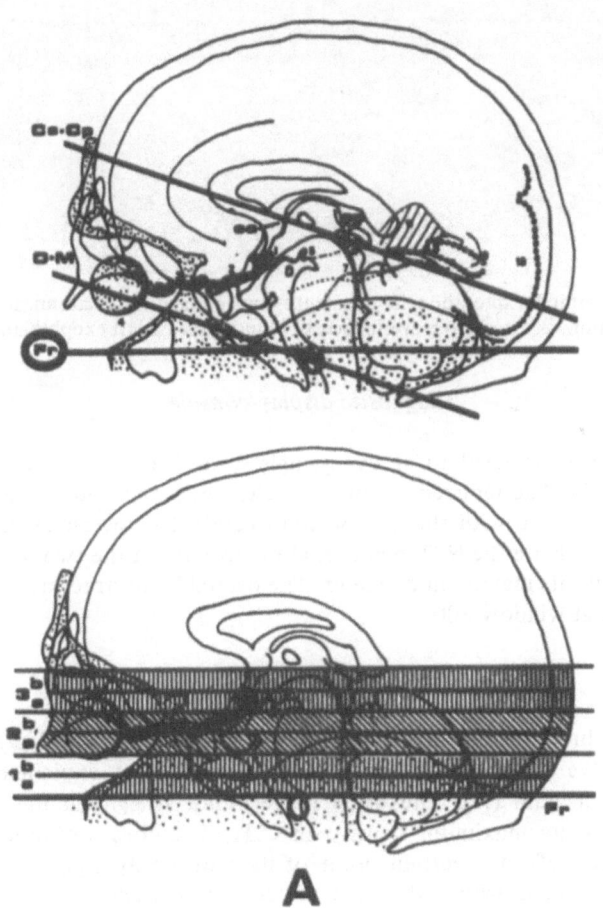

A

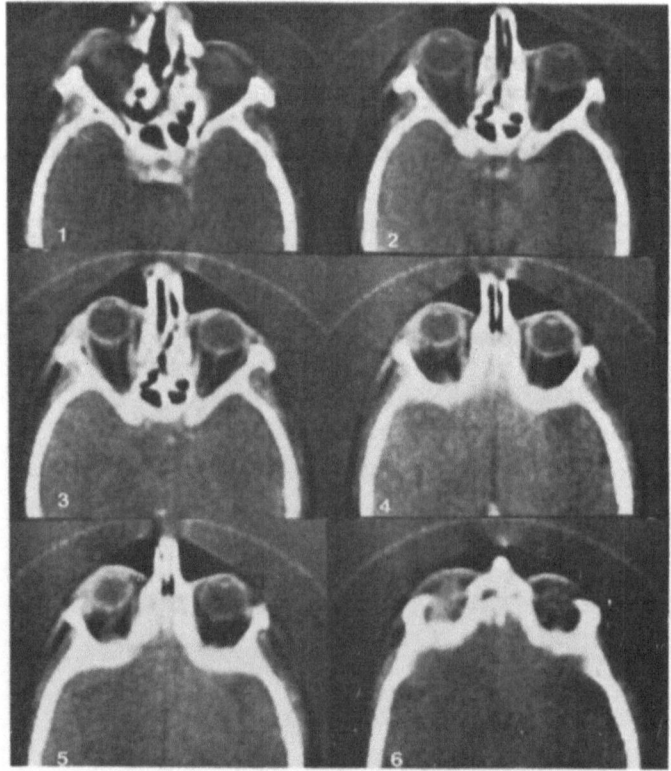

Fig. 2. C.T. orbital exploration in the neuro-ocular plane. A. Anatomical planes and C.T. orientation. B. Successive overlapped C.T. in a case of left exophthalmos (hyperthyroidism).

Diagnostic display console

We emphasize the need to study a single scan at different levels and windows (Fig. 3). The reduced widths hide the optic nerve edges, the sizes of which are analysed with the wide window (200). The reverse readings aid in the diagnosis. Note the N.O. plane: slight convexity of the two optic nerves, lens seen with its maximum diameter. The orbital bone structures are clearly shown here at window 200.

Partial volume effect

The darker line in fig. 4, first described by Moseley, is known as Moseley's white line. We think that this is a partial volume effect, explainable on the right-hand diagram (A). The optic nerve is not straight in the orbit. It cannot show its maximum density in C.T., if it does not appear in full within a scan. If, at a certain point of its course only a part of the optic nerve's diameter is within the scan, its density will appear less or even be non-existent (B).

158

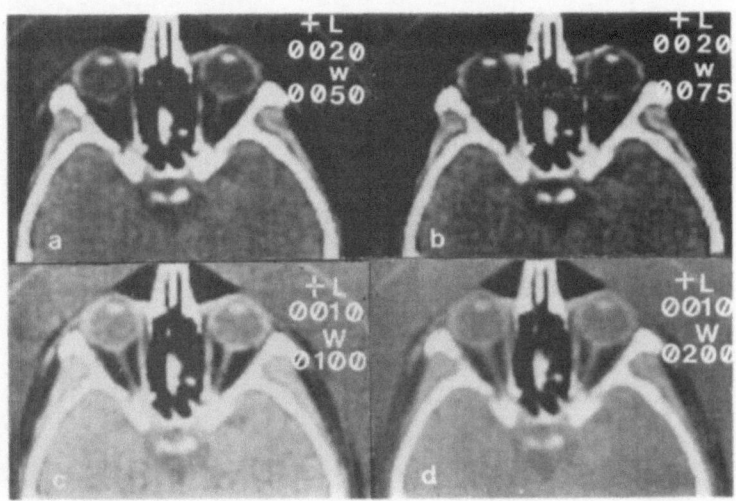

Fig. 3. Importance of the window choice. Note the different O.N. visualisation, from A to D.

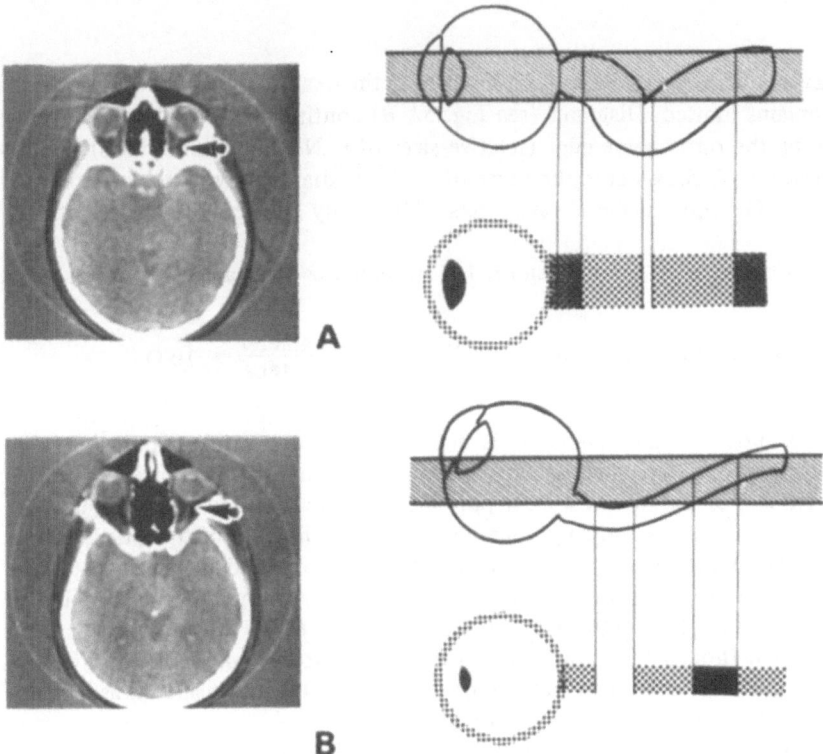

Fig. 4. Partial volume effect in O.N. C.T. A. In a case of papilledema with O.N. enlargement. B. In a case of vertical displacement of the eyeballs. (Possible explanation of the retrobulbar defects).

159

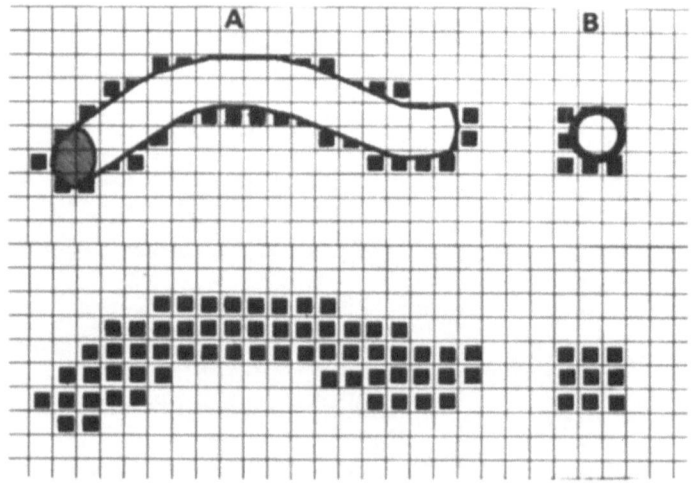

Fig. 5. Partial volume effect in O.N. C.T. a. Scheme of an axial O.N. view. b. Scheme of a frontal O.N. view.

Even with the precise criteria described, the examination of the optic nerve remains limited. Diagrams (see Fig. 5A,B) continue to leave doubt in evaluating the optic nerve edge (relative sizes of O.N. caliber and pixels). In our series, C.T. shows an optic nerve of 3—4 mm diameter with pixel size of 1.5 mm. The optic nerve always looks wider. Only the central densitometry is true.

We have tried to establish the following index of measurements (Fig. 6):

$$\text{Neuro-Ocular-Index (N.O.I.)} = \frac{\text{optic nerve diameter}}{\text{eyeball diameter}} \times 100$$

This index of measurements is not absolute but relative. Applied to the diagrams we were surprised to notice an indisputable difference between a normal population showing a pure Gaussian distribution and a population with papilledema showing a tendency towards the right of the index, with a second point which means something we do not understand as yet. The Gaussian distribution is limited by the small number of measurements. Nevertheless, Student's test shows its value (Fig. 6).

Even though the index is not a measurement but an estimation, it is, in our opinion, an instrument important enough to be considered as a reference. We have noticed wider optic nerves in:
— anterior, middle and posterior intracranial lesions;
— hydrocephaly;
— benign intracranial hypertension.
In short: in raised intracranial hypertension.

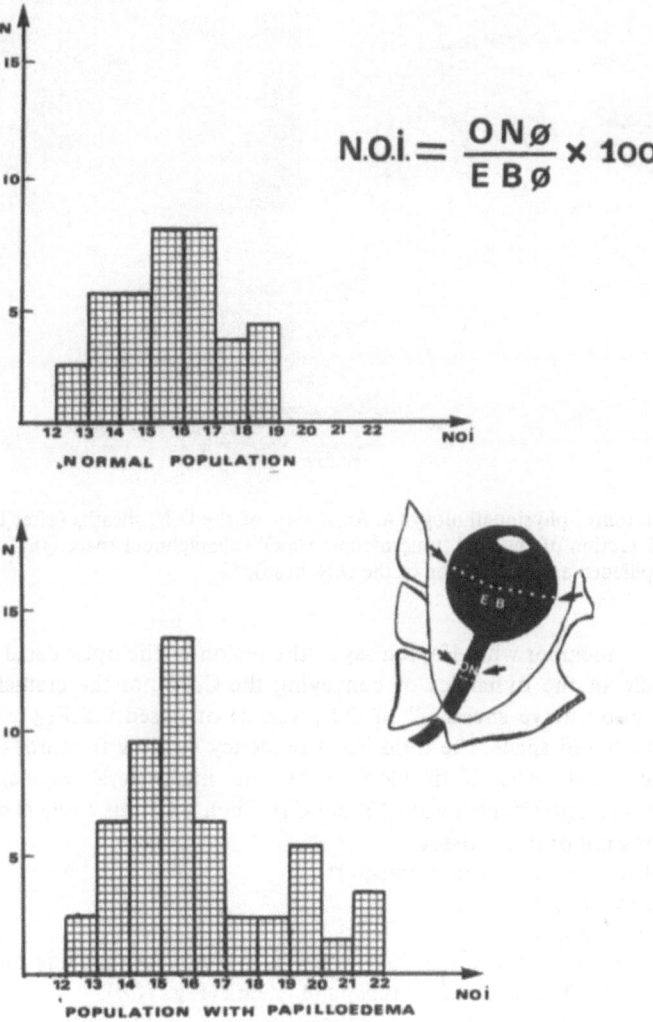

$$N.O.i. = \frac{ON\varnothing}{EB\varnothing} \times 100$$

NORMAL POPULATION

POPULATION WITH PAPILLOEDEMA

Fig. 6. Neuro-ocular index (N.O.I.). a. Evaluation in a normal population (histogram). b. Evaluation in a population with papilledema.

DISCUSSION

Why an enlarged optic nerve picture (Fig. 7)? The optic nerve travels through the orbit within the optic nerve dural sheaths:
— dura mater (5) (in A, redrawn after Hayreh);
— pia mater;
— between them, the arachnoid trabeculum (clearly seen in B on this optic nerve frontal section), which allows for the passage of the cerebrospinal fluid (C.S.F.).

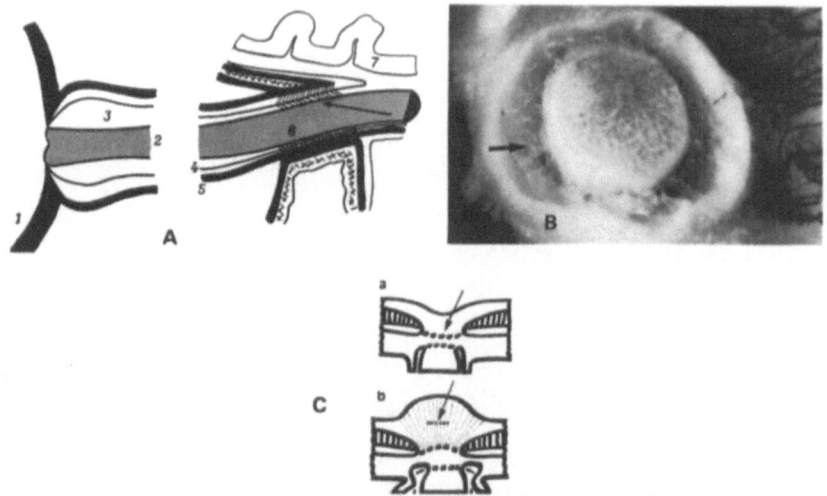

Fig. 7. Anatomy, physiopathology. A. Axial view of the O.N. sheaths (after Hayreh).
B. Frontal section of the O.N. (microscopic view); subarachnoid space (/). C. Production of papilledema (strangulation of the O.N. head).

Let us remember what Hayreh says: 'the region of the optic canal plays a crucial role in the dynamics of conveying the C.S.F. of the cranial cavity into the optic nerve sheaths." In the presence of raised C.S.F. pressure in the subarachnoid space, the fluid has a tendency to flow forwards through the optic canal (A6), until blocked by the intra-scleral vaginal space, squeezing the optic nerve head (A3 and Ca). Then a vicious circle is created:
− compression of nerve tissue
− disturbance of axoplasmic transport
− axonal swelling
− vascular stasis.
When oedamatous, the optic disc swells in the only expandable direction, which is the prelaminar area. This is papilledema (Fig. 7Cb).

Hayreh has experimentally produced oedema of the optic disc in the rhesus monkey by introducing and distending intracranial ballons, thus simulating a growing intracranial spaceoccupying lesion. The occurrence of optic disc oedema depends on the raised C.S.F. pressure in the cranial subarachnoid space and not in the ventricle alone and its free extension into the optic nerve dural sheaths. This is suggested by the disappearance of optic disc oedema on decompression of the sheaths.

Practical application

The practical application of the above is as follows:
− after clinical diagnosis (fluorography. neuro-ophthalmological examination);
− standard X-rays;

162

– the C.T. must be studied for (a) space occupying lesion (always contrast injection), (b) ventricular size, (c) optic nerve size;
– in bilateral papilledema, if an enlarged optic nerve apparently exists without other symptoms, always measure ventricle size;
– in unilateral papilledema first look for a local cause, but keep in mind the optic canal adhesions which may prevent the appearance of a nerve enlargement.

It may be necessary to make further examinations by means of arteriography and encephalography. If necessary, surgery for tumor removal, valve or optic nerve decompression may follow. In some cases a simple follow-up may be sufficient.

CONCLUSION

We could summarize the above as follows:
1. If papilledema exists (without local cause), always measure for optic nerve size;
2. if the optic nerve is widened, always look for a raised I.C.P.
It means that in papilledema, when C.T. is performed, if possible an orbital study must follow a cerebral study and an orbital study must be accompanied by a ventricular C.T.

Authors' addresses:
Servisio de Radiologie
Ospedale Civile 'Umberto 1°'
Ancona
Italy

Centre National d'Ophtalmologie des Quinze-Vingts
Service de Radiologie
Paris
France

Reprint request to Dr U. Salvolini (Ancona)

Proc. 3rd Int. Symp. on Orbital Disorders, Amsterdam 1977

COMPUTED TOMOGRAPHY IN OPHTHALMOLOGY

A. ROUSSEAU, J. MICHIELS, G. CORNELIS & H.H. VANDRESSE

(Brussels, Belgium)

In order to examine the orbitary cavities and the ocular globe as a whole, we already had recourse to different techniques that were more or less usual or more or less aggressive.

Common radiology of the skull and of the orbitary phlebography and angiography enabled us to support the ophthalmologic radio-diagnosis. The very smart technique that was perfected by the engineer, Mr. Hounsfield, of England, made it possible to display a certain number of orbitary lesions, for instance of tumoral origin, thanks to the weak density of the retro-ocular fat. When required, we can utilize the iodized product of contrast by I.V. in order to better visualize the soft structures that are of interest. Testing without pain and without drawbacks for the patient, with perhaps a possible risk of allergy induced by any contrast product, as we shall see in the following clinical cases, there is no denying the superiority of this technique as a diagnostic means, with regard to tumoral pathology tumors of the nerve, of the muscles, of the retina, of the globe as a whole or tumoral flood coming from neighbouring structures.

However, even with the injection of a contrast product, we are not able to visualize satisfactorily and securely the localized infections, pathologies, type irridocyclitis, or even the traumatic detachment of the retina.

Traumatic ruptures of the optical nerve are also difficult to discover with certainty.

This reservation which we enter today will undoubtedly be reconsidered tomorrow. For then we shall have at our disposal a better definition of the densities, and be able to lessen the thickness of the section that is at present 8 mm for the eyes, which also explains the non-visualization of extraneous elements measuring less than 8 mm in diameter.

We are unable to express an opinion regarding the traumatic haemorrhages (intra or extraocular); our experience in this field is inadequate. If the T.C. of the orbit is a particularly smart examination and even, let us say it, preferential, it does not do away with the other methods of angiographic or even phlebographic examinations which are henceforth complementary, but give better information thanks to the mere existence of this T.C.

To conclude, the computerized tomography is most advantageous, not only to the radiologists and the ophthalmologists, but also to the patients.

The elegance of this method, the absence of traumatic troubles for the sick, the quicker turnover of the patients in the neuro-radiology service and the control services, enable a faster adjustment and a more rapid diagnosis than when going through conventional ways. Besides and above all, it enables us to diagnose better the indications towards complementary examinations. Let us hope that the unceasing technical prograss will enable us to quickly obtain extremely fine definition and cross-sections, in order to still improve an accurate study of the delicate structures of the eyes.

Authors' address:
U.C.L.Saint Luc
Avenue Hippocrate 10
1200 Brussels
Belgium

Proc. 3rd Int. Symp. on Orbital Disorders, Amsterdam 1977

TECHNETIUM SCANNING IN ORBITAL DISORDERS

G. BLAAUW, W.H. BAKKER, P.P.M. KOOY & R. WIJNGAARDE

(Rotterdam, The Netherlands)

The advent of new and sophisticated techniques makes reappraisal of established methods necessary time and again. Although orbital arteriography and phlebography have gained widespread use only recently, these studies are now largely being supplanted by computerized axial tomography (CT-scan) and ultrasonography due to their increased reliability. As these tests will probably decrease the need to perform radioisotope investigation of the orbits as well, it seems fit to examine the value of radioisotope examinations of the orbital contents at present.

METHODS

A series of 82 patients with clinical evidence of unilateral orbital disease were studied by gamma-ray scintigraphy. They ranged in age from 3 to 82 years.

We used 15 milliCurie of technetium-99 m (pertechnetate) in all cases. The patients received 400 mg of potassium perchlorate one hour before the examination orally to minimize uptake of the radiopharmaceutical by lacrimal and salivary glands, choroid plexus, thyroid gland, and stomach. The head was extended to an en-face position, so that the orbits were placed in front of the cerebral hemispheres during scanning (Kramer & Polcyn, 1970). The orbits were frontally scanned one (F_1-scan). ten (F_2-scan), and sixty minutes (F_3-scan) after injection respectively (Grove & Kotner, 1973). Lateral scans were made approximately one hour after injection.

Reevaluation of the scintiphotos was performed without previous knowledge of diagnosis or side of proptosis. The patterns of radioactivity were classified as follows:

grade 0 — a pattern of symmetry seen in normal subjects.

grade 1 — a pattern of equivocal asymmetry.

grade 2 — a pattern of focal intense collection of radioactivity, or an abnormal pattern without the focal quality.

As the number of scans, which were judged to be positive, increased on successive scans, the F_3-scans were considered to be the most representative. Therefore the results from the interpretation of the F_3 scans were used for the study only, although both the F_1 and F_2-scans were complementary in some of the cases as will be shown later.

166

Table 1. The results of 82 orbital scans and the relation of the diagnosis and the pattern of collection of the radioactivity.

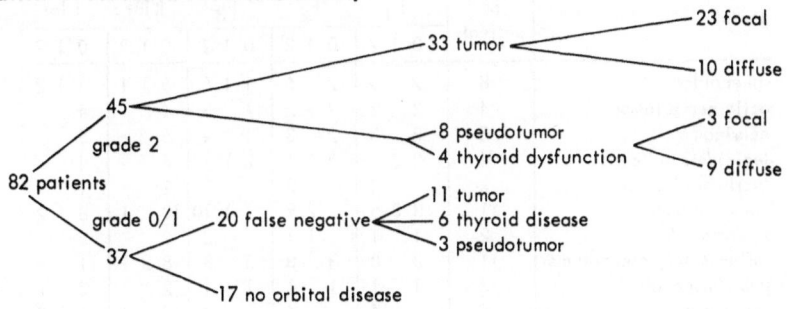

RESULTS

The grading in relation to the diagnosis is depicted in Table 1. Positive scans were derived from 45 patients. These constituted thirty-three tumor cases and twelve patients, who had either an inflammatory pseudotumour or thyroid dysfunction.

A pattern of focal intense collection of radioactivity is thought to be associated with tumors (Trokel, Schlesinger & Beaton, 1972). Consequently, we thought it worthwhile to differentiate between focal and diffuse patterns in the tumour cases and in the group of patients who had either an inflammatory pseudotumor or thyroid dysfunction. Focal patterns were present on twenty-three scans from the tumor group, and ten of these patients had diffuse patterns. In seven of the latter cases the diffuse pattern may have been caused by the extent of the tumor.

Twelve patients had a generalized orbital disease, i.e. an orbital pseudo-tumor or thyroid dysfunction. Focal patterns existed in three of these patients, so that a diffuse pattern was presented in nine cases, of which some are of special interest. Fig. 1 shows the successive scans of a patient with an inflammatory pseudotumor. While the F_1 and F_2-scans produce a

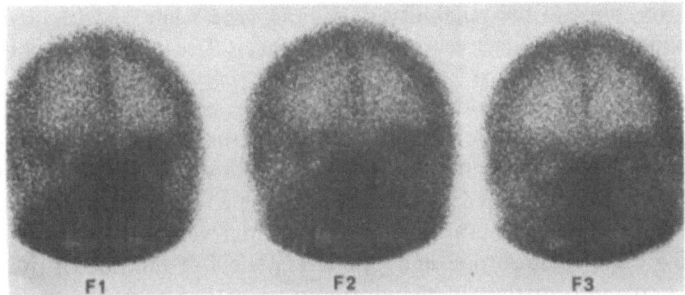

Fig. 1. Successive scans of a patient with an inflammatory orbital pseudotumor. The evolution from a more circumscribed pattern early after injection to a diffuse pattern of collection of the radioactivity one hour after injection may be seen.

Table 2. The grading in relation to the diagnosis of 82 orbital technetium scans.

grade	no patients	F$_1$			F$_2$			F$_3$			R lat			L lat		
		0	1	2	0	1	2	0	1	2	0	1	2	0	1	2
sphenoidal	8	2	6		2	6		1	1	6	6	1	1	5	1	2
optic nerve tumor	4	2	2		2	2		1	3		4			4		
neurinoma	5	2	3		2	3		1	4		5			5		
(epi-)dermoid cyst.	4	2	2		2	1	1	2	1	1	4			4		
lacrimal gland tumor·	2			2			2			2	2			1	1	
haemangioma	11	3	3	5		2	9		1	10	10	1		8	1	2
sarcoma	2	1	1		1	1				2	2			2		
inflammatory pseudotumor	11	3	8		3	8		3	8		8	2	1	11		
pyo-/mucocele	2	1	1		1	1		1	1		2			2		
metastasis	4			4			4			4	3	1		1	1	2
thyroid dysfunction	10	6	1	3	6	1	3	4	2	4	10			10		
lipoma/osteoma	2	2			2			2			2			2		
"no orbital" disease	17	14	2	1	15	1	1	16	1		17			17		

picture of a more circumscribed lesion, the F$_3$-scan contains a pattern, which must be judged to be diffuse. The same applied to some of the positive scans derived from patients with thyroid disease. Ten lateral views of the side of the orbital disorder were graded abnormal, but in all of these cases definite abnormalities were present on frontal scans as well.

In one of the cases the 'early' scans were positive, while the late scan was equivocal. Screening for thyroid disease was negative, and ultrasonograms, arteriograms, phlebograms, and CT-scans were normal.

In seventeen patients an orbital disease was not present upon further examination. These included patients with unilateral high axial myopia, optic neuritis, facial asymmetry and glaucoma. From twenty patients with an orbital disorder a negative scan was obtained. Table 2 shows their eventual diagnosis. These figures make the reliability of radioisotope scanning for the detection of orbital disorders 75 per cent.

DISCUSSION

Since we acquired the opportunity for CT-scanning only recently, we were not able to compare the reliability of radioisotope scanning with computer tomography. Preliminary results are such that CT-scanning is superior to radioisotope scanning.

The patterns of collection of radioactivity on the consecutive scans supplied further information on the nature of the disorder in the pseudo-tumor cases, thyroid disease, and in some of the vascular lesions. Furthermore the early scans helped us to choose the side for the biopsy in pseudo-tumor cases. A greater number than one frontal view one hour after the injection of the radioisotope and one lateral view of the side of proptosis yielded extra information in pseudotumor cases and thyroid dysfunction only.

Radioisotope scanning seems to be of definite value for the diagnosis in patients, who are suspected of having an orbital pseudotumor. Although scanning was performed in 4 patients who had an orbital metastasis, only, in all these cases the scans were highly positive. This may stress the significance of radioisotope scanning in these cases as well.

SUMMARY

Results of serial orbital technetium-99 m scanning were evaluated in 82 patients. The reliability for the detection of orbital diseases appeared to be 75 per cent. A distinction was made between focal and diffuse patterns. The serial examination produced a rather typical evolution from focal to diffuse patterns in pseudotumor cases.

REFERENCES

Grove, A.S. & L.M. Kotner. Orbital scanning with multiple radionuclides. *Arch. Ophthal.* 89: *301–305* (1973).
Kramer, S.G. & R.E. Polcyn. Extension of the head for orbital scanning in proptosis. *Amer. J. Ophthal.* 69: *284–286* (1970).
Trokel, S.L., E.B. Schlesinger & H. Beaton. Diagnosis of orbital tumors by gamma-ray orbitography. *Amer. J. Ophthal.* 74: *675–679* (1972).

Authors' address:
Departments of Neurosurgery, Nuclear Medicine and Ophthalmology
Academic Hospital
Erasmus University
Rotterdam
The Netherlands

Proc. 3rd Int. Symp. on Orbital Disorders, Amsterdam 1977

PLATE THERMOGRAPHY: ANGIOGRAPHIC CORRELATION IN ORBITAL AND CEPHALIC DISORDERS

M. PASSOT, P. BONNIN, M.T. IBA-ZIZEN & E.A. CABANIS

(Levallois, France)

We report here the results of comparison between thermographic and angiographic studies on patients with orbital and cephalic disorders. This comparison led us to think that thermographic abnormalities visualize the repercussions of orbital and cephalic disorders on local surface vascularization.

PRINCIPLES: LIQUID CRYSTALS

The purpose of thermography is to draw a thermic map of cutaneous areas studied. We did not use infrared telethermography but plate thermography with liquid crystals. But the results of both methods seem to be similar.

Liquid crystals are an intermediate state between solids and liquids. The molecules of the liquid cholesteric crystals are arranged in parallel planes. The axes of these molecules make a constant angle from one plane to the next. This angle varies with temperature, which produces changes of the selective reflexion of light by liquid crystals and modifications of their color.

This property of visualizing thermic changes by color modifications is the reason why liquid crystals are used in thermography.

MATERIAL AND METHODS

Our material is very simple:
- The thermographic plates were kindly provided by Pr. Tricoire.
- We used a plain camera to record the observed pictures as color slides.

The thermographic plates have a given sensibility and, for example, a thirty-three degrees plate is brown at 33 degrees centigrade, green at 34.5 degrees, blue at 35.5 degrees, and violet at 36 degrees (Fig. 1). This thermographic plate can be used for cutaneous temperatures between 33 and 36 degrees centigrade. Fig. 2 shows the diagram of the sensibility of the 31, 32, 33, 34 plates.

Thermographic technique

Our purpose was to study the eye by plate thermography. We first tried applying the plate directly to the eyeball, but we encountered some diffi-

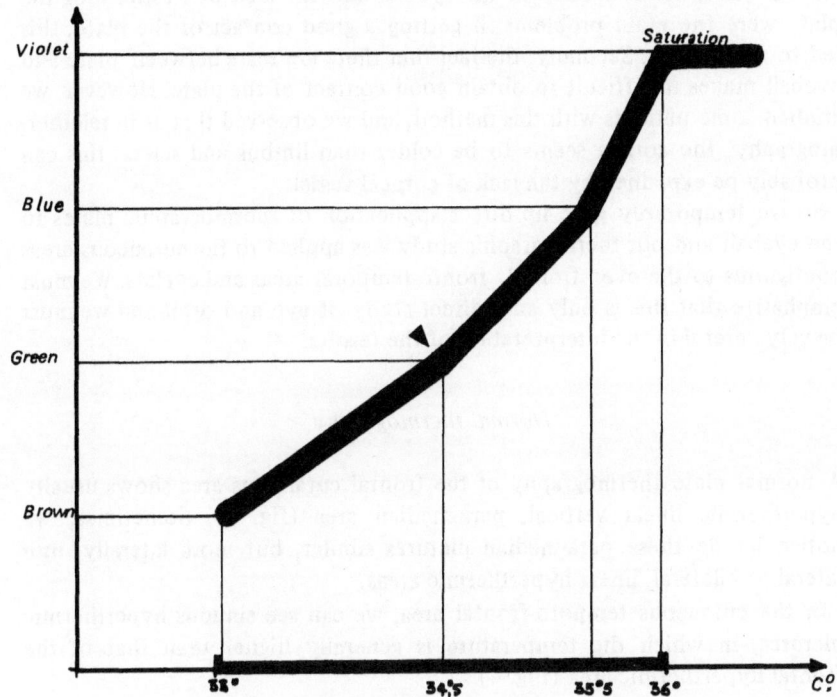

Fig. 1. Diagram of thermic sensibility of a 33° thermographic plate.

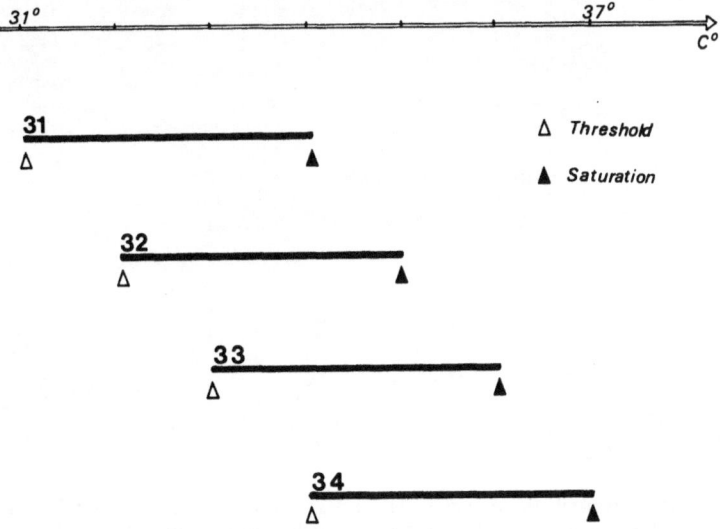

Fig. 2. Diagram of sensibility of 31°, 32°, 33°, and 34° thermographic plates.

culties. First, the convexity of the eyeball and the lack of elasticity of the plate were the main problems in getting a good contact of the plate; this led to radial folds. Secondly, the fact that there are tears between plate and eyeball makes it difficult to obtain good contact of the plate. However, we studied some patients with this method, and we observed that as in telethermography, the cornea seems to be colder than limbus and sclera; this can probably be explained by the lack of corneal vessels.

So we temporarily gave up direct application of thermographic plates to the eyeball and our thermographic study was applied to the cutaneous areas contiguous to the eye: frontal, fronto-temporal areas and eyelids. We must emphasize that this is only an indirect study of eye and orbit and we must be very careful in the interpretation of the results.

Normal thermography

A normal plate thermography of the frontal cutaneous area shows usually hyperthermic linear vertical, para-median area (fig. 3). Sometimes, we notice beside these para-median pictures similar, but more laterally, unilateral or bilateral, linear hyperthermic areas.

In the cutaneous temporo-frontal area, we can see sinuous hyperthermic pictures, in which the temperature is generally higher than that of the frontal hyperthermic area (Fig. 4).

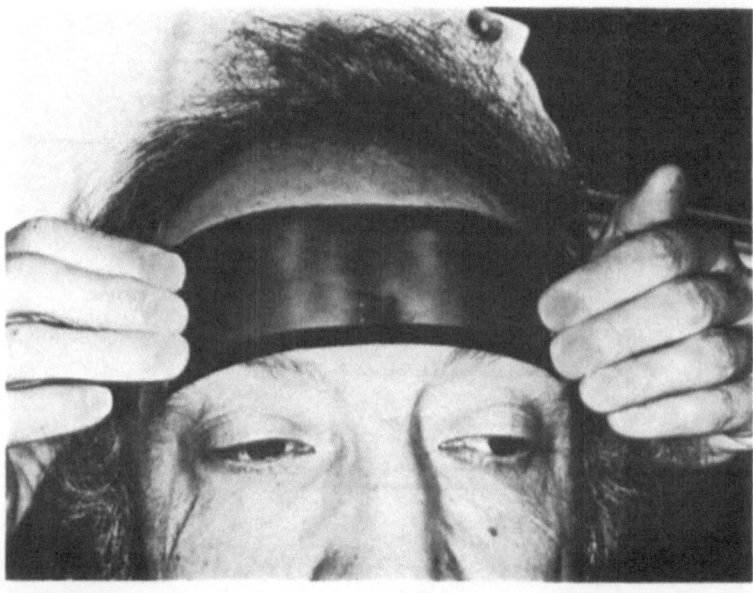

Fig. 3. Normal frontal thermogram. The linear vertical, para-median hyperthermic pictures are the visualization of the arterias medialis frontalis, branches of the ophthalmic artery, which is a branch of the internal carotid.

172

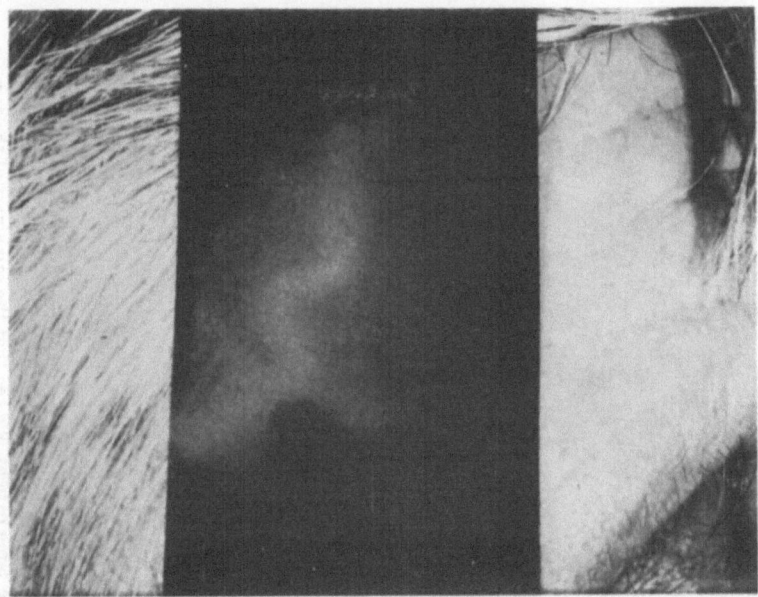

Fig. 4. Normal temporo-frontal thermogram. The sinous hyperthermic area is the visualization of the temporo-frontal branch of the superficial temporal artery, branch of the external carotid.

From the beginning, our opinion was that these pictures yielded thermic visualization of vessels and their topography led us to think that para-median frontal hyperthermic linear areas are thermic cutaneous projection of the arteria frontalis medialis. The frontal lateral hyperthermic areas seem to be the thermic cutaneous projection of the arteria frontalis lateralis (or supra-orbitalis). These two arteries are branches of the ophthalmic artery which is a branch of the internal carotid. We also think that the temporo-frontal hyperthermic area visualizes the thermic projection of the temporo-frontal branch of the superficial temporal artery, a terminal branch of the external carotid artery. Moreover one can easily palpate the arterial pulsa-tions in this area; and this was confirmed by correlating the temporo-frontal thermography with the external carotid angiography in a same patient (Fig. 5–6). In spite of head bending which is not the same on the two pictures, we can see that the same part of the temporo-frontal branch of the superficial temporal artery is visible.

PATHOLOGICAL EXAMPLES

We report here some pathological results in orbital or cephalic disorders.

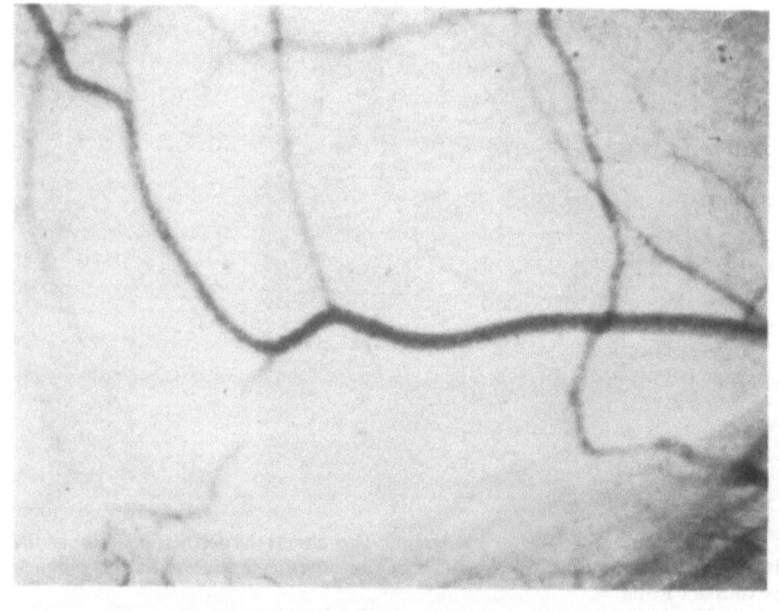

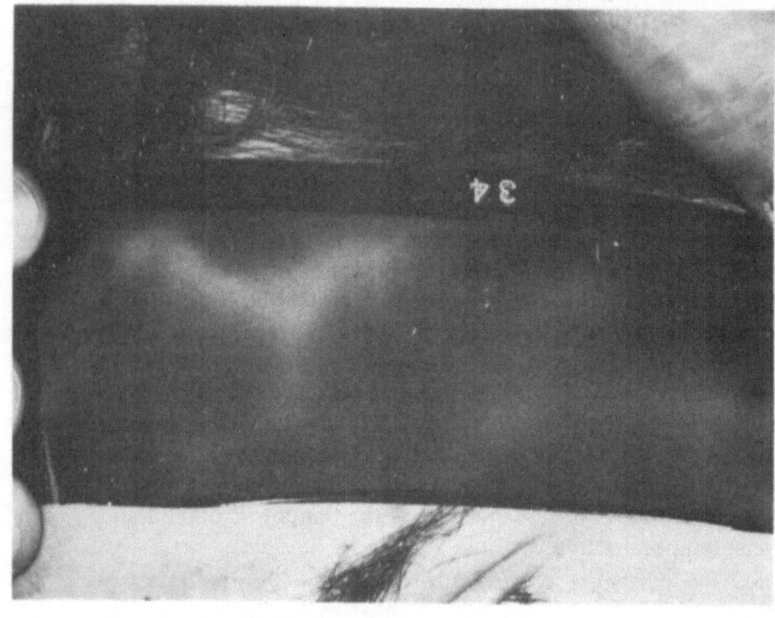

Fig. 5–6. Tempero-frontal thermography and external carotid angiogram of the same patient. We see that the same part of the temporo-frontal branch of the superficial temporal artery is visible.

Central retinal artery occlusion

Case 1

A 50 year old man had had, some days previously, a central retinal artery occlusion in the left eye. The plate thermography showed an important hypothermy in the left frontal area and the lack of visualization of the left arteria frontalis medialis. The carotidal angiogram showed a very tight stenosis of the left internal carotid.

Case 2

A 49 year old woman had, some weeks previously, a central retinal artery occlusion in her right eye and some symptoms of occlusion of most of the ciliary arteries which are also branches of the ophthalmic artery. The plate thermography showed no visualization of the right arteria frontalis medialis (Fig. 7). The right eyelids are hypothermic. The right naso-genial area is hyperthermic. (It is perhaps the sign of the compensation of the blood supply by the angularis arteria.) The angiogram of the right common carotid artery of this patient shows an occlusion of the right internal carotid and stenosis of the right external carotid (Fig. 8). So tight stenosis or occlusions of the internal carotid often produce a frontal hypothermy, but it does not appear every time and this is demonstrated by case 3.

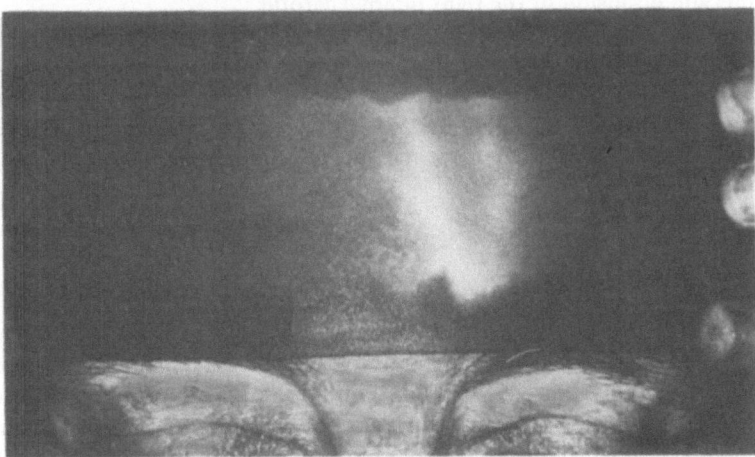

Fig. 7. Frontal thermogram of case 2. We see that there is no visualization of the right arteria frontalis medialis.

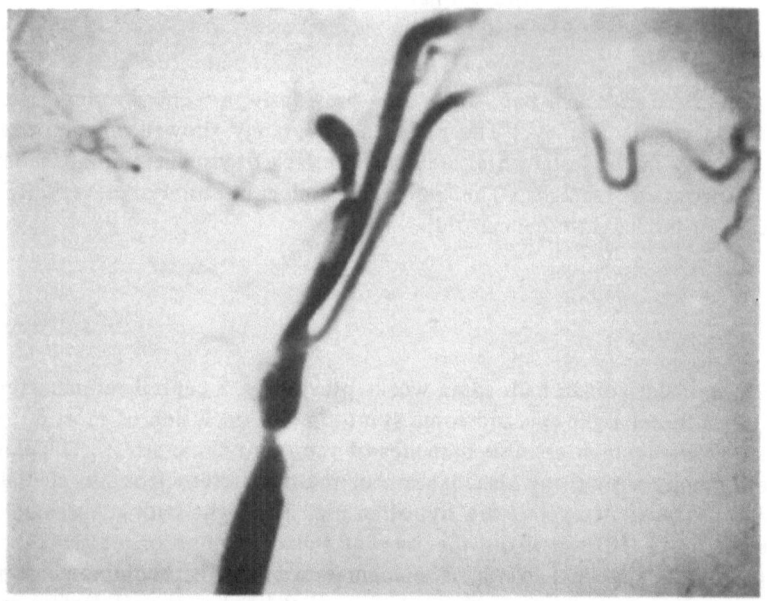

Fig. 8. Angiogram of the right common carotid of case 2. We see an occlusion of the internal carotid and a stenosis of the external carotid.

Case 3

A 65 year old man had a tight stenosis of the left internal and external carotids and occlusion of the right internal carotid.

The frontal thermography (Fig. 9—10) shows the picture of supplying of the right ophthalmic artery by the homolateral superficial temporal artery with an inversion of the internal frontal thermic gradient; the upper part of the right internal frontal hyperthermic area is warmer than the lower part. On the contrary, the whole left frontal area is hypothermic.

Carotido-cavernous fistula

Case 4

A 25 year old man had a right carotido-cavernous traumatic fistula. The carotid angiogram showed the filling with contrast of the right superior ophthalmic vein which is very enlarged and of a size even greater than that of the internal carotid. The thermography shows an important right palpebral hyperthermy. After closing of the fistula, the exophthalmos and the palpebral hyperthermy disappeared.

176

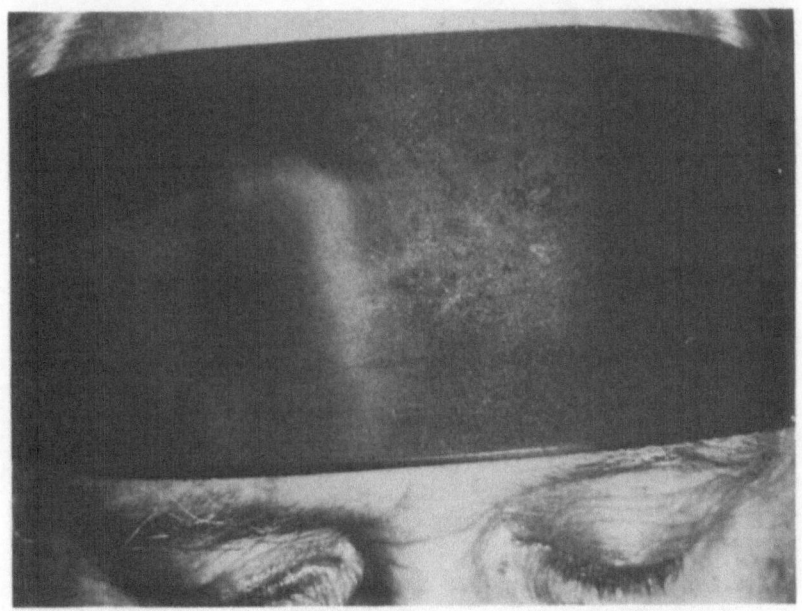

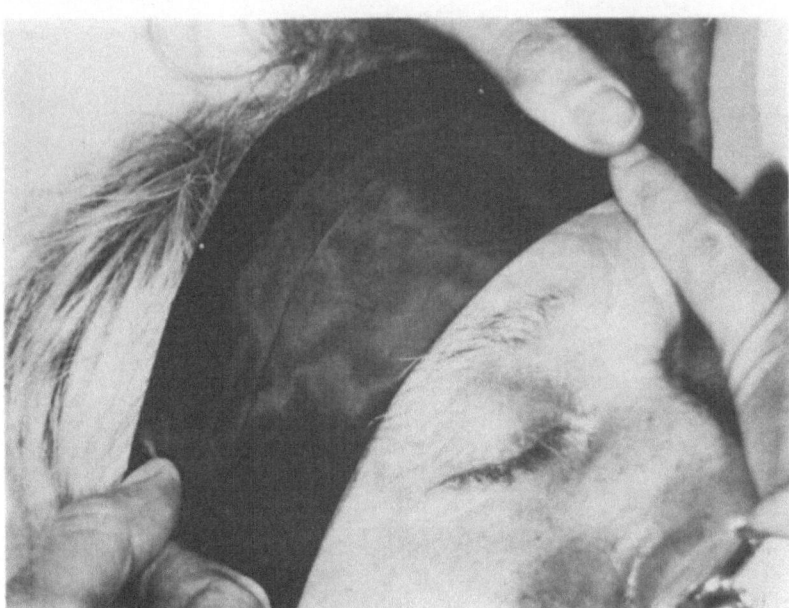

Fig. 9–10. Frontal thermogram of case 3. A 65 year old patient who had a tight stenosis of the left internal and external carotids and an occlusion of the right internal carotid. We see that there is an hypothermy of the left frontal area but an hyperthermy of the right frontal area with the picture of supplying of the right ophthalmic artery by the right superficial temporal artery with an inversion of the internal frontal thermic gradient: the upper part of the visualization of the arteria medialis frontalis is warmer than the lower part; which means probably an inversion of the flow in the arteria medialis frontalis.

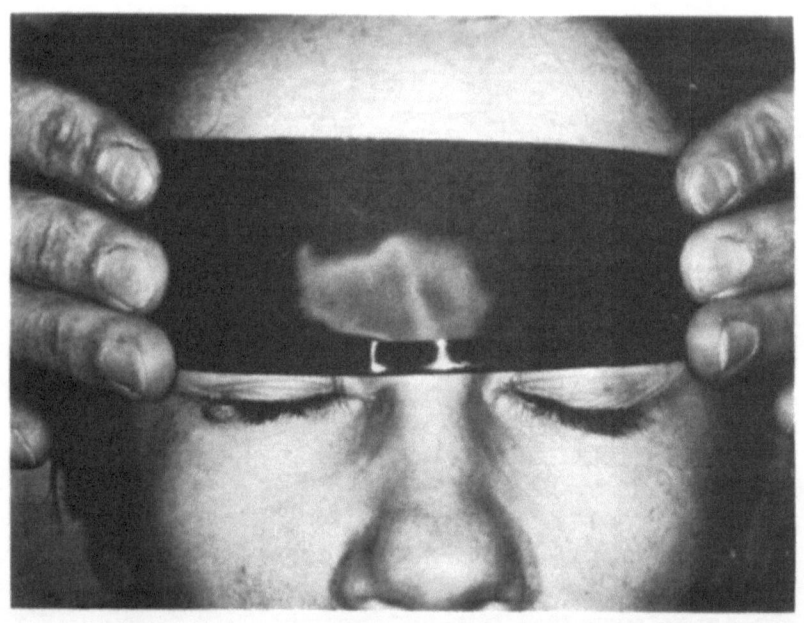

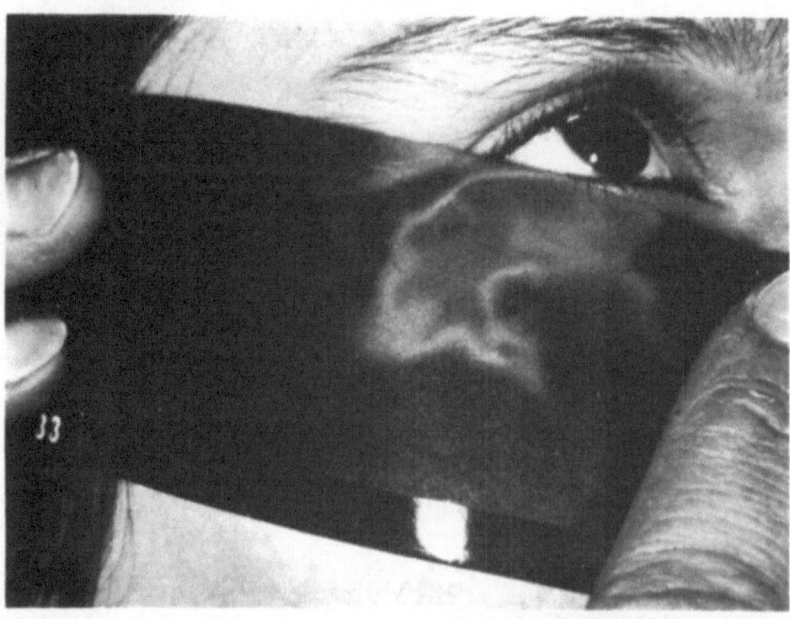

Fig. 11–12. Angioma of right eyebrow and of the lower eyelid. The thermogram shows an important hyperthermy.

Exophthalmos

We studied some cases of exophthalmos with plate thermography but the results of this study are not yet very easy to systematize. It appears in fact that the endocrine exophthalmos generally presents a normal thermography; that the inflammatory exophthalmos are of course hyperthermic (our case 5 was a phlegmon in the right orbit with a considerable palpebral hyperthermy). But thermography of tumoral exophthalmos is much more difficult to interpret because we must remember that we observe only the repercussions of the tumor on the local surface vascularization, and these repercussions may very greatly.

Case 6 is a 40 year old woman who had a right exophthalmos due to intra-conic tumor which was an hemangioma. The frontal thermogram is normal. The palpebral thermogram is normal too. The phlebography shows the deformation of the right angiogram by an intra-conic tumor. But the carotid angiogram shows no arterial abnormalities and this is perhaps the reason why the thermogram is normal.

Angiomas

Case 7

A 26 year old woman had an angioma of the right eyebrow, of the lower eyelid and the upper lip. A carotid angiogram showed arterio-venous abnormalities. The thermography shows a marked hyperthermy of the cutaneous area of the angiomas (Fig. 11–12). So we may see that plate thermography can be useful in the follow-up study of the cutaneous angiomas, before or after treatment.

In conclusion, we think plate thermography is easy to perform, not expensive, very safe, easy to repeat and reliable; our opinion is that it can sometimes be of interest in the study of vascular oculo-orbital disorders.

Authors' address:
Service d'Ophtalmologie
Hôpital N.D. de Perpétuel Secours
2, rue Kléber
92 309 Levallois
France

Requests for reprints to Dr. M. Passot at the above address.

Proc. 3rd. Int. Symp. on Orbital Disorders, Amsterdam 1977

C.T. ECHOGRAPHY AND THERMOGRAPHY IN THE DIAGNOSIS OF UNILATERAL EXOPHTHALMOS

G. BONAVOLONTÀ, G. CENNAMO, P. ROCCO, F. MENICHELLI, U. PASQUINI & U. SALVOLINI

(Napoli/Ancona, Italy)

Although Computerized Tomography (CT) is the most exciting recent discovery on the diagnosis of orbital diseases, it is sometimes necessary to resort to some risky neuroradiological procedures in order to clarify the diagnosis. To ascertain whether it is possible to avoid such methods, we decided to combine CT with other non-invasive techniques on a group of patients suffering from unilateral proptosis.

MATERIAL AND METHODS

Since September 1976, by combining CT, Echography (A-mode) and Telethermography, which in our opinion are the most complementary techniques because of their theoretical characteristics, we have studied 52 patients, of which 32 were neoplastic and 20 non-neoplastic. The patients were, of course, submitted to this group of examinations on the basis of a complete clinical examination and after a direct radiological study of the skull and orbits, if necessary even with tomography. CT was carried out at the General Regional Hospital 'Umberto I' of Ancona with an EMI-Bran Scanner Mark-1; ultrasonography was performed at the Eye Clinic of the 2nd Medical School of Naples' University with an Echograph KRETZ 7200 MA, A-mode, using a probe of 8 Mhz; telethermography at the Department of General Surgery of the same University, using an AGA-Thermovision 680 medical. In the group of neoplastic cases six recurrences after surgery have been included.

RESULTS

On the basis of these studies wer noted that the principal advantages of CT can be summarized as follows:
1. It provides an accurate diagnosis on the presence of an expanding lesion (EL), giving an excellent view of the whole anatomical area. We believe that a negative examination with CT can exclude an EL within the orbit.
2. In cases of positive EL it provides helpful information on its tissue density.
3. In cases of infiltrating lesions it provides information on the relations of the EL with the surrounding anatomical structures.
4. In cases of negative EL it can give precious information on muscular pathology.

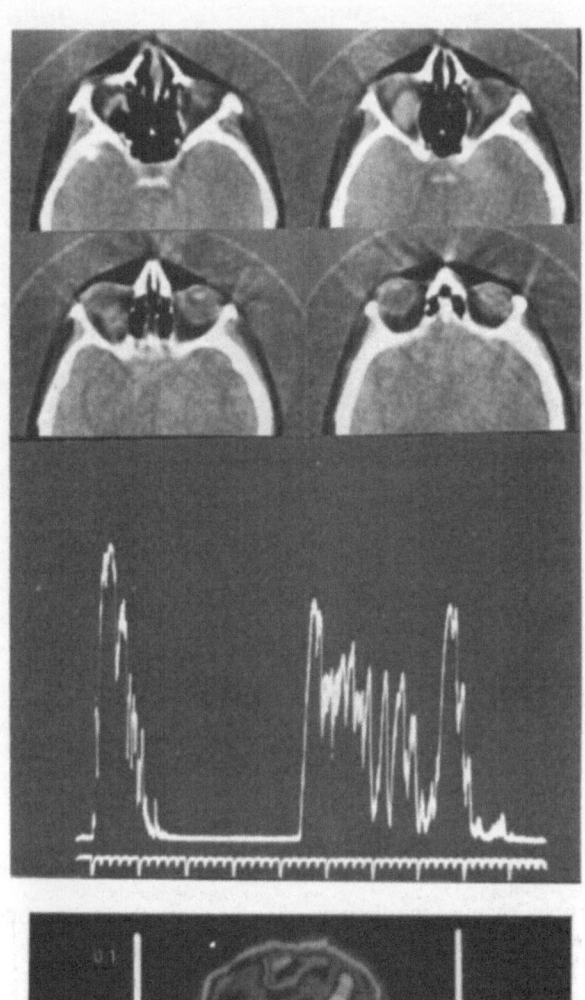

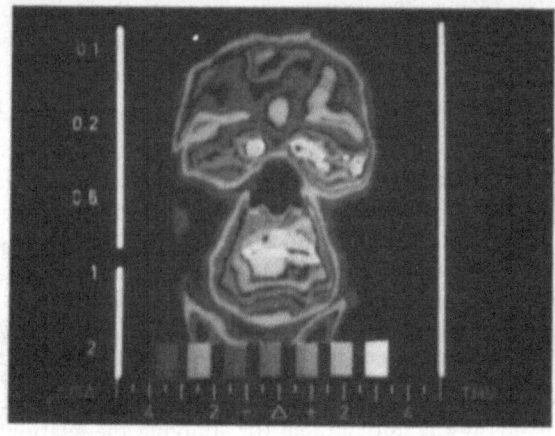

Fig. 1. (Case 6048). Top: CT shows a well circumscribed mass, medially to the optic nerve in the left orbit.
Middele: The echogram of this lesion is characteristic for a cavernous hemangioma.
Bottom: Hypothermy of $+2$ C$^{\circ}$ (C2) in the left orbit. Absence of facial asymmetry.

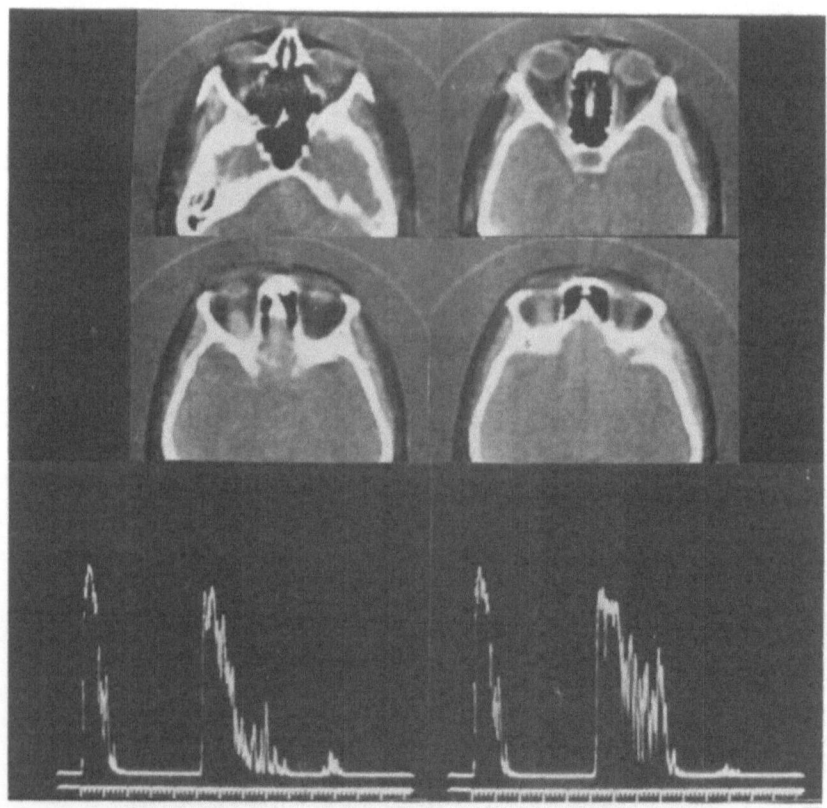

Fig. 2. (Case 4380). Top: CT shows a lesion in the left orbit which could be mistaken for an expanding lesion.
Bottom: Echography charified the diagnosis, showing only a thickening of the superior rectus muscle.
(Thermography was negative).

On the other hand, the limits of CT are that in cases of an orbital tumor it does not provide a diagnosis on the type of tissue involved, sometimes even a mistaken interpretation of the results is possible. We have had two cases in which CT showed a thickening of a muscle which was referred to an EL, but on surgical exploration no EL was found but a myositis.

The advantages of ultrasonography are that it confirms the presence of an orbital neoplasm providing information on tissue density as well, and, even when the CT is negative, this could be corrected in second instance. On the other hand, this method is not suitable for studying the relationship of the EL with the extra-orbital structures. CT and ECHO combined give accurate information on the presence and the tissue diagnosis of an expanding intra-orbital lesion, but they are inadequate for verifying whether the lesion is benign or malignant.

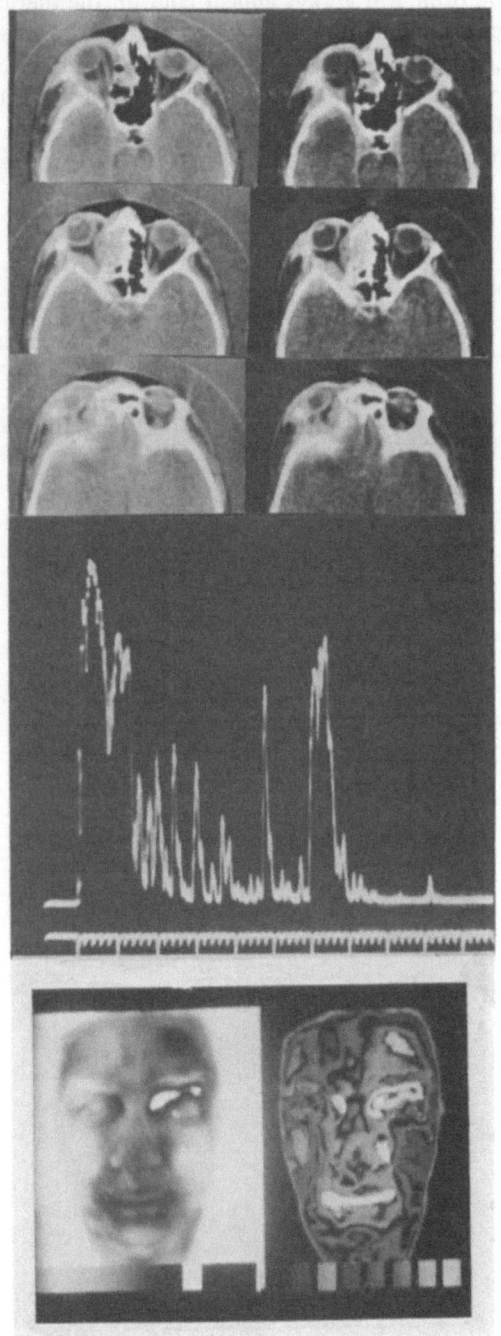

Fig. 3. (Case 7369). Top: CT shows an expanding lesion within the left orbit involving the surrounding anatomic areas.
Middle: The echogram shows the tissue acoustical dyshomogeneity.
Bottom: Hyperthermy of $+4$ C° ($\Delta 2$) in the left orbit. Hyperthermy of the left emiface.

We tried to fill in this lack of information with Telethermography. In negative cases the orbit will always appear cold on the thermography, as in cases of a benign expanding lesion. It will appear hot in cases of an inflammatory process, a vascular process or malignant neoplasms. With our previous experience on Telethermography we had a tool in hand that made it possible to distinguish between a malignant and a benign process while studying the whole emiface.

CONCLUSION

CT, ECHO and Telethermography combined can provide an accurate diagnosis in cases of unilateral proptosis without using invasive neuroradiological procedures.

Authors' address:
G. Bonavolontà
Instituto di Clinica Oculistica
Via Cappella dei Cangiani 5
Napoli
Italy

Proc. 3rd Int. Symp. on Orbital Disorders, Amsterdam 1977

INSTRUMENTAL VISUAL AXIS OPHTHALMODYNAMOMETRY

HAMPSON A. SISLER

(New York, N.Y.)

BACKGROUND

Ophthalmodynamometry is a clinical technique wherein intraocular pressure is artificially increased in graded fashion by applying a physical stress to the globe of the eye.

The first instrument in this category was made by Bailliart and Magitot, in 1917 (Bailliart, 1917). Bailliart's instrument was a calibrated spring pressure gauge with a round-tipped plunger for application against the globe of the eye, at the equator. Concurrent ophthalmoscopic examination of the optic disc was required and was often done by an assistant examiner.

Since ophthalmodynamometry is the only widely accepted non-invasive means we have for determining ophthalmic artery and intracranial vascular pressures, it is an important screening test in the evaluation of: suspected cerebral aneurysms; subclavian steal syndrome, or impending cerebrovascular accident of the carotid thrombosis type; low tension, or marginally controlled glaucoma; migraine headaches, or suspected increased intracranial pressure; hypertension, or pulseless disease, wherein sphygmomanometry on the arm may not be possible.

Suction, also applied at the equator of the eye is another method for increasing intraocular pressure for testing purposes, and was introduced in 1936 by Kukan. A recent derivative of this approach was developed by Gregus & Galen (1971). Disadvantages of these lie in the use of long pneumatic tubing which tends to collapse reducing actual transmitted suction, patient discomfort, and distortion of the globe by berniating it into the suction funnel. Such distortion is painful to the patient and also causes optical blurring of the disc, as seen with the examining ophthalmoscope.

The Bailliart unit has the disadvantage of lack of control and torque action of the long plunger. There is a tendency for slippage and shearing of the globe of the eye, with both leverage gain and vector loss of the actual applied force. Repeated readings tend to vary from each other.

All these units require the concurrent use of an ophthalmoscope.

The new instrument for ophthalmodynamometry, from American Optical Corporation, is called the 'Dynoptor' (Figs. 1 & 2). Invented by Sisler in 1972, the Dynoptor is used at the slip lamp, in a manner similar basically to applanation tonometry. No ophthalmoscope is used.

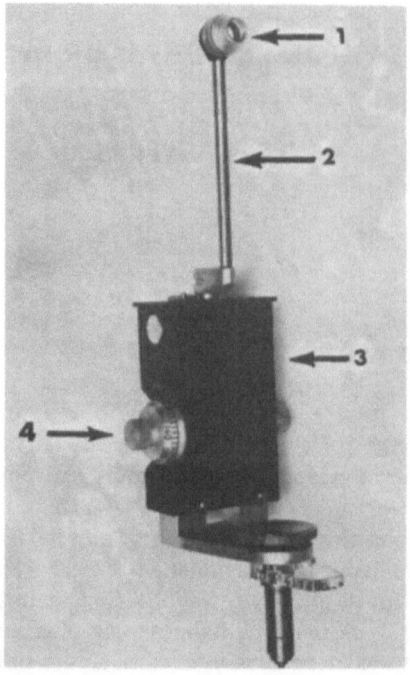

Fig. 1. Visual axis ophthalmodynamometer (dynoptor), resembling a Goldman-type slit lamp applanation tonometer. 1. High minus fundusviewing lens applicator tip, for visualizing the optic disc, 2. Support post for transmitting applied mechanical pressure, 3. Spring box, for applying graded pressures in grams of force, 4. Graded pressure dial.

The Dynoptor head (Fig. 1, 1) is a small, high-minus fundus viewing contact lens. The slit lamp's microscopic system focuses the image of the optic disc.

METHOD

After the patient's pupils have been widely dilated and topical anesthesia has been placed in the eyes and tonometry has been done, the Dynoptor is positioned. The slit beam is used in paracentral or paraxial position, as for all fundus viewing at the slit lamp. With the optic disc seen centrally in the field, the examiner focuses the image of the optic disc as seen with the slit lamp oculars.

The Dynoptor graded pressure dial is advanced until the first full-amplitude pulsation of the central retinal artery on the disc occurs. This is ophthalmic diastole. The examiner now returns to his view, turns the dial further, and stops when all pulsation ceases. He then pulls back on the joystick, reads the final dial position as systole, and records the data. 'Straddling' of the endpoints may be done for increased accuracy. Readings are then taken on the other eye.

186

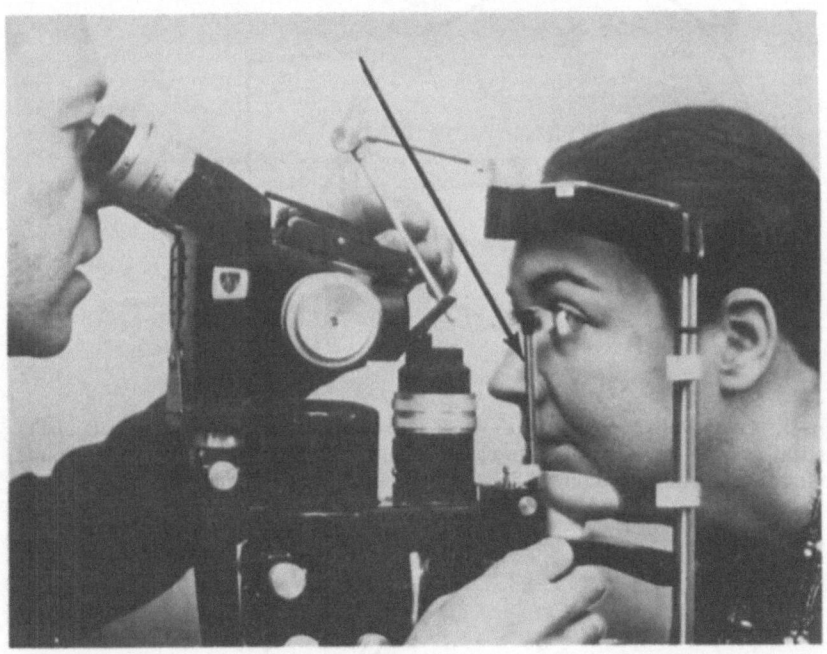

Fig. 2. Dynoptor (follow arrow), in use on American Optical slit lamp.

DISCUSSION

'Dynoptry' possesses several advantages over older forms of ophthalmo-dynamometry:

1. It is strictly a one-examiner instrument used at the slit lamp.
2. It is exactly radial in its pressure application, since the examiner views the optic disc along the same axis that he applies his pressure. Hence, it is more accurate (Figs. 3 & 4).
3. It involves less global distortion than is caused by the long shearing Bailliart plunger or the herniating suction cup.
4. Unlike the convex footplate of Bailliart or the suction cone of Kukan, the Dynoptor's concave contact lens tip conforms to the curvature of the eye.
5. It is not painful to the patient not only because of the reduced global distortion but because topical anesthesia is complete on the cornea but only partial at the equator, where other instruments are applied.
6. The need for an ophthalmoscope and for a second examiner are eliminated.
7. Patients are less fearful of this slit lamp procedure – akin to applantation tonometry – than they are of other dynomometric equipment.

   Adapter plates are available from the manufacturer (American Optical Corporation, Southbridge, Mass., U.S.A.) for use on the Haag Streit and Zeiss slit lamps.

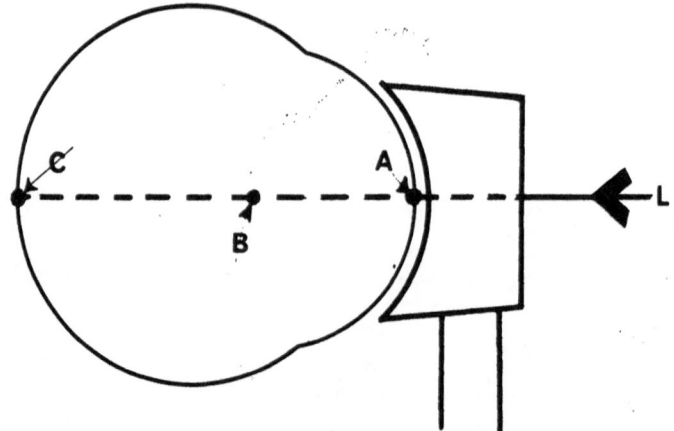

Fig. 3. Axis L-A-B-C represents (a) visual axis of the examiner, (b) visual axis of the patient, and (c) the axis of pressure application to the globe of the eye. Arrow points in the direction of (a) and (c)-(b) being in opposite direction to these.

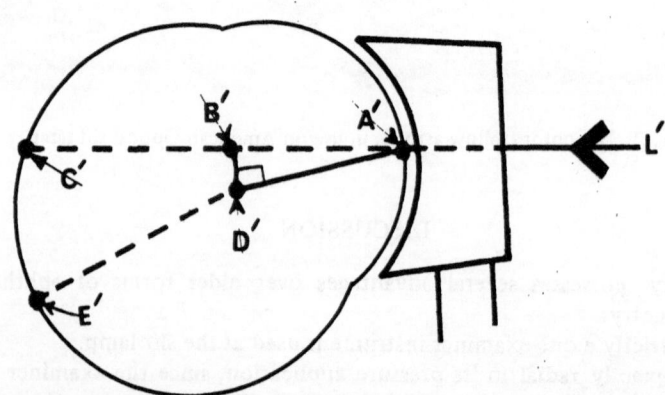

Fig. 4. This demonstrates the hypothetical situation of false, oblique application of pressure from poor technique. Axis L'-A'-B'-C' is the visual axis of the examiner, as well as the axis of pressure application, which must always coincide, with this method. D' is the optical center of the globe. Angle B'-D'-A' is a right angle. E' is the optic disc.

Under these circumstances, right triangle leg, A'-D' (shorter than hypotenuse A'-B') represents the *effective* applied force. Hence, some of the applied force is lost, and the instrument would read too high.

But, under these circumstances, the examiner would not see optic disc E' but some peripheral fundus area, C', and would realize his error. He would then re-start aligning elements exactly radially, to bring about the conditions illustrated in Fig. 3.

CONCLUSION

The Sisler unit for visual axis ophthalmodynamometry is the first such instrument to employ graded pressure to the globe of the eye along the visual axis of both patient and examiner, at the slit lamp. Without the possi-

188

bility of leveraging the force or applying it obliquely (as may occur with the Bailliart unit) or of losing suction in the long pneumatic tubing of the Kukan-related techniques, the visual axis method has proven to be significantly more accurate (Sisler, 1972).

REFERENCES

Baillart, P. La pression artérielle dans les branches de l'artère centrale de la rétine; nouvelle technique pour la déterminer. *Ann. Ocul.* 154: *648–652* (1917).

Gregus, P. & M.A. Galin. Suction ophthalmodynamometry via fluidic control. *Trans. Am. Acad. Ophthal. Otolaryng. 75: 647* (1971).

Kukan, F. Ergebnisse der Blutdruckmessungen mit einem neuen ophthalmodynamometer. *Z. Augenheilk.* 90: *166* (1936).

Sisler, H.A. Comparative ophthalmodynamometry using scleral pressure, suction and corneal pressure units. *Am. J. Ophthal.* 74: 964–966 (1972).

Sisler, H.A. Optical-corneal pressure ophthalmodynamometer. *Am. J. Ophthal.* 74: *987–988* (1972).

Author's address:
13 West 13th Street
New York, N.Y. 10011
USA

Proc. 3rd Int. Symp. on Orbital Disorders, Amsterdam 1977

PERI-ORBITAL ENDOSCOPY

C.T. BUITER

(Groningen, The Netherlands)

For a long time routine otolaryngological examination could give no more than a rather rough impression of that part surrounding the orbit which is covered by te E.N.T.-specialist, since a close visual study was impossible but for the anterior third of the nasal cavities. Posterior rhinoscopy can give some information about the nasopharynx and choanae, but it is often rendered impossible by the retching reflexes of the patient. Transillumination of the frontal and maxillary sinuses can give hardly any reliable information at all.

The need for better visualisation led to the development of endoscopes as early as 1880, when Zaufal (1909) modified Nitze's cytoscope, which was the first endoscope provided with distal electric illumination. Although various authors propagated their own modified versions of these endoscopes and succeeded in slimming down Zaufal's $\emptyset$ 6 mm telescope to $\emptyset$ 4 mm instruments, the endoscopy of the upper airways never received widespread recognition before the 1970's.

Nowadays the otorhinolaryngologist can give much more detailed and, therefore, more valuable information about a major part of the surroundings of the orbit since the endoscopes of the Hopkins® and Lumina® types have come at his disposal. These endoscopes combine the small 4 mm diameter with a high resolution and brightness and a wideangle viewing field. A quite adequate illumination of the areas to be examined is brought about by the use of 'cold light', i.e. light from a proximal light generator conducted to the tip of the endoscope by means of glass fibres, which are incorporated in the endoscopes along the optic system. The development of cold light, introduced by Hopkins, was an essential improvement, since the distal electric bulb of the endoscope could now be dispensed with; the instrument could be made slimmer without impairing the illumination, and the — now proximal — lamp could be made as powerful as was necessary.

Through the same glass fibres (electron-)flash light can be conducted to the examined area for photographic documentation, for which purpose the endoscope is coupled to a single lens reflex camera via an intermediate optics with a focal distance that is usually 95 mm. As the Hopkins® and Lumina® endoscopes have a very great depth-of-field, focusing is not required for photography. The exposure is controlled by the variable number of capacitors which are discharged with the (electron-)flash light. In the Wolf 5005 light-generator, which we use, both the lamp for the continuous light for endoscopic examination and the flash light-system are built in in such a way that these two kinds of light emerge from the same outlet, thus providing a system that is easy to handle (Buiter, 1974).

Nowadays a detailed endoscopic examination is possible of the superior, middle and inferior nasal meati (*nasendoscopy*), of the maxillary sinus (*antroscopy*), of the frontal and sphenoidal sinuses. For the endoscopy of the paranasal sinuses endoscopes with angles of vision of $0°$ or $30°$, $70°$ and $120°$ are required (straight forward = $0°$), for nasendoscopy two endoscopes with angles of vision of $30°$ and $70°$ are sufficient. Normally we use $\emptyset$ 4 mm Hopkins endoscopes, sometimes optics with a diameter of 2.8 mm are required for nasendoscopy, in the case of a very narrow nose.

Nasendoscopy and antroscopy can be carried out quite well under local anaesthesia with adults and children over 10 years old, whereas general anaesthesia is to be preferred for the endoscopic examination of the frontal and spheniodal sinuses and for all endoscopic examinations with small children.

The local anaesthesia in the nose is brought about by spraying with a surface anaesthetic (e.g. oxibuprocaine HCl 1% w/v). Extra space for manoeuvring is obtained by spraying with a mild decongestant as well (e.g. xylometazoline HCl 0.1%). If desired, a more profound effect of these two drugs can be obtained by inserting strips of cotton-wool soaked in these solutions into the nose instead of using the spray. The strips should be left in the nose for at least 10 minutes.

After the publications of Messerklinger (1970, 1972) *nasendoscopy* gradually became accepted as a full-grown method of examination. As it can easily be carried out under the local anaesthesia mentioned above in the out-patient departments, it is of great importance for every day practice. It enables the discovery of neoplasms (and/or the determination of their spread) that give no nasal symptoms and cannot be detected by means of anterior rhinoscopy, with patients suffering from proptosis, etc. Biopsies for histological examination can be taken from any place in the nose under visual control. The nasal opening of the nasolacrimal duct is now easily visualised and sometimes it is even possible to cure a dacryostenosis nasendoscopically. A close follow-up of the surgical anastomosis after dacryocystorhinostomy with photographic documentation of the findings has now become a standart procedure in our clinic. Once this anastomosis has become sufficiently wide it is even possible to perform endoscopy of the lacrimal sac, as has been described by Tajima & Ikegami (1973).

The endoscopic examination of the paranasal sinuses mentioned above is performed via a cannula.

With *antroscopy* this cannula is introduced into the maxillary sinus with the aid of a trocar by puncturing. The point at which the sinus is to be punctured is the same as that for routine rinsing of the maxillary sinus in the case of sinusitis, via the inferior meatus. An other way of approach is via the canine fossa, in which case a small depot of a local anaesthetic (e.g. lidocain 1% with adrenalin 1:100,000) has to be injected into the area concerned. Especially in the case of suspected or proven malignancy this approach should be avoided, however, in view of the possibility of thus causing an implantation metastasis in the puncture tract, which would then easily spread into the cheek.

Antroscopy is especially suited to discover small blow-out fractures, for which purpose it has proved to be superior to tomography. Apart from that there are more obvious possibilities, such as finding malignancies and inflammations.

Antroscopy has demonstrated that the normal X-ray photographs have a reliability of only 70% where it is a matter of demonstrating the presence of a sinusitis (Buiter, 1976). This may have its consequences in treating patients with iridocyclitis, etc.

Endoscopy of the frontal sinus is not needed frequently. It is generally performed under general anaesthesia, but local anaesthesia may prove to be sufficient. The cannula is inserted through a small hole with a diameter of approximately 5 mm, which is drilled into the sinus with the aid of an otological cutting burr, via a small incision of the skin parallel below the eyebrow.

Endoscopy of the sphenoidal sinus is hardly ever required. It can be performed by puncturing the cannula through the anterior wall with the aid of a trocar. In order to dertermine the right spot of the puncture, nasendoscopy can be performed. The use of a fluoroscope is to be recommended, however, to make it possible for the operator to find that place on the anterior wall which has a maximum depth of the sinus cavity behind it.

The C.T. scan is justly accepted widely now as a major improvement in radiographic diagnostics, and it is taking its place among the various methods of examination. However, it will never be able to show the tissues themselves or to provide material for a histological diagnosis. Thus it seems likely that in the future the combination of both the C.T. scan and the endoscopy of the upper airways will prove to be the most effective diagnostic method.

REFERENCES

Buiter, C.T. Photographic documentation with nasendoscopy and antroscopy. *ORL* 36 : *313–314* (1974).
Buiter, C.T. Endoscopy of the upper airways, p. 218. Excerpta Medica, Amsterdam/ American Elsevier publishing Company, Inc. New York, (1976).
Messerklinger, W. Die Endoskopie der Nase. *Monatschr. Ohrenheilkd. Laryngorhinol.* 104 : *451–456* (1970).
Messerklinger W. Technik und Möglichkeiten der Nasendoskopie. *HNO* 20 : *133–135* (1972).
Tajima, Y. & Ikegami. M. Endoscopic observations of the lacrimal sac following dacryocystorhinostomy. *Jap. J. Ophthal.* 17 : *175–182* (1973).
Zaufal. E. Zur endoskopischen Untersuchung der Rachenmündung, der Tuba en face und des Tubenkanals. *Archiv. Ohrenheilk.* 79 : *109–111* (1909).

Author's address:
E.N.T. Department
University Hospital
59 Oostersingel
Groningen
The Netherlands

Proc. 3rd Int. Symp. on Orbital Disorders, Amsterdam 1977

AN ACCESSORY MUSCLE IN THE LEFT ORBIT OF A FOETUS
OF 123 MM CROWN-RUMP LENGTH
(Str. 74030)

A.B. DE HAAN

(Amsterdam, The Netherlands)

An accessory muscle was found in the left orbit of one of a total of 60 apparently normal foetuses studied so far in an effort to obtain information on orbital development. This was a foetus of 123 mm crown-rump length. Its external features were normal, and frontal sections through the head disclosed no anomalies other than the accessory muscle in the left orbit. All sections are 25 microns thick.

The lower part of this muscle is encountered in a frontal section in which the posterior pole of the left eyeball is visible as well. The upper part of the muscle is seen in a plane immediately in front of the entrance of the optic canal.

The lower part of the accessory muscle arises from the rectus inferior muscle. In section 260 (Fig. 1) we observe a slight bulge on the cranio-

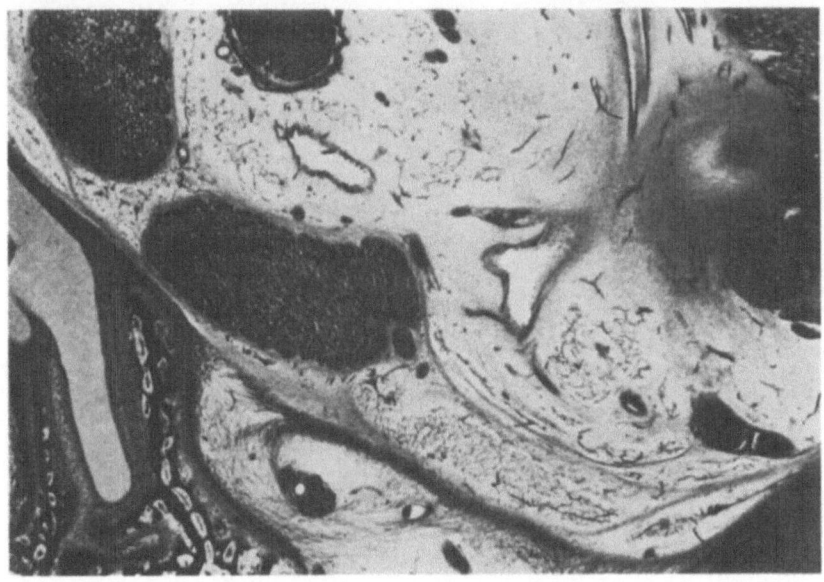

Fig. 1. Str. 74030 section 260. Upper right the posterior pole of the bulb.

lateral aspect of the rectus inferior muscle, while the more dorsal section 272 (Fig. 2) shows the accessory muscle detached from the rectus inferior muscle. In the next, more and more dorsal, sections we observe how the

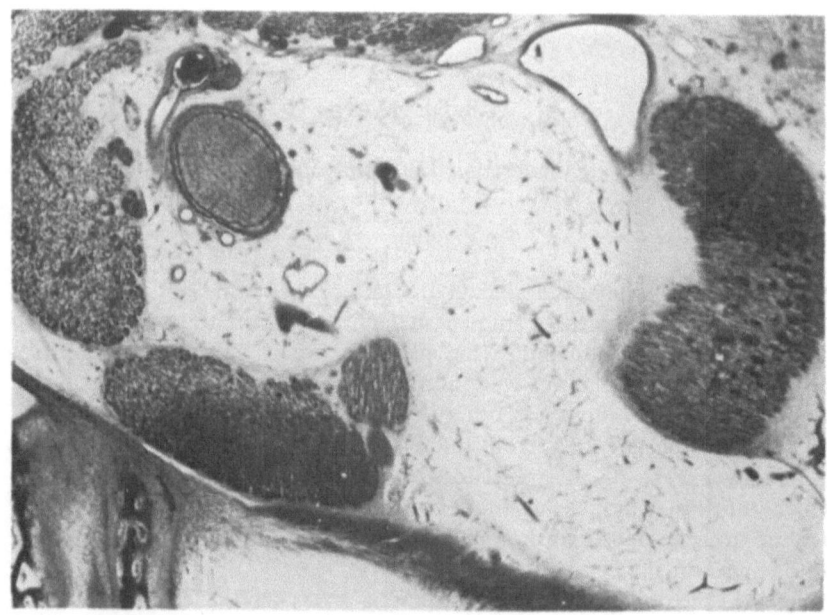

Fig. 2. Str. 74030 section 272.

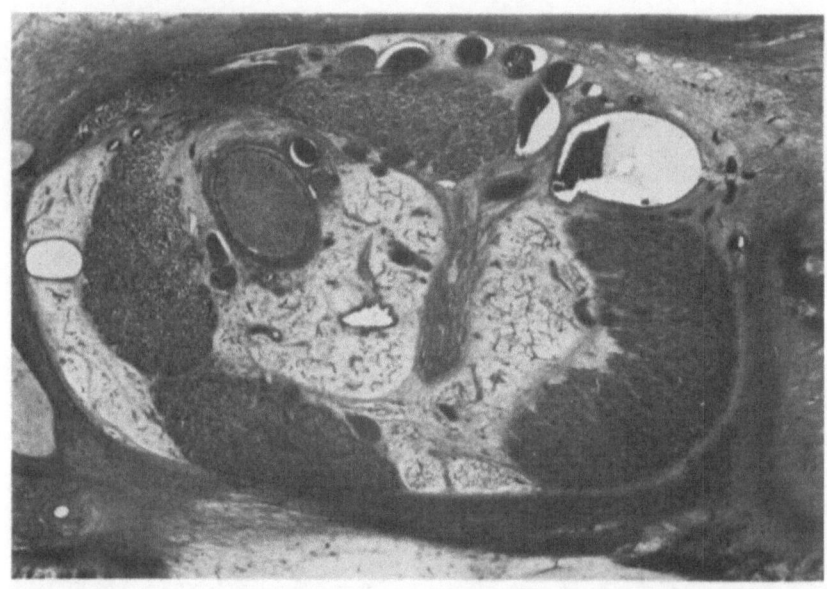

Fig. 3. Str. 74030 section 290.

accessory muscle departs from the rectus inferior muscle in a dorsocranial direction; its caudal and cranial parts are clearly surrounded by connective tissue, but this is less evident for the mid-portion.

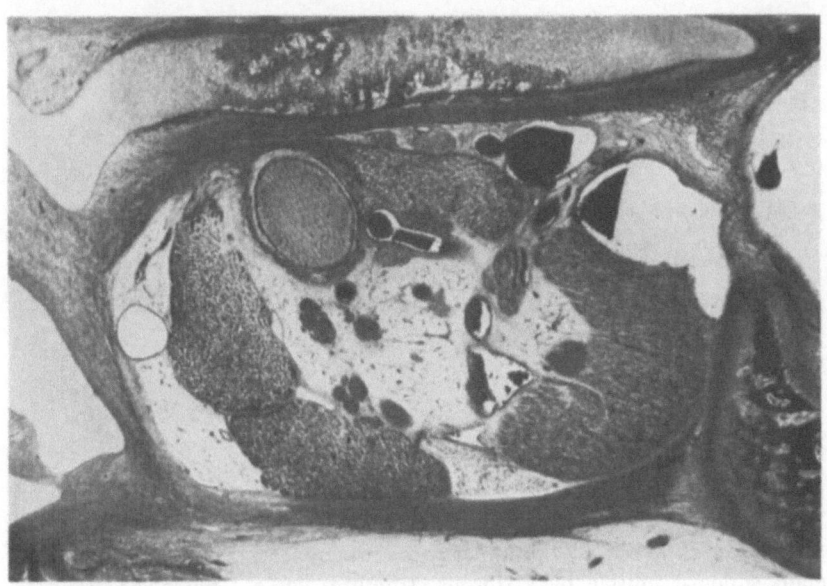

Fig. 4. Str. 74030 section 305.

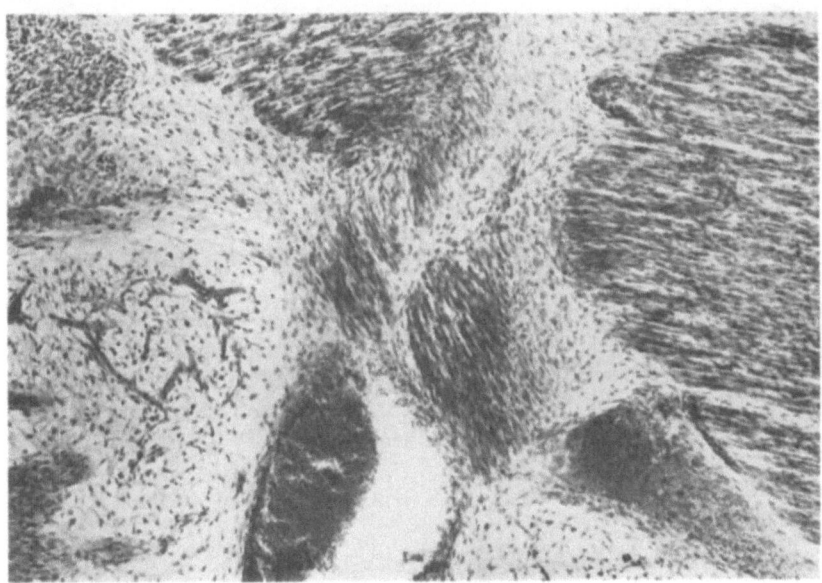

Fig. 5. Str. 74030 section 308.

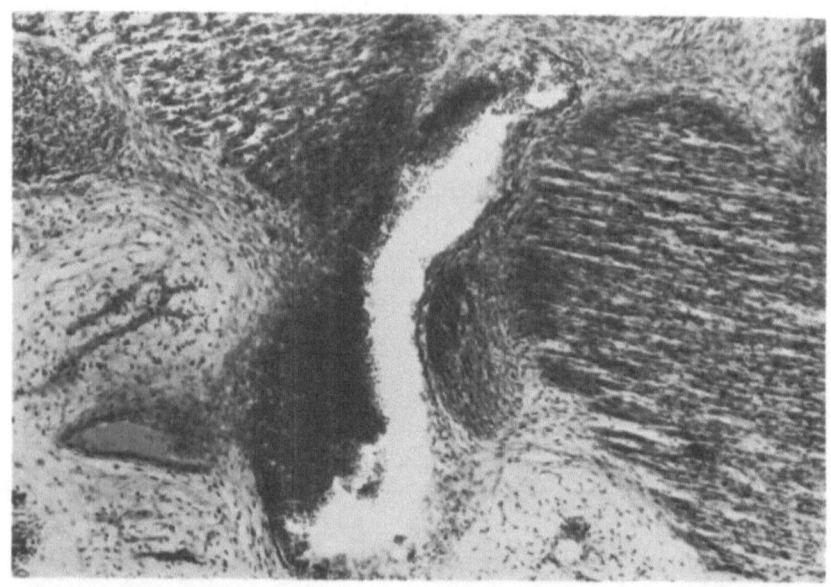

Fig. 6. Str. 74030 section 311.

In section 290 (Fig. 3) the upper part of the muscle is connected with the rectus superior muscle by a fibrous structure, while a narrower strand of connective tissue extends to the wall of the venous plexus in the latero-cranial part of the orbit. In a slightly more dorsal section, this strand is broader and curves below the venous plexus to the cranial aspect of the rectus lateralis muscle.

In section 305 (Fig. 4) the most cranial part of the accessory muscle is situated between the rectus superior and the rectus lateralis muscle, while section 308 (Fig. 5) shows a division of the accessory muscle. Only the lateral leg of this division is still visible in section 311 (Fig. 6).

SUMMARY

Demonstration of an accessory muscle in the left orbit of a foetus of 123 mm crown-rump length. The muscle arises from the rectus inferior muscle in the region of the posterior pole of the eyeball, and extends dorsocranially to the transition between the rectus superior and the rectus lateralis muscle; it is connected with these muscles by connective tissue.

Author's address:
Valeriusstraat 163
Amsterdam
The Netherlands

196

Proc. 3rd Int. Symp. on Orbital Disorders, Amsterdam, 1977

VASCULAR PATTERNS IN THE HUMAN ORBIT IN RELATION TO THE CONNECTIVE TISSUE SEPTA

M.P. BERGEN & J.A. LOS

(Amsterdam, The Netherlands)

INTRODUCTION

This study concerns the vascular patterns in the orbit, especially their relationship to the connective tissue system described by Koornneef (1974). First, some data from literature about orbital vascularization will be briefly recapitulated.

The orbit can be regarded as a cone. The apex of the cone lies at the optic canal and its base is formed by the bony edges of the eye-socket.

The ophthalmic artery, which forms the main supply for the arterial vascularization, enters the orbital cone at its apex, usually beneath the optic nerve (Hayreh & Dass, 1962). On its way to the base of the cone, the ophthalmic artery twists around the optic nerve (Salomon, Raybaud & Grisoli, 1971), via its lateral side to a cranio-medial position, where it divides into its terminal branches: the supra-orbital and the supra-trochlear arteries. These two, and most of the other arteries in the orbit, originate retrobulbarly from the ophthalmic artery and branch out to the adjacent structures of the eyeball. On the other hand, the arteries which supply the eyeball itself as well as the optic nerve keep an approximately central course.

The venous drainage of the orbital contents runs from central to peripheral. The large veins running peripherally along the surface of the cone leave the orbit either through the base of the cone, draining into the angular vein which lies medially, or through the fissures draining into the cavernous sinus (Seseman, 1869).

Strangely enough, there is hardly any information in the literature about the capillary system outside the eyeball.

MATERIAL AND METHODS

We used celloidine sections of 60 μ (Koornneef, 1974). In order to obtain a better idea of the spatial organization of the vessels, we also used thick transparent sections of about 5000 μ. These sections were from deeply

197

frozen heads in which the arteries were injected with contrasting silicone compound.*

RESULTS

At the point where the ophthalmic artery leaves the optic canal, it is still largely encased in the connective tissue surrounding the optic nerve: the optic sheath (Meyer, 1887). Shortly after leaving the optic canal, the ophthalmic artery loses contact with the optic sheath. Further on, the adventitia of the ophthalmic artery mingles with the optic sheath once more, just where the first large branch of the ophthalmic artery emerges, cranio-laterally to the optic nerve. From this branch the lacrimal artery originates. Beyond this, contact between the ophthalmic artery and the optic sheath is permanently lost. The central artery of the retina and most of the ciliary arteries have contact with the optic sheath over a longer distance than the ophthalmic artery.

As to the relationship between arteries and connective tissue septa (Koornneef & Los, 1975; Koornneef, 1974, 1977a,b), the arteries in general proved not to be enclosed in the connective tissue septa (Fig. 1). On the contrary, the arteries are confined within the adipose tissue compartments and only contact the connective tissue septa when they perforate these in passing from one adipose tissue compartment to another.

The interrelationship of the veins with the connective tissue apparatus is totally different. The large veins are in fact incorporated in the connective tissue septa (Fig. 1). The arrangement of the connective tissue septa and the configuration of the veins are both constructed along the same lines. In addition we found that laterally, in the rear part of the orbit, at the level of the fissures, the veins are encased in massive connective tissue.

Taking into account the general rule that arteries running between the septa and veins are enclosed within the septa, a more precise picture of their arrangement follows. At the back of the orbit, arterial density is high, especially in the center, where there is a great number of diverging arteries (Fig. 2). However, the arteries supplying the inferior oblique muscle maintain their central position up to the level of the back of the eyeball, where they enter the muscle. Arterial density decreases in the central region of the orbit towards the front, while, on the contrary, venous density increases. It is

* An injection technique was used to identify the vessels in the thick transparent sections. The injection compound was a Microfil silicone compound (reg. trade-mark of Canton Bio-medical Products, Inc.). Injections were made via the common carotid arteries. First the specimens were injected with a hypertonic NaCl solution, in order to dispose of blood-clots, and subsequently with the silicone compound. These injections were done under a pressure of about 120 mm Hg. The specimens were deeply frozen for 48 hours after which they were sectioned in the same way as described by Koornneef (1977), with the help of a 'biro electric sawing machine'. The sections were cleaned with running tap water to remove sawing dust. Next they were fixed in a 4% formaldehyde solution for a week. Clearing of the sections was performed according to modifications of the Spalteholz (1914) clearing method, described by Koornneef (1977), but in order to make the capillaries stand out the histological staining procedure was omitted.

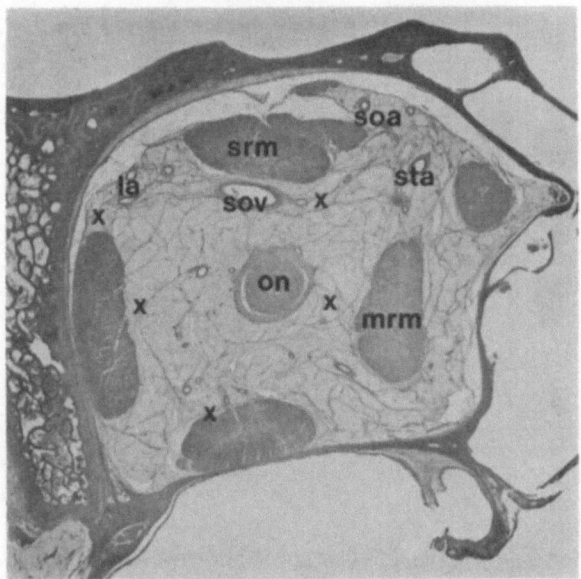

Fig. 1. Frontal 60 μ section, approximately 5 mm behind the back of the eyeball. Arteries are not enclosed in the septa, veins are.

o.n.: optic nerve, s.r.m.: superior rectus muscle, m.r.m.: medial rectus muscle, s.t.a.: supra-trochlear artery, s.o.a.: supra-orbital artery, l.a.: lacrimal artery, s.o.v.: superior ophthalmic vein, x: connective tissue septa.

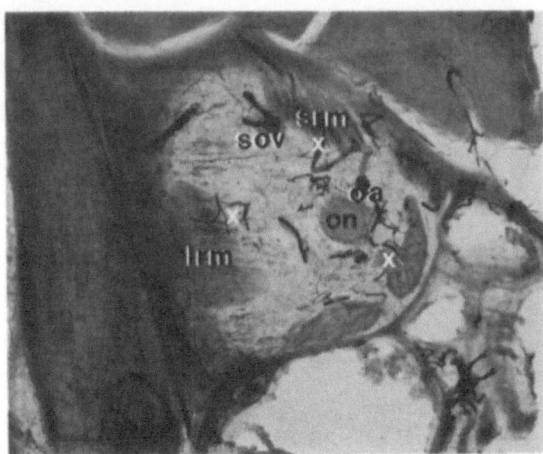

Fig. 2. Frontal 5000 μ section, approximately 17 mm behind the back of the eyeball, showing high arterial density. o.n.: optic nerve, s.r.m.: superior rectus muscle, l.r.m.: lateral rectus muscle, o.a.: ophthalmic artery, s.o.v.: superior ophthalmic vein, x: muscular arteries.

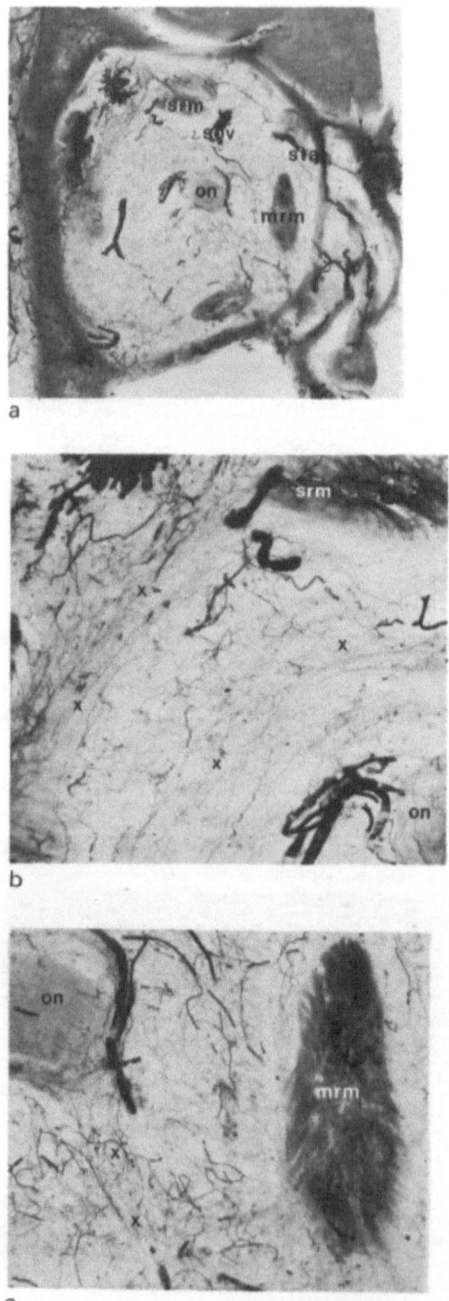

Fig. 3. Dense capillary networks just behind the eyeball. a. Frontal 5000 μ section, approximately 2 mm behind the back of the eyeball. b. Detail craniolaterally. Long capillaries circular to the optic nerve peripherally. c. Detail medially. Long capillaries radial to the optic nerve centrally. o.n.: optic nerve, s.r.m.: superior rectus muscle, m.r.m.: medial rectus muscle, s.t.a.: supra-trochlear artery, s.o.v.: superior ophthalmic vein, x: connective tissue septa.

thus not surprising to find that generally the muscular arteries enter the extrinsic eye muscles relatively far back in the orbit, with the exception of the above-mentioned arteries supplying the inferior oblique muscle. On the other hand, the drainage of the extrinsic eye muscle takes place more to the front, approximately at the level of the rear of the eyeball. The arterial and venous vascularization of the extrinsic eye muscles is mainly provided by vessels of large calibre.

We found that the capillary system in the orbit mainly originates straight from vessels of middle and large calibre, e.g., the muscular arteries. Going from the apex of the orbital cone in the direction of its base, density of the capillary network increases up to the level of the eyeball (Fig. 3), after which there is a gradual decrease in density. Frontally the orientation of the long capillaries corresponds with that of the connective tissue septa, that is, circular in the periphery and radial in the centre (Fig. 3b). These long capillaries run parallel to the connective tissue septa. Few of these long vessels perforate the septa. Capillary vascularization is compartment-bound. There seems to be little or no contact on the capillary level between the vascular networks in the extrinsic eye muscles on the one hand and in the adipose tissue compartments on the other.

CONCLUSION

In the orbit we find an orderly vascular pattern with a close and definite relationship to the connective tissue apparatus, notably to the connective tissue septa.

REFERENCES

Hayreh, S.S. & R. Dass. The ophthalmic artery. I. Origin and intra-cranial and intra-canalicular course. *Br. J. Ophthal.* 46: *65–98* (1962).
Koornneef, L. The first results of a new anatomical method of approach to the human orbit following a clincial enquiry. *Acta Morphol. Neerl.-Scand.* 12: *259–282* (1974).
Koornneef, L. & J.A. Los. A new anatomical approach to the human orbit. Mod. Probl. Ophthal. 14: *49–56*. Karger, Basel (1975).
Koornneef, L. Details of the orbital connective tissue system in the adult. *Acta Morphol. Neerl.-Scand.* 15: *1–34* (1977a).
Koornneef, L. The architecture of the musculo-fibrous apparatus in the human orbit. *Acta Morphol. Neerl.-Scand.* 15: *35–64* (1977b).
Meyer, F. Zur Anatomie der Orbitalarterien. *Morphol. Jahrbuch* 12: *414–459* (1887).
Salamon, G., C. Raybaud & F. Grisoli. Anatomical study of the blood vessels of the orbit. In: Proc. 2nd Congr. Eur. Ass. Radiol., Amsterdam, 1971. pp. 284–289. Excerpta Medica, Amsterdam (1972).
Seseman, E. Die Orbitalvenen des Menschen und ihr Zusammenhang mit den oberflächlichen Venen des Kopfes. *Arch. Anat. Physiol. Wiss. Med.:* *154–173* (1869).
Spalteholz, W. Ueber das Durchsichtigmachen von menschlichen und tierischen Präparaten und seine theoretischen Bedingungen. Hirzel, Leipzig (1914).

Authors' address:
Department of Anatomy and Embryology
University of Amsterdam
Amsterdam
The Netherlands

Proc. 3rd Int. Symp. on Orbital Disorders, Amsterdam 1977

THE ORBITAL MUSCLE AND THE CAVERNOUS SINUS

Chr. VERMEIJ-KEERS

(Leyden, The Netherlands)

INTRODUCTION

In the literature the dimensions of the orbital muscle — according to Müller (1858) a collection of smooth muscle fibres and elastic tendon fibres closing off the inferior orbital fissure in man — and its relations to other structures in the orbit are matters of discussion. The same holds, of course, for its action. Some authors consider the muscle to be involved in exophthalmos, either indirectly by compressing the veins (Kraus, 1911) or directly as a pro-truder (Groyer, 1903). Fründ (1911) thought that both aspects might play a part. Hesser (1913) and others rejected the possibility of compression because of the free venous anastomoses in the orbit and the indirect rela-tionship of the orbital muscle with the veins. Ernyei (1934) and Rohen (1953b, 1964) saw no role of the muscle in the development of exophthal-mos. And more recent authors even do not mention the orbital muscle in connection with exophthalmos, except Mullin et al. (1977), who use the term orbital muscle instead of extra-ocular muscle, which is very confusing.

In our opinion, the significance of Müller's muscle can only be judged after its anatomical aspects have been appropriately investigated. We therefore used serially-sectioned heads of embryos and foetuses and compared our findings with observations made in adult heads.

MATERIAL AND METHODS

The studies were performed in micro-sectioned heads of 16 human embryos and foetuses with a crown-rump length (C-RL), ranging from 30 to 155 mm, five adult human heads used exclusively for dissection with the aid of a binocular dissection microscope (see Vermeij-Keers, 1973), and a sagittally sectioned frozen adult human head. This head was placed sagittally in a home-made watertight rectangular wooden box fitted to the head, after which the box was filled with water and placed in a deep-freezer (-20° C). The deep-frozen box with the front sawn off was placed in a specially made P.V.C. conducting system of a band-saw, and sagittal sections were sawn about 1 cm thick, as far as the back of the box. The sections were then defrosted at room temperature and fixed between glass plates in Kaiserling's solution.*

* The dissections were made by W. Reychard.

To obtain a spatial picture of the orbital muscle and its related structures, a cardboard reconstruction was made of a sagittally sectioned 155 mm C-RL foetus aged 20 weeks (Vermeij-Keers, 1973).

RESULTS

Embryologic and foetal material

After evaluating various planes of section, we chose the sagittal direction as the most favourable for the investigation of the orbital muscle in relation to the orbital bones bordering the inferior orbital fissure, the orbital contents (with e.g. the superior and inferior ophthalmic veins), and the structures in the pterygo-palatine and infratemporal fossae as well as those in the retro-orbital region. In the 155 mm C-RL foetus the orbit, consisting of bone, cartilage, or mesenchyme, is covered by periorbita. The orbital muscle extends between the periorbita and the periosteal lining of the pterygo-

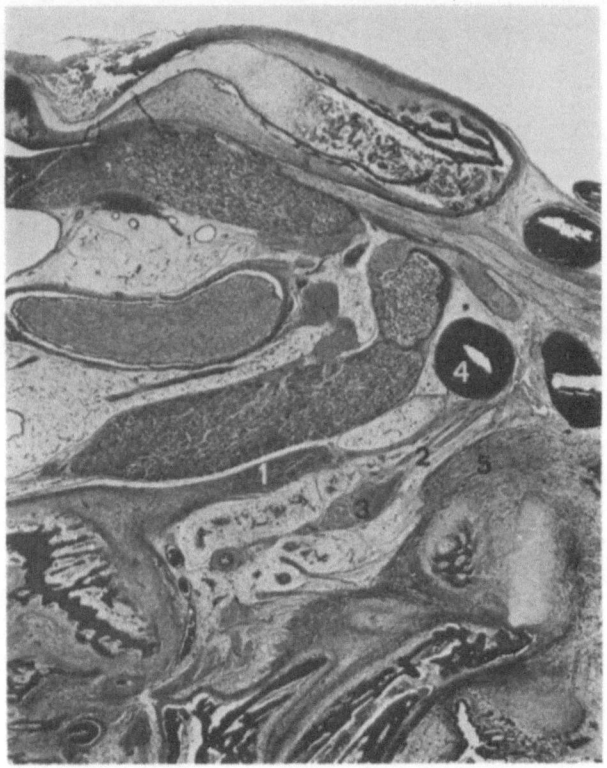

Fig. 1. Sagittal section of the left orbit of the 155 mm C-RL foetus. The orbital muscle (1) encircles most of the frontal part of the cavernous sinus (4). Rami orbitales (2) of the pterygo-palatine ganglion (3) are visible between the cavernous sinus (4) and the sphenoid bone (5). (X11,5.)

palatine and infratemporal fossae. In the frontal direction the orbital muscle extends in three slips: one behind the orbital process of the palatine bone, one above the infra-orbital groove, and a third behind the maxilla, where it is attached to the infratemporal facies of that bone.

Occipitally, the orbital muscle attaches to the sphenoid bone and extends as far as the annulus of Zinn. At the place where the annulus bridges the superior orbital fissure, the orbital muscle encircles most of the frontal part of the cavernous sinus. This part of the sinus occupies almost the entire caudo-medial sector of the superior orbital fissure beneath the annulus (Fig. 1). Due to this peculiar anatomical arrangement, there is a direct communication from the pterygo-palatine fossa to the retro-orbital region via the inferior orbital and superior orbital fissures in that order, without perforation of Müller's muscle. About eight rami orbitales, originating from the pterygo-palatine ganglion, and some small veins forming anastomoses between the pterygoid plexus and the cavernous sinus, use this specific route in leaving the pterygo-palatine fossa. On

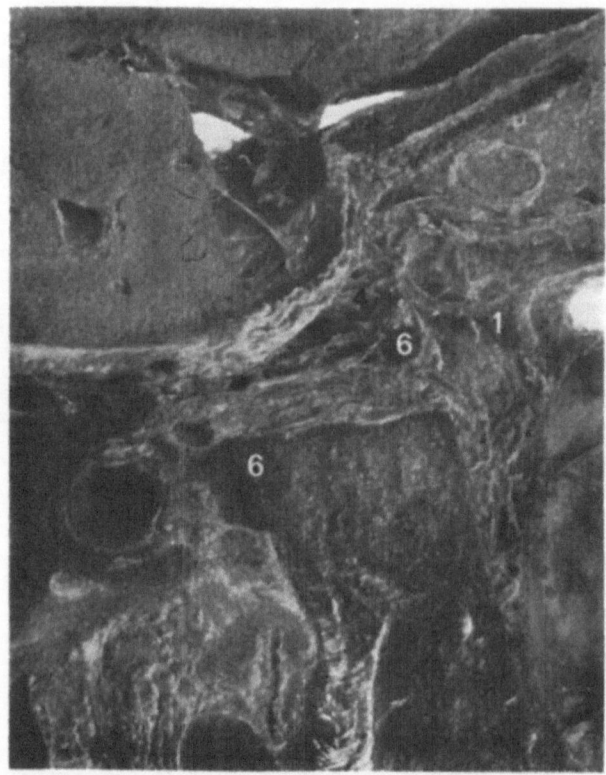

Fig. 2. Lateral view of a 1 cm thick sagittal section of the right orbit and retro-orbital region cut through the foramen rotundum (6) of an adult head. The spatial aspects of the orbital muscle (1) and the cavernous sinus (4) are comparable with those in Fig. 1. (X2.)

their way to the orbit, these rami orbitales join the frontal, lacrimal, and abducent nerves and the carotid plexus.

In all the embryos and foetuses starting with 34 mm C-RL, we found this direct relationship between the orbital muscle and the cavernous sinus. However, we found variations in the course of the ophthalmic veins and also a special canal in the sphenoid bone — just below the superior orbital fissure — used by some rami orbitales, as well as a rather large vein going to the retro-orbital region.

Adult human material

In principle, the macroscopical observations showed the same spatial relations in all specimens as were observed in our microscopical material (Fig. 2). The dimensions of the orbital muscle, however, varied between the different specimens and sometimes between the left and right side of one specimen. This finding and also those described for the embryologic and foetal material are probably ascribable to the enormous variations in the shape and size of the superior and inferior orbital fissures between different skulls but sometimes also between the left and right side of one skull.

DISCUSSION

Since Müller (1858) there has been general agreement that in man the orbital muscle closes off the inferior orbital fissure. Among other authors, Fründ (1911), Kraus (1911), and Duke-Elder (1961) describe some kind of relationship between the orbital muscle and the cavernous sinus. However, none of them noticed that at the site where there is a direct relationship between this muscle and the cavernous sinus, the orbital muscle has no attachment to the sphenoid. Thus, the inferior orbital fissure is not closed off in this area, and furthermore this arrangement makes it possible for rami orbitales and veins to pass from the pterygo-palatine fossa to the retro-orbital region through the inferior orbital and superior orbital fissures, successively, without perforating the muscle. Fründ (1911), Kraus (1911), and Hesser (1913) describe separate fascicles of smooth muscle fibres as part of the orbital muscle in close relationship with the superior and inferior ophthalmic veins. These smooth muscle fibres are probably those described by Koornneef (1977) in the orbital connective-tissue septa. We have not seen these fibres in continuity with the orbital muscle.

Because of the extensive contact between the orbital muscle and the cavernous sinus, it seems very likely that changes in the venous blood flow take place under the influence of the orbital muscle. Without further investigations we hesitate to conclude that contraction of the orbital muscle can cause exophthalmos by compressing the cavernous sinus; in any case, it seems probable that this muscle is too small in some individuals, and the right and left sides differ too much in others for such compression. However, more clinical attention to this phenomenon might solve the problem.

REFERENCES

Duke-Elder, Sir Stewart. System of ophthalmology. Vol. II. The anatomy of the visual system. Henry Kimpton, London (1961).

Ernyei, I. Die Rolle des Musculus orbitalis (Müller) beim Menschen. *Albrecht v. Graefes Arch. klin. exp. Ophthal.* 131: *398–400* (1934).

Fründ, H. Die glatte Muskulatur der Orbita und ihre Bedeutung für die Augensymptome bei Morbus Basedowii. *Beitr. klin. Chir.* 73: *755–775* (1911).

Groyer, F. Zur vergleichenden Anatomie des Musculus orbitalis und der Musculi palpebrales (tarsales). *S.-B.d.k.Akad. Wissensch.* Bd. CXII: *51–100* (1903).

Hesser, C. Der Bindegewebsapparat und die glatte Muskulatur der Orbita beim Menschen in normalem Zustande. *Anat. Hefte* 49: *248–290* (1913).

Koornneef, L. Spatial aspects of orbital musculo-fibrous tissue in man. A new anatomical and histological approach. Swets and Zeitlinger, Amsterdam and Lisse (1977).

Kraus, W. Über die Anatomie der glatten Muskulatur der Orbita und der Lider, speziell die Membrana orbitalis musculosa. *Münch. med. Wschr.* 58: *1993–1994* (1911).

Müller, H. Über einen glatten Muskel in der Augenhöhle des Menschen und der Säugethiere. *Z. wiss. Zool.* 9: *541* (1858).

Mullin, R.B., R.E. Levinson, A. Friedman, D.E. Henson, R.J. Winand & L.D. Kohn. Delayed hypersensitivity in Graves' disease and exophthalmos. Identification of thyroglobulin in normal human orbital muscle. *Endocrinology* 100 (2): *351–366* (1977).

Rohen, J.W. Die funktionelle Gestalt des Auges und seiner Hilfsorgane. Abh. der Mainzer Akad. der Wiss. u. Lit., Math.-nat. Kl., H.4 (1953b).

Rohen, J.W. Handbuch der mikroskopischen Anatomie des Menschen. Bd. III, Vierter Teil, Das Auge und seine Hilfsorgane. Springer, Berlin - Göttingen - Heidelberg - New York (1964).

Vermeij-Keers, Chr. Spatial aspects of the orbital muscle. *Z. Anat. Entwickl.-Gesch.* 141: *77–87* (1973).

Author's address:
Department of Anatomy and Embryology
University Hospital
Leyden
The Netherlands

Proc. 3rd Int. Symp. on Orbital Disorders, Amsterdam 1977

THE CONNECTIVE TISSUE APPARATUS OF THE HUMAN ORBIT. WHAT ABOUT IT?

LEO KOORNNEEF

(Amsterdam, The Netherlands)

As a consequence of some ununderstood motility and vascular disturbances encountered by our Orbital Centre, before and after surgery of blow-out fractures, a new anatomical and embryological approach to the human orbit was developed. This new approach revealed unknown connective tissue septa inside the human orbit which are highly. organized. These connective tissue septa lie between the eyeball and the orbital walls and are arranged in a specific spatial architecture (Koornneef, 1977*) forming a complex and ingenious connective tissue apparatus. This apparatus plays an important role during eye movements. Literature data support this view.

In 1960, Lang described a connective tissue system around the Achilles tendon, and states that the septa slide against one another and against fat cushions during movements. Considerable support is lend to this theory by the fact that he also found large quantities of hyaluronic acid around the septa. We know that hyaluronic acid is always present in places where friction and/or movements occur.

Recent histochemical investigations by Singh (Singh, 1976) equally show large quantities of hyaluronic acid in the human orbit. These two facts made us make a brief biomechanical study. In fresh post mortem material the medial rectus muscle was pulled backwards and fixed with a ligature, thus adducting the eye. Subsequently the orbit was deep frozen and sectioned in thick histological sections. The sections were stained with hematoxyline-azophloxine and clarified with methylsalicylate. Histological study of these sections revealed a quite normal and recognizable connective tissue apparatus. In other words, the normal architecture during eye movements is preserved but has changed its position, the septa sliding against one another and against fat cushions. Simultaneously performed embryological investigations (Koornneef, 1977) have pointed out that human orbital connective tissue starts its development about 3.5 months after conception. Humphrey (1959) has pointed out that foetal eye movements start approximately 3 months after conception. This time the relationship cannot be a coincidence. We believe that a normal development of human orbital connective tissue is dependent on normal eye movements. Eye movements inducing the

---

* Research done in the Department of Anatomy and Embryology of the University of Amsterdam (Head Prof. J. van Limborgh).

formation of septa, comparable e.g. with the direction of the trabeculae in human bone, which are equally dependent on the pressure vector in the bone.

How can this connective tissue system be fitted in the mechanism of a blow-out fracture? We believe that in a blow-out fracture not the inferior rectus and/or the inferior oblique muscles are trapped in the fracture hole. On the contrary, the entire motility apparatus around the fracture is caught (Koornneef, 1977). A motility apparatus consisting of muscles, orbital fat cushions and the connective tissue septa of the muscle is involved. If this complete motility apparatus is freed shortly after trauma, normal eye movements without diplopia can be obtained, because the possibility of normal eye movement is regained by operation. In their turn these eye movements induce the development of a normal connective tissue system. When the motility apparatus around the fracture hole is freed too late (the indication to operate should be considered carefully in each case and will not be dealt with in this paper) in the experience of our Orbital Centre poor results are obtained. This might be explained in the following way. When operating too late, organization of the connective tissue apparatus into aberrant scan connective tissue occurs.

Restoring the orbital floor and freeing the prolaps in the maxillary sinus will not bring normal eye movements back, because the scar clot around the muscles interferes. This explains the poor result obtained after operating on old blow-out fractures.

If posttraumic dilopia after a blow-out fracture persists an ordinary resection/recession procedure of the muscles can be performed on the eye involved in the fractured orbit or on the contralateral eye. These procedures are commonly accepted and can give satisfactory results. One should realize, however, that the real cause of the diplopia is not expelled or cured. I believe and plead that in certain cases, in which eye movements are considerably restricted by scar connective tissue, the eye muscles, being innocent, should be left alone. First connective tissue surgery should be given a chance.

In close cooperation with our Orthoptical Department we aim to select patients in order to perform connective tissue surgery. In these patients the muscles involved are loosened from the aberrant connective tissue; the scar clot is excentrated and intraorbital haemorrhage is avoided. Immediate post-operative eye movement practice is stimulated. Post-operative results, as reported by Oei (Oei, 1975) in this volume are encouraging.

RESULTS

Humphry, T. & D. Hooker. Double simultaneous stimulation of human fetusses and the anatomical pattern underlying the reflexes elicited. *J. Comp. Neurol.* 112: 75–162 (1959).

Koornneef, L. New insights in the human orbital connective tissue. *Arch. Ophthal.* 95: 1269 (1977).

Koornneef, L. Spatial aspects of human orbital musculo-fibrous tissue in man. Swets & Zeitlinger, Amsterdam, 168 pp. (1977).

Koornneef, L. Das Bindegewebe Apparat in der menschlichen Orbita. Proceedings of the D.O.G. Symposium, Freiburg, April 1977. Verlag J.F. Bergmann, München (1977).

Lang, J. Über das Gleitgewebe der Sehen, Muskeln, Fascien und Gefässe. *Z. f. Anat. u. Entw.* 122: *197–231* (1960).

Oei, T.H. Surgical approach of the orbital connective tissue in case of traumatic diplopia. Proc. 3rd Int. Symp. on Orbital Disorders, Amsterdam, 1977. Junk, The Hague (1978).

Singh, S.P. & M. Nikifosak. The biochemical composition of human retrobulbar connective tissue. Separate Experiments Vol. 32, pp. 395–396. Birkhäuser, Basel (1976).

Author's address:
Orbital Centre
University Eye Clinic
Wilhelmina Gasthuis
104, 1e Helmerstraat
Amsterdam
The Netherlands

Proc. 3rd Int, Symp. on Orbital Disorders, Amsterdam 1977

QUANTITATIVE APPROACH TO THE ESTIMATION OF THE RELATIONSHIP OF THE GROWTH PATTERNS OF EYE AND ORBIT

G. OUDHOF

(Baarn, The Netherlands)

During the 2nd International Symposium on Orbital Disorders held in Amsterdam in 1973, van Limborgh & Tonneyck-Müller reported on the relationship of ocular and orbital growth in chicken embryos. A close correlation of the growth of eye and orbit was found which indicated that the growing eye influences the orbital growth to a considerable extent. No definite answer could be given whether this relation was a causal one. Moreover, undersized orbits were seen in relation with deformities of other cranial components.

Not only a further factorial analysis but also an analysis of the interactions in the processes of endesmal and enchondral growth led us to extend the study to gain more insight into the developmental patterns and in the causality of the craniofacial morphogenesis. Therefore chicken embryos of 13–19 days of incubation were used in this investigation. Standardized X-ray photographs of the heads of the embryos were made with an X-ray projection microscope.

Measurements of angles between bones and measurements of the length of bones and groups of bones were the data for the mathematical calculation of the growth patterns and of the growth levels. The growth patterns of a group of normal embryos were compared with the data from sham-operated embryos and with those of a group of embryos with experimentally induced unilateral microphthalmia. The measurements in the normal embryos from 13–19 days showed a growth of the linear type for all bones, except for the interorbital septum, which had a still increasing quadratic type of growth and also the eyes and orbits, which showed a decreasing quadratic type of growth during this period.

In the sham-operated embryos the egg-shell was opened and the embryonic membranes overlying the head were removed at 68 hours of incubation. This intervention has a great influence on the development of the embryo in that the posthypophyseal cranial base consisting of the basi-sphenoid and basi-occipital bones showed an irregular growth; a linear growth type was found for the interorbital septum and lower levels of growth were seen for the measurements of the upper beak length.

In the experimental group of embryos in which the lens of the right eye was removed at 68 hours of incubation the posthypophyseal cranial base did not show alterations in comparison with the sham-operated group. This leads us to the conclusion that the posthypophyseal cranial base is characterized by a strongly regulated and intrinsically determined growth pattern, which is not influenced by factors emanating from the growing eyes.

The prehypophyseal area showed a lower mean level which was also lower than that of the sham-operated group. A lower level was also found for the palatal and the maxillary bones not only in comparison with the normal group but also in comparison with the sham-operated group. Neither the sidelong measurements of the premaxilla nor the width of the upper beak in this region showed alterations in growth type or in growth level in the group of microphthalmic embryos. It was concluded that the nasal capsule is not influenced by the removal of the eye primordium or, in other words, the growing eyes do not exert an influence on the nasal capsule nor on the premaxillary bone which ossifies intramembranously as a covering bone on the nasal capsule.

The sidelong measurements over the jugal arch on the left side showed the same level differences as in the sham-operated group. On the right side an extra level difference in comparison with the sham-operated group was found. The sutures between the quadrato-jugal, the jugal and the maxillary bones did not show an innate capacity to develop themselves to their normal length, nor are they capable of maintaining the direction of growth as the normal convexity of the zygomatic arch on the right side was changed into a straight rod of bones in the microphthalmic embryos; on the left side the convexity was greater than in the normal embryos. The form of the arches both in an antero-posterior direction as well as in a transverse direction is dependent on the regulating factors emanating from the environment.

The correlation coefficients, calculated for the relation between the eyes and orbits show a strong correlation on the left side in all three groups; on the right side there is a high correlation in the normal and the sham-operated groups, but in the experimental group the correlation is much lower.

A direct influence of the growing right eye on the right orbital structures in the microphthalmic group cannot be substantiated. The orbit grows faster than the eye rudiment. It must be stated that the growth of the orbital cartilages is not dependent on the presence of an eye. Or in other words: the eyes are not a continuous source of local epigenetic factors for the growing orbital cartilages.

The eye is always surrounded by an orbit; the eye primordium is necessary for the molding of the mesenchyme and imposes on the mesenchyme cells its growth pattern. For a relatively short period during which the differentiation from mesenchyme into cartilage takes place the growth rate of the eye primordium is of utmost importance. That growth pattern is transferred to the cartilage cells and is maintained in the subsequent daughter cells.

This view combines the essentials of the opinions that genetic as well as epigenetic factors play a role. Genetic factors determine the growth rate of the eye primordium; epigenetically the growing eye primordium imposes a growth pattern on the mesenchyme cells, which intrinsically is maintained after they have differentiated into cartilage cells.

Independent of the source that imposed the growth pattern, the orbital cartilages develop themselves in close correlation with the growing eye until the growth of the eye decreases.

The epigenetic factor emanating from the eye cup causes a curtailment of the polyvalued function of the mesenchyme to a causally correlated mono-valued function, resulting in a parallelism of both growth patterns of the eye and of the orbit in the time and in normal developmental histogenesis.

In their turn, the growing chondrocranial elements influence epigenetically the growth rates of the desmocranial elements. The process of differentiation of mesenchyme cells into osteogenic cells involves a decrease of intrinsic genetic control. The sensitivity to epigenetic and environmental influences remains the same as that in mesenchymal cells or becomes even greater. One may safely suppose that the process of division of a preosteoblast into two different daughter cells – a new preosteoblast, remaining as a maternal cell for subsequent cell divisions, and an osteoblast, able to deposit bone – is fully under the control of epigenetic and environmental factors. Since the osteocytes inside the bone and the osteoblasts on the outside are connected with each other as well as with the sutural and periosteal pre-osteoblasts, all these cells can receive continuous information about the changes in the tensions and pressures to which bone, during growth and function, is subjected.

Hence, the basic difference between cartilaginous growth and intramembranous bone growth can be defined as follows: cartilages follow a stabilized growth pattern whereas in the membranous bone growth the matric formation is dependent on epigenetic factors; ossification and calcification are processes of stabilisation of the acquired form.

REFERENCES

Limborg, J. van & I. Tonneyck-Müller. Orbital growth pattern in experimental microphthalmia. pp. 1–4 in: Proc. 2nd Int. Symp. on Orbital Disorders, Amsterdam 1973. Mod. Probl. Ophthal., Volume 14. Karger, Basel (1975).

Oudhof, G. Development and growth of the cranium. A quantitative experimental study in the chick embryo. Thesis, Amsterdam (1975).

Author's address:
Ferd. Huycklaan 46
Baarn
The Netherlands

Proc. 3rd Int. Symp. on Orbital Disorders, Amsterdam 1977

CYSTS OF THE OPTIC NERVE SHEATHS

J. BRIHAYE, M. VAN GEERTRUYDEN, R. HERZEEL, & B. WILLEKENS

(Brussels/Amsterdam)

Cysts of the optic nerve sheaths are exceptional, and the differential diagnosis with a slow evolutive tumor is very difficult. In the case of cysts of both optic nerves, with the progressive loss of vision that we are reporting, the possibility that its origin lies a coloboma of the optic disc is suggested by pathological examination.

CASE REPORT

J.C.R. progressively developed a left exophthalmos, since he was 3 years old. At the age of 21, he noted loss of vision in this eye, and reduction of vision in the right eye. At our first examination, in September 1973, the best corrected acuity was 6/10 in the right eye and less than 1/50 in the left. Pupils were symmetrical but the left pupillary reflex was slightly slower than the right one. The left eye was proptosed 7 mm and deviated to the temporal and inferior side; there was neither adduction nor elevation. Right visual field was full, but the blind spot was slightly enlarged. A rather complete temporal hemianopsia field defect was found in the left eye (Fig. 1). Ophthalmoscopy revealed a grey bulge in both discs; the left disc was slightly paler than the right one: both were normally vascularized (Fig. 2

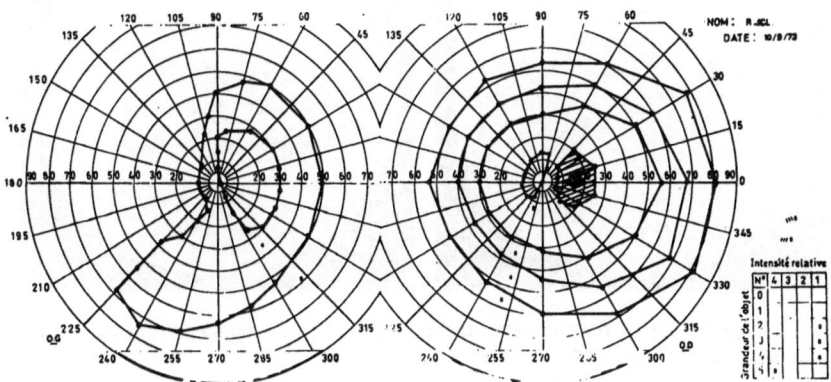

Fig. 1. At our first examination, right visual field showed an enlarged blind spot; left visual field revealed a temporal hemianopsia.

213

and 3); a few retinal folds were visible in the left posterior pole; in the right macula slight irregular pigmentation was observed; there was an area of chorio-retinal atrophy of approximately one half papillary diameter under the left macula.

Neurological examination was normal. X-rays of the skul and orbit demonstrated a slightly enlarged left orbit. Orbital echography showed waves suggesting a tumor in the posterior segment of the orbit. The brain isotopic scan and E.E.G. were normal.

General examination showed no other malformation.

A left orbital surgery by anterior approach revealed, behind the eyeball and in contact with it, a huge cystic tumor, larger than the eye itself; the optic nerve was not visible. Puncture produced a decrease in the size of the cyst and facilitated the orbital exploration; the liquid had a similar appearance and composition as the C.S.F. Enucleation and removal of the cystic mass was performed seeing that the left eye was quite blind: in addition the slowing decrease of the visual acuity of the right eye incited us to have a correct histological diagnosis. The post-operative course was uneventful.

Nine months later, visual acuity in the right eye decreased to 2/10. X-rays of the right orbit showed a superior orbital fissure slightly enlarged. Visual field examination demonstrated a central scotoma. Eye fundus was unchanged. Pneumo-orbitography did not reveal any retro-ocular lesion. Orbital echography indicated that the posterior wall of the eyeball was larger at 3 and 9 hours than at 6 and 12.

We concluded that a cyst was likely developing in the meningeal sheaths of the right optic nerve and we tried to puncture it, but we could hardly obtain any liquid.

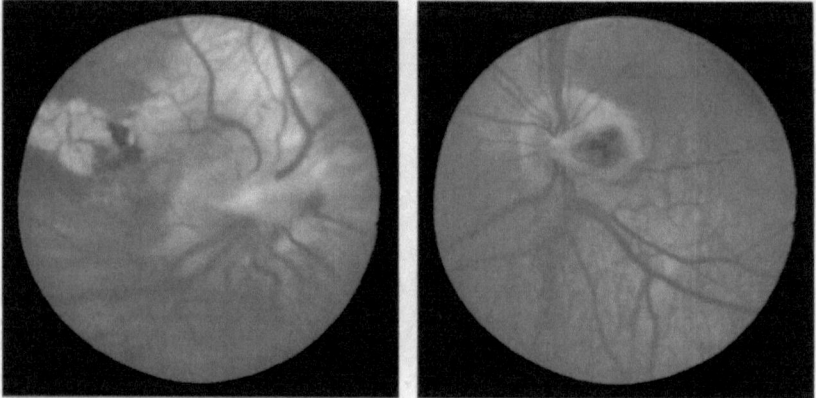

Fig. 2. Eye fundus of the right eye; there is a grey bulge extending in the central and temporal part of the optic disc.

Fig. 3. Eye fundus of the left eye; a grey bulge is visible in the center and nasal part of the optic disc which was slightly paler than the right one; in the posterior pole there are a few retinal folds, and under the macula an area of chorio-retinal atrophy.

Following corticosteroid therapy the visual acuity progressively increased to 5/10. This clinical condition has remained unchanged during the last three years.

HISTOLOGICAL EXAMINATION

The distal part of the optic nerve was fixed in paraffin and cut in a frontal plane. The eyeball and the proximal part of the optic nerve were fixed in celloidine and cut in a sagittal plane.

The optic nerve was surrounded by an empty space between the nerve fiber bundles and the meninges. On one side the space was forming a cyst lined by unicellular layer, stained red with Alcian blue. The optic nerve itself was decreased in volume, the bundles of nerve fibers were markedly reduced in size, and in certain areas they had almost completely disappeared; septa were enlarged; glial cells infiltrated the nerve fiber bundles. Serial sections were made; we found on a few slides the cyst extending into the sheath through a hiatus of the sclera to the level of the head of the optic nerve; it was separated from the posterior chamber of the eye only by a few layers of fibrous tissue; at this level acellular material, P.A.S. negative, was protruding into the cyst (Fig. 4 and 5).

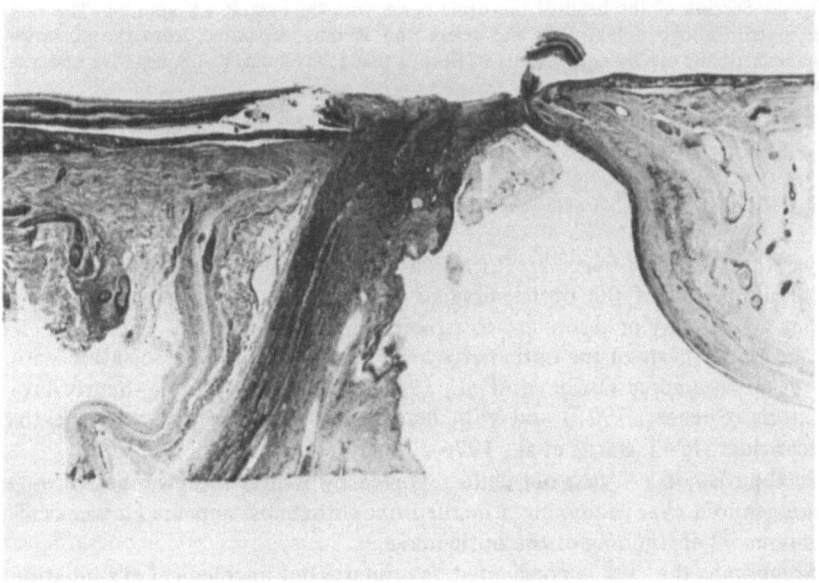

Fig. 4. Section of the optic nerve with an empty space in the sheaths forming a cyst. The optic nerve is markedly decreased in volume. The cyst extended into the sheaths to the level of the optic nerve head. Hematoxylin-eosine staining.

215

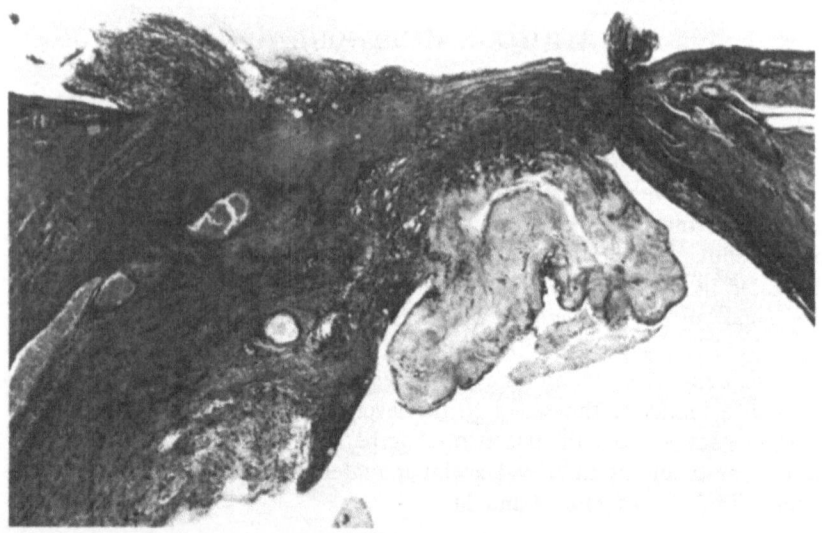

Fig. 5. Section of the head of the optic nerve with the cyst. P.A.S. staining. The cyst extended through a hiatus in the sclera and is only separated from the posterior chamber of the eye by a few layers of fibrous tissue. Acellular, P.A.S. negative material is protruding into the cyst.

COMMENTS

Cysts of the optic nerve are localized either in the intracranial or in the orbital portion of the optic nerve or close to the disc (Agatston, 1944). They are primary or secondary to a tumor or a hemorrhage.

Secondary cysts of the optic nerve have been described in association with optic nerve glioma (Brihaye et al., 1961), craniopharyngioma, neurofibromatosis (Spencer, 1972) and with hemangioma of the optic nerve sheaths (Schneider, 1942; Harris et al., 1976).

In the case of a 4 year old child reported by Wolter & McKenney (1964) an arachnoid cyst producing a marked exophthalmos, appeared 2 weeks after removal of a glioma of the optic nerve.

Sometimes the cyst is considered as primary, but histological examination suggests a tumor. Bane, in 1918, described a cyst behind the globe, containing rudimentary blood vessels, which could have been a meningioma. Walsh (1956) reported the case of a woman, 33 years old, who had loss of vision with optic atrophy of the left eye and bitemporal field defect: surgery revealed an intraneural cyst in the left optic nerve and chiasma; according to Zimmerman, the cyst, lined by stratified sqamous epithelium, was an epithelial cyst, maybe associated with craniopharyngioma.

Primary cysts of the optic nerve sheaths are exceptional; we only found 6 cases described in the literature of which 3 were intraorbital and 3 intracranial. cranial.

A chiasmatic intraparenchymal arachnoidal cyst was described by Chowdury (1976) in a 44 year old man: since three months his vision was deteriorating in both eyes, especially in the left; optic discs were atrophic, and the visual fields were remarkably constricted. After discision of the cystic membrane the vision improved.

Holt (1966) observed two cases of cyst of the chiasm and intracranial portion of the optic nerve: one patient, 33 years old, had incongruous homonymous hemianopsia and surgery showed a cyst of the intracranial portion of one optic nerve and chiasm; the other patient, 50 years old, had unilateral decrease of vision with papilloedema, enlarged blind spot and later on inferior hemianopsia; at exploration, the optic nerve was indented near the optic canal by a cyst. In both cases the cyst was incised; examination of the fluid did not disclose any tumor cell; nevertheless preventive X-ray therapy was applied; after 7 years in one case and 9 months in the other, there was no evidence of recurrence.

Among the intraorbital cysts, there are 2 cases reported by Miller & Green (1975): a 33 year old woman had unilateral visual field loss and papilloedema; histopathological examination showed that the optic nerve was atrophic and surrounded by enlarged subdural and subarachnoid spaces. The second case concerned a 56 year old woman with a left congenital frontotemporal cyst; she had bilateral optic atrophy and right homonymous hemianopsia; pathological examination revealed optic atrophy and saccular enlargement of the optic nerve sheaths with meningoendothelial proliferation.

A third case was reported by Smith, Hoyt & Newton (1969): a woman, 45 years old, had transcient obscurations of the vision in the left eye for 11 months, with a chronically swollen optic disc; she developed slight exophthalmos and a constriction of the visual field with increased blind spot of this eye. The sella turcica was enlarged, and pneumoencephalography demonstrated the image of an empty sella turcica. Surgical exploration of the orbit showed an enlargement of this optic nerve of 1.5 times the normal diameter. The optic nerve sheaths were opened and clear fluid emerged. The ophthalmic symptoms resolved shortly afterwards. Histopathologic examination showed that the optic nerve sheath was normal. The final diagnosis was: intra-sellar arachnoidal cyst combined with an arachnoidal cyst of the optic nerve sheaths.

With regard to our patient, the exact nature of the cyst and the cause of its progressive development remain uncertain. However, we have reason to believe that the cyst could be in relation with a coloboma of the disc.

Clinically we did not observe a real coloboma of the optic disc but the histological study demonstrated that, at the level of the optic disc, the cyst was extending in a hiatus of the sclera and was only separated from the vitreous cavity by a thin layer of fibrous tissue. At the same level, we saw acellular material protruding in the cavity of the cyst like an appendix which could have originated in the vitreous body. After years, accumulation of liquid has

217

provoked a compression of the optic nerve.

Mullaney (1973), in one of her cases of coloboma of optic disc in Edward syndrome, described failure of sclera with formation of a pouch behind the globe; meniscus tissue covered the opening in some slides; but, in this case, the pouch was localized outside the optic nerve and sheaths.

The case we report is. of special interest because of its rarity and the long evolution of the cyst since the proptosis was present for 20 years. We would also like to emphasize the exceptional appearance of both fundi which, histologically, seem to be a coloboma. The surgical and histological demonstration of a cyst in one of the optic nerves made that the decrease of vision of the other eye was probably caused by a similar lesion. This assumption incited us to simply puncture the right orbit as a treatment.

Considering the verified characteristics of the lesion, it appears that a drainage of the cyst, either by a retro-bulbar puncture or by a surgical approach, is sufficient to obtain an improvement of the clinical signs. An enucleation is only indicated when a tumor is suspected to be associated to the cyst.

SUMMARY

Report of a case of a young man, 21 years old, with left unilateral exophthalmos and progressive loss of vision since childhood. Compression by a huge cyst in the optic nerve sheaths caused atrophy of the optic fibers. A reduction of vision in the other eye may indicate that the lesion is bilateral.

Ophthalmoscopy revealed a very exceptional picture of a grey bulge in both discs, which histopathologically seems to be a coloboma of the optic nerve head; this could be the origin of the cyst in the optic nerve sheaths.

RESUME

Observation d'un jeune homme de 21 ans, atteint d'exophtalmie unilatérale gauche avec perte visuelle progressive évoluant depuis l'enfance. Les fibres optiques sont atrophiées suite à la compression exercée par un volumineux kyste développé dans les gaines du nerf optique. Une baisse visuelle de l' autre oeil fait suspecter l'existence d'une lésion similaire du nerf optique droit.

Le fond d'oeil présente des deux côtés une image très particulière des papilles: le centre de couleur grisâtre est surélevé. L'examen histologique est en faveur d'un colobome de la tête du nerf optique qui serait à l'origine du kyste.

REFERENCES

Agatston, S.A.. Congenital cyst of the optic nerve. *Am.J.Ophthal.* 27: *278-281* (1944).
Brihaye, M., G. Graff, J. Brihaye & P. Danis. Volumineux gliome kystique du chiasma à symptomalogie cérébrale prédominante. *Acta Neurol. Psychiatr. Belgica* 61: *525-538* (1961).
Burde, R.M., J.S. Karp & R.N. Miller. Reversal of visual defecit with optic nerve decompression in long-standing pseudotumor cerebri. *Am.J.Ophthal.* 27: *770-772* (1974).

Chowdhury, A.M.. Cyst within the parenchyma of the optic chiasm. *Brt.J.Ophthal.* 60: *581-582* (1970).

Danis, P., D. De Gandt, J. Dodion & P. Petit. Trisomie E (16-18) et malformation congénitale juxta-papillaire: étude anatomique. *Bull. Soc. belge Oph.* 152: *497–506* (1969).

Drews, R.C., Heterochromia iridum with coloboma of the optic disc. *Arch. Ophthal.* 90: *437*(1973).

Goldhammer, Y. & J.L. Smith. Optic nerve anomalies in basal encephalocele. *Arch. Ophthal.* 93: *115-118* (1975).

Harris, G.J., J.G. Sacks, P.E. Weinberg & R.B. O'Grady: Cyst of the intraorbital optic nerve sheaths. *Am.J.Ophthal.* 81: *656-660* (1976).

Hittner, H.M., M.N. Desmond & J.R. Montgomery. Optic nerve manifestations of human congenital cytomegalo-virus infection. *Am,J.Ophthal.* 81: *661-665* (1976).

H. Holt, Cysts of the intracranial portion of the optic nerve. *Am.J.Ophthal.* 61: *1166/226-1170/230* (1966).

Kindler, P. Morning glory syndrome: unusual congenital optic disk anomaly. *Am.J. Ophthal.* 69: *376-384* (1970).

Levitt, J.M. & R.I. Lloyd. Congenital prepapillary cyst containing a moving vascular loop. *Am.J.Ophthal.* 22: *760-764* (1939).

MacGregor, B.J.L., J. Gawler & J.R. South. Intracranial epithelial cyst. *J. Neurosurg.* 44: *109-114* (1976).

Manschot, W.A., Primary tumours of the optic nerve in von Recklinghausen's disease. *Br. J.Ophthal.* 38: *285-289* (1954).

Miller, N.R. & W.R. Green. Arachnoid cysts involving a portion of the intraorbital optic nerve. *Arch. Ophthal.* 93: *1117-1121* (1975).

Mullaney, J. Ocular pathology in trisomy 18 (Edwards' syndrome). *Am.J.Ophthal.* 76: *246-254* (1973).

Payne, B.F. Coloboma of the optic nerve in the human embryo. *Am.J.Ophthal.* 24: *395-402* (1941).

Pedler, C. Unusual coloboma of the optic nerve entrance. *Br.J.Ophthal.* 45: *803-807* (1961).

Savell, J. Optic nerve colobomas of autosomal-dominant heredity. *Arch. Ophthal.* 94: *395-400* (1976).

Smith, J.L., W.F. Hoyt & T.H. Newton. Optic nerve sheath decompression for relief of chronic monocular choked disc. *Am.J.Ophthal.* 68: *633-639* (1969).

Spencer, W.H. Primary neoplasms of the optic nerve and its sheaths: clinical features and current concepts of pathogenetic mechanisms. *Trans.Am.Ophthal.Soc.* 70: *490-528* (1972).

Walsh, F.B., J.W. Chambers & L.A. Lloyd. The ocular signs of tumors involving the anterior visual pathways. *Am.J.Ophthal.* 42: *247-377* (1956).

Walsh, F.B., J.W. Chambers & L.A. Lloyd. The ocular signs of tumors involving the anmore, Williams and Wilkins, pp. 2093-2095, (1969).

Willis, R., L.E. Zimmerman, R. O'Grady, R.S. Smith & B. Crawford. Heterotopic adipose tissue and smooth muscle in the optic disc. *Arch. Ophthal.* 88: *139-146* (1972).

Wolter, J.R. & M.J. McKenney. Collateral hyperplasia and cyst formation of orbital leptomeninx, secondary to optic nerve glioma. *Am.J.Ophthal.* 57: *1037-1042* (1964).

Authors' addresses:

Department of Ophthalmology
University of Brussels
Bosstraat
B-1090 Brussels
Belgium

Eye Clinic of the University of Amsterdam
and of the Netherlands Ophthalmic Research
Institute
104, 1e Helmerstraat
Amsterdam
The Netherlands

Requests for reprints to Dr M. Brihaye van Geertruyden at the Brussels' address.

Proc. 3rd Int. Symp. on Orbital Disorders, Amsterdam 1977

OPTIC NERVE HYPOPLASIA

D. LEBUISSON, P. DICONSTANZO, J.J. ARON & D. ARON-ROSA

(Paris, France)

ABSTRACT

Optic nerve hypoplasia is not a rare eventuality in children. How to distinguish it from optic nerve tumor, optic atrophy and complete optic nerve aplasia is reviewed from a multiple point of view, including optic canal tomography, fluorescein angiography and CAT examination.

Authors' address:
rue Manin 25
Paris
France

FACIAL CLEFTS IN COMBINATION WITH ANOPHTHALMUS ON TEAR DUCT ANOMALIES
The possibilities of plastic reconstruction

B. D. DE JONG & K. E. W. P. TAN

(Utrecht, The Netherlands)

INTRODUCTION

Both large facial clefts and anophthalmus are rare clinical entities. However, excellent studies have been carried out on both topics. Ask & van der Hoeve (1921) wrote a classic study on facial clefts, and Mann (1957) wrote one on anophthalmus.

The main purpose of the present study is the presentation of a number of very peculiar cases:
— one with bilateral facial clefts, and bilateral anophthalmus,
— one with a unilateral facial cleft, and a contralateral anophthalmus,
— one with bilateral facial clefts, tear duct anomalies, and deformities of the fingers and toes,
and to discuss the outlook for a plastic reconstruction.

CASE REPORTS

Case 1 (K.B.) (Fig. 1a & 1b)

Girl, born 1967, first child from healthy parents. Birth weight 3300 g.
This child has a complex deformity, consisting of
— a median palatum defect,
— bilateral oro-ocular clefts,
— bilateral clinical anopthalmus,
— severe mental retardation.
Otherwise the child seemed to be normal. The extremities did not show any deformity.

Case 2 (G.V.) (Fig. 2a & 2b)

Boy born 1975, the youngest child of 4 children from healthy parents. Birth weight 3900 g.
The other children did not show abnormalities.
The deformity in this child consisted of
— a lateral facial cleft on the right side (superior canaliculus was present),
— a clinical anophthalmus on the left side.

221

Otherwise the child seems to be healthy and has a good intelligence. The extremities are normal.

Case 3 (W.L.) (Fig. 3a. 3b & 3c)

Boy born 1972, first child of healthy parents, after one miscarriage. Birth weight 3000 g.
The deformities in this case consisted of
— a lateral facial cleft,
— bilateral cheilo-gnato-palatoschizis,
— hands and feet were highly abnormal with many constrictions of fingers and toes, and possibly intra uterine amputations,
— a fibrocutaneous appendix on the back of the head,
— lacrimal puncta were absent on the right side.
During surgery, a mucous-cyst was found in the lacrimal fossa on the right side.
— On the left side normal canaliculi were present. The nasolacrimal duct was obliterated, however.

DISCUSSION

What can we learn from these patients?
First of all, the aetiology of the last case (W.L.) seems to be different from those of the first two cases.
In the last one 'amnion bands' could well explain the facial cleft, the constriction of fingers and toes, and the fibrocutaneous appendix on the back of the head. In the first two cases there are no indications that 'amnion bands' play a role in the pathogenesis, and here a defective growth in embryonic life is propably responsible for the deformity.
The presence of a right superior canaliculus in the second case proves that the nasofrontal and maxillary processes fused more or less normally before the cleft originated. This supports the theory that facial clefts develop secondarily on the basis of an unbalanced growth.
The cases presented here were of particular interest to us and we have done a thorough study to lay down the priorities in reconstruction.
We agree with Gunter who published his results in 1963 that our first objective should be the protection of the eyeball by restoring the supportive function of the lower lid. Our second objective is the repair of the lining of the nasal and oral cavities and closure of the clefts by transportation of available tissues. Repair of the lacrimal passage was delayed until a later stage and has been performed in one case where epiphora or recurrent infections required it.

Case 1

This is the case with the bilateral oro-ocular clefts with hypoplasia of the

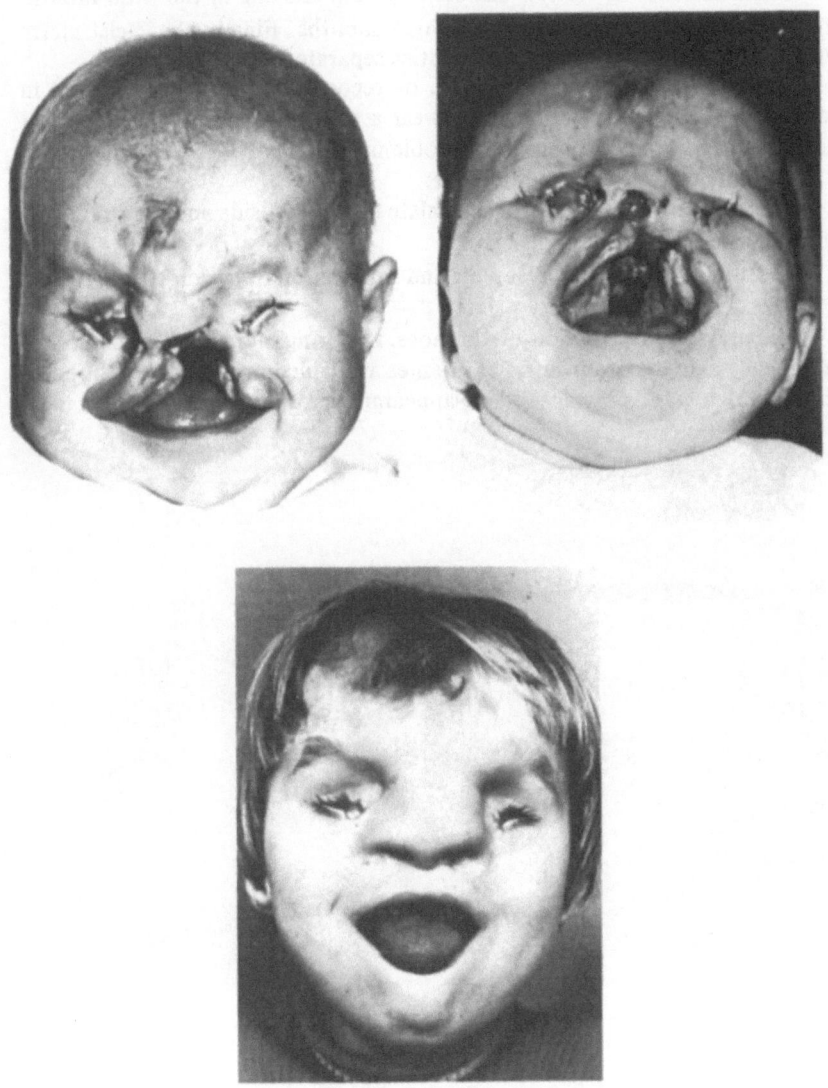

Fig. 1. Case 1. a & b Before surgery, 4 months old. c. After surgery, 6 years old.

(median) structures derived from the naso-frontal processus, and with the bilateral anophthalmia.

Closure of the facial clefts was attempted at the explicit wish of the parents, based on their religious beliefs. Although we hesitated to perform the operation we had no further arguments against, since the condition of the child proved to be excellent.

Reconstruction was carried out step by step starting in the third month, and was repeated after that every three months. Finally the facial clefts were closed and the nasal and oral cavities separated.

Although we are strong supporters of reconstructing the orbits even in cases of anophthalmia (in order to wear a suitable prothesis), this has not been done so far, due to behaviour problems of the child.

The following steps were carried out:

1. Closure of the lip and primary palate on the left side and removal of the choanal atresia in the naso-pharynx;

2. Closure of the naso-ocular cleft and removal of atresia on the right side;

3. Closure of the secondary palate;

4. Finally a reconstruction of the nose, requiring indirect transposition of (forehead) skin due to insufficient tissues available in the neighbourhood.

In this way a reasonably acceptable appearance was achieved (Fig. 1).

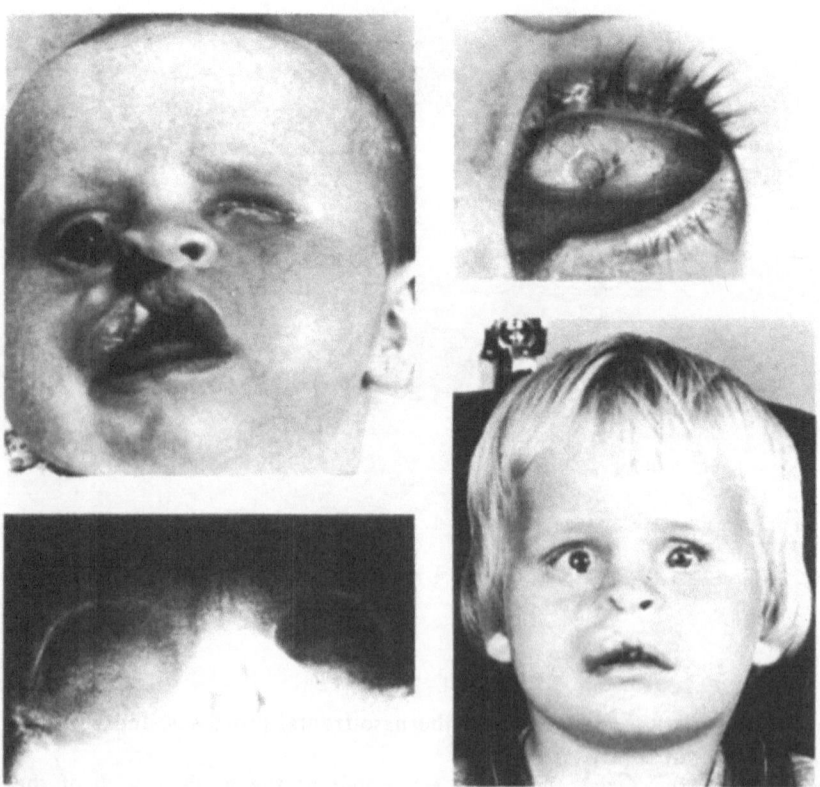

Fig. 2. Case 2. a. Before surgery, 3 months old. b. Left orbit showing 'clinical anophthalmus' c. X-ray of the skull, showing hypoplasia of the left orbit. d. After surgery, 2½ years old.

Case 2

In this case with the oro-naso ocular cleft on the right side and anophthalmia on the left side, surgical closure of the cleft has been carried out in two stages: eyelid reconstruction and closure of the upper end of the nasal cleft, by shifting available periosteal, mucosal and cutaneous flaps; closure of the oro-maxillary cleft according to a modified method of Le Mesurier; this was followed by the introduction of a gutta percha mould in the left orbit, which had to be renewed in quick succession due to a favourable expansive growth of the orbit, which resulted in a good pocket to wear a prosthesis.

The results are acceptable though the inner canthal ligament has to be reconstructed in a leter stage (Fig. 2b, 2d).

The expansion of the maxilla was satisfactory, except for the cleft between the central and lateral incisors and doubling of all the front elements.

Case 3

This case presented a coloboma of the lower eyelid as a manifestation of a oro-ocular cleft. He further showed a bilateral cleft of lip, primary and secondary palate.

As a first measure the lower lid was treated by shifting mucosa, tarsus and skin in such way that it resulted in lengthening in the vertical direction. The cleft in the orbital floor was covered by a periosteal flap mobilised out of the cleft.

We are not supporting bone transplantation as a primary measure as advocated by Mustardé, since we fear a disturbance of expansive growth of the orbit.

After closure of the lip and palate clefts in three sessions, a secondary procedure was necessary to shape the lower eyelid, by transpositon of a skin-flap.

Epiphora proved to be a troublesome complication. A similar procedure will be done on the left side. Recently a kind of conjunctivo-dacryo-rhinostomy was done, by placing a Jones tube in a canal lined subsequently by conjunctiva, the walls of a mucocyst lying in the lacimal fossa, and nasal mucosa.

There seems to be a bilateral hypoplasia of the maxilla. Probably this is induced by operative closure, and will require orthodontic measures later on.

We have the conviction that an early repair of the eyelids and reconstruction of the orbital floor has priority over other surgical procedures, such as closure of the palate and maxillary clefts.

A reconstruction of the tear ducts can be performed at a later stage.

Although rudiments of the lacrimal passages may be present, they will probably be hypoplastic, so that an operation using a Jones tube will be the best and the safest way.

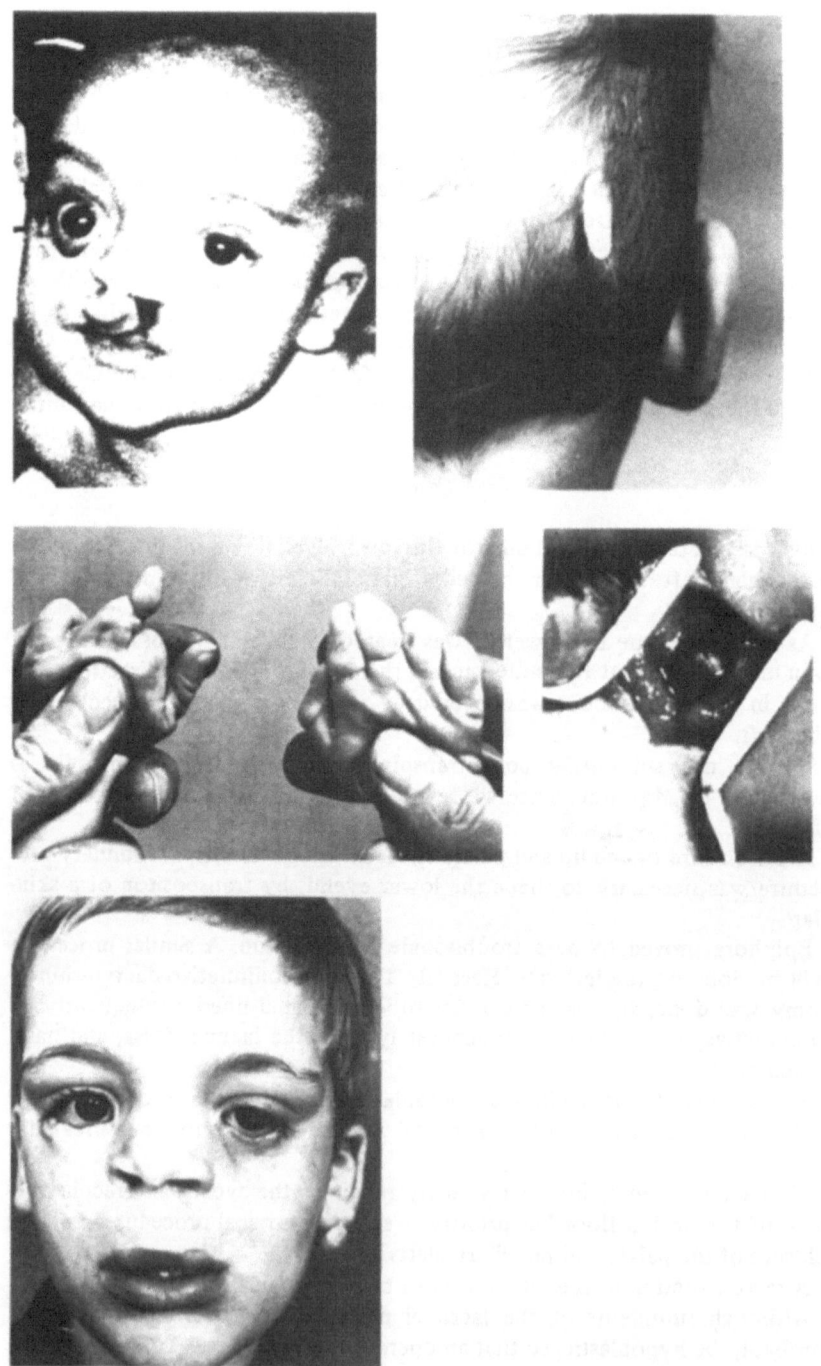

Fig. 3. Case 3. a. Before surgery, 2 months old. b. Fibrocutaneous appendix on the back of the head. c. Hands showing constriction of the fingers. d. Mucous cyst in the right lacrimal fossa. e. After surgery, 4½ years old, wearing an ocular prosthesis on the left side.

REFERENCES

Ask, F. & J. van der Hoeve, Beiträge zur Kenntnis der Entwicklung der Tränenröhrchen unter normalen und abnormen Verhältnissen, letzteres an Fällen von offener schrägen Gesichtsspalte. *A.v. Graefes Arch. Ophtal.* 105: *1157-1196* (1921).

Gunter, G. Nasomaxillary cleft. *Plast. Reconstruct. Surg.* 32: *637* (1963).

Mann, I. Developmental abnormalities of the eye, 2nd ed. Londen (1957).

Mustardé, J.C. Vertical and oblique facial clefts (orbitofacial fissures. pp. 94-101, in: Plastic surgery in infancy and childhood. Livingstone (1971).

Authors' addresses:
B.D. de Jong
Dept of Plastic Surgery
University Hospital
State University of Utrecht
Utrecht
The Netherlands

K.E.W.P. Tan
Royal Dutch Eye Hospital
Utrecht
The Netherlands

Proc. 3rd Int. Symp. on Orbital Disorders, Amsterdam 1977

EYELID RECONSTRUCTION IN FACIAL CLEFTS

B.D. DE JONG

(Utrecht, The Netherlands)

ABSTRACT

Priority is given to operative closure of the defects in the orbital floor and the lower lid, in order to guarantee a functional protection for the eyeball. Defects of the cheek, the upper lip and the palate can be operated in a separate session.

The operative results are demonstrated and developmental problems of the maxillo-facial area are discussed.

Author's address:
Dept of Plastic Surgery
University Hospital
State University of Utrecht
Utrecht
The Netherlands

228

Proc. 3rd Int. Symp. on Orbital Disorders, Amsterdam 1977

DIAGNOSTIC PROBLEMS IN CASES WITH BLOW-OUT FRACTURES AND MOTILITY DISTURBANCES OF OTHER ORIGIN

H. MÜHLENDYCK & D. LEITHÄUSER

(Giessen, W. Germany)

The concept of an orbital 'blow-out' as a mechanism of orbital floor fracture, has been widely recognized and accepted since the classic paper of Smith & Regan (Smith & Regan, 1957; Reny & Stricker, 1969; Hollwich et al., 1970; Lerman, 1970). The diagnostic and therapeutic problems were thoroughly discussed during the 1969 Symposium (Bleeker & Lyle, 1970). It should be remembered, however, that depending on the type of accident, we often find additional disturbances of ocular motility. These can be caused by a posttraumatic Brown's syndrome, central or peripheral nerve palsies and/or changes in the orbital soft tissue.

For the exact analysis of these different patho-etiological factors, meas-

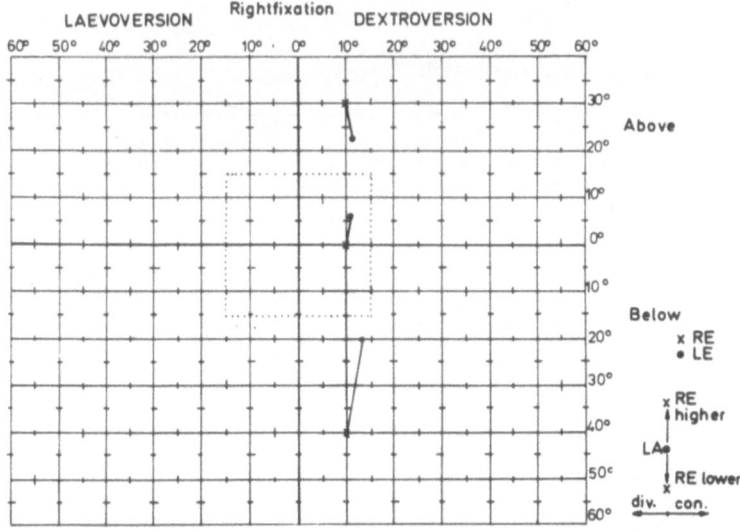

Fig. 1. Diagram of Synoptometer measurements. Intersections of vertical and horizontal lines correspond to the position of the fixing eye. X = right eye, ● = left eye. The gross lines connect the corresponding symbols of each measurement. For comparison the field of gaze which is usually examined with other methods is marked with a punctuated line.

urements of the deviations should be taken every $10°$ in as wide a field of gaze as possible, always under identical examining conditions. The Synoptometer designed by Cüppers is best suited for this purpose (Cüppers, 1972; Cüppers & Mühlendyck, 1976; Mühlendyck, 1975). The measured deviations are plotted on a diagram, in which the intersections of vertical and horizontal lines correspond to the position of the fixing eye (Fig. 1). The right eye is symbolized by a cross and the left eye by a point. The two symbols for each measurement are connected by a straight line.

For illustration, we took three measurements of a patient looking $10°$ to the right. In horizontal gaze, there is a left hypertropia of $6°$ with a slight esotropia. When looking down $40°$, the left hypertropia increases to $20°$. In upward gaze of $30°$ it converts into a right hypertropia of $8°$.

A similar deviation was seen in a twenty year old male patient who had a ski-accident and suffered multiple soft tissue injuries, including lacerations of the left upper eyelid and a typical blow-out fracture. Ten days after the accident the Synoptometer measurements demonstrated a general limitation of motility of the left eye, most pronounced in the upper right gaze (Fig. 2). The forced duction test showed limitation of ocular movement in all directions. The extensive floor fracture was repaired by a combined orbital and transmaxillary approach. After the operation the forced duction test was negative except for elevation in adduction. The Synoptometer measurements revealed a remaining deviation in the upper gaze and especially in the upper right one (Fig. 3). The patient complained of pain in the region of the left trochlea when looking up and to the right and a small thickening of the superior oblique tendon was palpable. These findings indicated that the

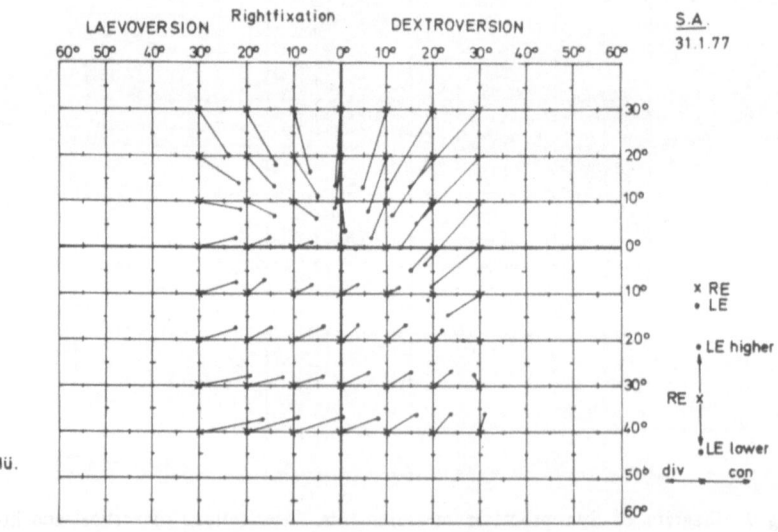

Fig. 2. Case 1, 10 days after blow-out fracture of the left eye. The position of the points demonstrates a general limitation of the movement of the left eye, most pronounced in the upper right gaze.

230

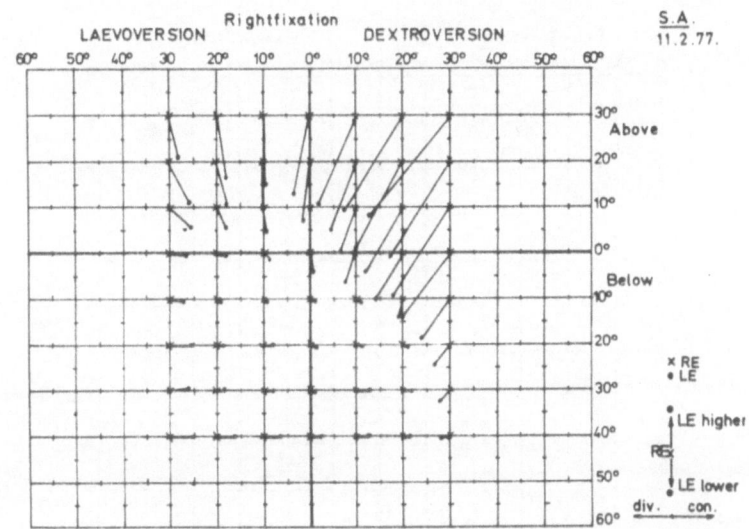

Fig. 3. Case 1, 3 days after repair of the left orbital floor. The lower field of gaze has returned to normal whereas the upper one has not changed at all. This situation indicates a Brown's syndrome.

accident led to injury of the tendon of the left superior oblique muscle, leading to a posttraumatic Brown's syndrome as previously described by Stein (1965). A planned surgical revision was rejected by the patient, so that only anti-inflammatory therapy was given. In contrast to Stein we observed a slow but steady improvement, so that three months later practically no restriction of motility remained (Fig. 4).

Less favourable results were seen in the following case with skull injuries in which an ocular nerve palsy occurred in combination with mechanical limitation of movement. The twenty-three year old female patient had had a car accident and suffered lacerations of her right upper lid and forehead, and was unconscious for one week. Two months later our examination demonstrated a head turn and tilt to the right (Fig. 5), an excyclotropia and a positive Bielschowsky test, indicating a left trochlear nerve palsy. The Synoptometer measurements in right gaze confirmed these findings. Surprisingly, in left gaze there was a left hypertropia on looking upwards which converted to a right hypertropia on looking downwards (Fig. 6).

This deviation could best be explained by an incarceration of the right inferior oblique muscle. This diagnosis was further supported by a hypaesthesia of the infraorbital region, although the tomograms failed to reveal a floor fracture. The forced duction test demonstrated a limitation of both elevation and depression in adduction and an incarceration, as cause of the restriction, was confirmed during surgery. One month later the deviation in the left gaze had markedly improved and after another three months had returned to normal (Fig. 7). The deviation in the right gaze, caused by the

231

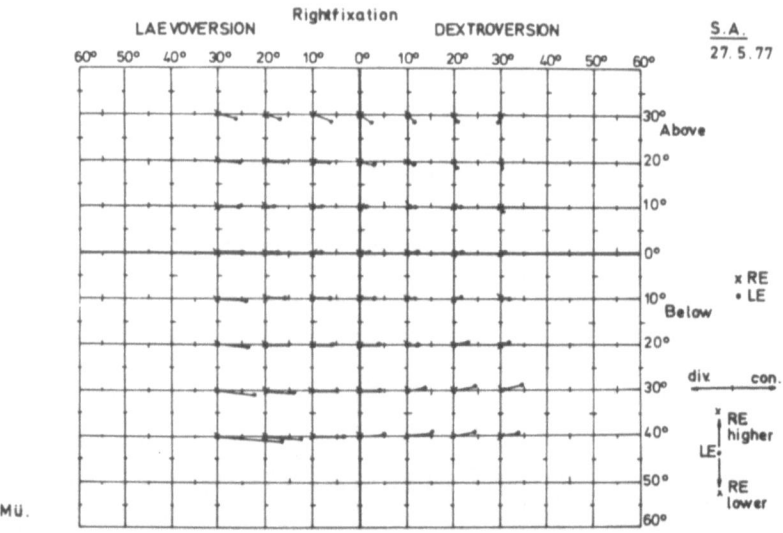

Fig. 4. Case 1, three and a half months later. No restriction of motility remained.

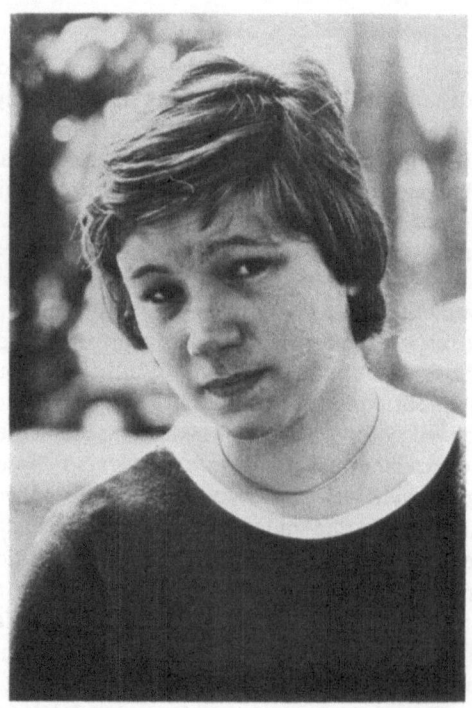

Fig. 5. Case 2, head tilt two months after skull injury mainly due to a left trochlera nerve palsy.

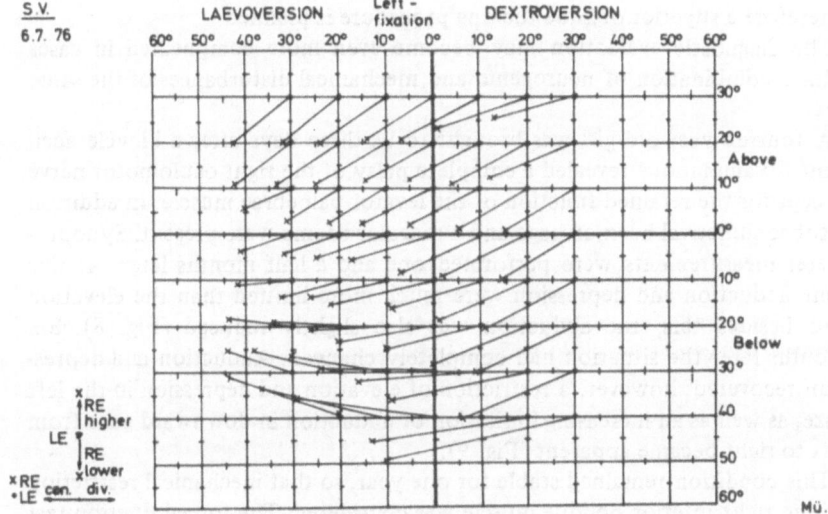

Fig. 6. Case 2, left fixation, the deviation in the right gaze corresponds to the left trochlear nerve palsy.

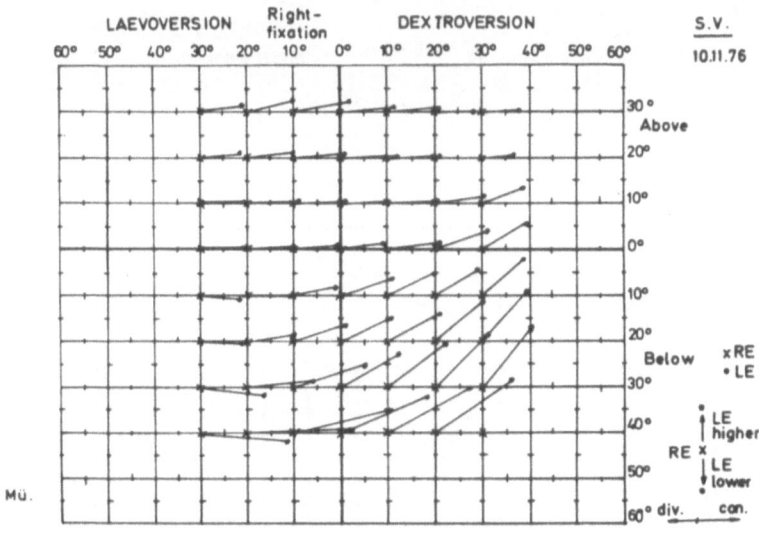

Fig. 7. Case 2, right fixation, four months after surgical exploration of the right orbital floor. The vertical deviations in the left gaze have returned to normal whereas the deviation in the right gaze caused by the left trochlear nerve palsy is unchanged.

left trochlear nerve palsy was unchanged and has remained for one year. Therefore a superior oblique tucking procedure is planned.

The diagnostic evaluation may become even more complicated in cases with a combination of neurogenic and mechanical disturbances of the same eye.

A fourten year old girl was brought to us three days after a bicycle accident. Examinations revealed a complete palsy of the right oculomotor nerve except for the retained function of the levator palpebrae muscle. In addition a subconjunctival haemorrhage and a macular edema were present. Synoptometer measurements were performed one and a half months later. At this time adduction and depression were much more limited than the elevation and besides this, the abduction was also slightly reduced (Fig. 8). Six months later the situation had completely changed. Adduction and depression recovered; however, a restriction of elevation and depression in the left gaze, as well as an increasing limitation of abduction in downward gaze from left to right became apparent (Fig. 9).

This condition remained stable for one year, so that mechanical restriction of the right inferior oblique muscle was considered. The forced duction test confirmed this diagnosis, although no orbital floor fracture could be demonstrated on X-ray, and no incarceration was found on surgical exploration. Postoperatively the forced duction test remained the same and there was a slight increase in the restriction of the movement, especially in upward gase (Fig. 10). This condition did not change over the next two years.

Before discussing possible explanations of this problem, another, similar, case will be presented.

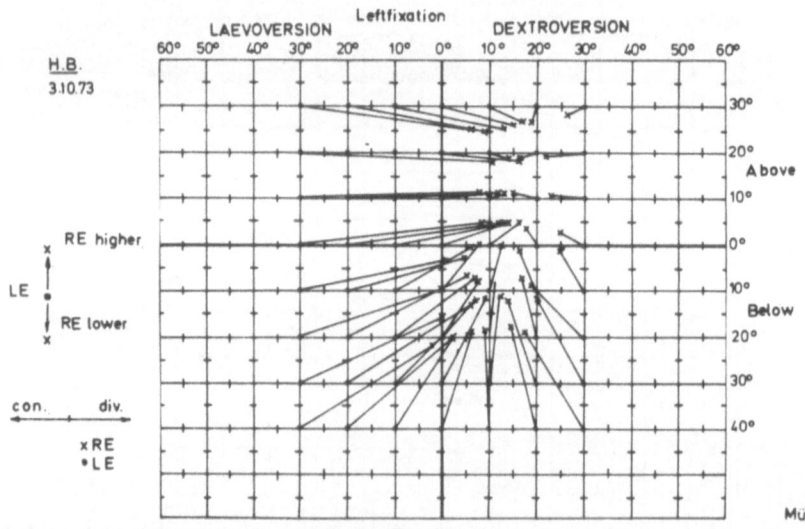

Fig. 8. Case 3, one and a hlaf months after right orbital trauma; uncomplete oculomotor nerve palsy and restriction of abduction is found.

234

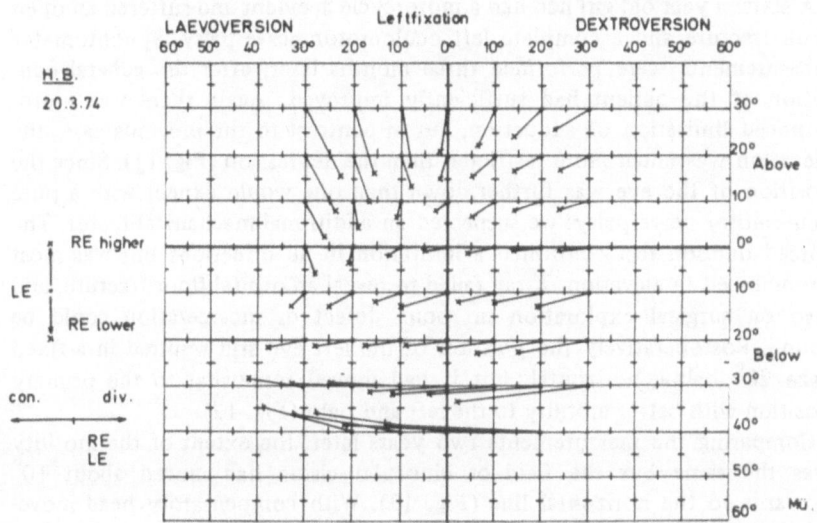

Fig. 9. Case 3, six months later, spontaneous recovery of adduction and depression is found. In left gaze a restriction of elevation and in downward gaze an increasing limitation of abduction of the right eye becomes apparent.

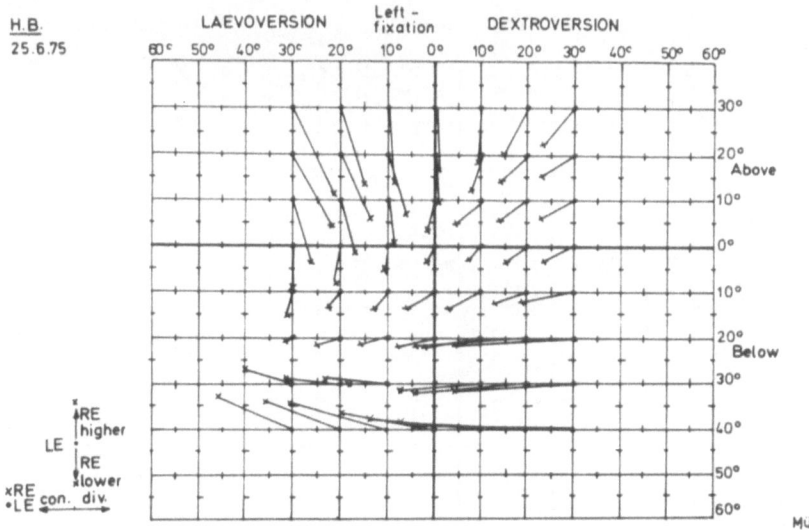

Fig. 10. Case 3, condition after surgical exploration of the right orbital floor. There is a slight deterioration of the motility in upward gaze.

A sixteen year old girl had had a motorcycle accident and suffered an open skull fracture and a complete left oculomotor nerve palsy. Synoptometer measurements were performed three months later, after the general condition of the patient had sufficiently improved. Again there was a pronounced limitation of adduction, but in contrast to the previous case, the elevation was much more restricted than the depression (Fig. 11). Since the position of the eye was further down than one would expect with a pure oculomotor nerve palsy; we suspected an additional mechanical factor. The forced duction test confirmed a limitation in all directions but was most pronounced in elevation. X-ray failed to reveal an orbital floor fracture, and also on surgical exploration no bone defect or incarceration could be found. Postoperatively the position of the left eye still resulted in a fixed gaze $20°$ below horizontal, but it had moved somewhat to the primary position with better motility to the left and right (Fig. 12).

Comparing the measurements two years later, the extent of the motility was the same but the field of binocular vision had moved about $10°$ upwards to the horizontal line (Fig. 13). With compensatory head movemetns the patient is able to get around quite well now. However, an aberrant regeneration of the oculomotor nerve had led to a paradoxical lid innervation (Fig. 14).

Although in the last two cases no orbital floor fractures could be demonstrated, there is no question that a substantial orbital compression trauma took place which is indicated, for instance, by the pronounced macular edema in the first case. Since the bony structures did not fracture there was a concentration of pressure at the apex of the orbit (Fig. 15). We feel that

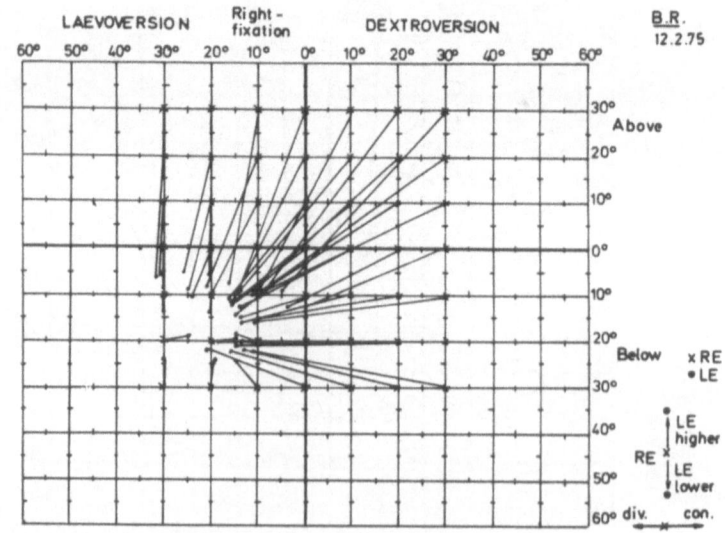

Fig. 11. Case 4, three months after open skull fracture with a complete left oculomotor palsy.

236

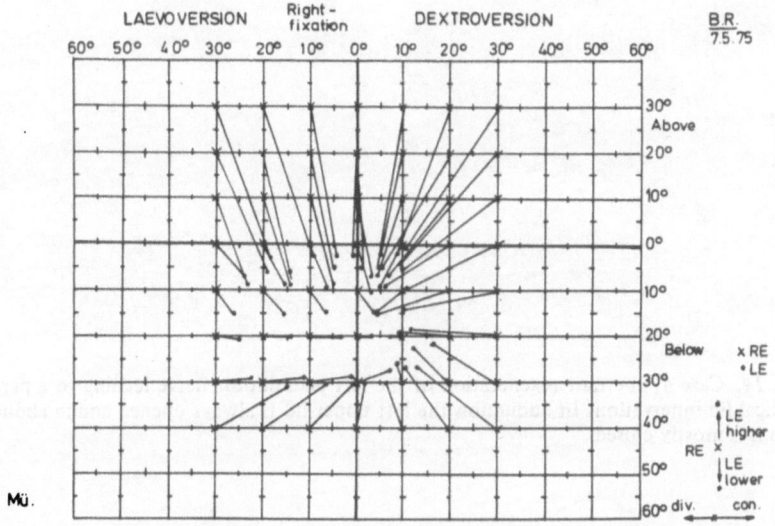

Fig. 12. Case 4, one month after surgical exploration of the left orbital floor, better motility to the right and left.

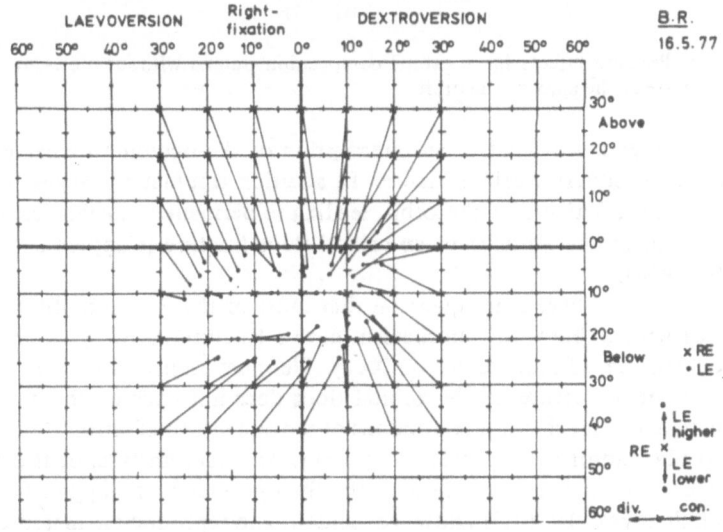

Fig. 13. Case 4, two years later, the extent of motility is the same but the field of restricted motility has moved about 10° upward to the horizontal line.

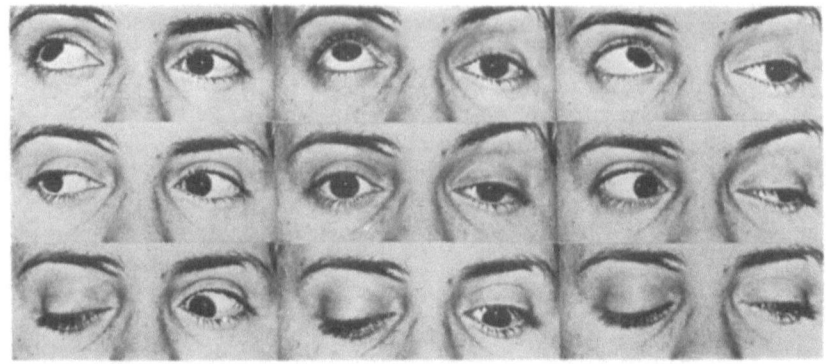

Fig. 14. Case 4, aberrant regeneration of the left oculomotor nerve leading to a para-doxical lid-innervation. In adduction the left upper lid is always opened and in abduc-tion it is mostly closed.

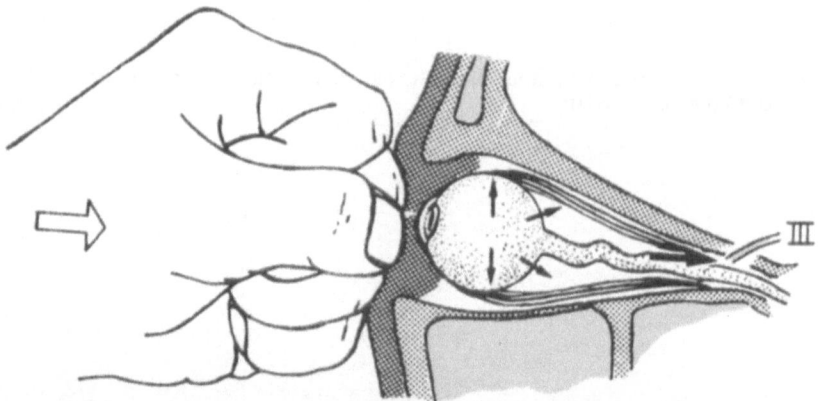

Fig. 15. Pressure effects in an orbital compression trauma without blow-out fracture concentrate at the apex of the orbit.

this compression has led to an interruption of the oculomotor nerve at the level of the superior orbital fissure. In addition traumatic changes occurred within the soft tissue of the orbit, leading to permanent mechanical restrictions even in the absence of an orbital floor fracture (Cüppers & Mühlen-dyck, 1976).

In summary, there is no question that most of the orbital motility distur-bances with a 'blow-out' mechanism have a fracture, although such a frac-ture might be difficult to see on X-ray. We must realize, however, that the absence of a fracture of the orbital floor does not exclude the possibility of permanent mechanical restrictions of movement. In addition a damage to the ocular motor nerves might be present. An exact analysis of these com-plicated cases is best possible with the Synoptometer of Cüppers (Cüppers & Mühlendyck, 1976). It allows continuous and reproducible measurements of eye movements in all directions to the most extreme positions of gaze (Cüppers, 1972; Cüppers & Mühlendyck, 1976; Mühlendyck, 1976).

REFERENCES

Bleeker, G. & M.T. Keith Lyle. Fractures of the orbit. In: Proc. Symp. on Orbital Fractures, Amsterdam 1969. Excerpta Medica, Amsterdam (1970).

Cüppers, C. Determination of the objective angle. *Orthoptics: 65–71* (1972).

Cüppers, C. & H. Mühlendyck. Die Verwendung des Synoptometers zur Differential-diagnose und postoperativen Verlaufskontorlle von sog. 'Blow-out' Frakturen. pp. 50–70, in: Das Kopftrauma aus augenärztlicher Sicht (W. Ehrich & O. Remler, eds.). Bücherei des Augenarztes 68. Enke Verlag, Stuttgart (1976).

Hollwich, F., G. Jünemann & E. Damaske. Klinischer Beitrag zur 'Blow-out Fraktur'. *Klin. Mbl. Augenheilk.* 156: *864–873* (1970).

Lerman, S. Blow-out fractures of the orbit. Diagnosis and treatment. *Br. J. Ophthal.* 54: *90–98* (1970).

Mühlendyck, H. Der Synoptometer als Grundlage von Operationsindikationen und Verlaufskontrolle bei komplizierten Augenmuskelstörungen. *Klin. Mbl. Augenheilk.* 167: *892–899* (1975).

Reny, H. & M. Stricker. Fractures de l'orbite. Masson et Cie, Paris (1969).

Smith, B. & W.F. Regan. Blow-out fracture of the orbit (mechanism and correction of internal orbital fracture). *Am. J. Ophthal.* 44: *733–739* (1957).

Stein, R. Posttraumatische intermittierende Pseudoparesen des Musculus obliquus inferior. (Bemerkungen zum Sehnenscheiden-Syndroom des Musculus obliquus superior). *Klin. Mbl. Augenheilk.* 147: *712–720* (1965).

Authors' addresses:
H. Mühlendyck
Abteilung für Orthoptik, Pleoptik und Motilitätsstörungen
Friedrichstrasse 18
6300 Giessen
W. Germany

D. Leithäuser
Abteilung für Hlas-Nasen-Ohrenheilkunde
Feulgenstrasse 10
6300 Giessen
W. Germany

Proc. 3rd Int. Symp. on Orbital Disorders, Amsterdam 1977

MECHANISMS, TOLERANCE LIMIT CURVE AND THEORETICAL ANALYSIS IN BLOW-OUT FRACTURES OF TWO AND THREE-DIMENSIONAL ORBITAL WALL MODELS*

TOYOMI FUJINO & TAKESHI B. SATO

(Tokyo, Japan)

According to Converse & Smith (1957), the orbital blow-out fracture is caused by a sudden increase of intraorbital pressure resulting from the application of a traumatic force to the soft tissue of the orbital area. This concept is supported by a classical experimental study by Smith (1957). His original description is as follows.

A baseball was placed over the closed lids of a cadaber orbit and the baseball was struck sharply with a hammer. Exenteration of the orbit revealed the fracture in its entirety. No fracture of the orbital rim or zygomatic arch was observed. In a second experiment, the opposite orbit of the cadaver was exentrated. The soft tissue of the rim was excised to allow a direct contact between the bony orbital circumference and the surfacing of the baseball. Repeated blows of similar force with the hammer failed to fracture the floor or the rim of the orbit. When the striking force was sufficiently increased, the orbital floor and the orbital rim collapsed simultaneously.

On reviewing this description, one would think that presence of the orbital contents is essential for development of the orbital blowout fracture. In other words, the orbital blowout fracture should not occur in the absence of the orbital contents. However, our experimental study on the dried human skull in the absence of the orbital contents showed clearly a typical punched out fracture of the orbital floor (Fujino, 1974). This phenomenon cannot be explained by Smith & Converse's concept.

In addition, the weakest point in Smith's study is that he drew his conclusion from pre and postoperative findings only, not from the experimental processes. In order to clarify the experimental process and result, we designed a two-dimensional eye model, resembling a cut section of the dried human skull from the mid-portion of the infraorbital margin to the optic canal, and a three-dimensional eye model, resembling a full sized orbit.

TWO-DIMENSIONAL EXPERIMENTAL EYE MODEL

A full sized two-dimensional eye model consisting of epoxy resin for the

* This study was supported by grants of the Yukichi Fukuzawa Memorial Fund (1975), the Takahashi Research Foundation for Industry and Economics (1975–76) and the Keio University Education and Research Development Fund (1976).

240

orbital walls, filled wtih 25% gelatin solution as the orbital contents, and with a 2.5 cm sized soft silastic eyeball. The sides of the eye model were covered by a thin silicone membrane with crossed mesh pattern, 0.5 cm apart (Fig. 1).

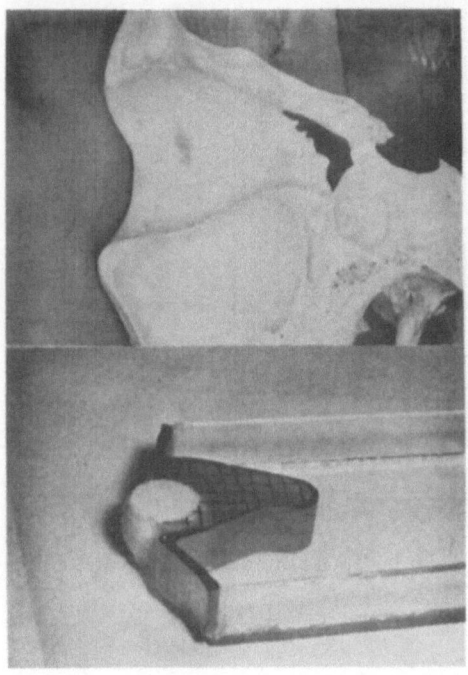

Fig. 1. Two-dimensional eye model. The upper part shows a section of the human dried skull from the mid-portion of the infraorbital margin to the optic canal. The lower part shows a full sized two-dimensional eye model, simulated with the above cut section.

Experiments

A swing type of impact tester was used (Fig. 2). The striker or a baseball dropped from the height desired. All movements of the eye model were recorded by a high speed camera, ranging from 500 to 1000 frames per second. Acceleration of the impacter was also recorded.

Three series of impact tests were performed. Test 1 was the impact on eyeball alone, and the direction of the impact was from the midpoint of the eyeball to the optic canal. Test 2 was the impact on the infraorbital margin, and the direction of the impact was from the infraorbital margin to the optic canal. Test 3 was the impact on both the eyeball and the infraorbital margin and the direction of the impact was between that of tests 1 and 2.

In order to confirm the experimental results mentioned above, the numerical calculation with a digital computer in the two-dimensional mathematical eye model formed by the masses, the springs, and dash pots was performed.

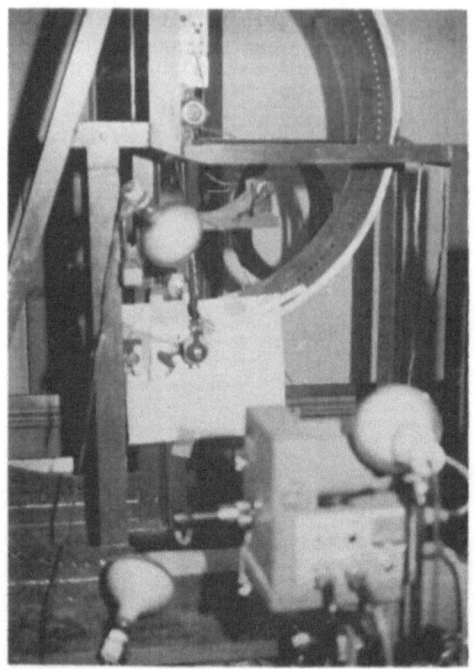

Fig. 2. Total picture of the impact tester.

Results

Test 1: Impact on eyeball alone

After taking the high speed movie films, each movement of the orbital walls and crossed mesh patterns were traced. The movement of the eyeball and the deviation of the crossed mesh patterns, especially behind the eyeball, were great, indicating an increased orbital pressure (Fig. 3a,b). However, this happened when the baseball hit the eyeball alone, without making contact with the orbital bony circumferences at the same time. This is different from Smith's experimental result. In this case, only a linear fracture of the orbital floor occurred. When the kinetic energy was increased, the baseball struck the frontal and zygomatic bones, but still only a linear fracture was noted.

A computer analysis confirmed the experimental result (Fig. 3c).

Test 2: Impact on infraorbital margin

Mesh patterns moved posteriorly in almost the same distance at each point (Fig. 4a,b,c). This means that the pressure of the orbital contents was not so high as in Test 1, but the orbital contents were pulled posteriorly by the deviation of the orbital walls, especially of the orbital floor. Finally, the orbital floor was fractured, as if the pole had buckled. When the kinetic energy was increased, a second fracture of the orbital floor posterior to the

242

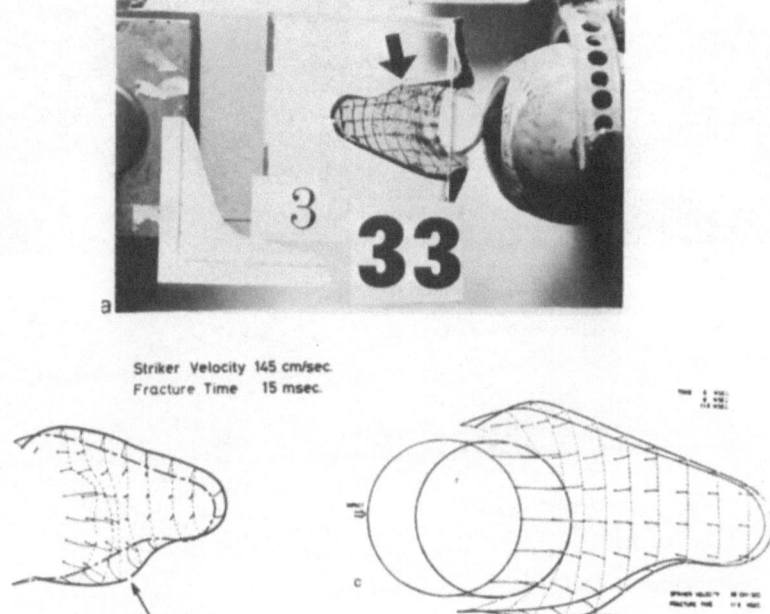

Striker Velocity 145 cm/sec.
Fracture Time   15 msec.

Fracture

Fig. 3. Impact on the eyeball alone. (a) An arrow indicates a linear fracture of the orbital floor. (b) Analysis of mesh pattern. Note a remarkable distortion of mesh pattern, especially behind the eyeball, indicating an increased hydraulic pressure of the orbital contents. (c) Computer analysis of the mathematical eye model. Note a similar pattern of the intraorbital distortion with (b).

first fracture was observed. Immediately after the first fracture occurred, both ends of the anterior and posterior segments were still in contact with each other. Further impact force to the anterior segment pushed the posterior segment upwards, twisting the far posterior portion of the posterior segment and finally fracturing it into two sections. This phenomenon was only observed in Tests 2 and 3, not in Test 1.

The computer analysis showed similar patterns, indicating the buckling force of the orbital floor as the main cause of the fracture (Fig. 4d).

Test 3: Impact on both eyeball and infraorbital margin

The result showed a similar pattern to that of Test 2, confirmed by computer analysis (Fig. 5).

Tolerance limit curve

The tolerance limit curve is obtained by placing the maximum impact force (peak acceleration x mass of the impactor) in the ordinate, and the rise time in the abscissa.

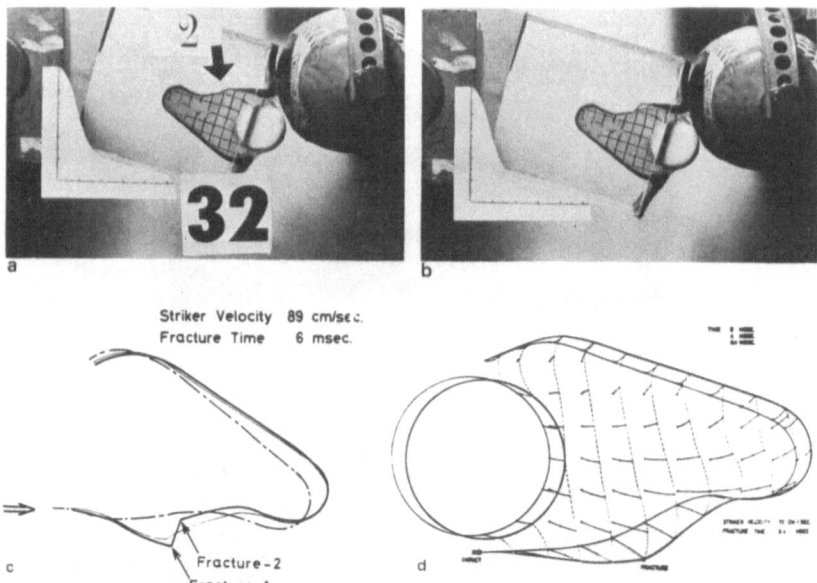

Striker Velocity 89 cm/sec.
Fracture Time 6 msec.

Fracture-2
Fracture-1

Fig. 4. Impact on the infraorbital margin. (a) Note a linear fracture of the orbital floor. (b) Note the two points fracture of the orbital floor by further impact force, followed by a linear fracture. (c) Movement of the orbital walls through the impact. The dotted line is the pre-experimental position of the orbital walls, the narrow solid line shows when a linear fracture occurred, and the wide solid line indicates when the two points fracture occurred. (d) Computer analysis of the mathematical eye model. Note the posterior transposition of mesh pattern.

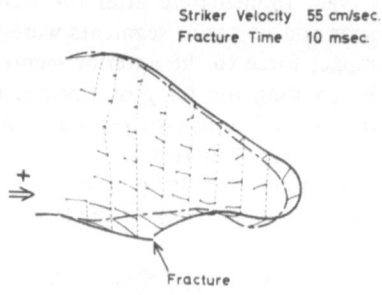

Striker Velocity 55 cm/sec.
Fracture Time 10 msec.

Fracture

Fig. 5. Impact on the eyeball and infraorbital margin. Note a similar pattern of mesh movement as in Figure 4.

More impact force was necessary in order to produce the orbital floor fracture in the case of impact to the eyeball alone. Less impact force produced an orbital floor fracture in the case of impact on the infraorbital margin, and both the eyeball and infraorbital margin (Fig. 6).

244

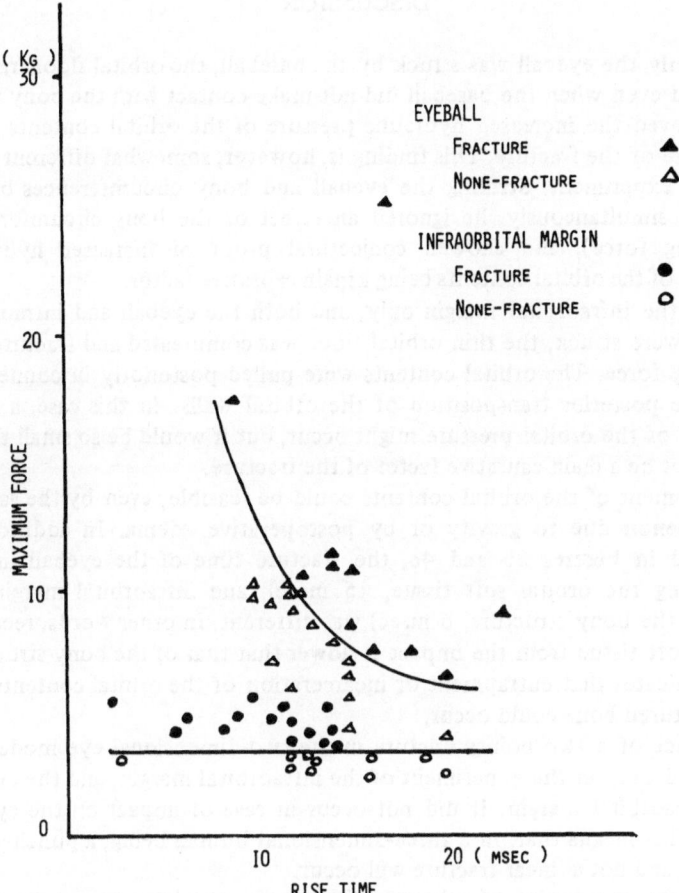

Fig. 6. Tolerance limit curve of two-dimensional eye model. The orbital floor is fractured by less impact force than the infraorbital margin, and both the eyeball and infraorbital margin were struck, and are fractured by more impact force when the eyeball alone was struck.

THREE-DIMENSIONAL EYE MODEL AND MATHEMATICAL MODEL

In order to confirm the results from the two-dimensional eye model, a three-dimensional eye model study was performed. In addition, simulations were carried out by digital computer, utilizing a three-dimensional mathematical eye model, composed of the rahmen elements for the orbital bones, and the voigt models and lumped masses for the orbital tissues, in order to investigate the behaviour of the orbital walls and contents, and its tolerance limits.

RESULTS

The three-dimensional experimental eye model studies confirmed the findings of the experiments with the two-dimensional model.

DISCUSSION

When only the eyeball was struck by the baseball, the orbital floor fracture occurred even when the baseball did not make contact with the bony walls. This proved the increased hydraulic pressure of the orbital contents to be the cause of the fracture. This finding is, however, somewhat different from Smith's experiment. Striking the eyeball and bony circumferences by the baseball simultaneously, he ignored an effect of the bony circumferences (buckling force), and showed conjectural proof of increased hydraulic pressure of the orbital contents being a main causative factor.

When the infraorbital margin only, and both the eyeball and infraorbital margin were struck, the thin orbital floor was compressed and fractured by buckling force. The orbital contents were pulled posteriorly in connection with the posterior transposition of the orbital walls. In this case, a slight increase of the orbital pressure might occur, but it would be so small that it could not be a main causative factor of the fracture.

Entrapment of the orbital contents could be feasible, even by the sagging phenomenon due to gravity or by postoperative edema. In addition, as observed in Figures 3b and 4c, the fracture time of the eyeball impact (reflecting the orbital soft tissue, 15 msec), and infraorbital margin (reflecting the bony structure, 6 msec) was different. In other words, recovery of the soft tissue from the impact is slower that that of the bony structure. This indicates that entrapment or incarceration of the orbital contents into the fractured bone could occur.

The fact of a two points fracture in the two-dimensional eye model was produced only in the experiment of the infraorbital margin, and the eyeball and infraorbital margin. It did not occur in case of impact on the eyeball alone. This means that, in a three-dimensional human being, a punched out fracture and not a linear fracture will occur.

From the standpoint of tolerance limit curve, the later two experiments require only a fraction (less than 1/3 in 3 dimensional eye model) of the buckling force, as compared with the former experiment. In daily traumatic cases, less impact force to the face will more likely occur.

According to the findings mentioned above, the orbital blow-out fracture is more likely to occur through the impact on the infraorbital margin, and the buckling force on the orbital floor.

Throughout the experiments, an interesting finding was observed. Even in the case of non-fracture experiments, the orbital contents were equally distorted as in cases of fractures. This phenomenon explains the clinical pictures of bizarre and multiple symptoms of the orbital trauma.

CONCLUSION

The orbital blowout fracture is more likely to be produced by a buckling force on the orbital floor in our two- and three-dimensional eye model and mathematical eye model experiments.

REFERENCES

Converse, J.M. & B. Smith. Enophthalmos and diplopia in fractures of the orbital floor. *Br. J. Plast. Surg.* 9: *267* (1957).

Fujino, T. Experimental blowout fracture of the orbit. *Plast. & Reconstr. Surg.* 54: *81* (1974).

Fujino, T., T. Harashina, Y. Yoshimura, M. Ohshima & T.B. Sato. Mechanism, tolerance limit curve and theoretical analysis in blowout fracture of two dimensional orbital wall model. *Jap. J. Plast. & Reconstr. Surg.* 19: *43* (1976).

Fujino, T., T. Nakajima, Y. Maruyama, Y. Moribe & T.B. Sato. Tolerance limit curve in blowout fracture of the orbit with eye models. *Jap. J. Plast. & Reconstr. Surg.* 18: *244* (1975).

Fujino, T., C. Sugimoto, S. Tajima, Y. Moribe & T.B. Sato. Mechanism of orbital blowout fracture. II. Analysis by high-speed camera in a two-dimensional eye model. *Keio J. Med.* 23: *115* (1974).

Fujino, T., S. Tajima, R. Tanino. C. Sugimoto, F. Aoyagi, Y. Moribe & T.B. Sato. Mechanism of orbital blowout fracture. Dynamic impact test with a two-dimensional eye model. *Jap. J. Plast. & Reconstr. Surg.* 17: *247* (1974).

Sato, T.B., T. Fujino, H. Nakajima & Y. Moribe. Theoretical analysis of mechanism of orbital blowout fracture with a digital computer. *Jap. J. Plast. & Reconstr. Surg.* 17: *550* (1974).

Smith, B. & W.F. Regan, Jr. Blowout fracture of the orbit. Mechanism and correction of internal orbital fracture. *Am. J. Ophthal.* 44: *733* (1957).

Authors' address:
Department of Plastic and Reconstructive Surgery
School of Medicine
Keio University
Tokyo 160
Japan

STABLE FIXATION OF FRACTURES OF THE ZYGOMATIC BONE WITH THE USE OF AO COMPRESSION PLATES

G.J. KUSEN, H.P. VAN DEN AKKER & M. BAZUIN

(Amsterdam, The Netherlands)

ABSTRACT

Until recently fractures of the zygomatic bone with caudal and dorsal dislocation were, after reduction, fixated with wire osteosynthesis at the fronto-zygomatic suture. In some cases endorotation of the zygomatic bone necessitated additional wiring in the infra-orbital rim.

To avoid the infra-orbital approach we used 4 hole AO 'mini' compression plates for fixation at the fronto-zygomatic suture. With this method endorotation of the zygomatic bone and flattening of the cheek was prevented, which proved to be of considerable value especially in old or infra-orbital comminuted fractures.

Authors' address:
University Hospital
104 1e Helmerstraat
Amsterdam
The Netherlands

Proc. 3rd Int. Symp. on Orbital Disorders, Amsterdam 1977

THE BLOW-OUT FRACTURE IN THE VIEW OF AN OPHTHALMOLOGIST

F. HOLLWICH, H. BUSSE & H.P. SCHIFFER

(Münster, W. Germany)

Blow-out fractures are of special interest to ophthalmologists, as they often cause diplopia. Reviewing the history, it is interesting to note that the first reports of blow-out fractures were reported by ophthalmologists. Already in 1892, before radiography had been introduced, the Austrian Theodor Beer reported 15 cases of traumatic enophthalmos, including two personal observations. Lederer, also an ophthalmologist, published another report in 1902, including 49 cases – 3 observations of his own – and postulated a cleft-like fracture of the orbital floor as the underlying cause.

This interest of ophthalmologists in blow-out fractures is primarily based on the diplopia which is often the consequence of this condition. It is vertical diplopia that is the alarming sign which brings the ophthalmologist on the scene. However, vertical diplopia is often noted by the patient only after the accompanying signs and symptoms of edema, haematoma and inflammation have subsided. This means that the patient has often left the hospital before vertical diplopia appears. Once this diplopia appears, the picture is quite characteristic allowing an easy diagnosis.

In this paper we would like to discuss two aspects of blow-out fractures: first, the surgical approach in recent injuries, and, second, the management of late cases. Our discussion is based on the observation of 68 of our own cases. Fig. 1 lists the ocular symptoms observed in these 68 patients at their admission to our eye clinic. Enophthalmos is not an early sign in uncom-

Primary
Ocular Symptomatology (68 patients)

1)   Periorbital edema, hematoma, pseudo-ptosis   36

2)   Motility disturbance: vertical diplopia   28 ⎫
                            hypotropia   2 ⎬ 32
                            hypertropia   2 ⎭

3)   Hypesthesia of the infraorbitalis nerve
     and hyposphagma   14 ⎫ 26
     Reduced vision   12 ⎭

4)   Enophthalmus

Fig. 1. Ocular symptomatology observed in 68 patients at admission to our clinic.

plicated blow-out fractures without a fracture of the orbital rim; it is seen after the swelling and edema of the orbital tissue have been reabsorbed.

In the next figures we would like to demonstrate which muscles were affected (Fig. 2). Quite naturally the inferior rectus muscle was most frequently involved. Fig. 3 shows the causes of accident. As other authors, we also found that the great majority of our blow-out fracture patients had been involved in traffic accidents. Fig. 4 shows the cases in which inter-disciplinary surgery was indicated. The surgical results of 49 patients included in Fig. 1) who were admitted with a delay of 14 days are shown in Figure 5.

We would now like to point out two aspects concerning the surgical procedure:
1. The surgical approach.
2. The management of late cases with diplopia.

Pareses after accident   (68 patients)
                          1968 - 1977

1) isolated paresis: 35
   M. rectus inferior   24
   M. obliquus inferior   11

2) combined pareses: 32
   M. rectus sup.a.obl.inf.   1o
   M. rectus inf. and internus   6
   M. rectus ext.,int.a.obl.sup.   5
   M. rectus inf. a. obl. inf.   3
   M. rectus int. a. obl. sup.   4
   M. rectus int.,inf.,obl.sup.   2
   M. rectus inf.,ext. a. sup.   2

3) ophthalmoplegia totalis: 1

            total   68

Fig. 2. Demonstration of the affected muscles (68 patients).

Causes of accident   (68 patients)

Traffic   3o persons   (44,1 %)

Work   12 persons   (17,6 %)

Fight/Play   12 persons   (17,6 %)

Sport   4 persons   (5,8 %)

others   1o persons   (14,7 %)
(i.e. hoof beat)

Fig. 3. Various causes of accidents.

250

<u>Ophthalmological or interdisciplinary wound-dressing</u>
(68 patients)

Ophthalmological   44
Interdisciplinary   24

Fig. 4. Cases requiring interdisciplinary surgery.

<u>Results of operations</u>

I. **49 patients – admission in the delay of 14 days:**

   44 **good results, in the field of use of binocular
      visualisation, monocular vision**
   2 **no binocular visualisation**
   2 **loss of vision in one eye (optic atrophy, detachment)**
   1 **no objectivation possible**

Fig. 5. Surgical results of 49 patients after operation.

THE SURGICAL APPROACH

Incision

The incision for the repair of blow-out fractures may be done in three
different ways (Fig. 6):
a) *The conjunctival approach:* The incision opens the lower conjunctival sac,
bringing the surgeon in the neighbourhood of orbital tissues: fat and muscle

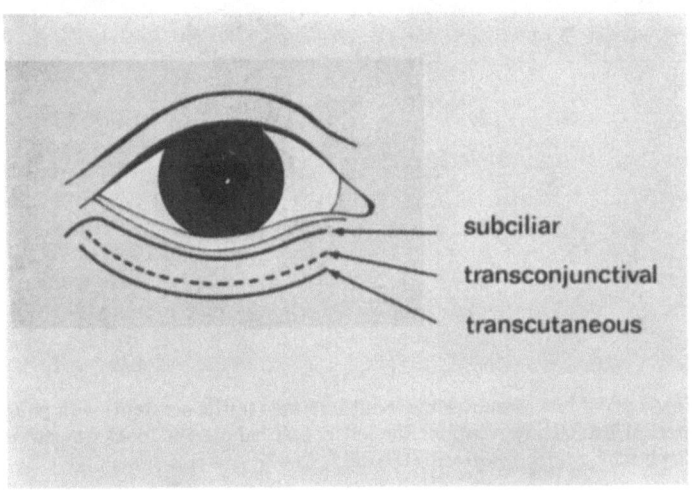

subciliar

transconjunctival

transcutaneous

Fig. 6. Three different possibilities of incision for the repair of blow-out fractures.

251

sheaths. After wound closure a scar develops extending throughout the lower part of the conjunctival sac.

b) *The subciliary incision:* Sometimes the surgeon interferes with the tarsal plate and the adhering fibres of the orbicularis muscle. Subsequently an ectropion may rarely develop.

c) *The transcutaneous incision:* We prefer this easy access to the periostium at the orbital rim, avoiding interference with the tarsal plate and the globe. If the wound is closed layer by layer and the orbicularis muscle is sutured carefully without including other tissues, persisting or remittent postoperative edema can be avoided.

THE MANAGEMENT OF LATE CASES WITH DIPLOPIA

The other aspect is the management of late cases, in which surgical intervention did not happen or was not successful in restoring binocular vision because of fibrosis and shrinkage of the incarcerated muscles.

In these cases a mechanically induced squint problem and, consequently, diplopia persists. These cases require evaluation of the ocular motility with the red glass test or, as we do, by Lees-screen observation. A combined resection and recession of the involved muscles is performed. This procedure has a good chance of success if the patient has exact normal retinal correspondence and sufficient amplitude of fusion.

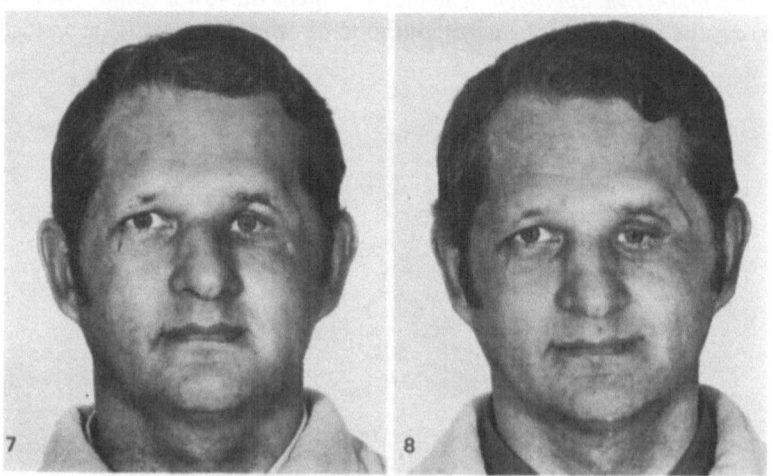

Fig. 7. First case of late diagnosed blow-out fracture (traffic accident) with poor result of late surgical orbital intervention: the left enophthalmic eye looks downwards and diplopia is present.

Fig. 8. The same patient after muscle surgery (recession of the inferior rectus (10 mm)) with normal primary position of the eyes.

252

PERSONAL OBSERVATIONS

In our 68 cases we observed five cases wth mechanically induced paralytic squint. After muscle surgery in 4 patients, who had binocular single vision prior to injury, we got a restricted, but sufficient binocular field of vision.

Case reports

The following two cases may demonstrate the procedure and the result of muscle surgery.

The *first case* is that of a 49 year old male patient who had multiple fractures with a late diagnosed blow-out fracture (traffic accident, 23.1.70) with poor result of late surgical orbital intervention (23.4.71). The left enophthalmic eye looked downwards and he had diplopia (Fig. 7).

After muscle surgery (19.5.71), recession of the inferior rectus (10 mm), he regained a normal primary position of the eyes (Fig. 8) with a limited binocular single vision (Fig. 9) and a field of fixation, adequate for his requirements (Figs. 10 and 11).

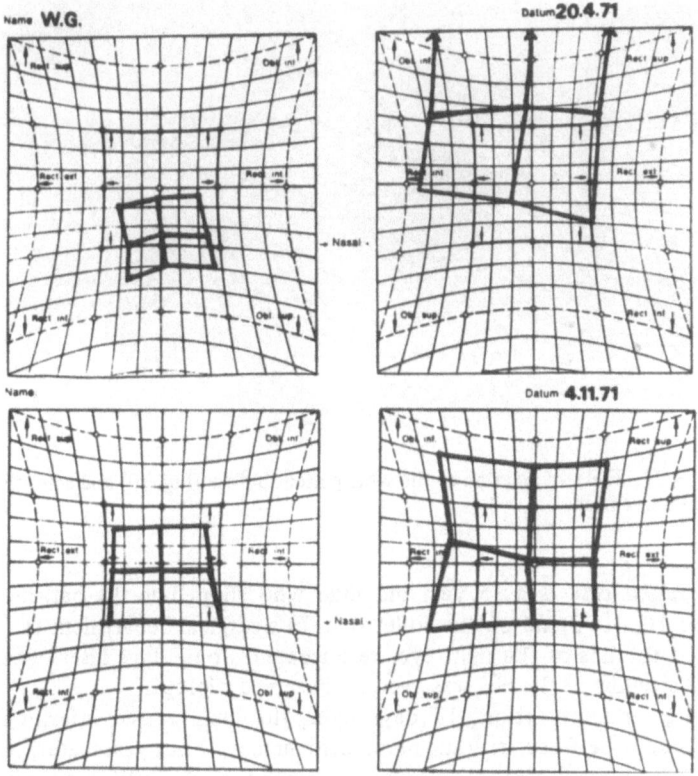

Fig. 9. Lees-screen of the above-mentioned patient before (20.4.71) and after (4.11. 71) surgical intervention: limited binocular single vision after surgery.

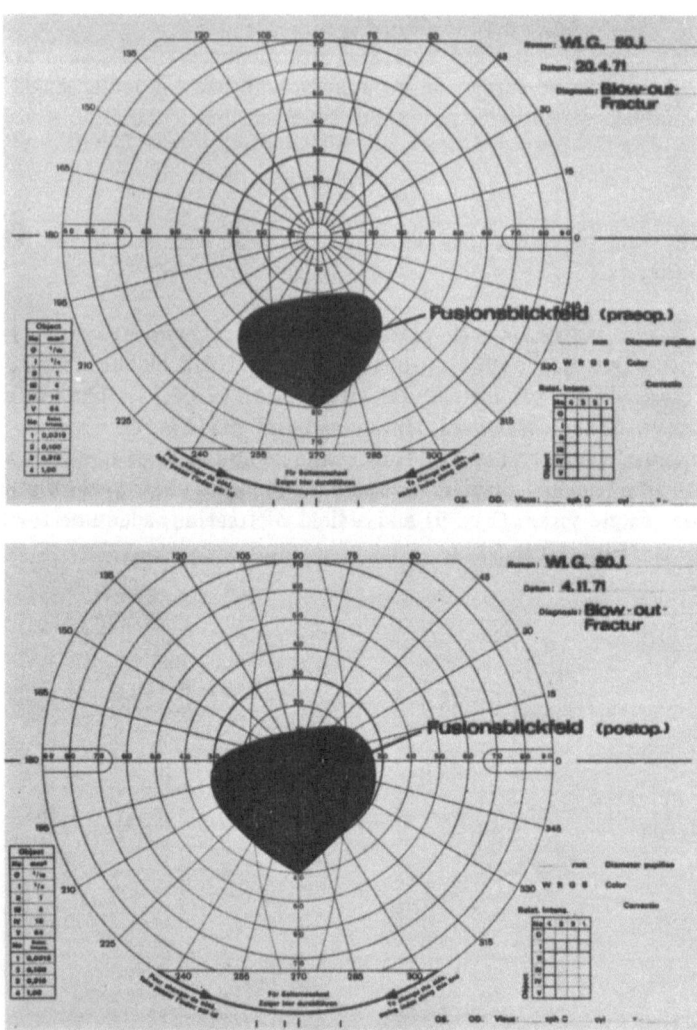

Figs. 10 + 11. Field of fixation of the same patient before (Fig. 10) and after (Fig. 11) surgical intervention.

The *second case* is a 35 year old man who slipped in the bathroom on October 10, 1973 and on the toilet seat. In a surgical department the lacerations of the lids of the right eye were treated. Some days later, when the marked swelling of the lids was over, he observed diplopia.

By surgical intervention, 18 days later, the incarcerated inferior rectus muscle could be freed without permanent success. Four years later, on May 3, 1977 the patient came to our clinic: a secondary paralytic strabismus had developed (Fig. 12). The right traumatized eye was deviated, the internal rectus and the inferior rectus were paretic.

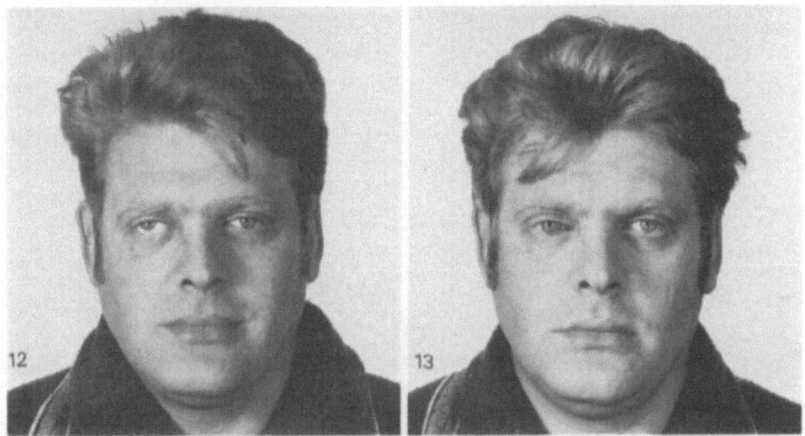

Fig. 12. Second case of late diagnosed blow-out fracture with secondary paralytic strabismus, deviation of the right traumatized eye, the internus rectus and the inferior rectus are paretic.

Fig. 13. The same patient after muscle surgery (20 days later): binocular vision is regained.

We performed the following muscle surgery on the 4 recti on May 4 and 17, 1977:
1. Tenotomy of the right externus.
2. Resection (6 mm) of the right inferior rectus.
3. Recession (3.5 mm) of the right superior rectus.
4. Thirteen days later on May 17, 1977: resection (6 mm) of the right medialis rectus of the right eye. Twenty days after surgery (Fig. 13), binocular vision was regained and now the Lees-screen before and after surgery (Fig. 14).

In this case of severe posttraumatic paralytic squint with diplopia a sufficient field of central binocular vision could be restored.

CONCLUSIONS

In conclusion we would like to say that the decisive point of blow-out surgery is to regain the binocular motility. The early investigation of ocular motility during the first two weeks, is of importance to decide whether or not surgical intervention is indicated. Furthermore, we discussed the different possibilities of approach to the orbit. In cases with permanent diplopia, generally due to late coming and therefore unsuccessful orbital surgery, muscle surgery may be helpful, provided that binocular single vision existed prior to injury. In these cases a combined procedure of surgery on the paretic muscle, and, if necessary, on his antagonistic as well as on his synergistic muscle, is indicated. We had 4 cases in which we could restore stereopsis with a restricted binocular field of single vision, adequate for most professional duties.

255

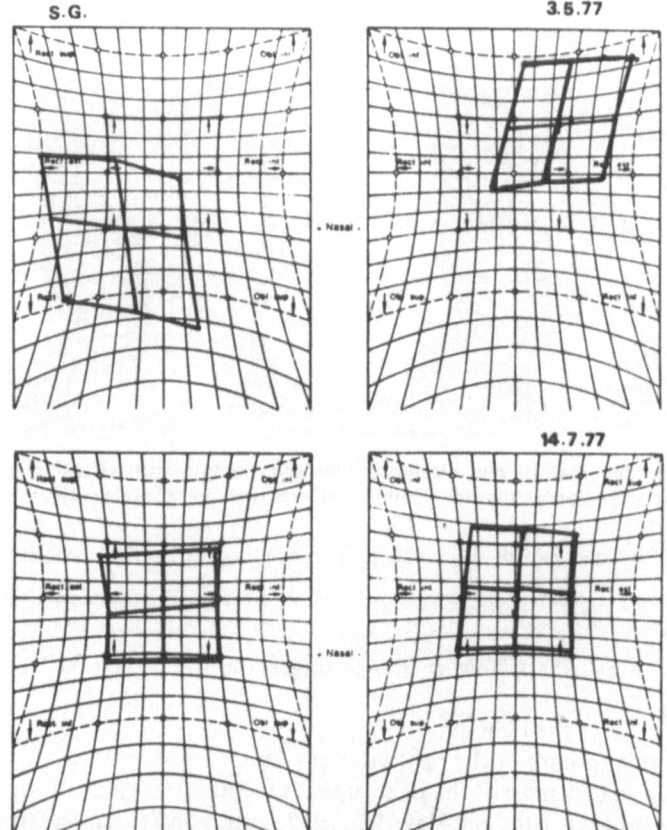

Fig. 14. Lees-screen of the same patient: On the left (3.5.77) before and on the right (14.7.77) after muscle surgery: Restoration of a sufficient field of central binocular vision after operation.

REFERENCES

Beer, Th. Studien über den traumatischen Enophthalmus. *Arch. Augenheilk.* 25: *315* (1892).

Hollwich, F. Late surgical correction of traumatic paresis of the right superior oblique muscle. p. 215, in: Bleeker & Lyle, Fractures of the Orbit. Proc. Symp. on Orbital Fractures, Amsterdam, 1969. Excerpta Medica, Amsterdam (1970).

Hollwich, F. & G. Jünemann. Klinischer Beitrag zur Blow-out Fraktur. *Klin. Mbl. Augenheilk.* 156: *864* (1970).

Hollwich, F., A. Boeteng & A. Wilke. Die Blow-out Fraktur aus ophthalmologischer Sicht. In: Naumann & Kastenbauer, Plastisch-chirurgische Massnahmen nach frischen Verletzungen. Verh. 11. Jahrestagung Dtsch. Ges. Plast. u. Wiederherstellungschirurgie, München 1973. Thieme, Stuttgart (1974).

Hollwich, F., A. Wilke & A. Boateng. Surgical reconstruction of blow-out fracture. Proc. 2nd Int. Symp. on Orbital Disorders, Amsterdam, 1973. Mod. Probl. Ophthal. 14, p. 646. Karger, Basel (1975).

Lederer, A. Über traumatischen Enophthalmus und seine Pathogenese. *Graefes Arch. Ophthal.* 53: *242* (1902).

Authors' address:
University Eye Hospital
Westring 15
D-4400 Münster/W
W. Germany

Proc. 3rd Int. Symp. on Orbital Disorders, Amsterdam 1977

SURGICAL TREATMENT OF BLOWOUT FRACTURE

YOSHINAO FUKADO

(Kawasaki, Japan)

Blowout fracture is the commonest fracture of the orbital floor resulting from blunt eye injury. It has special clinical criteria in the orbital fracture due to unusual eye movement. The disturbance of the eye movement upward and downward is caused by the herniation of the orbital contents into the gap of the orbital floor. Treatment of this fracture is considered as a very easy technique for repositioning of the orbital tissues. During the past 4 years we have had 166 cases of blowout fractures and all were treated with surgical repositioning of the orbital tissues under the operation microscope. This paper will report the clinical aspects of these 166 cases and some problems of their treatment.

All cases were divided into 2 groups: linear fractures and bone defect types, according to the protocols. The linear fractures were seen in 64 cases (39%) and bone defects were recognized in 102 cases (61%). Division into 2 groups is necessary for the choice of surgical method and for assessment of prognosis.

In investigation of the age distribution of the linear fracture type, 58% of the cases occur in the first and second decades. In the bone defect type, 48% of the cases are found in the first and second decades. The frailty of the bone may cause fracture of this type in young people.

On the other hand, the grades of the forced duction test were investigated on the protocols. The records of the grade were obtained only on 37 cases in the linear fracture and on 51 cases in the bone defect type. These cases were divided into 4 groups according to their grade, i.e., minus, one plus, two plus and three plus. In the linear fracture, the strongest resistance to passive eye movement was seen in the largest percentage, 35%. The number of cases with two and three plus resistance account for 54%. In the bone defect group, the largest number of cases was seen in the one plus group with 47%. In addition to the no resistance group, they account for 55%. In comparison, the linear fracture group shows a greater resistance than the bone defect group. In general, the bone defect group shows a rather mild resistance to passive eye movement but massive enophthalmos.

The treatment of the linear fracture, especially along the inferior orbital nerve, is very difficult. X-ray photographs of this type show a small dark shadow in the middle part of the upper area of the antrum. It involves a disorder of the inferior orbital nerve. To distinguish the orbital fat tissue from the inferior orbital nerve is not easy, even if the surgery is done under the operation microscope. Traction on the inferior orbital nerve causes sensory loss in the medial parts of the cheek and upper lip. Therefore, the repositioning of the orbital tissues may be insufficiently achieved. The poor post-operative results of blowout fractures are usually seen with these linear fractures in the line of the inferior orbital nerve. In the linear fracture type, the case where the fracture line runs in the direction of a right angle to the inferior orbital nerve, is not rare. An X-ray photograph of such a case shows a small dark shadow spread over a whole area at the upper limit of the antrum. The treatment of this type is rather easy and most of this type of case do not need the insertion of some artificial plate to avoid the further herniation of the orbital contents.

In the bone defect type, the technique of the surgery is very easy. The repositioning of the orbital tissues in this group is not difficult except in a large bone defect. X-ray photography of a large bone defect shows a large dark shadow filling almost the whole area of the antrum. Two stage procedure is necessary for the treatment. The surgery must be done under general anesthesia. First, the orbital floor is opened. The herniated orbital tissue is pulled up and a thin teflon plate is placed over the bone defect. Secondly, the alveolar mucous membrane is incised and the anterior wall of the antrum is exposed. A small bone window is opened to permit insertion of a gum balloon catheter into the antrum. The balloon is enlarged with about 10 ml of contrast medium. Finally, the orbital floor is reopened and careful examination is done to make sure of a complete repositioning of the orbital tissues. The balloon catheter is retained for 2 weeks. The results of the surgery in 4 cases are satisfactory.

It is desirable to use this two-way procedure more widely. To obtain a good result, careful investigation and complete repositioning of the herniated orbital tissues is essential. The silicon or teflon plate which is inserted over the bone defect area of the orbital floor must be as thin and small as possible.

Author's address:
Department of Ophthalmology
Kanto Rosai Hospital
Kizukisumiyoshi-cho, Nakahara-ku
Kawasaki 211
Japan

Proc. 3rd Int. Symp. on Orbital Disorders, Amsterdam 1977

SURGICAL DECOMPRESSION OF BLOWOUT FRACTURE

Y. FUKADO

(Kawasaki, Japan)

ABSTRACT

Treatment of blowout fracture is the repositioning of orbital contents and the reconstruction of the orbital floor. The complete repositioning of orbital contents between fractured bone fragments is not so easy. It is rather difficult, especially when the fracture lies in a deep area of the orbital floor and spreads out wide, even under the operation microscope.

During the past three years we have had about 100 cases of blowout fracture and surgical treatment was done under the operation microscope. Post-operative cure is obtained in only 50% of cases.

The surgical results refer to the severity of trauma and to the interval between trauma and surgery. The surgical technique, however, should be changed per case. The orbital approach is not always effective. Sometimes a two way, orbital and antral, approach is necessary.

Author's address:
Department of Ophthalmology
Kanto Rosai Hospital
Kizukisumiyoshi-cho, Nakahara-ku
Kawasaki 211
Japan

PROPTOSIS DUE TO PARASITIC INFESTATIONS

ALY MORTADA

(Cairo, Egypt)

Duke Elder & MacFaul (1900) described in detail the parasitic infestations of the orbit. Protozoa may give rise to proptosis as in the case of retrobulbar haemorrhage due to malaria or pseudo-tumor due to entamaeba histolytica (Mortada, 1968). Nemathelminths in the form of Filariasis (Sobhy Bey, 1922) (Figs. 1 and 2), Ascaris Lumbricoids, or Trichinosis (Fig. 3) may affect the orbit. Platyhelminthes affecting the orbit giving proptosis are Schistosoma (Bilharzia (Badir, 1946) or Cestodes as Taenia Echinococcus (Attiah, 1947; Handousa, 1949, Mortada, 1977), Taenia solium (Ayoub & Kamel, 1967; Hamed, 1968) or sparaganosis. Orbital myasis due to infection by some arthropod maggots is rare. In one of my cases larvae of oestrus ovis each about 1 x 1/4 cm with characteristic posterior respiratory openings (Fig. 4) produced an acute proptosis which resolved when the maggots appeared through a fistula in the upper lid.

In unilateral proptosis of unexplained origin (Mortada, 1962, 1963, 1965, 1968) and superior orbital fissure syndrome of uncertain aetiology

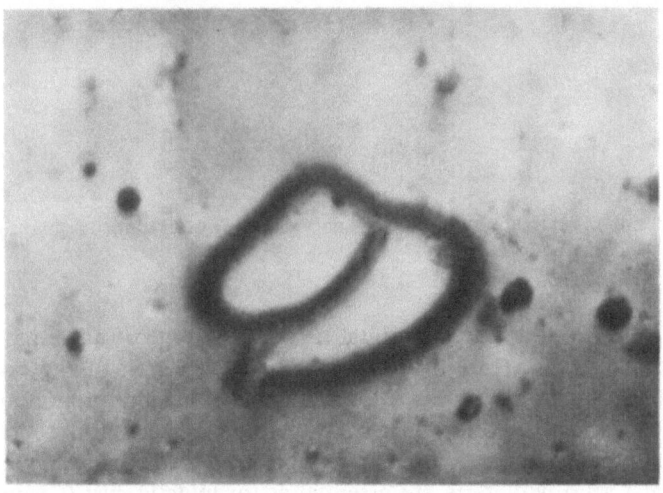

Fig. 1. Microfilaria Loa Loa in nocturnal blood (X 750) (does not cause proptosis).

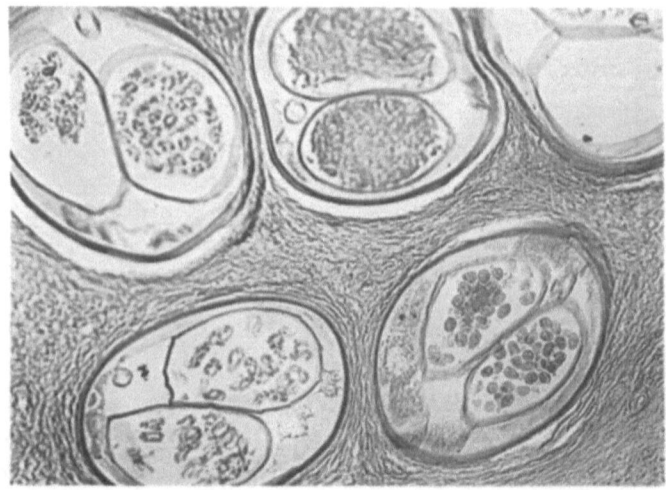

Fig. 2. Section in subcutaneous tissue showing sections of body of Onchocerca volvulus surrounded by fibrous tissue (X 120) (not reported from Egypt).

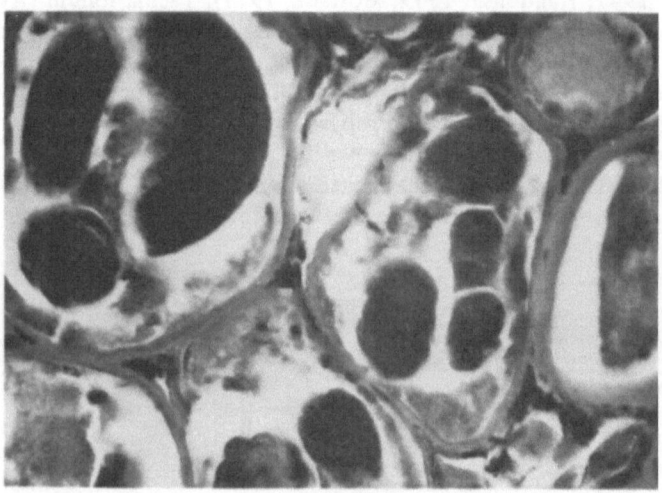

Fig. 3. Section in orbital muscle showing encysted larvae of Trichinella spiralis (X 540) (not reported from Egypt).

(Mortada, 1961) and superior orbital fissure syndrome of uncertian aetiology (Mortada, 1961) investigations must include search of the body for parasites. The blood is examined for eosinophilia, malaria and microfilaria, urine is examined for Bilharzia Haematobium eggs and stools for entamaeba histolytica and for eggs of Bilharzia Mansoni, Ascaris and ankylostoma. Intradermal sensitivity tests are essential as for hydatid cyst (Casoni test), Bilharzia, Ascaris, Toxoplasma, trichinella and cysticercus cellulosa.

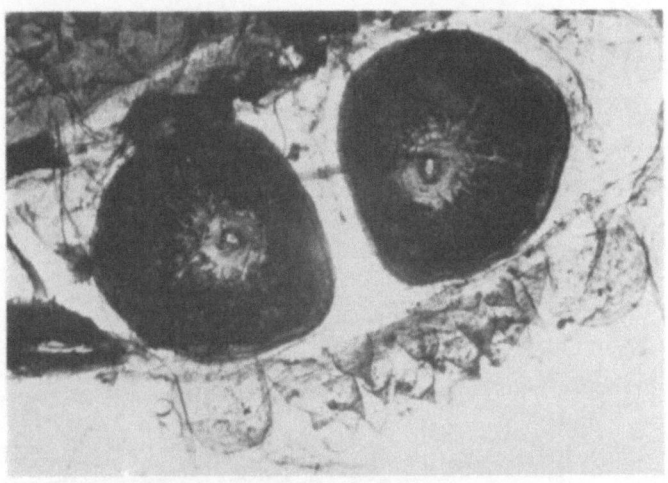

Fig. 4. The size of maggots of Oestrus ovis is 1 x 1/4 cm. Figure showing characteristic posterior respiratory openings (posterior spiracles) (X 20).

Although in some villages of Egypt one may find diseases due to Bilharzia, Ascaris, ankylostoma, filaria, malaria and amaebic dystentry, yet their reported orbital lesions are very rare. Among my one thousand cases of histopathologically diagnosed orbital tumours the following 5 cases were caused by parasitic infestation of the orbit.

Case 1

A 12 years old boy had right proptosis of 3 months' duration. The left eye was normal, visual acuity 6/6, fundus normal. The right eye showed oedema of lids, chemosis of conjunctiva, proptosis 20 mm. Hertel (left eye 16 mm) and limitation of ocular movements. Fundus showed optic atrophy but no error of refraction. Visual acuity was 1/60. An orbital mass was felt above the globe.

Urine was positive for the Bilharzia ova. Faeces were normal. Blood count showed: Haemaglobin 74%; W.B.C. 6,900; Eosinophils 9%; Basophils 0%; Lymphocytes 29%, Monocytes 4% and Neutrophils 58%. The removed orbital mass was soft, 1 x 2 cms, non-capsulated, adherent to the superior rectus muscle. The orbital roof showed no abnormality. Histopathological examination showed an inflammatory granuloma composed of a large number of nodules containing Bilharzia ova in different stages of degeneration. A group of terminal spined Bilharzia haematobium ova were found surrounded by inflammatory reaction (Fig. 5) composed of foreign body giant cells, eosinophils, plasma cells and fibroblasts. The aduly worm was not found in the sections. Antibilharzial treatment was given and the proptosis regressed enormously.

263

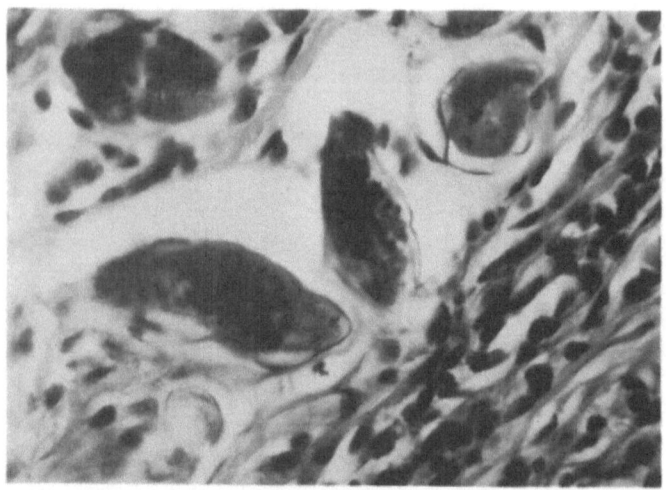

Fig. 5. (Case 1.) Bilharzia haematobium eggs (with terminal spine) surrounded by orbital pseudo-tumour (C 540).

Case 2

A 9 years old boy complained of right proptosis of 2 months' duration. The left eye was normal, fundus normal and visual acuity 6/9. The right eye showed oedema of lids, chemosis of conjunctiva, proptosis 21 mm (left side 15 mm) and limitation of ocular movements down. The fundus was normal and visual acuity 6/12. An abnormal mass was felt below the globe. Orbital exploration showed below the globe attached to inferior rectus, a 2 x 1.5 cms, pinkish, soft, non-encapsulated mass. The orbital floor was normal. Urine was negative for parasites. Faeces showed Ascaris ova. Blood was negative for parasites. Blood count showed HB. 60%; W.B.C. 5,600; Eosinophils 10%; Basophils 0%; Lymphocytes 30%; Monocytes 5%; and neutrophils 56%. Histopathological examination of the removed orbital mass showed a non-specific chronic inflammatory mass with lymphocytic follicular aggregations but no caseation. As all investigations showed nothing but Ascaris in faeces, the orbital pseudo-tumour was considered to be due to Ascaris toxins. With elimination of Ascaris infection the proptosis regressed.

Case 3

A 50 years old man complained of left proptosis of 3 months' duration. The right eye was normal, fundus normal and visual acuity 6/6. The left eye showed oedema of lids, chemosis of conjunctiva, proptosis 21 mm (right eye 16 mm), normal fundus, no error of refraction, visual acuity 6/9 and limitation of ocular movements. An orbital mass was felt between the eye and the nose. Left orbital exploration showed an inner orbital mass partly hard and

264

partly soft 2 x 1 cm adherent to medial rectus but the medial orbital wall was intact.

Urine was negative for parasites but faeces showed only binucleated and quadrinucleated entamaeba histolytics cysts. Blood was nagative for parasites. Blood count showed Hb 70%; W.B.C. 6,100; Eosinophils 6%; Basophils 0%; Lymphocytes 30%; Monocytes 4%; and Neutrophils 61%. Histopathological examination of orbital mass showed a chronic inflammatory mass with lymphocytic perivascular arrangement and fibrosis. The cause of orbital psuedo-tumour was considered to be amaebic dysentry. Treatment of the latter caused a great improvement in the degree of proptosis.

Case 4

A 21 years old male had left proptosis of unexplained origin of 3 months' duration. Intradermal Casoni test was positive. Urine and stools were negative for parasites. Orbital exploration showed in muscle cone space a cyst of 2 cm diameter adherent to the surrounding muscles. The removed cyst wall was composed of an external cuticular laminated ectocyst; a germinal syncytial endocyst and a cavity containing fluid and scolices, characteristic for hydatid cyst (Fig. 6) of Taenia Echinococcus.

Case 5

A 12 years old boy had right proptosis of unexplained origin of four months duration. Urine and stools were negative from parasites. Orbital exploration revealed in muscle cone space a small cyst of one centimeter diameter. Histo-pathological examination of the removed cyst showed section of larva

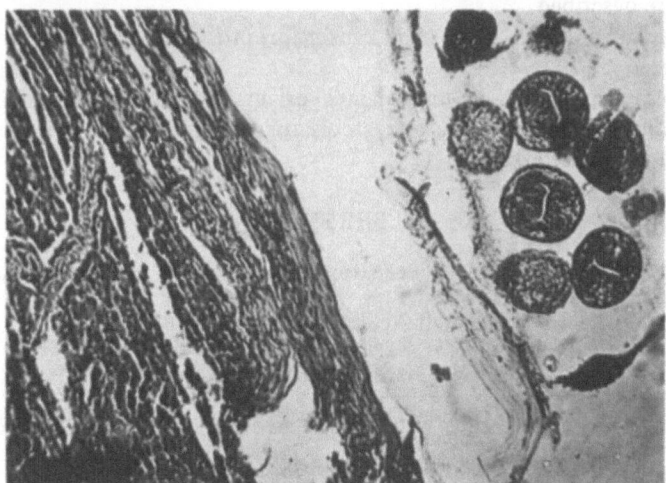

Fig. 6. (Case 4.) Hydatic cyst of the orbit showing an external cuticular laminated ectocyst; a germinal syncytial endocyst and a cavity containing characteristic scolices (X 150).

265

of Taenia solium, i.e. a cysticercus cellulosa (Fig. 8) showing a cyst wall, invaginated scloex with characteristic hooklets. The cyst was surrounded by granulation tissue rich in eosinophils.

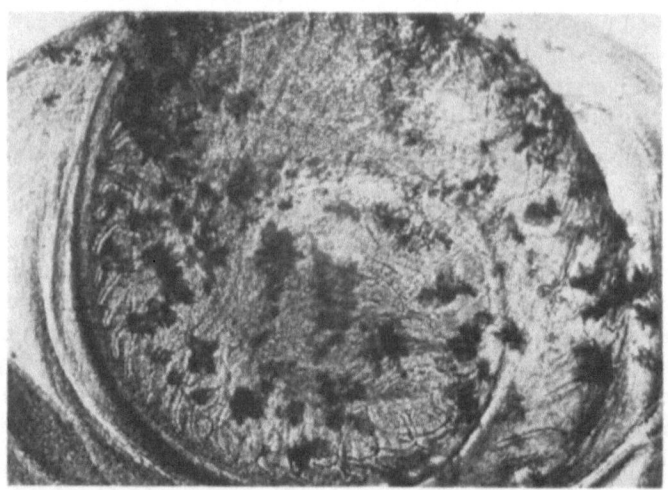

Fig. 7. (Case 5.) Cysticercus cellulosa showing cyst wall; invaginated scolex with characteristic hooklets (X 20).

SUMMARY

Five cases of unilateral proptosis due to hydatid cyst, cysticercus cellulosa, and pseudo-tumours due to Bilharzia ova, amaebic dysentry and toxins of ascaris are described.

Parasitic infestations of the orbit causing proptosis, especially in Egypt, are enumerated.

In cases of proptosis of unexplained origin, investigations must include examination of blood, urine and stools for parasites. Specific intradermal sensitivity tests are essential.

REFERENCES

Attiah, M.A.H. & M.A.M. Labib. Echinococcus infection. Hydatid cyst of the orbit. *Bull. O.S. Egypt* 40: *67* (1947).

Ayoub, M. & I. Kamel. Ocular cysticercosis. *Bull. O.S. Egypt* 60: *231* (1967).

Badir, G. Bilharzia of the orbit. *Br. J. Ophthal.* 30: *215* (1946).

Duke-Elder, S. & P.A. MacFaul. System of OPhthalmology. Vol. 13, Part 2, p. 21. Kimpton, London (1974).

Hamed, H.A. Orbital affectation with cysticercous cellulosa. *Bull. O.S. Egypt* 61: *253* (1968).

Handousa, A.S. Proptosis. *Bull. O.S. Egypt* 42: *32* (1949).

Mortada, A. Superior orbital fissure syndrome of uncertain aetiology. *Br. J. Ophthal.* 45: *662* (1961).

Mortada, A. Unilateral proptosis of unexplained origin. Part I. *Br. J. Ophthal.* 46: *369* (1962).

Mortada, A. Unilateral proptosis of unexplained origin. Part II. *Br. J. Ophthal.* 47: *445* (1963).

Mortads, A. Unilateral proptosis of unexplained origin. Part III. *Br. J. Ophthal.* 49: *547* (1965).

Mortada, A., Orbital pseudo-tumour and parasitic infections. *Bull. O.S. Egypt* 61: *393* (1968).

Mortada, A. Unilateral proptosis of unexplained origin. Part IV. *Br. J. Ophthal.* 52: *419* (1968).

Mortada, A. Unilateral proptosis of unexplained origin and unilateral superior orbital fissure syndrome of uncertain aetiology 'Mortada orbital syndromes' and some rare orbital lesions. Part 6. *Bull. O.S. Egypt* (accepted for publ. 1977).

Sobby Bey, M. Filaria affecting the orbit. Br. J. Ophthal. 30: 215 (1946).

Author's address:
Chairman and Senior Professor of Ophthalmology
Faculty of Medicine
18A 26 July Street
Cairo
Egypt

Proc. 3rd. Int. Symp. on Orbital Disorders, Amsterdam 1977

ACUTE INFECTIONS OF THE ORBIT

IVOR LEVY

(London, England)

Acute infections of the orbit now receive little attention in the literature, especially when compared with that given to orbital tumours. Yet they are common, potentially threatening not only to sight but also to life and are sometimes treated inadequately. In the pre-antibiotic era they were rightly regarded with considerable gravity. Birch-Hirschfeld's large series from the beginning of this century had a mortality of 19%, and of the patients described in Ehler's classical paper (1937), 5 of 35 died. In all series, of the patients who survived, Duke-Elder (1974) states that 'some 20% were left with blindness of the affected eye and a further 13% remained with a grave impairment of vision'. Antibiotics have transformed the situation though it is interesting to note that of the first 5 patients ever to receive penicillin, 2 died and both had orbital infections; the first had severe septicaemia when treatment was started, and the second, a young boy, died of a ruptured mycotic aneurysm.

Scott (1960) compared the outcome of acute orbital inflammation in the pre-antibiotic period 1930–1939 with that of 1950–1959. Interestingly the results were very similar; there were 4 deaths in 23 cases in the first period and 2 deaths in 14 cases in the second period. Furthermore in the latter series 4 of the 12 cases who recovered were blind and one who died was blind before death. Scott used combinations of benzyl penicillin, streptomycin and aureomycin; he had 2 cases of penicillin resistant organisms. At the London Hospital in the 5 year period 1932–1936, approximately forty patients were admitted with acute orbital infections and 4 died. They died of cavernous sinus thrombosis, meningitis and septicaemia.

The present series is from the in-patient records of The London Hospital and the Orbital Clinic, Moorfields Eye Hospital during the 5 year period June 1972 to June 1976. There were 82 patients with adequate follow-up. At the London Hospital there were on average 7 cases a year compared with one case of orbital tumour a year; in contrast at Moorfields there were more tumour cases than acute infections, reflecting the large number of tumour cases being referred to the Orbital Clinic. No patient died and none had permanent visual loss as a result of their infection. However, three had ocular palsies and 2 lid deformities. Thirty-five cases had recurrent infection or a slow resolution. The commonest organism was staphylococcus aureus though in the majority of cases no organism was isolated. The sinuses were the usual primary site of infection. Nine cases occured after surgery; 5 due to infected detachment implants one case following squint surgery, one was secondary to an infected graft and 2 cases followed surgery for infected sinuses.

Acute orbital infections should be admitted to hospital for the following reasons: the condition is a serious one and requires parenteral antibiotics, an underlying source of infection should be sought and finally a case which initially is considered to be one of acute bacterial infection may be something quite different. Of the thirty-five cases who had recurrent infection or a slow resolution the majority received minimal doses of oral antibiotics. Absorption of orally administered antibiotics is haphazard so that intravenous or intramuscular antibiotics in adequate doses are essential. To treat the possible range of organisms involved at least two antibiotics are required. There is a wide choice available but any combination must be active against penicillinase-producing staphylococci and B-haemolytic streptococci. A suitable regime is cloxacillin and ampicillin each in a dose of one Gram every six hours. This is given intravenously for 48 to 72 hours after which one can change to oral administration for a further five days; flucloxacillin is absorbed better than cloxacillin when given orally. In penicillin hypersensitive patients a suitable combination is Lincomycin 600 mgs twice daily intramuscularly and Cephaloridine 1.5 gms. every six hours intravenously.

If patients are given large doses of parenteral antibiotics not only will they recover more rapidly with fewer long term complications but any diagnostic dilemma is resolved for if such doses fail to produce a rapid resolution serious consideration should be given to the other causes of acute painful proptosis.

ACKNOWLEDGEMENTS

I would like to thank my colleagues at The London Hospital and Moorfields for allowing me to study the case notes of their patients and Mr. John Wright for his help and advice.

REFERENCES

Birch-Hirschfeld. Graefe-Saemisch Hb.d.ges. Augenheilk. 2nd ed. Berlin. volume 9 (1) pp 251 (1907–1930).
Duke-Elder, Sir Stewart. System of Ophthalmology. Volume 13 (ii) London (1974).
Ehlers, H Acta Ophthal., Suppl. 12., Copenhagen (1937).
Scott, G.I., Orbital Cellulitis and Cavernous Sinus Thrombosis. *Trans. O.S.U.K.* 80: *435–450* (1960).

Author's address:
The London Hospital
Dept. of Ophthalmology
London E.1
England

Proc. 3rd Int. Symp. on Orbital Disorders, Amsterdam 1977

MUCORMYCOSIS OF THE ORBIT

E. WEIGELIN & U. KLEHR

(Bonn, W. Germany)

Mucormycosis, an opportunistic Phycomycosis, is an acute, frequently fatal fungus disease characterized by the occurrence of broad, non-septate hyphae in tissues which tend to grow into arteries and produce thrombosis and infarction. This is the definition given by R.D. Baker in the 'Handbook of Special Pathology'. The disease is rare, the symptoms and signs for the cranial form, which interests us here, have been clearly described by many authors. So it seems unnecessary to discuss it here in detail. Clinical experience, however, shows that in most cases Mucormycosis is diagnosed too late for successful treatment, which is possible with antimycotic medicaments like Amphotericin B. Fleckner & Goldstein reviewed the 19 survivors between 1955 and 1969 and found that all but three were treated in this way and it is significant that the majority of fatal cases had either not received these drugs at all or taken antimycotics too late.

The rhino-orbital Mucormycosis was first described by Gregory et al. (1943). Other forms have been known since the second half of the last century (the pulmonary form, gastrointestinal, disseminated, cutaneous, focal and cranial form). For the diagnosis of all types of mucormycosis it is important to know that the infection nearly always develops in persons whose resistance is lowered by metabolic disorders.

The most important subgroups of fungus for the cranial form, which is combined with rhino-orbital affectation in 68% of the cases, is Rhizopus. (According to Baker the more detailed species identification of Rhizopus is beyond the scope of the average hospital or even medical school microbiologist or mycologist.) The genus is characterized by small sporangiophores which arise singly or in clusters opposite small rhizoids and bear also small spherical sporangia with amber spores between the sporangial wall and the columella (Baker, 1971).

These saprophytes live on the ground, in houses, are abundant in old bread and spoiling fruit and are frequently inhaled by healthy persons. In the person with a predisposing condition, such as diabetic acidosis, leukemia, renal insufficiency, which is often combined with uremia, in patients treated with corticosteroids, the fungus proliferates in the mucosa of the nose, nasal sinuses or bronchi and spreads locally and is found usually in vessel walls or infarcts within the tissue. This means, that we must consider the diagnosis of rhino-orbital Mucormycosis in patients with such a predisposing condition, if we find a unilateral orbital cellulitis with proptosis, ptosis, and internal and external ophthalmoplegia. If this clinical picture is combined with an obstruction of the central retinal artery, the diagnosis Mucormycosis is very probably. The typical case history in such subject begins with facial pain and headache, rhinitis with epistaxis and lid edema. Then the features which were just mentioned develop, the patient lapses into coma and dies after some days. The pathway of entry of the fungus into the orbit is the nasal cavity and the accessory nasal sinuses.

Infection of the orbital tissue may be complicated by infection of the interior of the eye, the bony orbit and the tissues of the face and nose. Extension through the roof of the orbit to the meninges and parenchyma of a frontal lobe of the brain produces mucormycotic meningitis and encephalitis. Very typical is the involvement of the ophthalmic artery and, from there, the extension to the artery of origin, the internal carotid artery.

The case we saw in December 1976 shows the typical symptoms and signs of the cranial form of Mucormycosis. Our patient had been in a chronic haemodialysis program for seven years, necessitated by chronic bilateral nephrocirrhosis with severe arterial hypertension. As far as we know this kind of case has not yet been described in the literature. The disease had begun in the week before hospitalization with headache and double vision. This was caused by a palsy of the 6th nerve on the right side. EEG and ultrasonic-echogram were normal at that time.

Two days later the pains were located in and around the right eye. The ophthalmologist found a slight swelling of the lids, no pathological changes of the eyeground and normal vision. The X-ray photography of the orbit was also normal. The pains in the right orbit were increasing markedly during the subsequent days. After hospitalization, six days after the onset, we found ocular symptoms such as ptosis, proptosis of 6 mm, immobility, occlusion of the central retinal artery and blindness of the right eye. The bodytemperature was 39.2°C, sedimentation rate 144/155, the number of leucocytes 20,200 and potassium in the blood serum was increased to 7.3 mEqu/1. X-ray photographs showed clouding and some fluid level in the right maxillar sinus and an unsharp borderline of the optic canal. All the blood cultures for bacterias were negative. An antibiotic and antimycotic therapy was started in a high dosage (Aminoglycotide, Cephallosporin and a derivative of Clotrimazolum). Except for the ocular symptoms, which corresponded to the syndrome of the apex of the orbit, there were no nervous complications at that time. But some hours later the same day, we found also a palsy of the 6th nerve on the left side and left side internal ophthalmoplegia. Therefore we diagnosed a thrombosis of the sinus cavernosus and also, because the ophthalmic blood pressure was clearly decreased, a beginning occlusion of the left ophthalmic artery. A heavy cerebral attack and meningism followed. Correspondingly the EEG showed a fronto-precentral δ-focus at the right and left with involvement of the temporal region of the right side too. In the slightly xanthochrome spinal fluid were 200/3 cells.

On the next day an occlusion of the external and internal carotid artery and thrombosis of the cavernous sinus were documented by angiography and cerebral scintigram (Fig. 1–3). The patient was comatose and died one day later. In the culture of the maxillary sinus tissue, fungi belonging to the Mucor group were growing.

Finally, I would like to say a few words about the therapy. Most patients with Mucormycosis who died have received rigorous antibiotic therapy in addition to the treatment of their general disease. Most survivors went through a systemic antifungal therapy. The data of these cases suggests the importance of early antifungal therapy like Amphotericin B or Oralnystatin. Chick et al. (1958) have shown that Amphotericin B has a definite fungistatic effect in experiments with rabbits and rats.

Fleckner & Goldstein (1969) give details of the precise medication with Amphotericin B. The initial dose of 5 mg Amphotericin B was increased over a four day period to 25 mg/day and after that until a peak dose of 0.2 mg/kg body weight was reached and administered every other day until a total dose of 2 g had been given.

McIntyre Gass suggests that systemic antifungal agents and antibiotics should be administered immediately if the diagnosis of Mucormycosis is suspected. Once the diagnosis is secure the antibiotics should be discontinued.

According to Baker's experimental research the use of corticosteroids in fungus infections is contraindicated. Surgical treatment, enucleation of an eye or exenteration of the orbit is probably onle useful as long as the disease has not yet affected the brain and the meninges.

Let me finally suggest that in cases of orbital cellulitis combined with local arterial occlusions in patients with severe chronic metabolic diseases one should alsway consider a diagnosis of Mucormycosis.

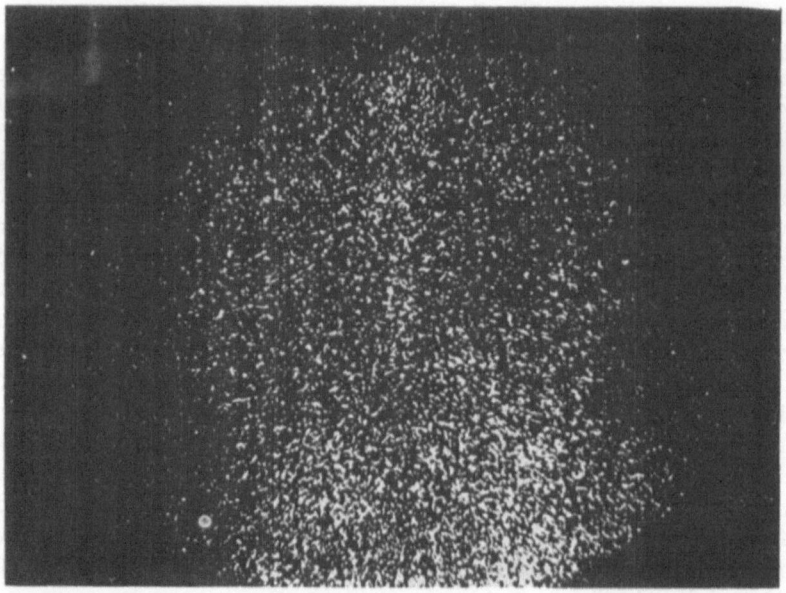

Fig. 1. Vascular pool scintigram of the head of our patient. Decreased blood-circulation in the right orbit.

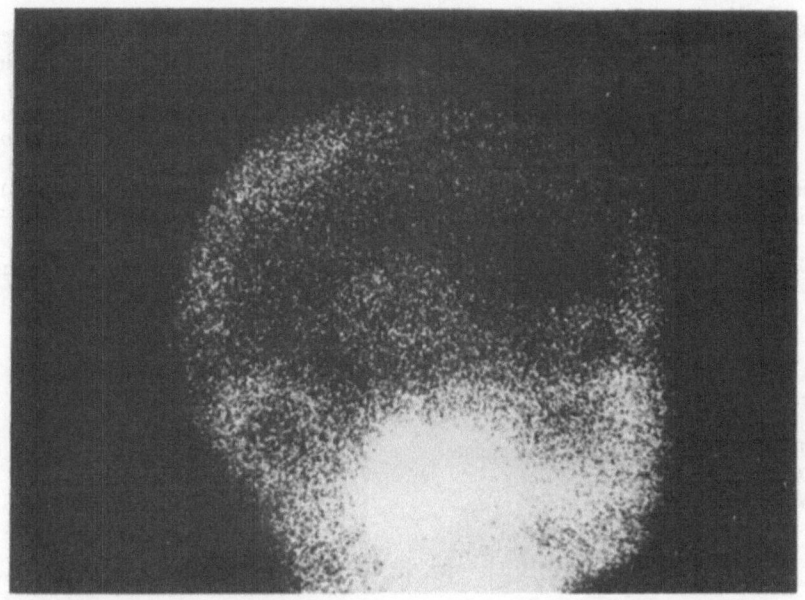

Fig. 2. Vascular pool encephalo-scintigram of our patient, side view after 5 min. Focus, right temporal, corresponds most likely to an infarctus.

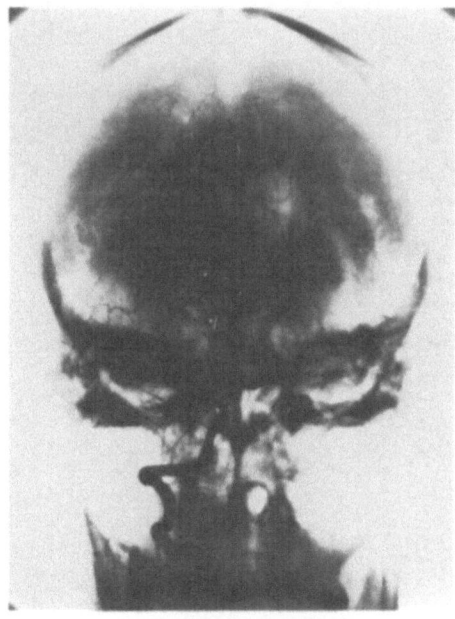

Fig. 3. Carotid Angiography shows occlusion of the right external and internal carotid arteries.

REFERENCES

Baker, R.D. The pathologic anatomy of Mucormycosis. pp. 832–918 in: Handbuch der speziellen Pathologischen Anatomie und Histologie, Band 3, Teil 5. Springer, Berlin (1971).

Chick, E.Q., J. Evans & R.D. Backer. Treatment of experimental Mucormycosis (Rhizopus oryzae infection) in rabbits with Amphotericin B. *Antibiotics & Chemother.* 8: *394–399* (1958).

Fleckner, R. & J.H. Goldstein. Mucormycosis. *Br. J. Ophthal.* 53: *542–548* (1969).

Gass, I.D.M. Ocular manifestations of acute mucormycosis. *Arch. Ophthal.* 65: *226–237* (1961).

Gregory, J.E., A. Golden & W. Haymaker. Mucormycosis of the central nervous system. *Bull. Johns Hopkins Hosp.* 73: *405* (1943).

Authors' address:
Institute of Experimental Ophthalmology
University of Bonn and
University Clinic for Internal Medicine
D-5300 Bonn-Venusberg
W. Germany

OPTO-CHIASMATIC ARACHNOIDITIS COMBINED WITH AN INTRA-ORBITAL INFLAMMATORY MASS LESION (CASE REPORT)*

GIORGIO IRACI, LAURA TOMAZZOLI GEROSA
& MASSIMO GEROSA

(Padova, Italy)

The case of a woman with slight diencephalic disturbances, a right exophthalmos caused by an intra-orbital inflammatory mass lesion, and a surgically proven opto-chiasmatic arachnoiditis is reported. Surgery (removal of the intra-orbital mass and of the arachnoiditic adhesions) failed to produce any beneficial effect on the vision of the right eye, which eventually became blind.

The coincidence of an intra-orbital inflammatory process and of intracranial arachnoiditis and the role of compression of the intracranial carotid artery on the ipsilateral optic nerve in the production of a nasal field defect are discussed.

In our series of opto-chiasmatic arachnoiditis (82 patients since 1951) we found some cases worthy of a separate description, as the one reported here.

CASE

A.M.C. (Clinical record No. 5695), a 33 year old woman, was first admitted to our Neurosurgical Department in 1968. Family history was normal: her past personal history showed a tubercular infiltration of the right lung (long ago cured with medical treatment) and several bouts of sinusitis. About one year prior to admission, she had noticed some menstrual irregularities and occasional frontal and right orbital headaches. Four months later, a slight protrusion and some impairment of sight appeared in the right eye. These symptoms progressed for some months, and then became stationary.

Upon admission, the right eye showed a 2 mm exophthalmos, barely reducible; visual acuity 4/10; a large defect (practically a hemianopsia) in the nasal half of the visual field, together with a relative central scotoma; and a very slight ptosis. Funduscopic examination showed papilledema (Fig. 1, top) Neuroophthalmologic findings were quite normal in the left eye which retained a visual acuity of 11/10. The general neurological examination was normal.

---

* The figures in this paper are reproduced, with permission, from Figure 11 of the paper presented at the Fifth Intern. Congress of Neurogenetics and Neuro-Ophthalmology, Nijmegen, 1977 (Junk, The Hague, 1978).

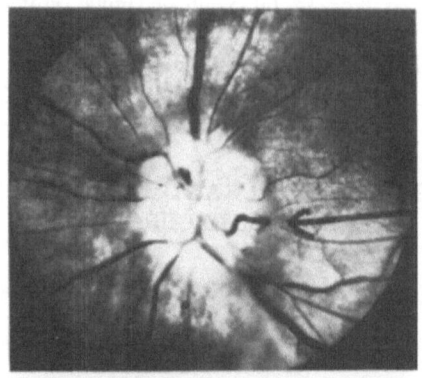

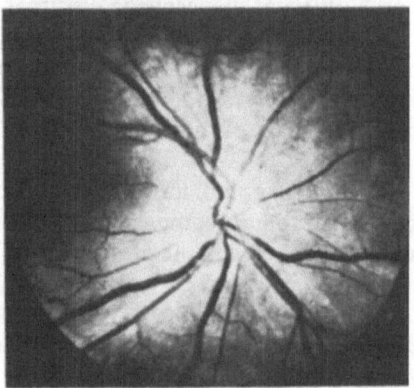

Fig. 1

No abnormalities were found with X-rays of the skull or with a right common carotid arteriogram. A total lack of filling of the right orbital veins showed on orbital phlebography (Fig. 2).

The patient was scheduled for exploration of the right orbit. However, after some days of intensive medical treatment with dexamethasone (Decadron, Merck Sharp & Dohme of Italy SpA, Rome), chymotrypsin, vitamin B/1-6-12, there was a marked improvement of sight in the right eye, with restoration of visual acuity up to 8/10, and disappearance of the visual field defect as well as improvement of the funduscopic alterations (Fig. 1, bottom). The patient signed herself out of hospital and went home with a prescription to continue her medical treatment.

Barely six months later, however, she was readmitted complaining of intense pain in the right orbit and further impairment of sight in the right eye. Visual acuity was down to 3/50, with optic atrophy and some venous distention. There was again a nasal hemianopsia, with an initial involvement of the temporal half. The right exophthalmos had increased to 4.5 mm. No changes of the right carotid arteriogram, nor of the orbital phlebogram, were found.

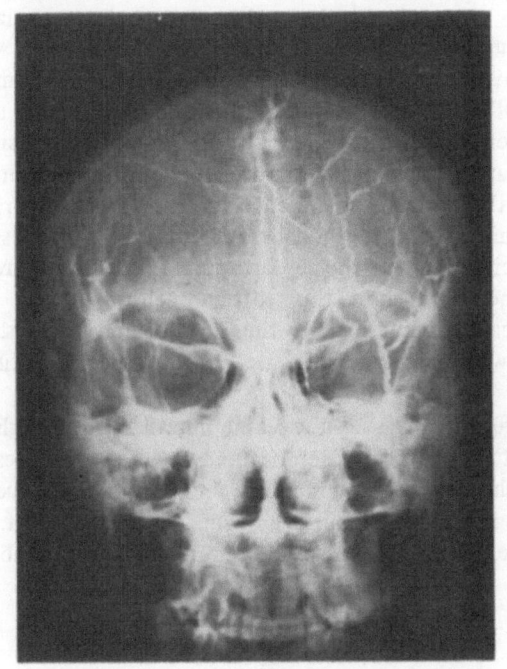

Fig. 2

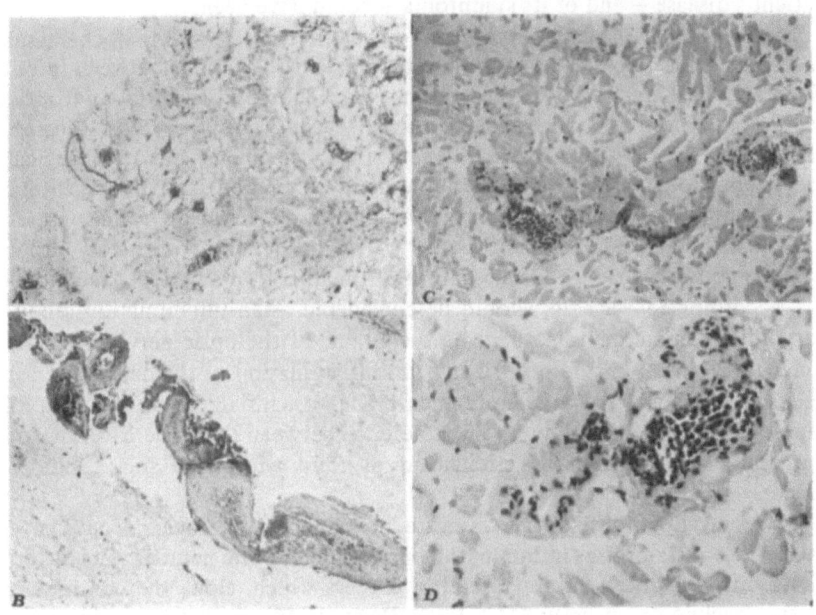

Fig. 3

Right frontal craniotomy (October 1968), and exploration of the right orbit led to the removal of a mass with the approximate size of a grape, situated between the upper and external rectus muscles. It was, however, doubted that this lesion could account for the severe impairment of visual acuity and visual fields, and an intradural exploration of the anterior optic pathways was performed. The right optic nerve and the chiasm were found embedded in a rather thick meshwork of arachnoiditic adhesions, which also pulled together the optic nerve and chiasma structures of the right side with the ipsilateral intracranial internal carotid artery. The adhesions were removed and the circulation of the cerebrospinal fluid was restored to normal. The right optic nerve was short, thin, soft and yellow-grayish.

The histological examination of the intra-orbital mass showed fibro-adipose tissue with circumscribed aspects of aspecific infiltration (Fig. 3A-D).

Upon discharge, there was no noticeable improvement of sight in the right eye. The patient's visual acuity deteriorated slowly and progressively during the follow-up: she has become practically blind in the right eye (where only light perception is preserved) and has normal sight in the left. The patient, despite hormone treatment, has also become amenorrhoic about one year after surgery.

COMMENTS

The interesting feature of this case seems to be the combination of opto-chiasmatic arachnoiditis and an intra-orbital inflammatory mass lesion. The first question that comes to one's mind is what the pathogenesis of this patient's disease — and of its symptoms — could have been.

After Onodi (1934) called attention to the general relationship of the nasal accessory sinuses to the surrounding structures, the relations between infectious and inflammatory diseases of the head (notably sinusitis) and optic neuritis has been a much debated issue (Walsh & Hoyt, 1969). Redslob (1939), in a study of 'normal' anatomical specimens and pathological specimens from patients with optic neuritis, concluded that the arachnoid membrane is a well-defined sheath, which follows the intra-orbital part of the optic nerve and can be the site of an inflammatory process, either isolated or together with inflammation of the dura or pia mater. Arachnoid-itis, according to Redslob, should be considered as an inflammation secondary to inflammatory disorders of the brain, of the optic nerve or of the sphenoidal sinus. On the other hand, an inflammation of the dura does not necessarily involve the arachnoid membrane. An inflammatory process of the arachnoid sheath produces an adherence between the three coverings of the brain, interrupting the circulation of fluid within the sub-arachnoid spaces.

If we may hypothesize, the severe recurrent bouts of sinusitis could have caused the intra-orbital inflammatory mass and an optic neuritis. The latter, in its turn, produced an arachnoiditic process which, along the continuum of the arachnoidal structure (Muller & Deck, 1974), spread to the intracranial anterior optic path ways. The menstrual irregularities could thus have been due to a diencephalic involvement.

According to the concept of natural predisposition to arachnoiditis as accepted by some authors, one further interpretation could be that arachnoiditis was the consequence of the intra-orbital inflammatory process but, in the meantime, the cause of optic neuritis or, anyway, of damage to the optic nerve through an impairment of the normal hydrodynamics of the cerebro-spinal fluid, of its circulation and blood supply or of its nutritional and metabolic requirements.

Whether the nasal hemianopsia of the right eye was caused by the right optic nerve neuritis or by pressure from adhesions is not clear. Another possibility could be compression by the right internal carotid artery. Similar cases with pressure on the optic nerves or chiasm by arteries lying nearby, like the carotid artery or the A/1 tract of the anterior cerebral artery, have been described in the literature and were found in our own series of opto-chiasmatic arachnoiditis (Iraci, 1974). O'Connell & DuBoulay (1973) showed that single space-occupying lesions can produce a 'true' binasal hemianopsia. O'Connell's anatomical studies (1973) confirmed that binasal hemianopsia can be due to compression of the uncrossed fibers in the optic nerve or chiasm by these arteries. The crossed nasal, and uncrossed temporal fibers of the optic chiasm do not only differ anatomically in the areas of the retina they arise from, but also physically. According to O'Connell, tension is the force that produces bitemporal hemianopsia, while pressure produces nasal field defects. Bergaust (1963) reported a case where a bilateral malposition of the internal carotid artery (with normal walls) had produced bitemporal field defects.

The poor functional result of surgery in our patient appears to confirm, however that the inflammatory process was primarily involving the optic nerve and that the arachnoiditis was secondary to neuritis. The fact that the contralateral eye has remained unaffected throughout the years (an unusual event in opto-chiasmatic arachnoiditis, where a bilateral involvement of sight at some time during the natural course of the disease is customary) can be due to a primary role of the intra-orbital inflammatory mass, or can be ascribed to a partial success of the exploration and lysis of the adhesions in the prevention of an irreversible damage to the optic structures of the left side.

REFERENCES

Bergaust, B. Unusual course of internal carotid artery accompanied by bi-temporal hemianopsia. *Acta Ophthal.* (Kbh.) 41: *270–274* (1963).

Iraci, G. Opto-chiasmatic arachnoiditis. Report of 2 cases with unusual apparent etiologic features. *J. Neurosurg. Sci.* 18: *142–149* (1974).

Migliore, A., M. Massarotti, G. Ettorre, et al. L'aracnoidite ottico-chiasmatica. Revisione critica di 108 casi operati. *Ann. Ottalmol. Clin. Ocul* 96: *221–232* (1970).

Muller, P.J. & J.H.N. Deck. Intraocular and optic nerve sheath hemorrhage in cases of sudden intracranial hypertension. *J. Neurosurg.* 41: *160–166* (1974).

O'Connell, J.E.A. The anatomy of the optic chiasma and heteronymous hemianopsia. *J. Neurol. Neurosurg. Psychiat.* 36: *710–723* (1973).

O'Connell, J.E.A. & E.P.G.H. DuBoulay. Binasal hemianopsia. *J. Neurol. Neurosurg. Psychiat.* 36: *697–709* (1973).

Onodi, A. The general relations of the accessory sinuses of the nose to the surrounding structures. Catalogue of the Onodi Collection, Royal College of Surgeons, Beadley Bros., London (1934).

Redslob, E. Arachnoidite intra-orbitaire. *Rev. Oto-neuro-ophtal.* (Paris) 17: *161–163* (1939).

Walsh, F.B. & W.F. Hoyt. Clinical neuro-ophthalmology. 3 Vols (see Vol. 1 pp. 621ff). The Williams & Wilkins Co., Baltimore (1969).

Authors' addresses:
G. Iraci & M. Gerosa
Institute of Neurosurgery
and
L. Tomazzoli
Institute of Ophthalmology
University of Padova
Via Giustiniani 5
35100 Padova
Italy

Requests for reprints to Dr G. Iraci at the above address.

Proc. 3rd Int. Symp. on Orbital Disorders, Amsterdam, 1977

METASTATIC ORBITAL ABSCESS, AN UNUSUAL OBSERVATION

A. HUBER

(Zürich, Switzerland)

In the orbit infectious diseases, whether due to bacteria, viruses or fungi, are seldom primary. Usually they reach the orbit by extension from adjacent structures like the paranasal sinuses, the globe, the teeth, the middle ear, face or cranial cavity. However, hematogenous spread from remote lesions (bacterial endocarditis, abscess of brain, pyemia, influenza, scarlet fever etc.) seems to be rather rare, probably due to the fact that the infectious metastatic emboli travelling by the blood stream are carried on past the ostium of the ophthalmic artery to lodge not in the orbit, but rather in the brain and the meninges.

Acute orbital inflammations occur in two different forms: the non-suppurative and the suppurative. The non-suppurative type or orbital cellulitis is characterized by pain, fever, lid edema, chemosis, proptosis and limitation of ocular movement. It may subside spontaneously or with the aid of antibiotics, but may also become either suppurative or a chronic inflammatory process. The suppurative form of acute orbital inflammation leads to necrosis of orbital tissue and to formation of pus. Frequently the necrosis is walled off by local tissue responses and typical abscess formation occurs.

This last form of orbital infectious disease will be discussed for an unusual case where the correct diagnosis was only made during surgical exploration and where all diagnostic procedures at our disposal beforehand pointed rather to a neoplasm than to an intraorbital abscess. This presentation will demonstrate how difficult the diagnosis of chronic abscess formation in the orbit can be,

The patient, a boy of 11 years old, had undergone a tonsillectomy in July 1976 because of recurrent tonsillitis. Three days later he developed a fever accompanied by intense pain in the left region of the neck. Six days after the tonsillectomy he showed symptoms of an acute shock due to pyemia with anaerobic green streptococci. After a while a parapharyngeal phlegmona developed on the left side, which needed surgical incision and extensive drainage. With intensive antibiotic treatment (gentamycin, ampicillin, penicillin) the general condition improved gradually and a fortnight after the tonsillectomy the fever disappeared completely. Two days later the patient complained of sudden diplopia. Ophthalmologic examination revealed a left-sided exophthalmos (Fig. 1) of 6 mm, a slight impairment of ocular

281

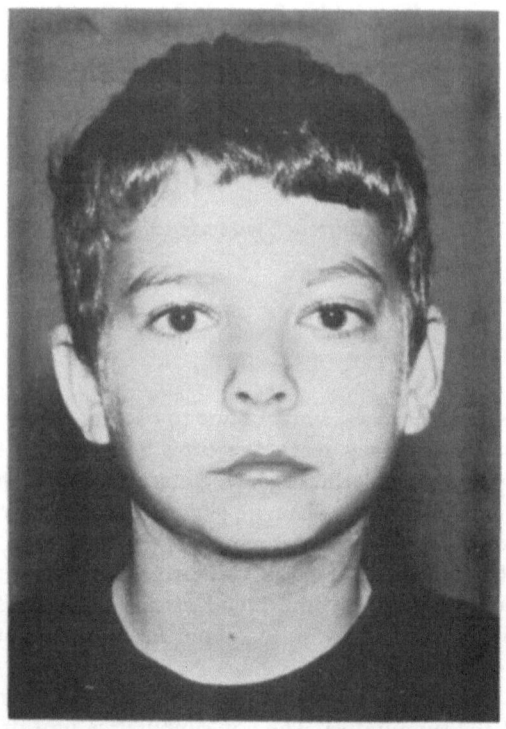

Fig. 1. Exophthalmos of 6 mm of the left eye (combined with distinct limitation of upward movement in the sense of superior rectus paresis).

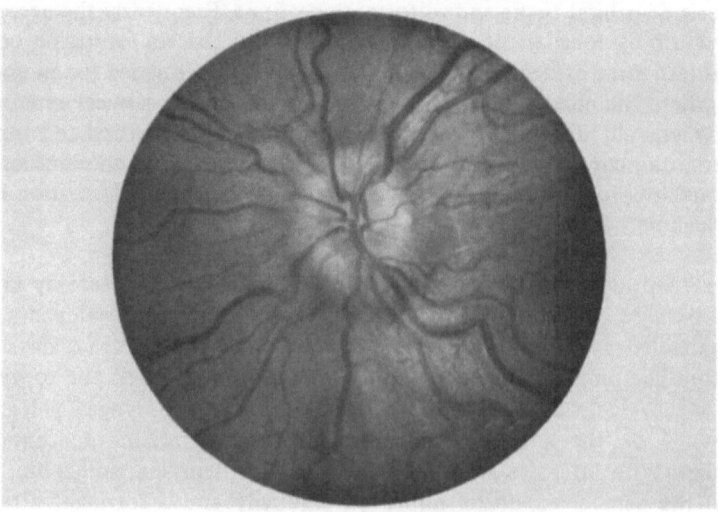

Fig. 2. Papilledema of the disc of the left eye with blurred disc margins, deflection of the vessels over the disc and capillary stasis of the disc tissue.

motility with consequent diplopia in all directions, a slight miosis of the left pupil, a normal aspect of both discs, normal visual fields and no defect of the central vision. Ultrasonography (A- and B-scan) showed a retrobulbar process of blurred outlines extending about 12 mm in the axial direction towards the apex of the orbit (Fig. 3); the A-scan pattern of low reflection was indicative of the pseudotumor/lymphoma/sarcoma group. In view of the preceding septic complications, an inflammatory pseudotumor was diagnosed finally, and treatment was performed with 50 mg prednison for ten days daily and every other day for the next fifteen days. Proptosis and the limitation of ocular movements improved slightly; however, with reduction of the prednison dose new symptoms occurred: pain in the left eye, especially during extensive movements, distinct limitation of upward movement in the sense of a superior rectus paresis, left-sided papilloedema of 2 diopters with blurred disc margins, deflection of the vessels over the disc and capillary stasis of the disc tissue (Fig. 2). A left carotid angiography showed a dorsally shifted ophthalmic artery in the posterior part of the orbit but no evidence of tumor stain or arteriovenous abnormality. Computerized tomography showed a round tumor-like mass in

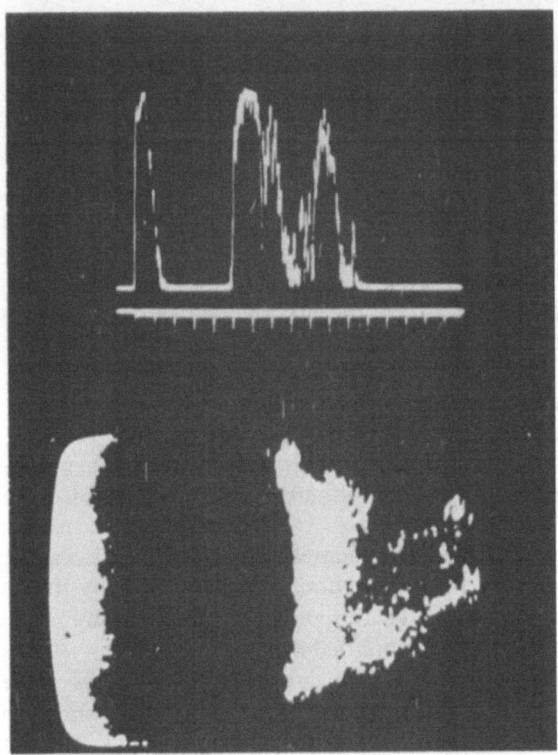

Fig. 3. Ultrasonography. A-Scan (above) manifests pattern of low reflection suggestive of the pseudotumor-lymphoma-sarcoma-group. B-scan (below) shows retrobulbar process of blurred outlines extending about 12 mm in axial direction towards the apex of the orbit.

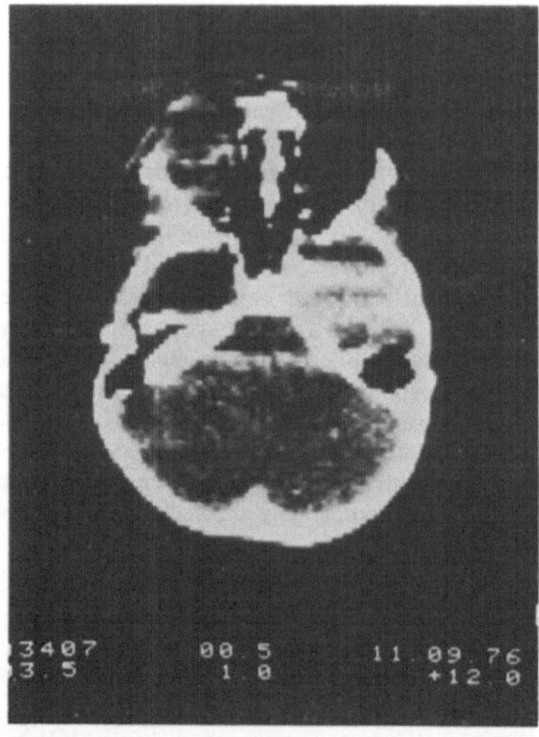

Fig. 4. Computerized tomography depicting in the middle and lateral region of the left orbit a round tumor-like mass of increased density of 10 to 12 mm diameter.

the middle and lateral region of the left orbit, with a 10—12 mm diameter. The computer tomogram was interpreted as a real intraorbital tumour and not as a pseudotumor (Fig. 4).

In view of this, three diagnostic possibilities were considered:

1. intraorbital tumor without relation to the preceding pyemia;
2. intraorbital abscess formation (with atypical ultrasonic pattern);
3. inflammatory orbital pseudotumor (again with atypical computerized tomogram).

This uncertainty in the pre-operative diagnosis was the reason for a transfrontal approach for the exploration of the left orbit by the neurosurgeon (almost three months after the primary tonsillectomy and about two months after the onset of exophthalmos).

During the operation the following observations were made: after the orbital roof and the periorbita were opened, a huge tumor-like solid mass appeared to fill out the whole length of the left orbit. The neurosurgeons thought they had found a typical neurinoma! When tissue was taken for bopsy, the incision in about 5—6 mm depth of solid avascular tissue suddenly entered into an abscess cavity from which yellowish-creamy pus was evacuated. This pus turned out to be sterile. Since the abscess membrane was adherent to the optic nerve, only its upper parts were resected and radical extirpation was disregarded. The bleeding granulomatous tissue in the depth of the abscess was carefully removed. The orbital roof was covered with peiorbital and dural tissue and the frontal bone replaced.

With antibiotic treatment, a gradual decrease of exophthalmos, total disappearance of extraocular muscle disorders and regression of the left-sided papilloedema occurred.

According to the literature as well as our personal experience, metastatic orbital abscess formation is rather rare. Orbital cellulitis occurs relatively frequently in children (due to the intensive development of the lymphatic and vascular system in the orbit) and this may result in the formation of free pus in the orbit, but with the aid of antibiotics this will generally subside before an abscess has been formed. The clinical picture with lid oedema, chemosis, proptosis, gross limitation of ocular movements and frequent impairment of visual function is not comparable with our case where such acute inflammatory signs have not been observed. Even orbital pseudotumor (inflammatory pseudotumor), characterized by lid oedema, conjunctival chemosis, proptosis and limitation of ocular movements, frequently with sudden onset, does not fit into the pattern of our abscess case.

The primary diagnosis of pseudotumor, mainly based on the ultrasonic findings and not on the clinical appearance, was certainly mistaken and led to the administration of high doses of prednison which obscured the orbital disease. In our case ultrasonography did not show the cystic abscess with thick membrane formation. It manifested echoes rather typical for the pseudotumor/lymphoma/sarcoma group. On the other hand, computerized tomography indicated a real tumor-like mass in the affected orbit and no specific signs for abscess (as, e.g., cavity formation). Yet, in view of the specific signs for abscess (as, e.g., cavity formation). The more so as the characteristic clinical signs and symptoms of orbital cellulitis or pseudotumor of the orbit were not present, and the computer tomogram distinctly pointed to a well-defined solid tumor in the affected orbit. Yet, in view of the preceding septicemia and the parapharyngeal phlegmona a metastatic abscess formation in the orbit seemed to be the best diagnosis. Certainly all necessary diagnostic procedures were applied to elucidate this tricky case. Whether incisional or needle biopsy would have contributed in this case to a correct diagnosis is doubtful. In view of the uncertain pre-operative diagnosis and the location of the process, the transfrontal approach proved to be fully justified.

REFERENCES

Cheney, R.C. A case of orbital abscess producing a clinical picture of separation of the retina. Pathological findings, including an anaemic infarct of the optic nerve. *Arch. Ophthal.* 52: *252–258* (1923).

Coop, M.E. Pseudotumor of the orbit. A clinical and pathological study of 47 cases. *Br. J. Ophthal.* 45: *513–541* (1961).

Dallow, R.L., K.J. Momose, A.L. Weber & S.H. Wray. Comparison of ultrasonography, computerized tomography (EMI scan) and radiographic techniques in the evaluation of exophthalmos. *Trans. Am. Acad. Ophthal. Otolaryng.* 81: *305–322* (1976).

Henderson, J.W., G.M. Farrow, K.D. Devine & R.H. Miller. Orbital tumors. Section 1, pp. 25–74. W.B. Saunders, Philadelphia (1973).

Hogan, M.J. & L.E. Zimmermann. Ophthalmic pathology, an atlas and textbook. 2nd ed., pp. 720–780. W.B. Saunders, Philadelphia (1962).

Iliff, C.E. & H.J. Ossofsky. Tumors of the eye and adnexa in infancy and childhood. Ch.C. Thomas, Springfield, Ill., pp. 131–135 (1962).

Moro, F. Les pseudotumeurs de l'orbite. *Ophthalmologica* 151: *349–389 (1966)*.

Papst, W., H.-G. Mertens & E. Esslen. Die chronisch-okuläre Myositis. I. Die exophthalmische okuläre Myositis. *Klin. Mbl. Augenheilk.* 133: *673–694* (1958).

Reese, A.B. Tumors of the eye. Hoeber Medical Division, Harper & Row, New York. 2nd ed., pp. 538–541 (1963).

Ullerich, K. Die gezielte Diagnostik raumfordernder Prozesse der Orbita. Büch. des Augenarztes 70. Enke Verlag, Stuttgart (1976).

Author's address:
Stadelhoferstrasse 42
CH-8001 Zürich
Switzerland

Proc. 3rd Int. Symp. on Orbital Disorders, Amsterdam 1977

INFLAMMATORY ORBITAL PSEUDOTUMOR
A CLINICAL-PATHOLOGICAL STUDY

RICHARD M. CHAVIS,* ALEC GARNER & JOHN E. WRIGHT

(Washington, D.C. / London, England)

We retrospectively studied fifty-five patients who presented at the Orbital Clinic at Moorfields Eye Hospital between 1969 and 1976 with a clinical picture consistent with inflammatory orbital pseudotumor. Although these findings, including proptosis, pain, diplopia, and lid swelling, may be mimicked by many conditions, no patient was included in whom a definitive etiologic diagnosis was possible. Our objective was to examine the extent to which the character of the cellular infiltrate correlated with the response to therapy and eventual prognosis.

CLINICAL AND HISTOPATHOLOGIC CORRELATIONS

Patients were divided into five clinical groups; the first resolving spontaneously, or responding well to steroids (groups one and two). However, of the and the fifth, biopsy suspected lymphoma. Significantly, no progression to systemic disease was documented in any patient either resolving spontaneously, or responding well to steroids (group one and two). However, of the patients responding poorly, or not at all to steroids (groups three and four), seven were found to develop a systemic or previously unsuspected disease on follow-up examination, three revealing disseminated lymphoma. In light of our observations of the respective clinical groups we reviewed the histology of biopsied tissue (Table 1). All biopsies were independently reviewed without knowledge of the original histologic diagnosis, pertinent clinical history or responses to therapy where prescribed. If the histological findings in the fourteen patients whose lesions resolved with or without steroids (groups one and two), are compared with those who responded transiently or not at all (groups three and four), it seems that the most distinctive differences relate to the presence and location of transformed lymphocytes or lymphoblasts. Where the lymphoblasts were within germinal follicles there was a uniformly favourable outcome whereas lymphoblasts spread diffusely through the cellular infiltrate were associated with a uniformly poor prognosis. Morgan (1975) reported a similar distribution in a review of disseminating lymphocytic neoplasms and benign (possibly reactive) lympho-

* Supported by the Friends of Moorfields Research Fellowship.

Table 1. Histopathologic-clinical correlation. Histopathologic findings in patients grouped according to clinical behaviour. Patients denoted with identification number

Histology	Group 1 8 patients	Group 2 6 patients	Group 3 4 patients	Group 4 10 patients	Group 5 6 patients
Massive (+++) lymphocytic infiltration	41	0	6	23, 40, 48, 45	67, 68, 69, 70, 71, 72
Germinal follicles	7, 16, 41, 59	0	0	0	0
Lymphoblasts (diffusely distributed)	0	0	6	17, 22, 23, 40, 48	67, 68, 69, 70, 71, 72
Plasma cells					
a. moderate or	7, 10, 16, 41, 59, 66	0	0	12, 17, 31, 40	0
b. minimal	26, 35	1, 8, 18, 49, 56	6, 11, 36, 47	20, 22, 23, 48, 50, 45	70
c. absent	0	27	0	0	67, 68, 69, 71, 72
Eosinophils					
a. present	16, 35, 41, 66	1, 8, 49, 56	0	20, 31, 45	68
b. absent	7, 10, 26, 59	18, 27	6, 11, 36, 47	12, 17, 22, 23, 40, 48, 50	67, 69, 71, 72, 70
Macrophages					
a. moderate or	7, 10, 35, 41, 59, 66	1, 8, 18, 49, 56	6, 36, 47	17, 22, 23, 40, 48, 50	67, 68, 71
b. minimal	16, 26	27	11	12, 20, 31, 45	70, 69, 72

cytic tumors. Although intense lymphocytic infiltration was most evident in the groups showing steroid resistence (five of fourteen patients) as against one of fourteen patients with remission, the difference is marginal. Eosinophils, although not confined to one group, were more frequent in the steroid responsive group (one and two) (eight of fourteen patients) than in the steroid-treatment group (three and four) (three of fourteen patients). Plasma cell and macrophage numbers, however, were not conspicuously different in either group which contrasts with other claims that the presence of such cells foretells a favourable prognosis (Zimmerman, 1964).

The limited number of cases involved in this study and the considerable overlap in the histological findings between clearly reactive lesions and presumed neoplasms preclude dogmatic statements. Nevertheless, the data does warrant some conclusions:

1. Germinal follicles are associated with a good prognosis and indicate a reactive lesion. These patients are not likely to appear with subsequent systemic or additional orbital diseases.

2. There is an association between diffusely distributed lymphoblasts, steroid-unresponsiveness and a probable neoplastic lymphoid lesion.

3. Eosinophils are more common in reactive lesions than in presumed lymphomas. Other cellular components do not show any preferential distribution in either neoplastic or non-neoplastic groups.

REFERENCES

Morgan, G. Lymphocytic tumors of the orbit. pp. 355–360, in: Proc. 2nd Int. Symp. on Orbital Disorders, Amsterdam, 1973. Mod. Probl. Ophthal. 14. Karger, Basel (1975).

Zimmermann, L.E. Lymphoid tumors. pp. 429–446, in: Ocular and Adnexal Tumors: new and controversial aspects (M. Boniuk, ed.). Kimpton, London / C.V. Mosby Co., St. Louis (1964).

Authors' addresses:

Richard M. Chavis
Washington Hospital Center
Department of Ophthalmology
110 Irving Street N.W.
Washington D.C. 20010
USA

Alec Garner & John E. Wright
Moorfields Eye Hospital and
Institute of Ophthalmology
London
England

Requests for reprints to R.M. Chavis at the above address.

Proc. 3rd Int. Symp. on Orbital Disorders, Amsterdam, 1977

EYE TUMORS IN DR. SOETOMO HOSPITAL
SURABAYA INDONESIA

R.K. TAMIN-RADJAMIN

(Surabaya, Indonesia)

INTRODUCTION

Everyone agrees on the importance of early detection and diagnosis of eye tumors for prompt and proper treatment. This is possible in developed countries, where people are sufficiently educated and know the dangers of the disease, but in developing countries like Indonesia the situation is very different. Patients usually visit the clinic at an advanced stage of the disease due to lack of knowledge or information.

To improve this situation we have started to collect data, and this paper is to show the present status of eye tumors in the Dr. Soetomo Hospital Surabaya.

MATERIAL AND METHODS

A retrospective study has been made of all patients who visited the eye clinic of Dr. Soetomo Hospital Surabaya during the period of 1972–1976. All kinds of eye tumors are included in this study. Diagnosis was made by clinical methods and if possible followed by histopathological examination.

The patients were grouped according to age, sex, localization of the tumors and malignancy.

RESULTS

Table 1. Incidence of eye tumors 1972–1976, at the eye clinic of Dr. Soetomo Hospital Surabaya.

period	eye tumors	new patients visiting the eye clinic	percentage
1972	63	17872	0.59%
1973	78	13197	0.59%
1974	57	13238	0.43%
1975	47	14206	0.33%
1976	116	15879	0.73%
total	361	74392	0.49%

During 5 years we have found a total of 361 eye tumors among 74392 new patients who visited the eye clinic which means an incidence of 0.49%.

Table 2. Incidence of eye tumors according to age and sex.

age in years	number of eye tumors		
	male	female	total
−10	57	68	125
−20	28	49	77
−30	26	33	59
−40	14	22	36
−50	14	19	33
−60	14	12	26
−70	1	4	5
total	154	207	361

Most eye tumors occur in people under 10 years of age: 125 patients (68 females and 57 males), followed by the age group between 10 and 20: 77 cases (49 females and 28 males). The lowest incidence occurs in people after the 6th decade. The youngest patient in our series is 10 days old (lipofibroma) and the oldest 70 years old (cystic basal cell Carcinoma).

Among 125 cases of the group under 10 years of age, there are 63 clinically diagnosed retinoblastomas of which the youngest patient is 2 months old and the oldest 6 years.

Table 3. Incidence of eye tumors according to localization.

localization	eye tumors
Eyelid	105
Conjunctiva	123
Cornea	−
Limbus	9
Lacrimal Sac	3
Uvea	2
Retina	63
Retrobulbar	56
Total	361

According to localization, most of the eye tumors are tumors of the eyelid and conjunctiva. There are no corneal tumors.

DISCUSSION

Our study shows that retinoblastoma constitutes an important part of all eye tumors, especially in the malignant group. Therefore most of our eye tumor patients admitted to the hospital are children. Their range varies

Table 4. Incidence of malignant eye tumors based on histopathological studies.

Retinoblastoma	27
Basal cell carcinoma	6
Epidermoid carcinoma	6
Undifferentiated epidermoid carcinoma	5
Adenoid carcinoma	5
Squamous cell carcinoma	2
Malignant melanoma	3
Lymphosarcoma	2
Suspect sarcoma	1
Total	57

Malignant eye tumors based on histopathological studies are mostly retino-blastomas (27 cases) and Carcinomas (24 cases).

between 2 months and 6 years of age, with an average age of 29 months (Reese (1977) 18 months). They mostly come in an extraocular stage and are very often inoperable. If something could be done, it is only an exenteration of the orbit, followed by radiation. In spite of this treatment these patients die a few months later (Figs. 1 and 2).

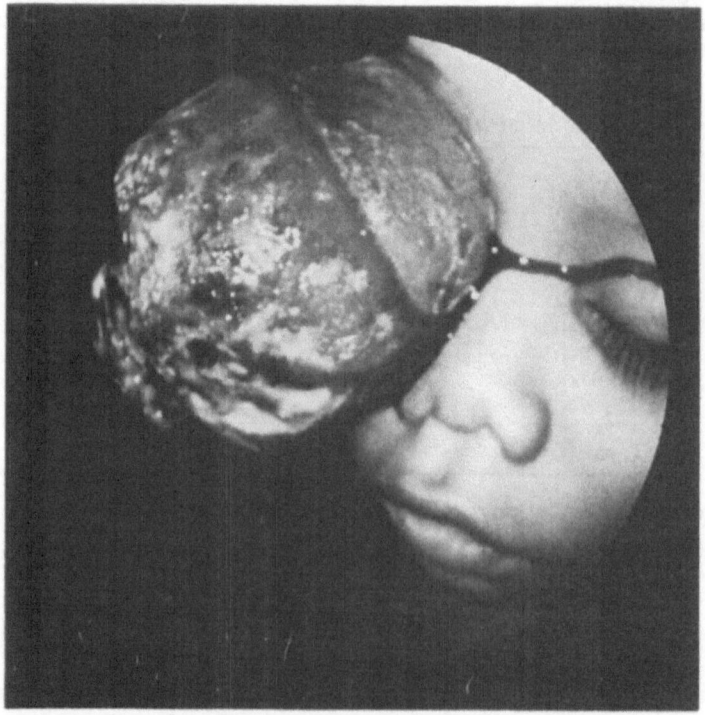

Fig. 1. Retinoblastoma

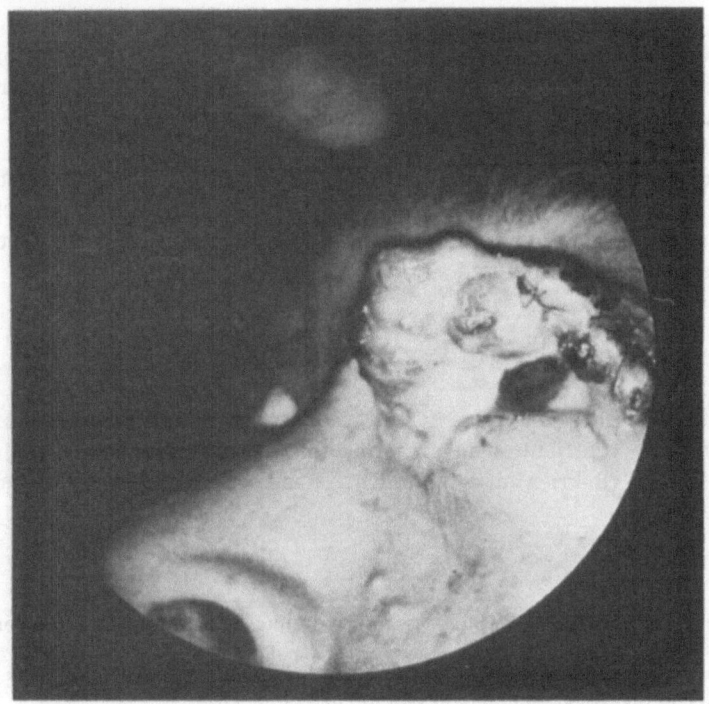

Fig. 2. Epidermoid carcinoma

The reasons of coming in a late stage are:
1. Many children are raised by grandparents who are very ignorant.
2. Financial problems prevent them from seeing a doctor.
3. Difficult transportation from remote villages to the nearest eye center.
4. Fear of the doctor's treatment.
5. Preference to go to a traditional medicine man (dukun).
Although some of them are seen by a doctor in an early stage, they refuse to undergo an enucleation

Routinely both eyes were examined, but we seldom found bilateral cases.

Concerning carcinoma cases, most of them are localized in the eyelid and since the majority of the cases come in a very advanced stage, we often have to excise the whole eyelid which creates serious problems for reconstruction. After operation they seldom return to the hospital for follow up.

We only found 2 cases of uveal tumors in 5 years. It means approximately 0.5%; this is in accordance with the statements of former investigators, for instance ten Doesschate, who found only one case in 20 years (Ten Doesschate, 1968).

Regarding retrobulbar tumors, diagnosis and management is difficult, due to lack of facilities and its inaccessibility.

SUMMARY

A report of 361 patients with eye tumors who visited the eye clinic of Dr. Soetomo Hospital Surabaya during the years 1972—1976 is presented. Among them are 154 males and 207 females. Their ages varied from 10 days to 70 years, with the average of 22 years.

Histopathological studies showed that 57 cases or 44,9% were found to be malignant and most of them were Retinoblastoma. This does not reflect the real pattern of eye tumors, since most of the cases came in an advanced or very late stage and/or refused any form of surgery.

ACKNOWLEDGEMENT

The author wishes to express her gratitude to the following members of her staff for the contribution in preparing this paper: Koentjoro Liman, P.N. Oka, J. Kadi, Bakri Abd. Sjukur, E. Aswan-Gumansalangi and Wisnujono Soewono.

REFERENCES

Doesschate, J. ten. Causes of blindness in and around Surabaya, East Java, Indonesia. Thesis (1968).

Reese, A.B. Tumors of the Eye. Harper & Row, Publishers Hagerstown, Maryland, New York, San Francisco, London, 3rd Edition, p. 91 (1977).

Author's address:
Dept. of Ophthalmology
School of Medicine
Airlangga University
Dr. Soetomo Hospital
Surabaya
Indonesia

Proc. 3rd Int. Symp. on Orbital Disorders, Amsterdam 1977

OCCURRENCE AND FREQUENCY OF EYE TUMORS
IN ETHIOPIA

BARBARA SCHMIDT

(Berlin, W. Germany)

Orbital tumors are much more frequent in Africa than in Europe (Templeton, 1967) and they constitute a high percentage of all malignant tumors in African pathological institutes. Children are much more afflicted than adults (Davies, 1968; Discamps, 1972; Templeton, 1967). There is a different distribution of tumors to what we find in Caucasians. Despite the highly pigmented African race, there are practically no intraocular melanomas. Basal cell carcinoma and hemangioma are rare (Discamps, 1972; Templeton, 1967). The retinoblastoma and neuroblastoma are of about the same incidence as in Europe. The epithelium cell carcinoma of the conjunctiva in adults and Burkitt's lymphoma seem to be due to the environment and associated bad hygienic conditions.

EPITHELIAL TUMORS

Papillomata of the conjunctiva are not rare. There seems to be a relationship between their frequency and the severity of conjunctival inflammations which are dependent on hygienic conditions. The papilloma of the conjunctive may be precancerous (Duke Elder, 1967; Reese, 1966). Papilloma may be seen at the lid margin and on the conjunctiva of the bulb, like contact metastases.

Dermoids are as common as in Europe. Sometimes one gets frightened because the dermoid is not of a yellowish color, but black. This is due to the local with doctor (wogesha) who has punctured it and caused a hematoma.

I never saw *Basal cell epithelioma* and *squamous cell carcinoma* of the skin.

The *squamous cell carcinoma of the conjunctiva* is rather common. Carcinomas of the conjunctiva deserve to be especially mentioned because of all other malignant tumors they are much more widespread in Ethiopia than in Europe. According to Hogan & Zimmerman (1962) and Reese (1966) there is a certain relation to frequency and severity of conjunctivitis which, on the other hand, depends on hygiene. Carcinomas of the conjunctiva offer a colorful external picture − sometimes they are hard marrow tumors and at other times they are soft and deteriorating (Fig. 1a,b,c). They may grow

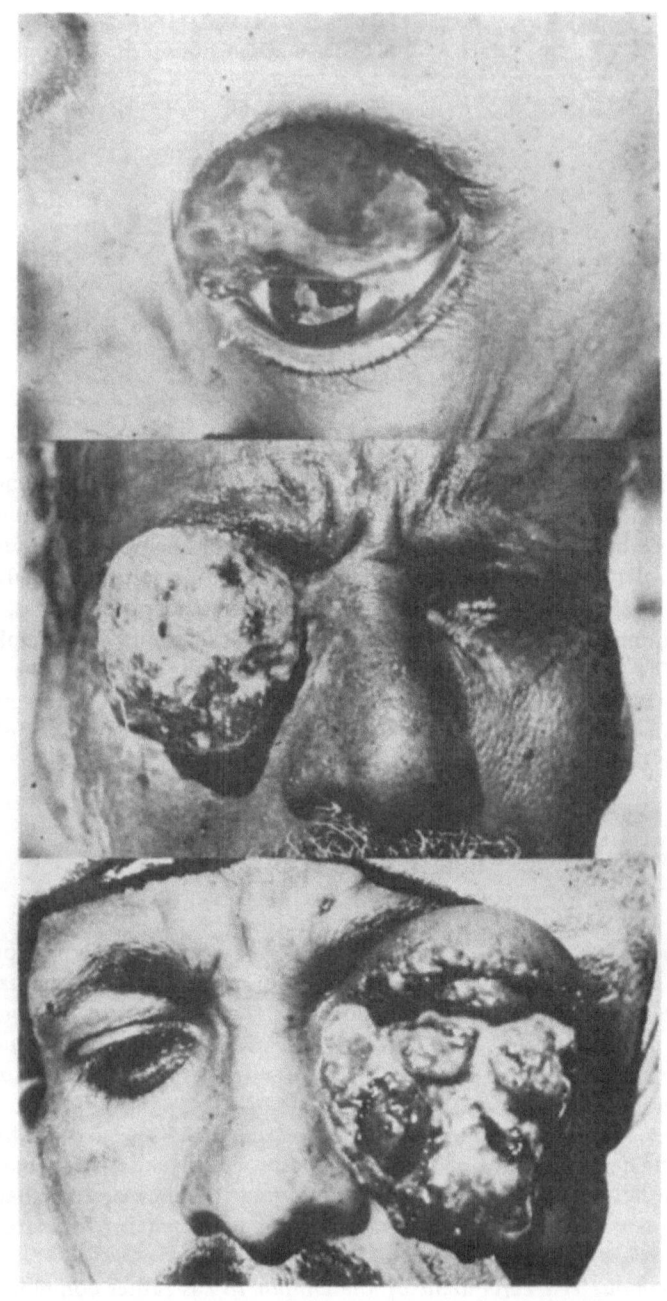

Fig. 1. a, b, c

absolutely exophytic so that the bulb remains completely intact in a tumor as big as a fist. In other cases they grow behind the bulb in such a manner as to cause proptosis together with lagophthalmic ulcers, resulting in perforation, or rupture of the bulb. Sometimes, only remaining parts of the sclera are then to be found in the tumor mass. They mostly metastasise only into the regional lymph nodes. Histologically, squamous cell carcinomas are to be expected but largely non-differentiated squamous cell carcinomas may occur, as well as basal cell carcinomas — the latter less frequently.

MESOBLASTIC TUMORS

Inflammations of the orbit, *orbital phlegmonas*, are rather common due to injuries by thorns and fighting injuries. A proptosis may be due to parasites, various fungus infections and, at times, one has to deal with an amoebic abscess.

Hydrops of the lacrimal sac is probably caused by trachoma and is frequent in trachomatous regions.

Mucoceles are a frequent occurrence. They dislocate the eyes either towards the corners of the mouth or in a far upward direction. I was able to observe osteomas which were of immense dimension.

One of the more frequent tumors, and up to now only described in Africa, is *Burkitt's lymphoma*. It amounts to about 50% of all orbital tumors. This is a rapidly growing tumor, its history is seldom longer than three months. This tumor mostly afflicts the jaw but in about 20% it involves the orbit (Fig. 2). It may occur uni- or bilaterally. Children are more often afflicted than adults (Discamps, 1972; Templeton, 1967). In advanced cases the

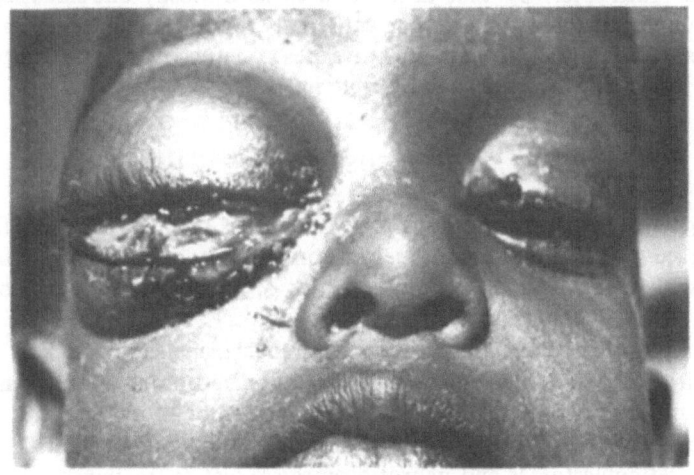

Fig. 2.

297

differential diagnosis from a retinoblastoma can be really difficult. Histologically, the tumor is composed of a homogenous population of primitive cells with vacuoles in the nucleus and cytoplasm, it also displays a scattering of histiocytes. An arthropod vectored virus has been taken into consideration as a possible cause of the tumor. There may be a correlation to the incidence of malaria. Also, the sea level seems to play a role. At any rate this tumor is occurring in Africa, in the so-called tumor belt, an area of high humidity.

VASCULAR TUMORS

Hemangiomata in the orbital region are rare. They are otherwise common in the bodies of Africans.

PIGMENTED TUMORS

Congenital melanosis, especially close to the limbus, is rather common. Artificial eyes, made in Europe, even those with a dark iris, never fit Ethiopians.

I have never seen *melanoblastomas*. The reports of Davies and Templeton do not even mention them.

NEUROGENIC TUMORS

Cephaloceles in the facial and orbital region exist. *Gliomas* of the optic nerve dilate the optical nerve canal causing a proptosis of gigantic dimensions.

Neurofibromas of the orbit are also of a very large size.

Retinoblastomas occur as often as in Europe. However, children are not brought to the physician's attention until at the stage of cat's eye amaurosis and much later. By that time there exists a mostly one-sided, apple-sized, suppurating and evil smelling tumor. As soon as the father enters the doctor's office, usually together with a peace corps worker, the diagnosis can simply be established by the horrible smell.

DISCUSSION

Alhtough the Ethiopians do not count themselves members of the African Negro race — they are of hamitic-semitic origin — my observations do correspond with those of other African statistics. My experiences are, of course, not a statistic evaluation.

It seems that the rare occurrence of intraocular melanoma and lid basal cell epithelioma are depending upon racial dispositions in contrast to Caucasians. Burkitt's lymphoma, as well as carcinoma of the conjunctiva seem to be due to environmental factors while all the other tumors known, such as retinoblastomas and neurofibromas are just as frequently observed in Europe.

SUMMARY

Orbital tumors are much more frequent in Africa than in Europe. They constitute a high percentage of all malignant tumors in African pathological institutes. Children are more afflicted than adults. Burkitt's lymphoma and the carcinoma of the conjunctiva seem to be due to environmental factors, while melanomas and lid basal cell epitheliomas seem to be less frequent than in Europe.

REFERENCES

Burkitt, D. Determining the climatic limitation of a children's cancer common in Africa. *Brit. med. J.: 1019* (1962)

Burkitt, D. & D. Wright. Geographical and Tribal Distribution of the African Lymphoma in Uganda. *Brit. med. J.: 568* (1966).

Davies, J.N.P. In: Tumours in Children, von H.B. Mardsen, J.K. Steward, Springer, Berlin (1968).

Discamps, G., J.C. Doury & M. Chovet. A statistical study of the cancers of eye and orbit in Africa, based on 460 pathologic observations. *Med. Trop.* 32: *385* (1972).

Duke-Elder, Sir St. System of Ophthalmology, 8. Kimpton, London (1967).

Duke-Elder, Sir St. System of Ophthalmology, 13. Kimpton, London (1974).

Hogan, M.J. & L.E. Zimmerman. Ophthalmic Pathology, Saunders, Philadelphia (1962).

Reese, A.B. Tumors of the eye, Harper-Row, Publishers, New York (1966).

Templeton, A.C. Tumours of the eye and adnexa in Africans of Uganda. *Cancer* (Philad.) 20: *1689* (1967).

Templeton, A.C. Orbital tumours in African children. *Brit. J. Ophthal.* 55: *254* (1971).

Ziegler, J.L. Burkitt's lymphoma and malaria. Trans. roy. Soc. trop.

Ziegler, J.L. Burkitt's lymphoma and malaria. *Trans. roy. Soc. trop. Med. Hyg.* 66: *285* (1972).

Author's address:
Augenklinik-Klinikum Steglitz
Hindenburgdamm 30
1 Berlin 45
W. Germany

Proc. 3rd Int. Symp. on Orbital Disorders, Amsterdam 1977

SIX HUNDRED AND EIGHTY-FOUR TUMORS OF THE EYE AND THE ORBIT TREATED IN THE FARABI EYE HOSPITAL OVER THE LAST FIVE YEARS

H. CHAMS & A. KHEYRIEH

(Teheran, Iran)

Since important statistical data on this subject have not been available recently from this part of the Middle East, we present this work, which is based on anatomopathological studies. A few rare cases which might be of some interest to this Symposium are included.

To prevent confusion it should be mentioned that the Farabi Hospital is the main ophthalmologic centre of Iran. During the last year we have received 116,976 patients. The anatomopathologic study has only been done in doubtful cases.

In our 84 cases of retinoblastomas there were twice as much males involved as females. The same distribution of the tumor was noted all over Iran with almost the same frequency each year. In our bilateral cases only one girl had two older brothers of 4 and 6 years, neither of them had retinoblastoma.

CASE REPORTS

Extraocular ectopic melanocarcinoma

Mr. H.E., aged 75 years, was seen for a proptosis of the right eye; the eye looked upwards and inwards. Eye movements were limited in all directions. A solid mass was palpable at the external and inferior side of the orbit. The vision was 7/10 E and the fundus was normal. At the operation, a pigmented mass of 3 bij 2.5 bij 2.5 cm was found which was very adherent to the

Table 1. Six hundred and eighty-four tumors treated over the last five years

	Number	Male	Female	Mean age years
Tumors	684	408	276	Adults 52
Malignant	386	241	145	Children 3*
Benign	298	167	131	29.5

* To calculate the mean age of children with malignant tumors, retinoblastoma and rhabdomyosarcoma have been taken into consideration.

300

Table 2. The malignant tumors

	Number	Male	Female	Mean age	Cases
Retino-blastoma	84	58	26	3	+ Optic N 15, Orbit 10, Bilat. 5
Rhabdomyo-sarcoma	7	5	2	6,5	Embryonal 6, Alveolar 1
Basal cell carcinoma Eyelid	124	72	52	51,5	12 were pigmented
Epidermoid carcinoma	81	51	30	50,5	Conj. 41, Orbit 20, Limbus 18, Cornea 2
Melano carcinoma	26	17	9	52,5	Eye & Orb. 13, Choroid 5, Eyelid 3, Conj. 2, C.B. 1, Iris 1, Ectopic 1
Lacrimal gland tumor	8	7	1	43	Mixed 5, Adenocar. 1, Anaplastic 2 1 child of 2 years

Table 3. Other malignant tumors*

	Number	Male	Female	Mean age
Sebaceous gland car.	8	3	5	57
Sweat glands carcinoma	14	7	7	53
Squamous cell car. Lids	8	4	4	57
Epith. in situ	14	9	5	51,5
Plasmocytoma	2	1	1	30,5
Metastatic	2	1	1	67,5
Lymphosar. Orbit	4	3	1	20
Lymphoreticulosarcoma	1	1		26
Lymphoma + CLL	1		1	60
Fibrosarcoma	2	2		43

* To facilitate classification we have placed all tumors of the lacrimal gland in the same table.

eye. The eye was enucleated. The sclera was indemned, the choroid normal and apparently this was a primary ectopic melanocarcinoma which was confirmed by anatomopathologic study (Figs. 1 and 2).

Anaplastic carcinoma of lacrimal gland

A.M. a boy of 2 years of age was brought to us for a proptosis of the right eye, which had started two months ago. He had no light perception. The eye was enucleated and the tumor was taken out. The anatomopathologic result was an anaplastic carcinoma of the lacrimal gland.

Ectopic meningioma of orbit

Mr A.D., 54 years old, was seen for a proptosis of the right eye, which had started two years ago. The eye was downwards and outwards. A solid mass,

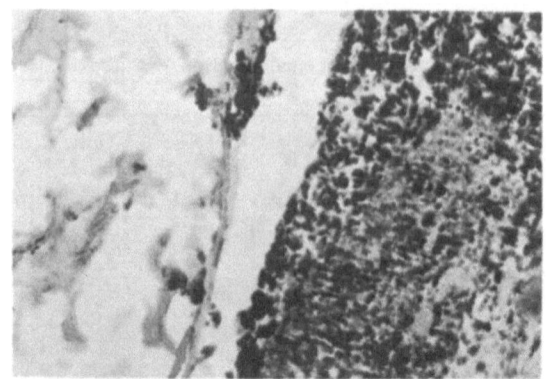

Fig. 1.

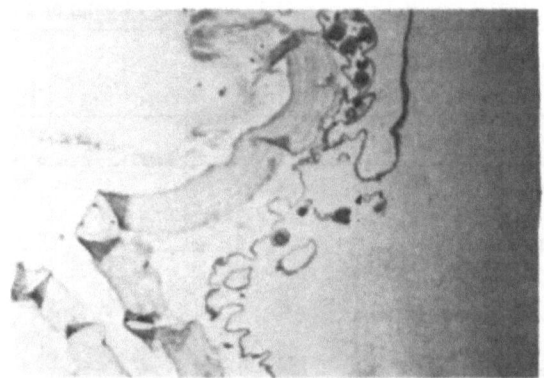

Fig. 2.

Table 4. Benign tumors

	Number	Male	Female	Mean age	Cases
Pigmented tumors	64	35	29	33,5	Eyelid 42, Conj. 21, Iris 1
Papilloma	52	37	15	38	Eyelid 34, Conj. 18, Keratoacanthoma 2
Hemangioma	22	9	13	27	Cap. 19, Cav. 3
Meningioma	5	2	3	38	Orbit 2, Optic N 2, Ectopic 1
Hamartoma	7	5	2	22	Limbus 5, Ext. 1, Int. 1

the size of a nut was palpable at the superointernal side of the orbit. The röntgebographic studies showed no abnormalities. The operation was done by the supra-orbital way. The optic nerve was indemned.

Table 5. Other benign tumors

	Number	Male	Female	Mean age
Pilomatrixoma	10	2	8	20 yrs
Lipoma & Fibrolipoma	14			22
Lymphoma & Lymphangioma	3	2	1	60
Glioma, Optic Nerve	3		3	26
Neurofibroma, Eyelid	2	2		12
Orbit	1		1	45
Osteoma	1		1	35

The meningioma of the optic nerve

Miss M.M., 5 years old, was brought to us for a proptosis of the right eye, which had started three years ago. She had an exposed keratitis. She was enucleated and two pieces of 12 by 10 by 6 mms of a solid mass were excised, with the optic nerve. The diagnosis of meningioma was confirmed.

Table 6. 114 benign cysts

	Number	Mean age		Number	Mean age
Dermoid	44	18 yrs	Mucocele	4	43 yrs
Epidermal	26	18.5	Lac. sac	3	40.5
Conjun.	15	31.5	Hydatic	3	8
Inclusion	10	48.5	Iris	1	0.5
Sebaceous	7	52	Lymphatic	1	22

During the last five years 114 cystic formations of the eye and the adenexa have been observed in the Farabi Hospital, 63 males and 51 females. The mean age was 25 years. The most frequent was the dermoid cyst, 44 cases. The hydatic cyst of the orbit is rare in Iran, only 14 cases have been ob-

Fig. 3.

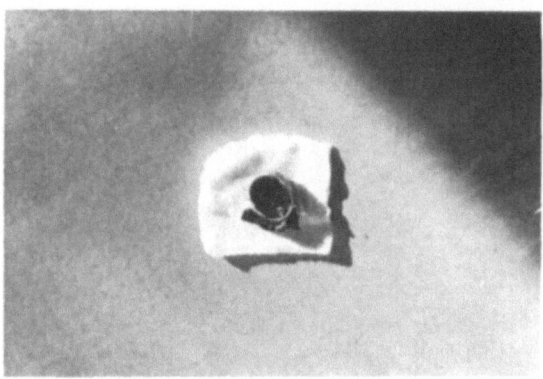

served since 1935. The three cases that we have had during the last five years were all children from 5 to 12, all from agricultural families. They all had a painful proptosis. The röntgenograms showed an enlarged orbit in all these cases. In one case the Casoni test was positive. The Weinberg-Parvu was always negative (Fig. 3).

CONCLUSION

Six hundred and eighty-fours tumours have been observed at the Farabi Eye Hospital of Teheran, during the last five years. The statistic data and a few rare cases of tumors are presented here.

REFERENCES

Chams, G. & G. Sadoughi. Les kystes hydatiques de l'orbite. *Sem. Hopit. (Paris)* 46: *201-203* (1955).

Drews, R.C. Primary malignant melanoma of orbit in a negro. *Arch. Ophthal.* 93: *335-336* (1975).

Jakobiec, F.A., R. Ellsworth & M. Tannenbaum. Primary orbital melanoma. *Am. J. Ophthal.* 78: *24-39* (1974).

Lopez, D.A., D.N. Silvers & E.B. Helwig. Cutaneous menigioma – a clinicopathologic study. *Cancer* 34: *728-744* (1974).

Pirouz, M.S. Kystes hydatiques de l'orbite observés a l'hopital Farabi. *Ann. Oculist. (Paris)* 209: *749-757* (1976).

Authors' address:
The Farabi Eye Hospital
Tehran
Iran

Proc. 3rd Int. Symp. on Orbital Disorders, Amsterdam 1977

LYMPHORETICULAR DISEASE WITH INVOLVEMENT
OF THE ORBITAL WALL?
THE VALUE OF SELECTIVE BONE BIOPSY

E.A. VAN SLOOTEN

(Amsterdam, The Netherlands)

Lymphoreticular disease, if pseudotumour is included, is one of the most frequent neoplastic affections in the orbital region. This is also true for the material collected by the Amsterdam working party on orbital disorders.

The limit between good and evil is notoriously vague where lymphoreticular affections are concerned. Examples of progression from benign lesions to agressive malignant disease and spontaneous regression of a condition that had been regarded as malignant occur in almost every large series of cases.

When confronted with a patient who has an orbital mass displacing the eyeball, one of the first possibilities one will have to consider is some form of lymphoreticular disease. When, however, the mass is firmly adherent to the orbital wall and changes suggesting destruction of bone structure can be detected, other possibilities have to be taken into account, in the first place metastatic malignant disease from the breast, kidney, thyroid, etc.

In case no signs or symptoms of distant malignancy can be detected by simple means, much time and energy can be saved by performing an early biopsy when cytological examination of aspirated material does not, as is very often the case, lead to a clear-cut diagnosis. It is generally known how carefully a biopsy must be planned if one wishes to avoid permanent injury to the function of the eye.

Many anatomical investigations, and recently the work done by Koornneef (1977), have provided a good insight into the microstructure of the peri- and retrobulbar connective tissue apparatus which keeps all orbital structures in their place. Damage, even to a small part of this intricate system, easily leads to permanent cosmetic and functional problems through disruption with resultant sagging and scar tissue retraction which hampers the movements of the eye.

Entering the orbit at any place from the front within the periorbita causes the greatest damage. The most sparing approach is usually from outside the orbital periosteum after optimal localisation of the lesion from which a biopsy is to be taken with echography and tomography. A short longitudinal incision into the periosteum gives good access at the same time causing little injury to the orbital contents. For a tumour situated behind the bulbus the best approach is through the lateral wall of the orbit unless the mass lies in the medial segment.

Whenever there exist radiographically demonstrated changes of the periorbital bones suggesting destruction or invasion, it is preferable to take the biopsy from the affected bone for several reasons:

1. Intraorbital structures remain unharmed.

2. Pathological examination of abnormal tissue within the marrow spaces very often allows a more exact diagnosis because the tissue is relatively well protected by the surrounding bone, whereas mechanical damage often results from trying to extract tiny pieces of soft tissue through a small incision far from the mass to be biopsied.

3. Radiological verification of the place from which the biopsy is being (was) taken, is possible and may be a great advantage.

Three cases illustrating these points were presented. All were initially regarded as a form of lymphoreticular disease. They were eventually diagnosed as cellular angioma, non-specific inflammation and fibrohistiocytic sarcoma on bone biopsies.

REFERENCES

Koornneef, L. Thesis, Amsterdam (1977).

Slooten, E.A. van. Lateral approach to the orbit. pp. 454–456 in: Proc. 2nd Symp. on Orbital Disorders, Amsterdam, 1973. Mod. Probl. Ophthal., Volume 14. Karger, Basel (1975).

Author's address:
Prinsengracht 573
Amsterdam
The Netherlands

Proc. 3rd Int. Symp. on Orbital Disorders, Amsterdam 1977

INTRA-ORBITAL TUMORS OF THE PERIPHERAL NERVES

J.P.A. GILLISSEN & H.J.F. PEETERS

(Amsterdam, The Netherlands)

According to some authors, about 10% of all orbital tumors are of neuro-genic origin. Of the last 444 orbital tumors seen at the orbital centre of the Amsterdam University Eye Clinic, 18 were diagnosed as tumors of the peripheral nerves (about 4%). The tumors of the peripheral nerves in the orbit are divided into:

1. neurofibroma
2. neurolemmona or Schwannoma
3. malignant Schwannoma.

The diffuse or multiple form of neurofibroma (the Von Recklinghausen disease) has several variants: diffuse or circumscribed, solitary or multiple.

In general, they are painless and they have a lumpy, rubber or a 'knotted cords' feeling. This kind of tumor manifests itself in every part of the orbit except in the lens. Often the eyelids are affected. In most cases they are congenital and some authors consider this tumor as a hereditary one.

Proptosis and displacement of the eyeball are the main symptoms. The proptosis may pulsate if the continuity of the bony orbit is disrupted and cranial pulsation is transmitted. In most cases the growth is very slow. 'Café au lait' spots are landmarks among the diagnostic signs. One can often see pendulous hypertrophy of the skin, be it regional or generalised.

The treatment is difficult since excision is frequently associated with con-siderable haemorrhage and total removal is impossible in most of the cases.

We have seen 10 cases of plexiform neurinomas in our series. In 8 cases diplopia, displacement of the eye or cosmetic reasons made it necessary to operate. In these cases we were aware of the fact that surgery was only palliative.

In two cases (a boy with a buphthalmos and a man with a large tumor) enucleation was performed. In another case, a boy who had used diphan-toin for years for epilepsy, the tumor was irradiated with high voltage X-rays of 1500 r as a growth inhibitor. It is known that diphantoin stimu-lates growth of neural tissues (neural crest syndrome) and in this case the X-ray therapy seems to have been effective. X-ray treatment was also per-formed in another patient with a large slow growing tumor in the orbit, with no results.

A solitary orbital form of neurofibroma can occur at any age. It forms a firm encapsulated mass, slowly growing with periods of intermittency lasting sometimes several years. Proptosis and impairment of eye muscle movements are the main symptoms.

In our series we have 6 patients with this solitary neurofibroma or neurolemmoma. Our pathologists made much effort to differentiate between these two types, which is very difficult. In one of these cases we considered it too dangerous to perform surgery, because operation would result in a loss of vision as the tumor was situated in the apex round the optic nerve. In the other 5 cases an operation was performed. In two cases the operation was radical, and the patients had no symptoms after surgery. Vision was good and no diplopia existed afterwards.

Several authors warn against malignant degeneration when this tumor is not completely extirpated. In our series we did not encounter it in the 3 cases where the operation was not radical on account of danger to vital structures, as one must excise the tumor 2 cm peripheral of its boundaries.

In one patient, having a neurofibroma in the orbit since 1959, 3 operations were performed in the last 18 years for recurrence of exophthalmus. The last one occurred two years ago, the patient having no complaints now.

Among the 444 orbital tumors we saw three patients with a neuroma. A neuroma is defined as a tumor of neural fibres. The first patient, a female of 22 years, had a tumor situated in the orbital roof which could be removed completely. There were no signs of a recurrence 1.5 years after the operation, and the patient has been free of double vision or other complaints.

The second patient developed an amputation neuroma of the infra-orbital nerve after an accident with facial injuries, 9 years ago. Three years later he complained of pain in the right side of his face. In X-ray pictures the infra-orbital canal was found to be fractured. After surgical decompression of the infra-orbital canal he was free of symptoms for the next 3 years. Then the patient returned and in the X-ray pictures a large defect was visible in the orbital floor. Surgical exploration revealed a large neuroma which penetrated into the orbit. The tumor was completely removed. After operation the patient suffered from phantom pains.

The last patient with a neuroma was a 64 years old lady who complained of severe facial pains and diplopia. Trigeminal neuralgia was diagnosed at first and the Gasserian ganglian was destroyed without any alleviation of the pains. Because of diplopia the patient was presented in our clinic. X-ray photographs revealed a large tumor of the orbit bulging into the maxillary sinus. After surgical extirpation of the tumor, which appeared to be a neuroma, the patient was symptomless.

None of our neurogenic tumors were malignant.
In the literature, malignant tumors are described as:
1. malignant Schwannoma
2. malignant epitheloid Schwannoma
3. malignant melanocytic Schwannoma
4. nerve fibre fibrosarcoma.

In all these cases radical surgery is advocated, if possible. Inoperable tumors should be attached with cytostatic drugs or x-ray therapy.

In summary, it is desirable to know the nature of every orbital tumor. Mostly they can be verified by biopsy or extirpation of the tumor and the subsequent pathological examination. However, the risk of surgical intervention, be it biopsy or a removal of the tumor, should always be evaluated against the advantages of surgical therapy.

In general, surgical intervention must be delayed if the process is situated near the apex and the vision is not endangered. On the other hand, if the visual capacity is threatened, it is permissible to open the orbit even at the risk of damaging vital structures.

In none of the cases of neurofibroma where we extirpated only a part of the tumor did we see growth stimulation due to the operation.

Authors' address:
Eye Clinic of the University of Amsterdam
Wilhelmina Gasthuis
104, 1e Helmerstraat
Amsterdam
The Netherlands

Proc. 3rd Int. Symp. on Orbital Disorders, Amsterdam 1977

BENIGN TUMORS OF THE BONY ORBITAL WALL

H.J.F. PEETERS & J.P.A. GILLISSEN

(Amsterdam, The Netherlands)

The benign tumorous malformations of the orbital wall are a relatively small group of the exophthalmos-causing factors.

For this paper, we exclude:
- the congenital anomalies such as the several forms of craniostenosis;
- the more extensive clinical pictures such as Crouzon's disease;
- Paget's disease;
- Apert's syndrome; and also
- the space-occupying lesions, dermoids, haemangiomas and neurofibromas, causing enlargement of the orbit.

If we confine ourselves to the tumors of the orbital wall, a group of slow-growing lesions presents itself, in which three are the most important: the osteoma, fibrous dysplasia and meningioma. In Reese's book (1963) this group forms 6% of 230 consecutive cases of clinically studied expanding lesions. In Henderson's book (1973) — of 465 orbital tumors — they make up 9%. In 444 cases presented to the Orbital Centre of the University Eye Clinic of Amsterdam the figure comes to 8% (Table 1).

Concerning symptoms (Table 2), it is understood that during the period of growth (from about 6 months to 30 years) they and the signs become more severe depending on the sites of tumefaction.

In short, the characteristics are the following:

Table 1.

Orbital tumors	A.B. Reese	J.W. Henderson	Orbital Centre Amsterdam
	1963	1973	1977
Total consecutive cases	230	465	444
osteomas	2	5	4
fibrous dysplasia	1	5	8
meningiomas	11	32	23
Group total	14 (± 6%)	42 (± 9%)	35 (± 8%)

Table 2. Symptoms in general of benign space-occupying masses*

---

displacement of the eye
diplopia
soft tissue swelling
sometimes palpable
pain is not common
seldom papilledema
      visual disturbance
      optic atrophy
slow growth

Osteoma
— mesodermal origin; embryonic rest
— predilection site: anterior ethmoid cells or frontal sinus; secondly: maxillary and sphenoid sinus
— age distribution: 2nd, 3rd and 4th decade of life
— sex ratio: male more than female
— growth: slow or not at all
— X-ray pictures are most important: abnormally dense, normal bone tissue gives a typical opacity.

Fibrous dysplasia (the term to be preferred for the one-bone and contiguous bone location)
— cause unknown (it seems that osteoblasts change into fibroblasts and back)
— location: sphenoid, ethmoid, frontal bone, maxilla and zygomatic bone;
— age distribution: 2nd, 3rd decade of life
— no sex preference (different reports)
— growth: slow or sometimes less slow (depending on age); tends to stop in older patients)
— X-ray pictures: (d.d. with the other two of the group) i.d. has more 'weak' parts in the mass shadows, a more 'smudgy' appearance (Blodi, 1976).

Meningioma
— originate from the neural crest (meningocytes in combination with a mesodermal factor); invasion of the marrow spaces with secondary osteoblastic proliferation (Blodi, 1976)
— site: inside (optic nerve) or outside the orbit (sphenoid ridge)
— age distribution: 4th, 5th decade of life (in general)
— sec ratio female : male = 3 : 1 (approx.)
— slow progression; possible hormonal influence (such as pregnancy) seems to speed up growth
— two types of growth: a) globular; b) flat ('en plaque')
— X-ray pictures: (difficult to interpret) meningiomas are at first not visible, later spongy bone-reaction, later dense shadows, later destruction; to differentiate with the others.

THERAPY

One can agree with the statement that surgical intervention has to wait until the clinical picture demands it. Total removal is almost possible; irradiation in fibrous dysplasia is even dangerous; malignant transformation is seen. Ophthalmologist, E.N.T. specialist and neurosurgeon together have to choose the best surgical route: anterior, lateral or transcranial.

Authors' address:
Eye Clinic of the University of Amsterdam
Wilhelmina Gasthuis
104, 1e Helmerstraat
Amsterdam
The Netherlands

Proc. 3rd Int. Symp. on Orbital Disorders, Amsterdam 1977

FIVE CASES OF NASAL SINUS MUCOCELES AND THEIR OCULAR SYMPTOMS

H. MATSUO & M. USUI

(Tokyo, Japan)

Nasal sinus mucoceles give rise to difficult problems: the symptoms depend on their location, their rate of growth and the direction of their growth. The purpose of this paper is to point out both the clinical and the diagnostic problems of mucoceles.

CASE REPORTS

Case 1

A 45 year old male was admitted to our Department on September 13, 1970, complaining of bilateral blurred vision and exophthalmos over a period of seven years.

Prior to admission to our Department, he had been diagnosed as an exophthalmic goitre and chronic choroiditis at another hospital, and he had been treated for two years. He had a history of bilateral frontal sinusitis which had been operated on at the age of 20. Physical examination revealed bilateral exophthalmos with significant Graefe's and Moebius' signs. Exophthalmometry gave a reading of 17.5 mm for the right eye and 18 mm for the left. Visual acuity was 0.2 for the right eye and 0.5 for the left, with correction. The left eye was 2 mm lower than the right. There were limitations of ocular movement of both eyes except for the downward gaze. Both anterior chambers were clear and there was no opacity in the vitreous bodies. Ophthalmoscopic examinations did not show any evidence of a specific disease and the thyroid function tests were normal. X-rays of the skull and sinuses showed an extreme enlargement of both frontal sinuses. In the upper wall of both orbits the margin had disappeared and bone destruction was present (Fig. 1 and 2).

Preoperative diagnosis of mucoceles of both frontal sinuses was made, and an external fronto-ethmoidal operation was performed for each sinus. During the operation defects of both orbital roofs were seen, but no hole was present in the septum. The mucoceles contained a large amount of mucopurulent material, measuring approximately 30 ml in the right sinus and 50 ml in the left. Culture of the aspirated material was sterile. After the operation the exophthalmos disappeared and the peculiar retinal folds diminished gradually and they had disappeared completely seven days postoperatively. Visual acuity in each eye improved to 0.6, with correction.

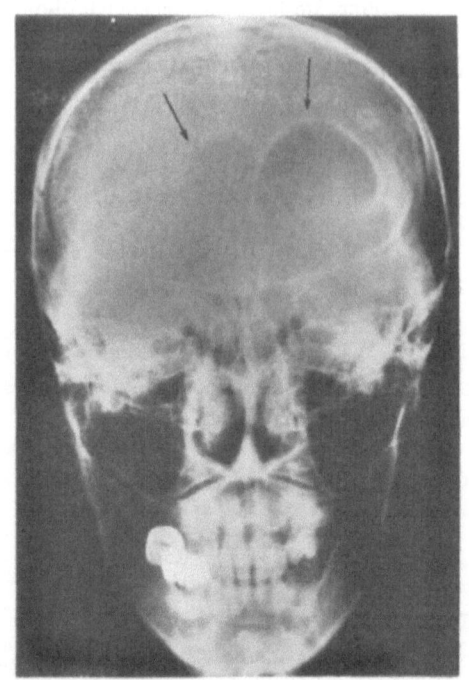

Fig. 1

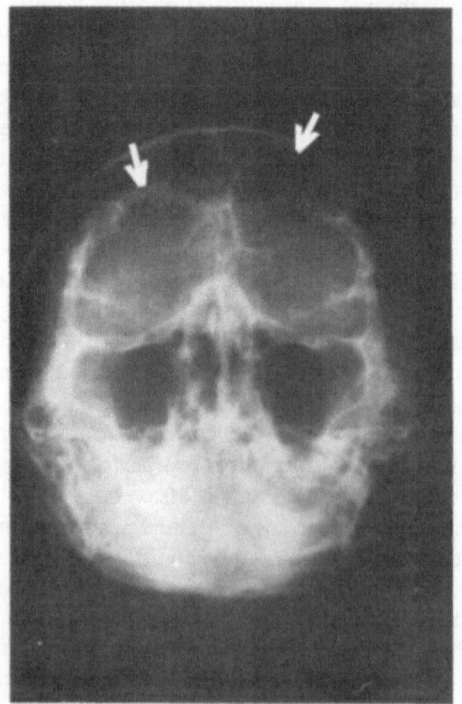

Fig. 2

A 27 year old male was admitted to hospital on May 15, 1976, with the chief complaint of left exophthalmos and diplopia. Six months prior to admission, proptosis of the left eye had become apparent with downward displacement of the globe. He had recognized asthenopia and dull pain of the frontal head for two months continuously. The visual acuity in each eye could be corrected to 1.2. The left eye was 3 mm lower than the right, and its movement remarkably limited in the upper gaze. A tumor the size of the tip of a small finger was palpable in the inner portion of the upper orbital margin. The exophthalmos of the left eye was remarkable as the scale was 16 mm for the left and 11 mm for the right eye. Orbitometry revealed a high intraorbital pressure of the left orbit, but this high pressure decreased with over 400 g compression. Funduscopic examination of the left eye showed peculiar retinal folds in the posterior pole. With ultrasonography (B-scan), there were two shadows that appeared massive. One of these was situated in the nasal side of the upper orbital cavity and the other behind the globe. X-rays of the skull and the sinuses by posterior-anterior and Waters' views showed a marked enlargement of both frontal sinuses with three antral formations (Fig. 3). Lateral view demonstrated a large protrusion of the sinus which extended towards the cranium, and the posterior wall of the sinus could not be identified due to erosion (Fig. 4). Arterio-

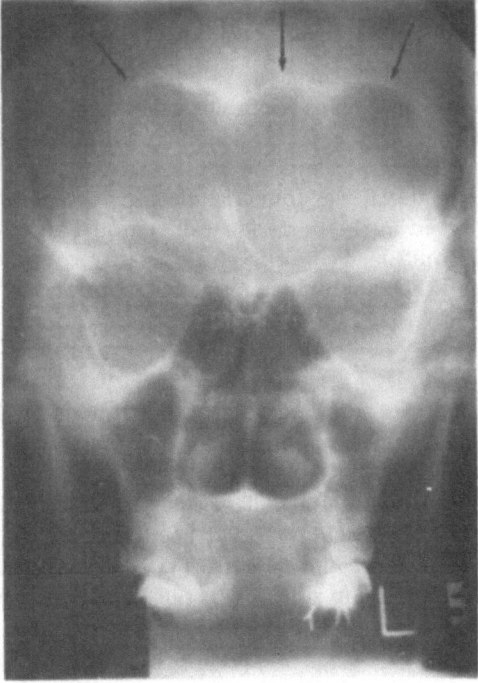

Fig. 3

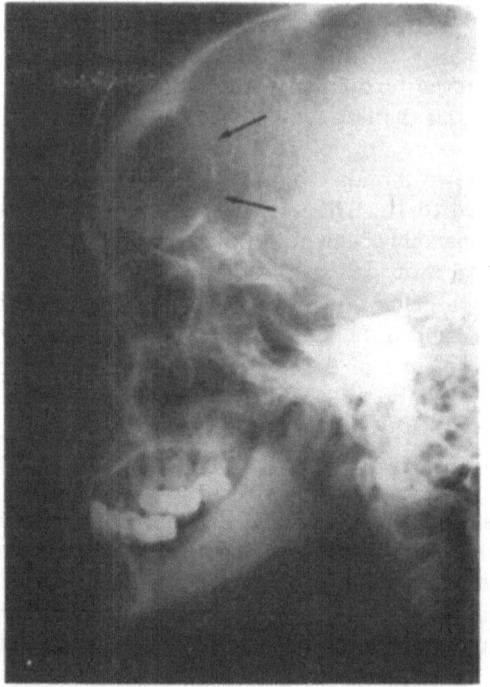

Fig. 4

graphy (CAG) showed no vascular leaks nor vascular invasion in the pro-
trusive area of the frontal sinus. Neurological examination did not significantly change. On June 9, 1976, Killian's operation was performed for a
mucocele of the left frontal sinus. In the cavity about 130 ml of yellow-
green non-odorous material was found, and a bony defect of approximately
3 x 3 cm was observed in the posterior wall. Through this defect, a section
of the dura mater could be seen. The post-operative course was uneventful
and the diplopia and the exophthalmos gradually improved.

Case 3

A 48 year old male was admitted to the Department on July 23, 1970,
because of marked conjunctival congestion of the right eye with diplopia in
downwards gaze for about four months.

Past history revealed bilateral maxillary sinusitis which had been operated
on at the age of 18. The right side had been re-operated 10 years later.
Visual acuity of each eye could be corrected to 1.2. On examination, the
right eye was displaced 1 mm superior to the left. Right ocular movement
was limited in downwards gaze. Conjunctival congestion and chemosis were
observed in the right eye, but in the cornea, the anterior chamber, the lens
and the fundus were normal. Exophthalmometry showed a reading of 15
mm for the right and 13 mm for the left eye.

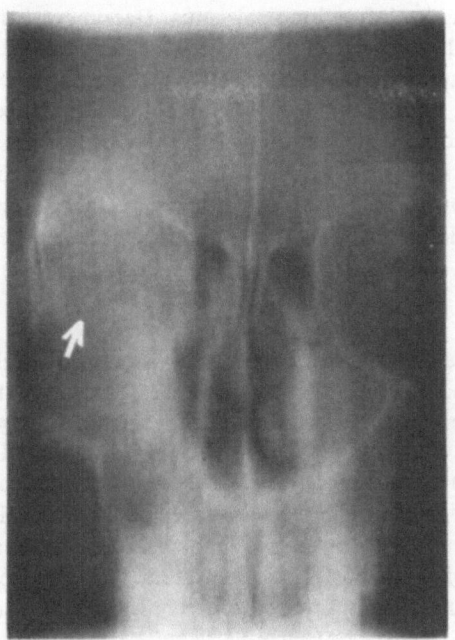

Fig. 5

On palpation, the external portion of infraorbital margin contained a mass the size of the tip of a small finger with slight tenderness. X-rays in the Waters' position revealed thin diffuse density in the right orbit, and there was a defect in the orbital floor detected by tomography of the skull at 4 cm from the front (Fig. 5). Once again sublabial antrostomy was performed. The orbital floor was absent to a great extent and the cavity contained 15 ml of chocolate-like material. Pathological examination of the mucous membrane did not reveal malignancy and the culture of the fluid showed no growth.

Post-operatively, the exophthalmos and the limitation of the right ocular movement improved and the diplopia disappeared completely.

Case 4

An 11 year old girl was referred to hospital on January 5, 1976, because of a left chronic dacryocystitis. About four months earlier, she had noticed a moderate swelling of the same region and the epiphora became increasingly significant during the past two weeks when she had suffered from a cold. The left conjunctival congestion was marked and the tear sac area was swollen and red. There was a very hard induration with slight fluctuation. Examination of the passage of the lacrimal fluid with stain material revealed a vealed a strong resistance in the canal, but the stain was detected in the inferior nasal meatus. The ocular position and eye movements were normal, as were the fundi. Rhinoscopic findings did not show abnormalities. Roentgen examination of the skull and sinuses by Water's view showed a small vague round shadow in the left ethmoidal sinus. Dacryocystography showed no enlargement of the tear sac, but contrast medium flowed into the meatus with a narrow line along the shadow (Fig. 6). During the operation the tear sac was found to be intact. A yellow-gray coloured mucocele was found beneath the sac, compressing it as well as the canal. An external fronto-ethmoidal operation was performed. The mucocele contained about 15 ml of aseptic muco-purulent material. Postoperative dacryocystography showed a satisfactory dilated tear sac and a good passage of the canals (Fig. 7).

Case 5

A 32 year old male had noticed a blurred vision of the right eye during the past seven months. Vision of the right eye was 1.2, with correction, and 1.5, without correction, for the left. Ocular movements and eye positions were normal. Slight exophthalmos of the right eye was noted. The fundus of the left eye was normal, but the right revealed a marked choked disc. Some kind of disturbance of the optic nerve was suspected by the critical fusion flicker frequence test, due to a lower frequency value. X-ray examination of the skull and the orbit with posterior and Waters'. view did not reveal a lesion, but optic foramina view showed the destruction of the surrounding bony

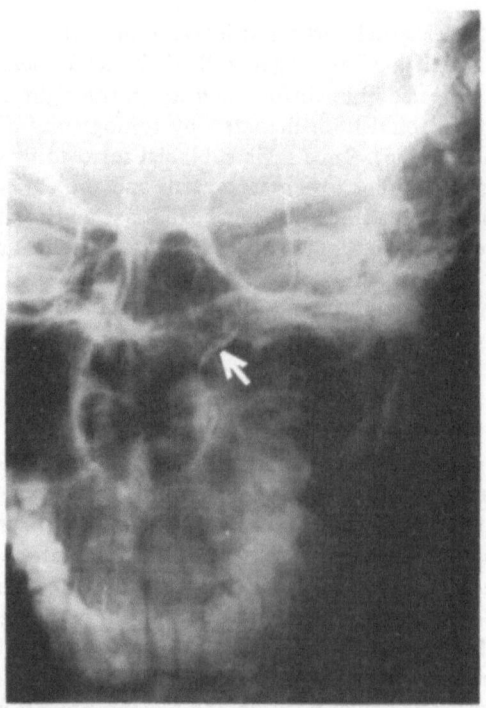

Fig. 6

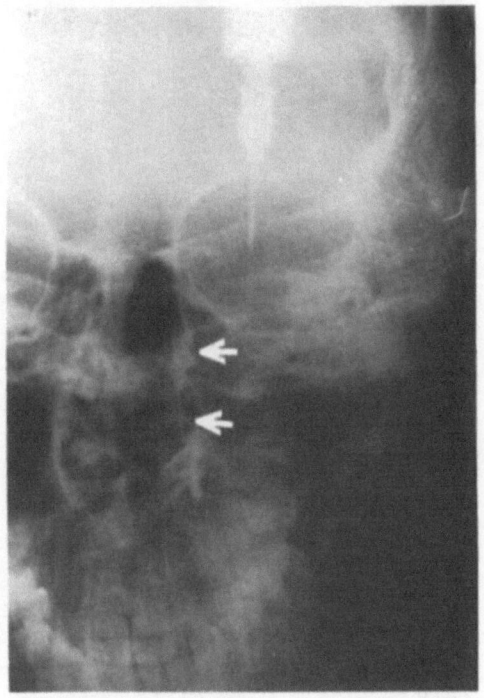

Fig. 7

wall of the optic canal and disappearance of septa in the sphenoidal sinus (Fig. 8). A frontal tomogram revealed a bulging of the roof of the sphenoidal sinus to the anterior fossa of the cranium with partial erosion (Fig. 9). After a pre-operative diagnosis of mucocele of the posterior ethmoid cells or sphenoidal sinus the transfrontal sphenotomy was performed. After removal of the posterior part of the ethmoidal bone, a whitish mucocele of the sphenoidal sinus was observed. The mucocele contained about 7 ml of aseptic viscous material.

The post-operative course was uneventful, and the retinal edema around the optic disc disappeared completely two weeks after the operation.

COMMENTS

Mucoceles arising from para-orbital sinuses are usually unilateral and their symptoms vary greatly depending on their location, rate of growth and extension into the orbit.

In Case 1 the mucoceles arose from the bilateral frontal sinuses and gave symptoms resembling exophthalmic goitre and choroiditis with retinal folds. Bilateral mucoceles of the frontal sinus are rare; therefore, it was necessary to make a differential diagnosis from thyroid disease and chronic choroiditis. Plain X-rays of the skull, the ocular examinations and the thyroid function test were essential to solve the problems in this case.

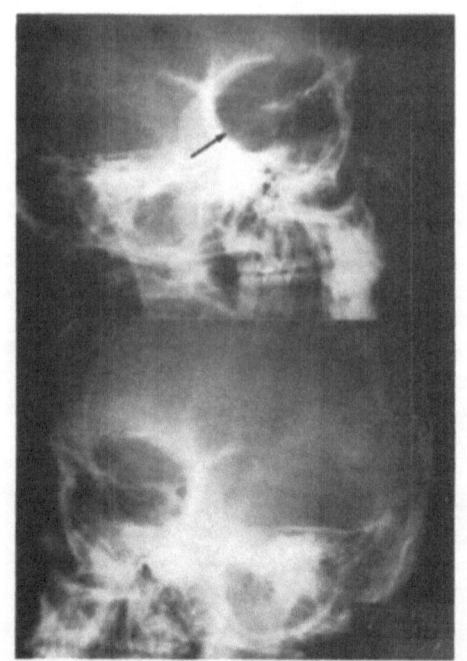

Fig. 8

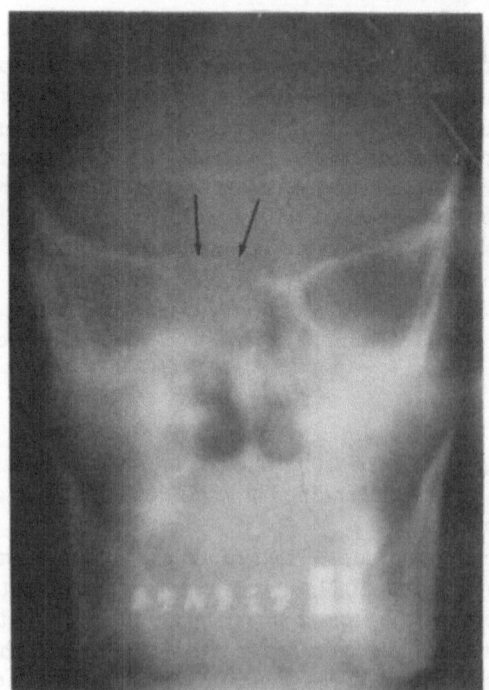

Fig. 9

Case 2 is a large mucocele of the frontal sinuses communicating with the intracranium. In general, an intracranial extension of the frontal mucocele is rare (Frenkel, 1968), but when it has existed for many years it may develop into a giant cyst. In our case there were two holes, between the mucocele and the orbit, and between the mucocele and extradural space of the intracranium. These findings may explain that the neurological and the ocular findings were not significant in spite of the huge dimensions of the mucoceles.

A mucocele of the anterior ethmoid cells, as found in Case 4, can sometimes produce symptoms similar to those of dacryocystitis. In such a case an operation may be undertaken with a diagnosis of dacryocystitis (Schlagenhauff, 1949). Epiphora without obliteration of the tear passages can be due to pressure of a mucocele behind the tear sac. Therefore, dacryocystography is of great importance to make a diagnosis for this type of lesion.

Maxillary sinus mucoceles are rare (Fukado, 1971), but occasionally we may encounter this type of mucocele, which gives rise to an obstruction of the canal of the sinus after a sinus operation. Ocular signs become apparent when the mucocele destroys the bone of the orbit floor and extends to the orbital cavity. A frontal tomogram is necessary to determine the lesion.

Sphenoid sinus mucoceles are also relatively rare. The diagnosis is usually difficult because a plain X-ray cannot always elucidate the lesion and the rhinoscopic examination shows only little change (Shiraiwa, 1976). However, plain X-rays, especially for the optic foramina views and the frontal tomograms are helpful in discovering these lesions (Calcaterra, 1974; Fugitani, 1975).

SUMMARY

Five cases of different mucoceles of the nasal sinuses, which presented relatively rare ocular symptoms, are reported. They are:

Case 1: Bilateral frontal sinus mucoceles presenting exophthalmos of both eyes. Ophthalmoscopic examination revealed peculiar retinal folds in both posterior poles.

Case 2: A unilateral frontal sinus mucocele, giving rise to a unilateral exophthalmos due to a large cyst extending into the anterior cranial fossa.

Case 3: A maxillary sinus mucocele accompanied by an upward displacement of the eyeball.

Case 4: Ethmoid sinus mucocele, showing a long-standing epiphora due to a compression of the dacryocystic duct.

Case 5: A sphenoid sinus mucocele manifested as a unilateral choked disc.

REFERENCES

Calcaterra, T.C., et al. The diagnostic evaluation of unilateral exophthalmos. *Laryngoscope* 134: *231–242* (1974).

Frenkel, M. Laminography in the management of mucoceles. *Am. J. Ophthal.* 65: *522–526* (1968).

Fugitani, T., et al. Cyst of sphenoidal sinus. Jibiinkoka, Rinsho. *Pract. Otolaryng.* (Kyoto) 68: *1127–1132* (1975).

Fukado, Y., et al. Ocular manifestations of mucocele of paranasal sinus. *Acta Soc. ophthal. jap.* 75: *979–987* (1971)

Schlagenhauff, K. Über die Mucocele des Siebbeins in der Tränensackgegend. *Wien. Klin. Wschr.: 716–718* (1948).

Shiraiwa, T., et al. Paranasal sinus cysts with ocular involvements. Jibiinkoka. *Otorhinolaryng.* (Jap.) 48: *375–379* (1976).

Authors' address:
Tokyo Medical College Hospital
6-7-1 Nishishinjuku Shinjuku-ku
Tokyo
Japan

Proc. 3rd Int. Symp. on Orbital Disorders, Amsterdam 1977

THE ORBITAL MANIFESTATIONS OF
VON RECKLINGHAUSEN'S DISEASE

D.J. COSTER & J.E. WRIGHT

(London, England)

INTRODUCTION

Frederick Daniel Von Recklinghausen described, in 1882, multiple neuro-fibromatosis, a condition characterised by multiple neurofibromata of the skin, abnormal pigmentation of the skin, and multiple neurofibromata of peripheral nerves. Orbital involvement is relatively common. The purpose of this paper is to review a group of patients who have presented recently to the Orbital Clinic at Moorfields Eye Hospital, City Road, London, with orbital manifestations of the disease.

CASE MATERIAL

Patients with six or more 'café au lait' spots exceeding 15 mm in diameter can be assumed to have the disease (Crowe & Schull, 1953; Whitehouse, 1966). This does not mean that patients with less spots do not have the condition; however, all the patients included in the review had an abundance of cutaneous manifestations. Twenty patients have recently been assessed in the Clinic with the orbital manifestations of Von Recklinghausen's disease. Their ages at the time of initial presentation ranged from six months to fifty-five years. However, all but three presented in the first decade of life. Fourteen were male and six female. Nine of the twenty had a positive family history with an autosomal dominant pattern of inheritance. However, negative family histories could not be confirmed.

CLINICAL FEATURES

The principal reasons for presentation were lid deformity with facial as-symetry, proptosis, or, less commonly, buphthalmos. Combinations of these occur, and in this group of patients twelve had lid deformities, ten had prop-tosis, and two had glaucoma. The lid deformity is due to the presence of plexiform neuromata, often associated with hypertrophy of otherwise normal bony skeleton and soft tissues. Proptosis can be due to optic nerve gliomata, isolated neurofibromata, or plexiform neuromata. There is a distinctly different pattern of disease in those presenting as children and those presenting later in adult life. All three patients presenting in adult life with proptosis had isolated neurofibromata of orbital nerves.

RADIOLOGY

Plain X-rays are important in confirming a clinical diagnosis. The most important signs seen in orbital views are orbital enlargement which was seen in thirteen cases, optic canal enlargement which was seen in eleven, and elevation of the sphenoidal wing as seen in six. Three cases had defects in the orbital apex and two had enlarged pituitary fossae. Of the three adults presenting with proptosis, all had essentially normal films, although one showed erosion of the orbital roof in relation to the tumour.

DISCUSSION

There are two groups of patients who present with the orbital manifestations of Von Recklinghausen's Disease. The first group comprises children with facial and periorbital abnormalities associated with plexiform neuromata, optic nerve gliomata or glaucoma. These children have abnormal radiology. The second group comprises patients presenting later in life who tend to have solitary neurofibromata on orbital nerves and have normally developed orbits on X-ray. The tumors can, however, be related to areas of

Patients with Von Recklinghausen's Disease are at risk of developing neoplastic disease in tissues derived from the neural crest (Heard, 1963). In this series of patients five children developed optic nerve gliomata and one died of sarcomatous change in a plexiform neuroma.

With such a wide range of orbital pathology related to Von Recklinghausen's Disease a search for café au lait spots is an important part of the assessment of any patient with an orbital mass. The pattern of disease varies with age in any one patient and serious complications can occur at any stage of a patient's life.

REFERENCES

Crowe, F.W. & W.J. Schull. Diagnostic importance of cafe-au-lait spots in neurofibromatosis. *Arch. Int. Med.* (Chicago) 91: *758–766* (1953).
Heard, G. Malignant disease in Von Recklinghausen's neurofibromatosis. *Proc. Roy. Soc. Med.* 56: *502–503* (1963).
Whitehouse, D. Diagnostic value of the cafe-au-lait spot in children. *Arch. Dis. Child.* 11: *316–319* (1966).

Authors' address:
Moorfields Eye Hospital
City Road
London EC1V 2PD
England

Reprint requests to D.J. Coster, F.R.C.S., at the above address

324

Proc. 3rd Int. Symp. on Orbital Disorders, Amsterdam 1977

OSSIFYING FIBROMAS OF THE ORBITAL ROOF

FREDERICK A. JAKOBIEC, GUY D. POTTER,
JOHN MITCHELL & IRA S. JONES

(New York, N.Y., USA)

INTRODUCTION

This paper reports on three cases of fibro-osseous tumors that created lytic defects in the orbital roof. Their clinical and radiographic appearances led to a pre-operative diagnosis of either a mucocele or an epidermoid cyst. Histopathologically, however, these lesions were interpreted as benign ossifying fibromas. Ossifying fibromas have received scant attention in the ophthalmic literature and are often subsumed with fibrous dysplasia (Jakobiec & Jones, 1976). The purpose of this paper is to present the clinical, radiographic, and pathologic differences between ossifying fibroma and fibrous dysplasia, and to highlight the 'cystic variant' of ossifying fibroma that our patients developed.

CASE REPORTS

Case 1

In June 1976 a 38 year old male radiologist discovered an asymptomatic osteolytic lesion in the roof of his left orbit on routine sinus x-rays taken for the evaluation of non-specific sinus congestion (Fig. 1). Vision was 20/20 (6/6) in both eyes and the ocular examination was completely unremarkable. Absent were displacement or proptosis, ocular motility disturbance, and a palpable mass. Frontal and lateral tomograms of the orbit revealed a well outlined defect involving the mid portion of the left supraorbital margin that extended posteriorly along the orbital roof. The major diagnostic possibilities were an epidermoid-dermoid cyst, a hemangioma, or an eosinophilic granuloma. The margin of the lytic defect was not considered to be as typically well corticated or sclerosed as is usually seen in epidermoid-dermoid cysts. Because of the fear of a more ominous problem, such as a reticulum cell sarcoma of bone, exploration and biopsy were deemed necessary. At surgery an incision was made under the left brow and carried down to bone. The periosteum was incised and separated from the roof of the orbit with a periosteal elevator. A small hole was reached in the orbital roof. Complete access was possible only after a portion of the superior orbital rim was removed with a Stryker saw; the intervening bone to the

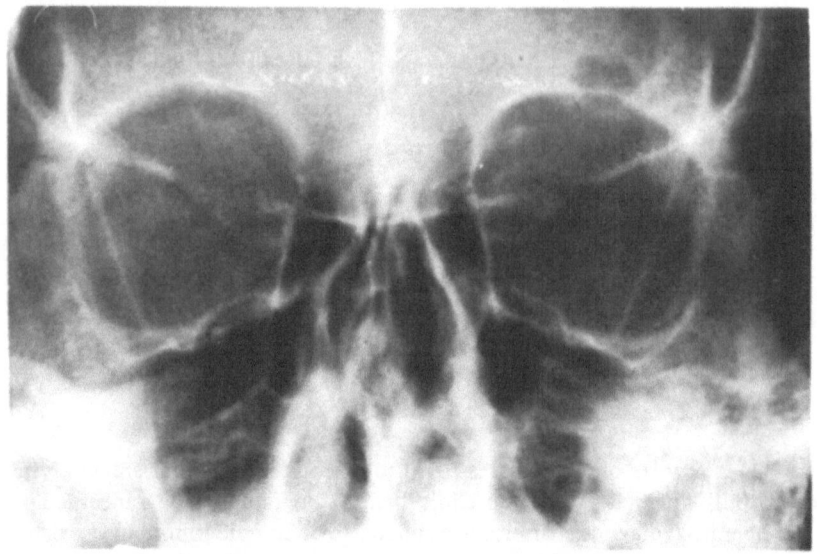

Fig. 1. Asymptomatic small osteolytic lesion in roof of left orbit without sclerotic margin, resembling an epidermoid.

defect was rongeured. The defect contained cheesy, yellowish, blood stained material consistent with the appearance of the contents of a dermoid cyst, and it was attempted to curette as much of this material as possible. Pathologic examination of the biopsy tissue disclosed a benign fibro-osseous tumor. During 15 months of follow up there has been no enlargement of the osseous defect, nor has it disappeared.

Case 2

A 57 year old male was seen in ophthalmologic consultation in June 1976 for evaluation of an anterior superonasal left orbital mass. Five years earlier the patient had sustained a facial fracture of undetermined extent. There had been multiple 'inflammatory episodes' ocurring about the left eye culminating in the appearance of proptosis. On examination the ocular status was unremarkable, but there were 3 mm of relative left proptosis caused by a firm, rubbery mass attached to the upper inner angle of the left orbit (Fig. 2). Routine skull and orbital x-rays disclosed absence of the cortical margin of the left supero-medial portion of the orbital rim. The medial portion of the frontal sinus was occupied by a mass of soft tissue density which on the Water's view was seen to be associated with an extensive displacement of the supero-medial orbital wall into the retrobulbar space. The osseous outlines of the uninvolved lateral portion of the left frontal sinus were normal appearing and not enlarged; its scalloped margins had been preserved. There was opacification of the left ethmoid and maxillary sinuses, as well as a retention cyst of the right antrum. Lastly, there was evidence of an old

326

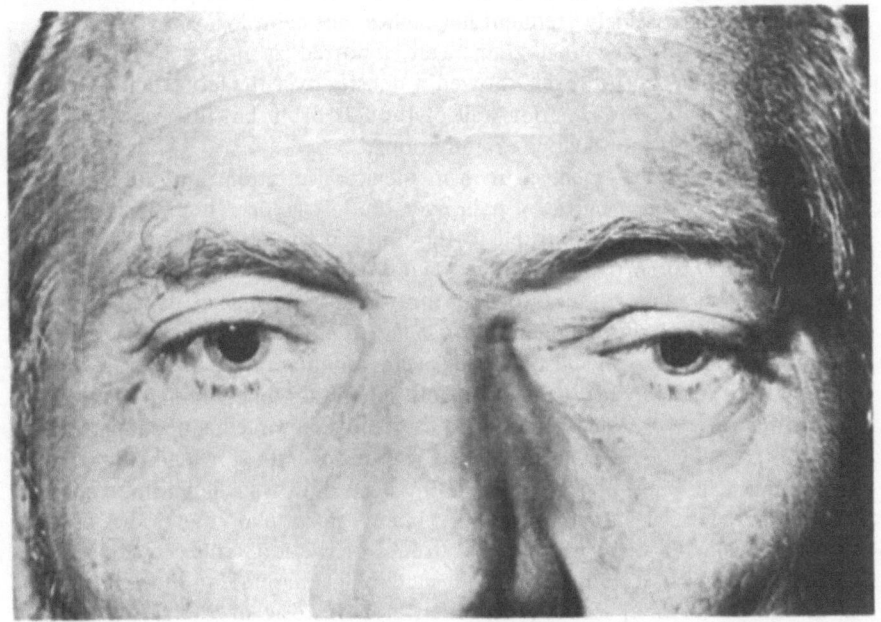

Fig. 2. Solid, rubbery left superonasal orbital mass mimicking a mucocele.

healed left orbital floor fracture. B-scan ultrasonography portrayed a rounded mass superonasally that had poorer sound transmission than that seen in mucoceles. The clinical and radiographic findings, however, suggested the diagnosis of a mucocele, and the orbit was explored. At surgery a calcific mass was encountered. The superficial shell of bone encasing the mass was broken with rongeurs until thickened boggy tissue was encountered that was thought to be sinus mucosa. This tissue was biopsied and as much as possible was removed. No pus or mucus discharged when this tissue was incised. The mass did not seem to be so calcific in its depth or in its more posterior extension into the orbit. The pathologic examination showed a fibro-osseous tumor. In 15 months of follow up the patient has experienced a recurrence of the superonasal tumor. Further surgery is planned.

Case 3

While living in Spain in 1962 a 36 year old white female developed generalized headaches that persisted with increasing severity and eventually accompanied by proptosis. Radiographic studies disclosed changes in the lesser wing of the sphenoid bone. After hospitalization a pneumoencephalogram was interpreted as showing a spheno-orbital meningioma, which was subsequently subtotally resected and read out histopathologically as a meningioma. Post-operatively visual acuity and ocular motor function were allegedly unremarkable, but the patient continued to complain of headaches.

327

Upon returning to the United STates in 1964 she was re-examined with the complaint of increasingly frequent headaches, but neurological examination and repeat pneumoencephalogram were reported as normal. The radiographic examination, however, showed a density over the left ethmoid with some thickening of the superior wall of the left orbit, but this was thought to be unchanged from previous examinations.

The patient was not seen again in medical consultation until July 1973, when she developed progressive pain over the left globe. There was vertical diplopia and she was re-admitted to the hospital for evaluation. The visual acuity was 20/20 (6/6) in both eyes, but there were 2 mm of left relative proptosis. The range of extraocular motion was normal at distance, but there was vertical dysconjugation on near gaze. The pupillary responses, fundus examination, and visual fields were unremarkable. The impression was that the patient had a recurrent left sphenoid wing meningioma. New skull films revealed destruction of the roof and superomedial portion of the left orbital wall (Fig. 3). The sinus itself was not overall expanded, and there were small scallopings present in the uninvolved sinus wall. The tomographic study also revealed intactness of the lateral portion of the floor of the frontal sinus without expansion. Polytomes of the left sphenoid showed a persistent surgical deformity of the sphenoidal margins of the left orbit from the previous operation. Persistent hyperostosis of the left planum sphenoidale and left wing of the sphenoid were noted. A left carotid arteriogram revealed a tumor blush, which received its vascular supply through an accessory meningeal artery from the maxillary artery. The patient was

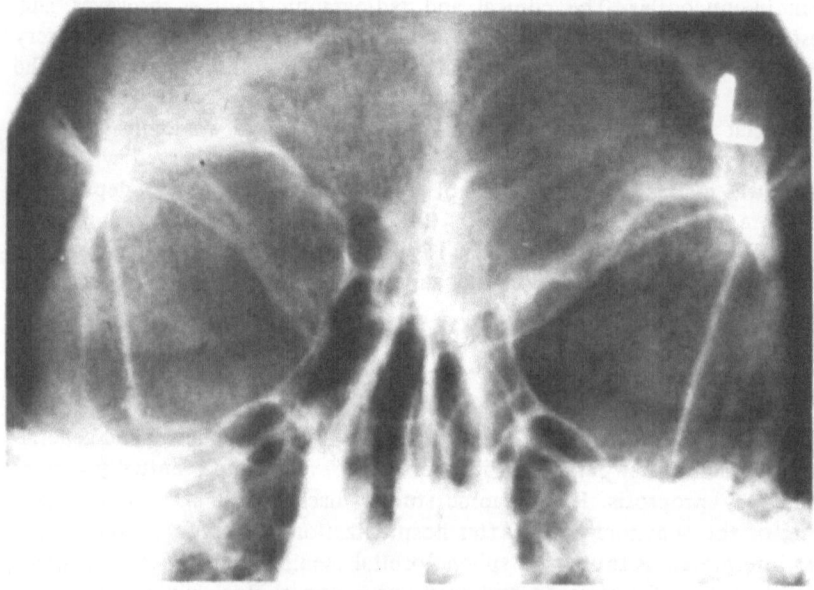

Fig. 3. The floor of the left frontal sinus is depressed. Note lack of enlargement of the sinus and preservation of the mural scallopings.

328

thought to have either a recurrent meningioma and/or frontal ethmoidal mucocele. At exploration through the left ethmoidal sinus region a mass was identified that had produced a hole in the floor of the left frontal sinus. This mass was dissected posteriorly into the orbit where 'copious amounts of mucous membrane were removed'. Post-operatively the patient retained excellent vision and oculomotor function and has not required additional surgery.

PATHOLOGIC FINDINGS

All three cases demonstrated essentially the same histopathologic findings. Within an outer shell of denser bone, trabeculae and small spicules of bone were scattered throughout a highly cellular and well capillarized fibrous stroma (Fig. 4). The trabeculae of bone were disconnected and ranged from curlicue patterns to spherules of bone suggestive of cementicles or psammoma bodies (Fig. 4). The bone was often heavily calcified (Fig. 5) and composed of irregular lamellae with entrapped osteoblasts. Many of the trabeculae were rimmed by actiev-appearing osteoblasts and multinucleated osteoclasts (Fig. 5, inset).

DISCUSSION

Lehrer (1969) reported three cases in the neurologic literature of ossifying fibromas of the orbital roof that created an expansile, distinctly marginated lesion with the radiographic pattern of a large 'balloon or bubble'. His

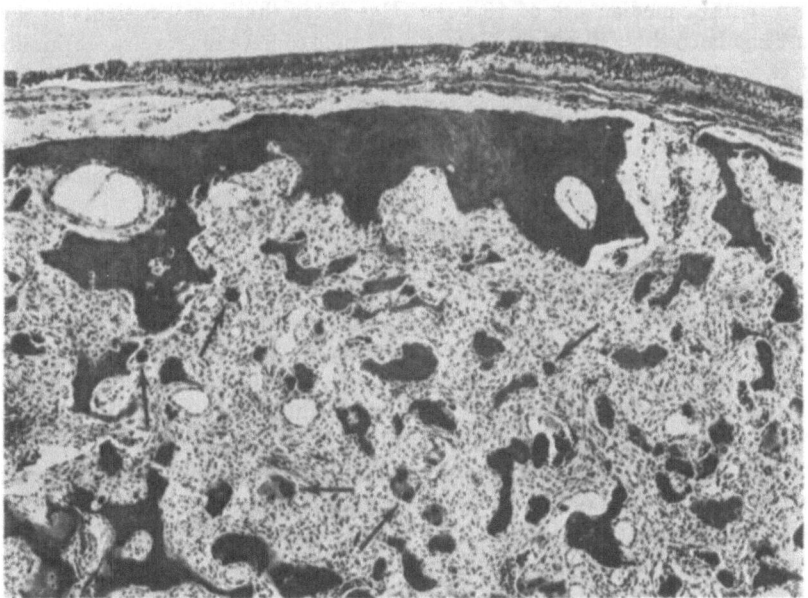

Fig. 4. Fibro-osseous lesion present under the mucosa of the frontal sinus. Arrows point to small 'cementicles' or pseudo-psammoma bodies that are actually composed of osteoid (H&E, x 48).

329

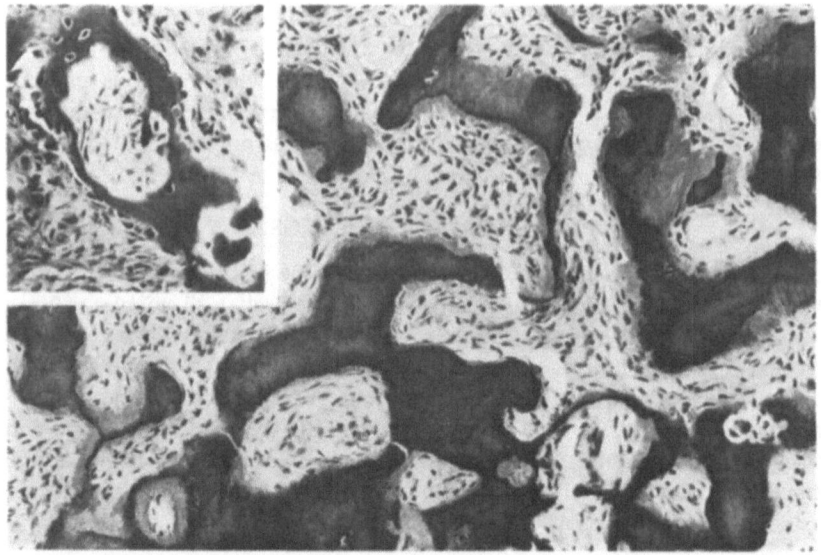

Fig. 5. Trabeculae are composed of well calcified lamellar bone. Inset shows spicules rimmed by osteoblasts and osteoclasts (H&E x 120; inset, H&E x 120).

patients were neurologically intact and aged 11, 20 and 50 years. He reviewed the literature and found eleven other reported cases similar to his own, with a median age of 13 years. Het noted that many patients in the past had been thought on radiographic grounds to have mucoceles, dermoids or cholesteatomas, an impression reinforced at surgery by the discovery of lesional tissue with a soft consistency and a greenish-yellow, hemorrhagic appearance. Pathologically, confusion often arose with meningioma, because of the presence of small calcospherites or 'cementicles' in the biopsied tissue which superficially resemble psammoma bodies.

Our case 1 is probably the smallest ossifying fibroma on record, since it was totally asymptomatic and discovered by a radiologist when he obtained sinus films for non-specific sinus congestion. The lesion had created a small lytic defect in the roof of the orbit; its lack of cortical sclerosis raised the possibility of a lesion other than an epidermoid, which was nonetheless the first radiographic diagnosis. The other two cases suggested a mucocele on clinical and radiographic examination, due to the displacement of the globe from depression of the roof of the orbit (i.e., the floor of the frontal sinus). In these two cases, however, there were subtle radiographic findings that in retrospect should have rendered the diagnosis of a mucocele suspect. The most important finding was the lack of overall enlargement of the involved sinuses, which away from the destroyed portion of the roof showed normal sinus architecture with persistent scalloping of the sinus outlines. It is not possible to have a partial mucocele of a sinus, since by definition the sinus opening is blocked and an expansion in all directions usually occurs, although overall expansion may occur predominantly in only one direction, e.g., antero-posteriorly, and be missed on routine films. The tomographic study performed on our third patient further indicated that there was no erosion in the lateral portion of the floor of the frontal sinus, which should have been rarefied or expanded had there been a generalized involvement of the sinus. Lastly, the involved area of the roof was irregular rather than smoothly contoured as in a mucocele.

Another pre-operative diagnostic finding of some value was the absence on B-scan ultrasonography of good sound transmission through the lesion, which one would not have expected in a mucocele. Mucoceles invariably have good sound transmission because they are filled with either air or low density mucoid material, whereas the second patient in our series who had an ultrasonogram failed to show sonolucency owing to the fibro-osseous tissue composing the lesion. Arteriography may be of help in ruling out the possibility of a mucocele. In our third patient an arteriogram disclosed a tumor blush, which should not be found in a mucocele which is devoid of mass. We are aware of other related cases of ossifying fibroma not included in this series in which arteriography revealed a conspicuous tumor blush. In our experience a tumor blush is not prominent in cases of fibrous dysplasia; this may be a useful way of distinguishing between the two lesions.

Fu & Perzin (1974) have stressed that it is worthwhile to segregate ossifying fibroma from fibrous dysplasia. They reviewed the clinical and pathologic characteristics of 7 patients with ossifying fibroma (5 females and 2 males) with an average age of 15 years (range 7 to 28 years). As in our cases, there was a variably radiodense or lytic lesion of the involved bones of the paranasal sinuses. These lesions appeared somewhat better circumscribed radiographically than cases of fibrous dysplasia. They noted a higher recurrence rate in patients with ossifying fibroma compared with fibrous dysplasia, and felt that ossifying fibroma was deserving of a more vigorous surgical attack. Our patient 1 with a small lesion has not yet experienced a recurrence, but patient 2 obviously has, and patient 3 presumably was misdiagnosed on first craniotomy 15 years ago as having a meningioma, because the small cementicles in her lesion might have misled the pathologist into thinking that she had a meningioma.

Fu & Perzin (1974) also emphasized the pathological differences between ossifying fibroma and fibrous dysplasia. The bone formation within fibrous dysplasia is of the poorly calcified, immature woven bone type, in which there are no lamellar lines or osteoblasts rimming the osteoid, which blends imperceptibly into the firbous stroma. In contrast, mature lamellar bone can almost always bee seen in ossifying fibroma in scattered fields. The impression created on low power scanning of ossifying fibroma is also different, inasmuch as there tends to be a more highly cellular and richly capillarized stroma and more of a balance toward the osseous element, particularly in maturing lesions. All three of our patients displayed the typical cementicles or rounded bony spherules that can easily provoke the pathologist into diagnosing a meningioma. The findings of entrapped osteoblasts in these cementicles and the presence of lamellar lines separating centrally ossified matrix from peripheral immature osteoid serve to distinguish them from psammoma bodies.

331

Table 1.

Lesion	Clinical and radiographic features	Pathologic features
Osteoma	Onset in middle age, slowly developing facial asymmetry, facial pain, headache, chronic sinusitis, exophthalmos, nasal obstruction, displacement of eye, papillededa, optic atrophy; frontal, ethmoidal, and maxillary sinuses more often involved than sphenoid; well-outlined, homogeneously dense, and calcified radiographically	Wide trabeculae of dense lamellar bone; three types recognized (ivory, mature and fibrous) depending on cellularity of the stroma between the trabeculae; fibrous variant may still be actively growing, since osteoblasts partially rim the trabeculae
Fibrous dysplasia	Cutaneous pigmentation and precocious menstruation in Albright's syndrome; orbital disease usually monostotic and nonsyndromic; children and young adults affected; proptosis, painless facial swelling, optic atrophy if sphenoid and optic canals involved; radiographically, ground-glass, poorly delimited, destructive lesion	Trabeculae of woven bone (no lamellar lines); 'arrest' of bone maturation; no osteoblasts rimming the trabeculae; moderately cellular banal fibrous stroma
Ossifying fibroma	Lesion peculiar to craniofacial bones; affects children and young adults; proptosis, painless facial swelling; aggressive clinical course; radiographically, bone destruction by circumscribed lesion with irregular faint calcification; may become radiodense with 'maturation' into osteoma	Trabeculae of lamellar bone and osteoid in various stages of maturation; osteoblasts present; cellular fibrous stroma; minimal mitotic activity may erroneously suggest osteogenic sarcoma; rounded bony spicules may be mistaken for psammoma bodies of meningioma of cementicles of cementifying fibroma, an odontogenic tumor
Osteoblastoma	Painless proptosis in young individuals; radiographically greater than 1 cm in diameter; destructive focus surrounded by sclerotic margin	Localized lesion, surrounded by sclerotic bone; trabeculae of lamellar bone with osteoblasts
Osteogenic sarcoma	Average age at presentation approx. 30 (older than second decade in tumors of long bones); may follow radiotherapy for retinoblastoma, less common as primary tumor; facial swelling, facial pain, epistaxis, poor healing after loose tooth extraction, proptosis; radiographically, poorly defined destructive lesion with increased bone density	Malignant stroma with pleomorphism, mitotic activity; malignant osteoid blends into spindle cells; some tumors may be highly fibrosarcomatous with need to search for osteoid

Besides meningioma and fibrous dysplasia, the differential diagnosis (Table 1) of ossifying fibroma includes fibrous osteoma, osteoblastoma, and osteogenic sarcoma. Fibrous osteoma is related to the mature ivory osteoma, except that the bony trabeculae in the former are thinner yet still interconnected, and the cellular stroma is more hypercellular. Such lesions usually evolve into ivory osteomas. There is also some evidence to suggest that ossifying fibromas may progressively mature into fibrous osteomas (Lehrer, 1969; Fu & Perzin, 1974). Osteoblastoma is composed of spicules of lamellar bone with osteoblasts rimming the trabeculae in common with ossifying fibroma, but there is additionally a sclerotic rim of dense bone visible radiographically and pathologically surrounding the active, central lesion. Osteoblastoma is related to the osteoid osteoma of long bones. Osteogenic sarcoma features a malignant stroma with atypia, hyperchromasia, mitotic activity, and malignant osteoid. These findings are never in evidence in ossifying fibroma.

The management of ossifying fibroma is complete surgical excision of the involved tissue, given the propensity of this tumor for recurrence. Lesions which are more radiolucent than radiodense suggest activity and perhaps should be treated more aggressively.

REFERENCES

Fu, Y.S. & K.H. Perzin. Non-epithelial tumors of the nasal cavity, paranasal sinuses and nasopharynx: a clinico-pathologic study. II. Osseous and fibro-osseous lesions, including osteoma, fibrous dysplasia, ossifying fibroma, osteoblastoma, giant cell tumor and osteosarcoma. *Cancer* 33: *1289* (1974).

Jakobiec, F.A. & I.S. Jones. Mesenchymal and fibro-osseous tumors of the orbit. Chapter 44 in: Clinical Ophthalmology (T. Duane, ed.), Hagerstown, Md. (1976).

Lehrer, H. Ossifying fibroma of the orbital roof. *Arch. Ophthal.* 20: *536* (1969).

Authors' address:
Departments of Ophthalmology and Radiology
Columbia-Presbyterian Medical Center
New York City, N.Y.
USA

Reprint requests to:
Dr Frederick A. Jakobiec
Director, Reese Laboratory of Ophthalmic Pathology
Edward S. Harkness Eye Institute
Box 57
New York, N.Y. 10032
USA

Proc. 3rd Int. Symp. on Orbital Disorders, Amsterdam 1977

IN VITRO AND IN VIVO DIAGNOSIS OF
ENDOCRINE OPHTHALMOPATHY

O. FISCHEDICK & K. ULLERICH

(Dortmund, W. Germany)

DIAGNOSTIC METHODS BEFORE THE
ERA OF NUCLEAR MEDICINE

From a statistical survey published by Reese in 1968 we have learned that endocrine ophthalmopathies make up 15% of all tissue-displacing disorders of the orbit; this is the biggest coherent entity among them. Many attempts were made during the last 25 years to find adequate endocrinological tests for diagnostically separating this group from the whole complex of orbital diseases.

As long as methods of nuclear medicine were not yet available we could only expect to arrive at a correct classification and diagnosis of these endocrine ophthalmopathies by a combined evaluation of the symptoms lid retraction, protrusion, and levator muscle block, in 30% of the cases. A further 20% were diagnosed by assessment of thyroid hyperfunction. The remaining 50% of the cases could only be diagnosed, at that time, by means of surgical biopsies from the orbit.

TWO-PHASE STUDIES OF RADIOIODINE UPTAKE

Diagnostics were substantially improved by the introduction of radioiodine techniques. Horst (1952), Ullerich & Horst (1954, 1955) Horst & Ullerich (1958) were able to ascertain that, and how endocrine ophthalmopathies are co-existing with certain disorders of the mechanism regulating the hypothalamic-hypophyseal-thyroid axis. Two-phase radioiodine studies helped to demonstrate that the thyroid gland, in this condition, does not respond in the usual way to stimulation by parenteral application of thyrotrophin. The feedback control of the hormonal iodine level in the blood is constantly blocked. Disconnection of the thyroid from its central regulatory system (hormonal control) provokes a pathological autoregulation in the organ itself with accelerated iodine metabolism which could be demonstrated by an increased 24-hour serum level of 131 iodine. Cases with hyperthyreodism showed, in addition, increased radioiodine uptake into the thyroid (Horst, 1952; Ullerich & Horst, 1954; Horst & Ullerich, 1958). When this regulatory disorder was identified as a constant phenomenon in endocrine ophthalmopathy, it became possible to improve the accuracy of diagnosis from a mere 50% to 98%. The absence of thyroid response to the suppressive influence of radioiodine which we had already demonstrated, was elaborated by Werner (1955) and employed for a specific test for endocrine ophthalmopathy.

Since the time of our publications (1954–1960) the two-phase study of radioiodine metabolism has gained general approval. For 17 years there was no modification of the technique. It was fully adequate to all cases of endocrine ophthalmopathy, whether associated with hyperthyreodism or primary euthyreodism, posttherapeutic euthyreodism or hypothyreodism.

A certain drawback of two-phase studies was found in the fact that patients have to subjected to irradiation, that they must go to a special laboratory for nuclear medical testing, and that the whole procedure takes about 48 hours. The suppression test after Werner involved another negative effect because the radiation dose is doubled by repeated measuring. In some cases, an additional application of hormonal iodine may not be without risk. This explains why many teams, including our own group, have always been looking for new methods to improve and supplement the two-phase study of radioiodine metabolism. It is hoped to substitute eventually another procedure that would avoid the exposure of the patient to radionuclides. Let me briefly review these attemps.

DETERMINATION OF THE SERUM EXOPHTHALMUS FACTOR DETERMINATION OF LATS FACTOR

We will first discuss the measuring of the exophthalmus factor in the patient's serum. Our group had outlined the difficulties of this diagnostic approach in 1958 (Ullerich, Gloer, Hoffmann-Konrads, 1958); hereafter the method was again demonstrated by several other teams, in particular by Horster (1967, 1970, 1971). Studies by Schemmel et al (1972) and Werner (1972, 1974) have shown, however, the inadequateness of experimental models with carp and goldfish: here the appearance of protrusion is nothing more than an unspecific reaction that can be provoked just as well by TSH fractions, and which may not be parallelled tu human endocrine ophthalmopathy. Therefore the section 'Thyroid' of the German Society for Endocrinology has recently decided to drop this method entirely.

Adams & Purves (1957) occasionally found a 'long-acting-thyroid-factor' in sera of patients with hyperthyreosis and endocrine ophthalmopathy. This protein complex which cannot be demonstrated in the thyroid, provokes delayed thyroid activity in mice. It is an immune body not directly related to endocrine ophthalmopathy and which is found in not more than 50% of all patients. On account of this poor accuracy the method is no longer in use.

CHEMICAL DETERMINATION OF PROTEIN-BOUND IODINE, COMPETITIVE PROCEDURES FOR T$_4$-DETERMINATION, T$_3$-GLOBULIN BINDING CAPACITY.

The decisive metabolic criterion of thyroid hyperfunction is an increased release of hormonal iodine into the circulating blood. At present, we still have no clinical test for assessing the kinetic process of hormone release. Chemical testing for iodine has been improved and competitive procedures for tracing minimal levels of triiodthyronine and thyroxine were developed, and it was thought that the measuring of hormonal iodine serum levels might provide another acceptable method. Between 1963 an 1974 we adopted this method to supplement our two-phase radioiodine metabolism studies and the suppression test.

The chemical test for protein-bound iodine is impaired by its failing specificity to hormonal iodine, moreover, it may be grossly vitiated by previous application of other iodine compounds in diagnostic or therapeutic procedures.

Determination of T_4 levels by competitive methods was found to be not sufficiently accurate, but rather susceptible to extrathyroid factors.

Determination of the T_3-binding capacity is influenced not only by hormonal iodine levels, but also by the quantity of carrier proteins.

Consequently, our search for more exact diagnostic procedures had to be continued.

RADIOIMMUNE ASSAYS
T_3-RIA, T_4-RIA, TRH STIMULATION

An entirely new approach was made possible by the introduction of the radioimmunoassay into hormone chemistry. This investigative procedure works on the principle of sensitizing experimental animals, mostly rabbits, against certain hormone compounds, in our case, T_3, T_4, and TSH. When antibodies of these animals are treated with the respective hormone compounds (additionally labelled with I_{125}) in known concentrations, and then subsequently treated with patient sera bearing hormone compounds of unknown concentrations, these patient serum hormones will replace the labelled compounds bound to the antibody complex. With the help of exactly defined concentration curves we are now able to identify and determine even minimal serum levels of T_3, T_4, and TSH.

Determination of thyrotrophin made it possible to show that endocrine ophthalmopathy is associated not with an increased, but with a severely depressed thyrotrophin level in the blood, which is contradictory to earlier opinions.

Our insight in the pathogenesis of the disease was further enlarged by Boler and his co-workers in 1974. They extracted a thyrotrophin-releasing hormone (TRH) from the hypothalamos of numerous animals and were also able to achieve its isolation as a tripeptide, and its synthetization. Not much later Ormston et al. (1971) showed that the effect of thyrotrophin on the pituitary is blocked in patients with hyperthyreodism in these patients parenteral application of TRH fails to provoke a rise in the blood level of thyrotrophin. We see how the regulatory system is blocked in endocrine ophthalmopathy at three points: hypothalamus-hypophysis, hypophysis-thyroid, and in the feedback control hormonal iodine-hypophysis. The blocking is probably provoked by the receptors' being occupied by immunologic processes.

336

From 1953 to this year, our three working groups have carried out diagnostic classification and therapy in more than 500 cases of endocrine ophthalmopathy. In 1976 and 1977 we definitely dropped the diagnostic methods of PBJ-determination, competitive T_4-testing, and T_3-binding reaction. They have been replaced by the new immunoassays, while two-phase studies of radioiodine uptake were continued for comparative evaluation. Until now we have performed this rather expensive double testing in 46 patients. Results may be summarized in three groups:

Twenty-three patients suffering from endocrine ophthalmopathy associated with thyroid hyperfunction showed the following picture: in 16 patients blood levels of triiodthyronine and thyroxine were increased, while the thyrotrophin level remained low and was not stimulated by application of TRH. In 7 patients triiodthyronine levels were normal, the thyroxine levels remained in the normal range, but serum TSH was lowered. TRH failed to induce a rise of TSH. Just one year ago, most clinical teams might have interpreted this set of symptoms as 'T_3-hyperthyroidism! Our latest experience, however, suggests that it is rather a transitory phase prior to the full picture of thyroid hyperfunction, because we know that T_4 is bound to rise subsequently in such cases.

The two-phase radioiodine study may only be dispensed with, in our opinion, in those cases of endocrine ophthalmopathy where all in vitro tests have definitely shown positive results. In our 23 cases two-phase studies yielded pathological results in 22 tests. The last case remained unclear because of previous iodine exposure (Table 1).

Endocrine exophthalmy and
Hyperthyroidism

T_3 - RIA	T_4 - RIA	TSH ⊥ TRH – RIA	
↑	↑	low no increase	16
↑	↔	low no increase	7
			23

Results in endocrine ophthalmopathy with primary euthyroidism. The percentage of endocrine ophthalmopathy associated with primary euthyreosis must have been somewhat overestimated formerly. In our series we found not more than two cases where we observed normal levels of triiodthyronine and thyroxine, but an absence of TRH-reaction. In cases of this kind thyroid regulation disorders are demonstrable by the two-phase study of radioiodine uptake. One of them was unilateral, and we used computerized tomography to exclude an orbital tumor (Table 2).

Results in endocrine ophthalmopathy with posttherapeutic euthyroidism or hypothyroidism. Our material includes 21 cases that were investigated subsequently to strumectomy or radioiodine therapy which had normalized thyroid hyperfunction or even induced hypofunction. In this group in vitro tests yielded results of such varied quality patterns that diagnostic classification absolutely demanded additional two-phase studies.

After treatment, 10 cases showed normal T_3 and T_4 levels, low values of TSH, and a blocked TRH reaction. 4 cases had a normal T_3, low T_4, one case had both values reduced.

In two of our cases hormonal iodine values were normal while TSH was strongly increased and THR reaction abnormally enhanced. These cases 4 subsequently developed thyroid hypofunction. Four cases showed lowered T_3 and T_4, but strong stimulation by TRH. Clinically, these cases manifested hypothyroidism. It was interesting to see how TRH/TSH studies were already indicating a beginning hypofunction at the time when hormonal iodine levels still remained in the normal range (Table 3).

Trusting the new invitro tests alone, these 21 cases could not be classified correctly as endocrine ophthalmopathies, but the two-phase test for radioiodine yielded a clear answer in 19 of them. Two cases could not be evaluated because they were under hormonal iodine substitution.

Endocrine exophthalmy
Primary euthyroid

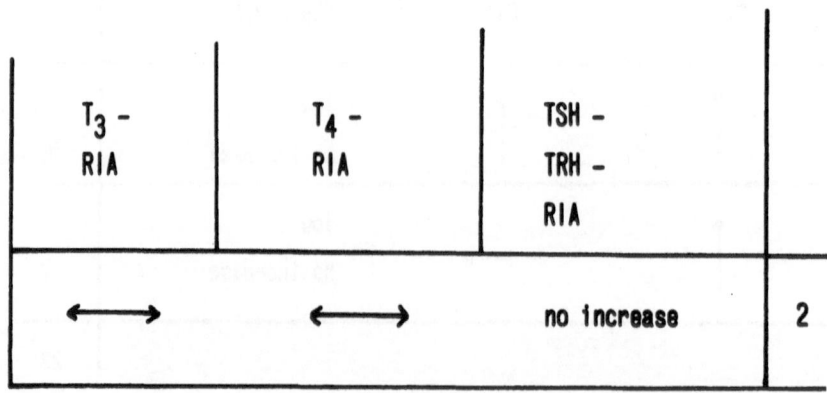

T_3 - RIA	T_4 - RIA	TSH - TRH - RIA	
←→	←→	no increase	2

Endocrine exophthalmy

Posttherapeutic euthyroidism or hypothyroidism

T_3 - RIA	T_4 - RIA	TSH - TRH - RIA	
$\longleftrightarrow$	$\longleftrightarrow$	low no increase	10
$\longleftrightarrow$	$\downarrow$	low no increase	4
$\downarrow$	$\downarrow$	low no increase	1
$\longleftrightarrow$	$\longleftrightarrow$	raised rapid increase	2
$\downarrow$	$\downarrow$	raised rapid increase	4
			21

To summarize our experience in 1976 and 1977, we may safely propose the following schedule:

In all cases of endocrine ophthalmopathy with thyroid hyperfunction, diagnostic procedures should begin with the in-vitro methods of the new radioimmunoassays for T_3, T_4, TSH, and TRH stimulation should follow. Some 50% of the results will be synonymous in all three tests, and then no two-phase study of radioiodine uptake is needed. In the remaining 50%, in all cases of primary or posttherapeutic euthyroidism, and in cases of hypothyroidism the in-vitro tests should be supplemented absolutely by the two-phase study.

Any hopeful conjecture that it might be possible to dispense with two-phase studies for thyroid diagnostics in the near future (Pfannenstiel, 1974) must be discouraged, for the time being, at least in the field of endocrine ophthalmopathies.

REFERENCES

Adams, D. & H.D. Purves. The chage in thyroid J 131 content between 8 and 48 hours as an index of thyroid activity. *Metabolism* 6: *26* (1957).

Albert, J.P. Der Initial-Suppressionstest in der Schilddrüsendiagnostik. *Diagnostik* 5 (8): *373–375* (1972).

Azizi, F., A.G. Vagenakis, G.I. Portnay, B. Rapoport, S.H. Ingbar & L. Braverman. Pituitary-thyroid responsiveness to intramuscular thyrotropin-releasing hormone based on analyses of serum thyroxine, tri-iodothyronine and thyrotropin concentrations. *New Engl. J. Med.* 292 (6): *273–277* (1975).

Boler, J., G. Enzman, K. Folkers, C.Y. Bowers & A.V. Schally. The identity of chemical and hormonal properties of the thyrotropin in releasing hormone and pyroglutamyl-histidylproline-amide. *Biochem. Biophys. Res. Comm.* 37: *705* (1969).

Brase, A. Schilddrüsen-Funktionsdiagnostik: T_3in vitro-Methode. *Diagnostik* 4 (6): *260–262* (1971).

Cassidy, C.E. Thyroid suppression test as index of outcome of hyperthyroidism treated with antihyroid drugs. *Metabolism* 19: *745* (1970).

Clifton-Bligh, P., G.E. Silverstein & G. Burke. Unresponsiveness to thyrotrophin-releasing hormone (TRH) in treated Graves' hyperthyroidism and in euthyroid graves' disease. *J. Clin. Endocrinol. Metab.* 38: *531* (1974).

Emrich, D. et al. Bedeutung und Treffsicherheit verschiedener Parameter der Schild-drüsenfunktion in der Praxis. *Dtsh. med. Wschr.* 98 (46): *2169–2174* (1973).

Frenco, P.S., J.M. Hershman, E.D. Haigler & J.A. Pittman. Response to thyrotropin-releasing hormone compared with thyroid suppression tests in euthyroid Graves' disease. *Metabolism* 22: *1357* (1973).

Glanzmann, C., Kl.P. Braun & W. Horst. Die Schilddrüsen- und Hypophysenfunktion im Radiojod-Dreiphasenstudium nach oraler Gabe von TRF. *Dtsch. med. Wschr.* 97: *132* (1972).

Glöbel, P., R. Berberich & E. Oberhausen. Periphere Umwandlung von T_4 zu T_3 beim Menschen. *Nucl. Med.* 14 (2): *106–118* (1975).

Graul, E.H. & H. Müller. Diagnostik der Schilddrüsenerkränkungen. *Der informierte Arzt* I: *365* (1973).

Graul, E.H. & H. Müller. Differentialdiagnostik der Hyperthyreose und des autonomen Adenoms. *Der informierte Arzt* I: *405* (1973).

Hall, R., J. Amos & B.J. Ormston. Radioimmuno-assay of human serum thyrotrophin. *Br. Med. J.* 1: *582* (1971).

Herrmann, R. & C. Schneider. Der Radioimmuno-assay für Trijodthyronin und Thy-roxin im Serum und seine Anwendung bei Hyperthyreosen. *Radiologie* 14: *156* (1974).

Hesch, R.D., M. Hüfner & A. von zur Mühlen. Erste klinische Ergebnisse mit einer radioimmunochemischen Bestimmuntsmethode von Trijodthyronin im Plasma (IT_3). *Dtsch. med. Wschr.* 97: *351* (1972).

Hesch, R.D., M. Hüfner, A. von zur Mühlen & D. Emrich. Trijodthyronine levels in patients with euthyroid endocrine exophthalmos and during treatment of thyroto-xicosis. *Acta endocrinol.* (Kbh.) 75: *514* (1974).

Horn, K., I. Marschiner & P.C. Scriba. Erster Ringversuch zur Bestimmung der Konzen-trationen von L-Trijodthyronin (T_3) und L-Thyroxin (T_4) im Serum: Bedeutung für die Erkennung methodischer Fehlerquellen. *J. Clin. Chem. Clin. Biochem.* 14: *353* (1976).

Horst, W. Methoden und Ergebnisse des Radiojodstoffwechselstudiums zur Diagnostik thyreoidaler und extrathyreoidaler Erkrankungen. *Klin. Wschr.* 30: *439* (1952).

Horst, W. & K. Ullerich. Hypophysen-Schilddrüsen-Erkränkungen und endokrine Ophthalmopathie. 31. Beih. der Klin. Mbl. Augenheilk. Ferd. Enke Verlag, Stuttgart (1958).

Horst, W. & K. Ullerich. Bedeutung des Radiojod-Stoffwechselstudiums für Diagnostik und Therapie der endokrinen Ophthalmopathie. Ber. 63. Zusammenkunft der DOG im Berlin, p. 136 (1960).

Horster, F.A. Endokrine Ophthalmopathie. Springer Verlag, Berlin/Heidelberg/New York (1967).

Horster, F.A. Zur Pathophysiologie und Therapie der endokrinen Ophthalmopathie. *Verh. dt. Ges. Inn. Med.* 76: *771* (1970).

Horster, F.A. & W. Wildmeister. Klinische Bedeutung des synthetischen TRH. *Dtsch. med. Wschr.* 96: *175* (1971).

Hüfner, M. & R.-D. Hesch. Radioimmunoassay for Trijodthyronine in human serum. *Acta endocrinol.* (Kbh.) 72: *464* (1973).

Ivy, H.K. Medical approach in ophthalmopathy of Graves' disease. *Mayo Clin. Proc.* 47. *980* (1972).

Klein, E., J. Kracht, H.L. Krüskemper, D. Reinwein & P.C. Scriba. Klassifikation der Schilddrüsenkrankheiten. *Dtsch. med. Wschr.* 98: *2362* (1973).

M.P. König, H. Borgi, H. Kohler, H. Rôsler & H. Studer. Wann ist eine Radioisotopen-diagnostik bei Schilddrüsenerkrankungen indiziert, wann überflüssig? *Schweiz. med. Wschr.* 105 (12): *361–367* (1975).

Lamberg, B.-A., A. Gordin, M. Viherkoski & G. Kvist. Long-acting thyroid stimulator (LATS) in toxic nodular goitre, toxic adenoma and Graves' disease. *Acta Endocrinol.* 62: *199* (1969).

Lerche, W. Zur Klinik der endokrinen Ophthalmopathie. *Fortschr. Med.* 92: *278* (1974).

Lieblich, J. & R.D. Utiger. Trijodthyronine radioimmunoassay. *J. Clin. Invest.* 51: *157* (1972).

Mahlstedt, J., K. Joseph & E.H. Graul. Suppressionstest der Schilddrüse nach einmaliger Gabe von 3 mg L-Thyroxin. *NUC-compact* 3: *4* (1972).

Maisey, M.N., T.K. Natarajan, P.J. Hurley & H.N. Wagner. Validation of a rapid computerized method of measuring pertechnetate uptake for routine assessment of thyroid structure and function. J. Clin. Endokrinol. Metab. 36: 317 (1973).

May, P. & R.K. Donabedian. A sensitive radioimmunoassay for thyrotropin releasing hormone. *Clin. Chim. Acta* 46: *371–376* (1973).

May, P. & R.K. Donabedian. Factors in blood influencing the determination of thyrotropin releasing hormone. *Clin. Chim. Acta* 46: *377–382* (1973).

Mitsuma, T., J. Colucci, L. Shenkman & C.S. Hollander. Rapid simultaneous radioimmunoassay for triiodothyronine and thyroxine in unextracted serum. *Biochem. Biophys. Res. Commun.* 46 (6): *2107–2113* (1972).

Mitsuma, T., M. Gershengorn, J. Colucci & C.S.Hollander. Radioimmunoassay of Trijodthyronine in unextracted human serum. *J. Clin. Endocrinol. Metab.* 33: *364* (1971).

Montz, R., C. Schneider & M.-L. Jürges. Kritik der Schilddrüsen-in-vitro-Teste (T_3 und T_4-Test). *Med. Welt* 22 (N.F.) (12) : *477-479* (1971).

Mühlen, A. von zur, R.D. Hesch, D. Emrich & W. Creutzfeldt. Wirkung von synthetischen 'thyreotrpin releasing factor' auf Plasmaspiegel von thyreotropem Hormon und Wachstumshormon bei Gesunden, Patienten mit Hyperthyreose und primärer Hypothyreose. *Dtsch. Med. Wschr.* 95: *2623* (1970).

Mühlen, von zur, A., D. Emrich, R.D. Hesch & J. Köbberling. Untersuchungen über die Beeinflussung der Thyreotrophin-Sekretion beim Menschen. *Acta endocrinol.* (Kbh.) 68: *669* (1971).

Ormston, B.J., J.R. Kilborn, R. Gurry, J. Amos & R. Hall. Further obserations on the effect of synthetic thyrotrophin-releasing hormone in man. *Br. Med. J.:* *199* (1971).

Ormston, B.J., L. Alexander, D.C. Evered, F. Clark, T. Bird, D. Appleton & R. Hall. Thyrotrophin response to thyrotrophin-releasing hormone in ophthalmic Graves' disease. Correlation with other aspects of thyroid function. Thyroid suppressibility and activity of eye signs. *Clin. Endocrinol.* 2: *369* (1973).

Pfannenstiel, P. Diagnostik von Schilddrüsenerkrankungen. Verlag der Byk-Mallinckrodt Radiopharmazeutika-Diagnostika, Dietzenbach/Steinberg (1974).

Pfannenstiel, P. & H.U. Pixberg. Erweiterte 131 J-Diagnostik von Störungen im Schilddrüsenreglerkreis durch Belastung mit TRH. *Münch. med. Wschr.* 115: *495* (1973).

Pittman, C.S., J.B. Chambers & V.H. Read. The extrahyroidal conversion rate of thyroxine to trijodthyronine in normal man. *J.Clin. Invest.* 50: *1187* (1971).

Schemmel, K., L. Weisbecker, H. Kahl, H. Uthgenannt, G. Kreysing & S. Zepf. Exophthalmogener Effekt durch endogenes und exogenes thyreotropes Hormon im Tierexperiment. *Schweiz. med. Wschr.* 102: *667* (1972).

Schneider, C., R. Montz & H. Kunstmann. Uber die Hypertyreose-Diagnostik mit der Gesamt-Thyroxinbestimmung (T_4-Test). *Dtsch. Med. Wschr.* 97: *327* (1971).

Schoen H.D. Die nuklear-medizinische Diagnostik der Schilddrüsenerkrankungen. *Fortschr. Med.* 88 (10) : *433* (1970).

Sellers, E., A.G. Awad & E. Schönbaum. Long-acting thyroid stimulator in Graves' disease. *9Lancet: 335* (1970).

Sterling, Kl., D. Bellabarba, E.S. Newman & M.A. Brenner. Determination of trijodthyronine concentration in human serum. *J. Clin. Invest.* 48: *1150* (1969).

Trapp, P. Nuklearmedizinische Untersuchungen zur Schilddrüsenfunktionsdiagnostik. *Münch. med. Wschr.* 114(26) : *1217-1222* (1972).

Ullerich, K., B. Glöer & E. Hoffmann-Conrads. Zur Frage des klinisch-experimentellen Nachweises einer thyreotropen Stimulierung bei endokriner Ophthalmopathie. *Arztl. Forschung* 10 (I): *480* (1956).

Ullerich, K. & W. Horst. Abgrenzung des einseitigen Exophthalmus durch ein spezielles Radiojodstoffwechselstidium. Ber. 58. Zusammenkunft der DOG Heidelberg, p. 269 (1953).

Ullerich, K. & W. Horst. Ergebnisse einer modernen Strahlentherapie des endokrinen Exophthalmus. Ber. 59. Tagung der DOG in Heidelberg, p. 267 (1955).

Ullerich, K. & W. Horst. Zur Typenlehre des endokrinen Exophthalmus. *Klin. Mbl. Augenheilk.* 128: *215* (1956).

Wallack, M.S., H.M. Adelberg & J.I. Nicoloff. A thyroid-suppression test using a single dose of L-thyroxine. *New Engl. J. Med.* 283: *402* (1970).

Wenzel, K.W. Variationen der Thyrotropin-Releasing—hormone (TRH) stimulierten Thyreotropin (TSH)-Antwort im Vergleich zum Schilddrüsensupressionstest und den Trijodthyronin (T_3)- und Thyroxin (T_4)-Serumspiegeln bei sogenannter euthyreoter endokriner Ophthalmopathie. *Endokrinologie* 66 (1): *67-73* (1975).

Wenzel, K.W., H. Meinhold & H. Schleusener. Different effects of oral doses of triiodothyronine or thyroxine on the inhibition of thyrotrophin releasing hormone (TRH) mediated thyrotrophin (TSH) response in man. *Acta Endocrinol.* 80: *42-48* (1975).

Werner, S.C. The thyroid. Hoeber Medical Division, Harper & Row, New York (1955).

Werner, S.C. The eye changes of Graves' disease. *J. Med. Assn* 177: *551* (1961).

Werner, S.C. The eye changes of Graves' disease. *Mayo Clin. Proc.* 47: *969* (1972).

Werner, S.C., G. Acebedo & I. Radichevich. Rapid radioimmunoassay for both T_4 and T_3 in the same sample of human serum. *J. Clin..Endocrinol. Metab.* 38: *493-495* (1974).

Williams, E S., R.P. Ekins & S.M. Ellis. Thyroid suppression test with serum thyroxine concentration as index of suppression. *Br. Med. J.* 5679: *338* (1969).

Authors' addresses:
Prof. Dr. K. Ullerich
Augenklinik der Städt. Krankenanstalten
Dortmund
W. Germany

Prof. Dr. O. Fischendick
Abt. f. Röntgenologie und Nuklearmedizin
Knappschafts-Krankenhaus
Dortmund
W. Germany

Proc. 3rd Int. Symp. on Orbital Disorders, Amsterdam 1977

MEDICAL INVESTIGATION OF DYSTHYROID EYE DISEASE

N.F. LAWTON, P. FELLS & G.A.S. LLOYD

(London, England)

In this paper we report on the results of medical investigation in 61 patinets with known or suspected dysthyroid eye disease seen in the Thyroid clinic at Moorfields Hospital.

The purpose of medical investigation in patients with dysthyroid eye disease is twofold. In the first instance it is important to establish thyroid status because hyperthyroidism and hypothyroidism require treatment in their own right, irrespective of the management of eye disease. The second purpose of investigation is to establish the diagnosis of dysthyroid eye disease in those patients whose clinical presentation is atypical. In this group of patients the diagnostic problem is usually that of unilateral proptosis. We may therefore divide modern tests of thyroid function into two groups.

INVESTIGATION OF THYROID STATUS

Serum TSH assay

This measurement is of no value in the diagnosis of hyperthyroidism. However, in hypothyroidism an increase in serum TSH is the first biochemical abnormality to occur and may precede a fall in thyroid hormone levels. Primary hypothyroidism is rare in patients with dysthyroid eye disease unless a previous thyrotoxic illness has been treated by surgery or radio-iodine. The chief value of TSH assay is therefore to preclude overtreatment with antithyroid drugs in a patient with eye disease and associated thyrotoxocosis.

Thyroid hormone assays

A major advance in the assessment of thyroid status has been the introduction of a readioimmunoassay for tri-iodothyronine (T3) as well as thyroxine (T_4). A significant proportion of patients referred because of ocular complaints to our clinic (25%) have associated thyrotoxicosis which has passed unnoticed. In many of these patients serum T4 assay alone does not provide biochemical confirmation of the diagnosis . In a group of 20 such patients the serum T4 was normal in 13 though often the value was towards the upper limit of normal. On the other hand the serum T3 was clearly elevated in all 20 patients and symptoms of hyperthyroidism, of which the commonest were tremor and irritability, responded well to antithyroid drugs. Because the thyrotoxicosis is often mild only short course of treatment may be required and in occasional patients the illness is self limiting without antithyroid drugs.

DIFFERENTIAL DIAGNOSIS OF DYSTHYROID EYE DISEASE

Thyroid antibodies

The presence of circulating antibodies to thyroid tissue remains a valuable aid to diagnosis (Hall et al., 1970). However, thyroid antibodies are present in only about 60% of patients and false positive results must occasionally occur since antibodies are present in 10–20% of the normal population.

Thyrotrophin releasing hormone (TRH)

TRH is normally present in the hypothalamus and its function is to stimulate the pituitary to release thyrotrophin (TSH). TRH therefore acts as a regulator to the normal servo system operating between the thyroid and the pituitary. In normal subjects TRH given intravenously causes a transient increase in serum TRH maximal 20 minutes after the injection. In hyperthyroid patients no such increase occurs presumably because the pituitary is suppressed by high levels of serum T3 and T4.

The value of the TRH test in the diagnosis of dysthyroid eye disease is based on the observation that euthyroid patients who suffer from the Graves, diathesis may also have an absent TSH response to the TRH injection (Lawton et al., 1971).

An absent TRH response therefore has a similar significance to the absence of thyroid suppression by exogenous T3 and there is a statistical correlation between T3 suppressability and TRH responsiveness in dysthyroid eye disease.

Furthermore, the TRH test is occasionally positive in patients whose T3 suppression test is normal. TRH also has the additional advantage of clinical safety and the test takes only 25 minutes of the patient's time.

A second type of abnormal TRH response may also occur in dysthyroid eye disease. This takes the form of an exaggerated rise in TRH and this response is always associated with circulating thyroid antibodies (Ormston et al., 1973). The exaggerated response is of rather less diagnostic significance than the absent response.

In our experience of 41 TRH tests in patients who were all euthyroid as judged clinically and by normal T3 and T4 levels, an absent response occurred in 22 and an exaggerated response in 9. The test is therefore abnormal in approximately 75% of patients.

In the majority of these patients it was possible to make the diagnosis of dysthyroid eye disease on clinical grounds. Nevertheless there is a small group of patients with no previous or family history of thyroid disease whose other investigations including T3, T4, TSH and thyroid antibody are

344

Thyroid Status	No.	High Serum T_3	High Serum T_4	T.R.H. Response	
				Absent	Exaggerated
Hyperthyroid	20	20	7	20	-
Enthyroid	41	-	-	22	9

negative. In 10 such patients of the present series who presented with unilateral proptoses without lid retraction, the TRH response was absent in 8. In the past such patients were inevitably extensively investigated often by carotid angiography without the diagnosis being made. In our experinece patients with unilateral proptosis ultimately developed bilateral disease. However, it is clearly important that full medical investigation including a TRH test is carried out at an early stage in this group of patients.

The advent of CT scanning of the orbits has greatly improved diagnostic accuracy and frequently shows characteristic thickening of several ocular muscles. However, these changes are not seen in all patients with dysthyroid eye disease and in a small number of difficult cases it is not possible to distinguish orbital pseudo tumour from dysthyroid eye disease on the basis of the CT scan alone. In our opinion the radiological diagnosis should always be combined with specific tests of thyroid function.

SUMMARY

Many patients who would previously have been diagnosed as ophthalmic Graves' disease or dysthyroid eye disease have an associated thyrotoxic illness which may be mild and pass unnoticed. Diagnosis in such cases depends upon the availability of T3 assay since many of these patients have a 'so-called' T3 toxicosis. In the diagnosis of dysthyroid eye disease the TRH test has proved confirmation in up to 75% of patients and has been particularly useful in distinguishing unilateral proptosis due to dysthyroid eye disease.

REFERENCES

Hall, R., K. Kirkham & D. Doniach. Ophthalmic Graves' disease: diagnosis and pathogenesis. *Lancet* 1: *375–378* (1970).
Lawton, N.F., R.P. Elkins & J.D.N. Nabarro. Failure of pituitary response to thyrotrophin releasing hormone in euthyroid Graves' disease. *Lancet* 2: *14–16* (1971).
Ormston, B.J., L. Alexander, D.C. Evered, F. Clark, T. Bird, D. Appleton & R. Hall. Thyrotrophin response to thyrotrophin releasing hormone in ophthalmic Graves' disease: correlation with other aspects of thyroid function, thyroid suppressibility and activity of eye signs. *Clin. Endocr.* 2: *369–376* (1973).

Authors' address:
Moorfields Eye Hospital
City Road
London E.C.1
England

THE RELEVANCE OF THE TRH-TEST IN THE
DIFFERENTIAL DIAGNOSIS OF EXOPHTHALMOS

W.M. WIERSINGA & J.L. TOUBER

(Amsterdam, The Netherlands)

The recent discovery of the hypothalamic releasing hormones has greatly advanced our knowledge of the hypothalamic-pituitary system. Each anterior pituitary hormone has its hypothalamic counterpart in a release stimulating and/or inhibiting hormone. Available for clinical use are the hypothalamic hormones TRH (thyrotrophin releasing hormone) and LHRH (luteinizing hormone releasing hormone, which also stimulates the release of the follicle stimulating hormone FSH). The pituitary thyrotrophin and gonadotrophin reserve can now be asssessed accurately by injecting TRH and LHRH, and measuring the thyrotrophin and gonadotrophin response respectively. The main clinical use of the TRH-stimulation test is however in the diagnosis of thyroid disorders.

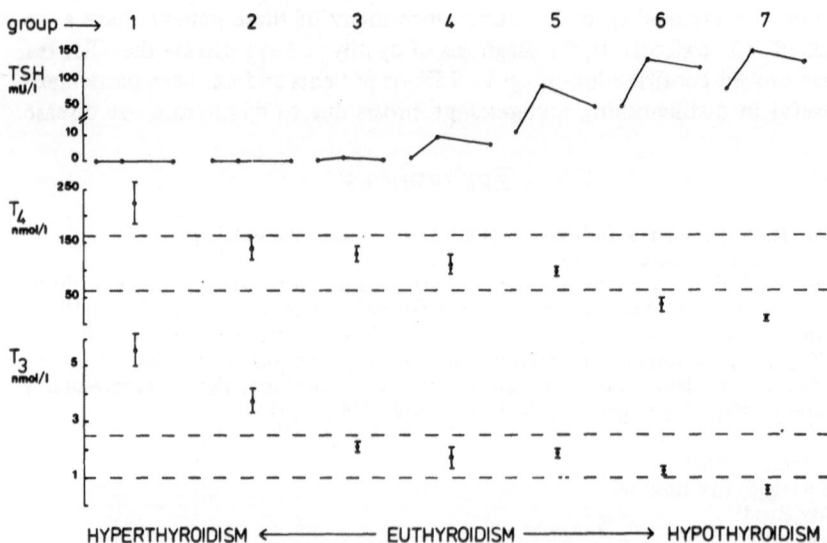

Fig. 1. Thyroid function tests in hyper-, eu- and hypothyroidism. (Upper part: TSH-response to 200 μg TRH i.v. at 0-20-60 minutes; middle and lower parts: basal plasma values of T_4 and T_3 ($\bar{x} \pm$ SEM) respectively, normal ranges between interrupted lines; composition of groups – see text).

The TRH-stimulation test as carried out in our laboratory. is performed by giving 200 μg TRH intravenously as a bolus injection. Blood samples are drawn through an indwelling venous catheter, and thyrotrophin (TSH), triiodothyronine (T3) and thyroxine (T4) are determined by radioimmunoassay.

Figure 1 depicts a simplified scheme of the results of the TRH-stimulation test in normal volunteers and in patients with a wide variety of thyroid function disorders. In normal volunteers (group 4) TRH-injection results in a TSH-response with a peak at 20 minutes.

Overt thyrotoxic patients (group 1) with elevated T4 and T3 values show an absent TSH-response due to the complete suppressive effect on the TSH-secretion by the circulating thyroid hormones, which cannot be overcome by the TSH-release stimulating effect of TRH.

Group 2 consists of hyperthyroid patients with elevated plasma-T3 values only; these patients have a so-called T3-toxicosis. The TSH-response to TRH in these patients is also absent.

In between groups 2 and 4 is a population of patients with normal T4 and T3 values and an absent or very severely blunted TSH-response to TRH. They can be seen as having subclinical hyperthyroidism.

Patients with overt hypothyroidism (group 7) have low T4 and T3 values; basal TSH-values are very much increased, and after TRH an exaggerated TSH response is seen.

In mild hypothyroidism (group 6) plasma-T4 is decreased while plasma-T3 is normal; basal TSH and TSH-response after TRH are still much elevated, although not as high as in group 7.

Finally, there are patients with normal T3 and T4 in whom basal TSH is either normal or slightly elevated and in whom the TSH-response after TRH is greater than in normals; these patients seem to have subclinical hypothyroidism (group 5).

Thus, the TRH-test enables us to fit the patient in the continuous spectrum from overt hyperthyroidism to overt hypothyroidism. The TRH-test has proved to be of extreme value especially for the diagnosis of hyperthyroidism, whatever the cause may be. A normal TSH-response to TRH excludes hyperthyroidism which makes the TRH-test the most sensitive indicator in the diagnosis of this disorder. An absent TSH-response without concomitant hyperthyroidism has been seen only in some patients with Cushing's disease and in severe inanition. Thus there are very few false negative results, and the specificity of 1 TRH-test in the diagnosis of hyperthyroidism is very high. Further advantages of the TRH-test are that the test is not influenced by iodine and that it is a reliable and safe alternative for the T3-suppression test.

In patients with exophthalmos endocrine causes must be differentiated from non-endocrine causes. Endocrine exophthalmos can be seen in the presence of hyperthyroidism, euthyroidism and − rarely − hypothyroidism. Hyper- and hypothyroidism can be readily diagnosed by measuring the basal values of T4, T3 and TSH; the TRH-test confirms the diagnosis if necessary. The main usefulness of the TRH-test lies in detecting those patients who seem to be euthyroid with normal basal T4 and T3 values, but who show an abnormal TSH-response. Both an absence of, or an exaggerated TSH-response strongly imply an endocrine nature for the exophthalmos. In general the finding of an absent TSH-response to TRH correlates with a non-suppressible ^{131}I-uptake by the thyroid gland in the T3-suppression test, although some discrepancies in this respect have been reported in the literature. It should be realized, however, that 20—25% of euthyroid patients whose exophthalmos is undoubtedly of endocrine origin, respond normally in both the TRH-test and T3-suppression test.

Authors' address:
Division of Endocrinology
Dept. of Internal Medicine
University Hospital
Wilhelmina Gasthuis
104, 1e Helmerstraat
Amsterdam
The Netherlands

Proc. 3rd Int. Symp. on Orbital Disorders, Amsterdam 1977

STUDY ON DYSTHYROID OPHTHALMOPATHY

YOICHI INOUE & TOYOKO INOUE

(Tokyo, Japan)

One of the most puzzling syndromes in ophthalmology has been the variable and capricious exophthalmos associated with endocrine disorder. But modern ophthalmology has been unveiling the mechanisms of exophthalmos one by one (Kroll et al., 1966; Coleman et al., 1972).

The discrepancy between exophthalmos and ophthalmic manifestations has not been investigated actively because the information concerning the character of the soft tissue in the orbital space is insufficient.

Lately it has been reported that the characteristic changes of the extra-ocular muscle(s) in endocrine exophthalmos are reflected by computed orbital tomography (Enzmann et al., 1976) (CT-scan). The purpose of this paper is to evaluate CT-scans of various types of dysthyroid ophthalmopathy and their relation to clinical findings from the ophthalmological point of view.

MATERIAL AND METHODS

The material comprises data on 135 cases with dysthyroid ophthalmopathy including 72 with extraocular muscle involvement, 45 with optic nerve involvement and others. Table 1 shows the distribution of ocular changes in the present series. The age and sex distribution of the present cases is presented in Fig. 1. Though each one was selected in order to investigate its CT-scan, the pattern of distribution was, unexpectedly, similar to that of common cases with dysthyroid ophthalmopathy in the Japanese population. All cases were examined with an EMI-scanner using the 160 x 160 matrix and 8 mm collimation.

RESULTS AND DISCUSSION

Extraocular muscle involvement

In order to clarify the explanation, attention has been given to clinical observation of disturbances of ocular movement. Ocular movement shows frequently limitation of elevation. This condition, caused by myopathy (Kroll et al., 1966) of the inferior group of muscles which exerts downward traction on the eyeball, results in hypotropia at an advanced stage.

349

Table 1

Materials (cases)

ocular changes	No. of case
extraocular muscle	72
optic nerve	45 (including 27 cases with EOM changes)
lid retraction alone	20
lid swelling alone	20
myasthenia	5
total	135

Age and Sex Distribution of 135 Cases with Dysthyroid Ophthalmopathy

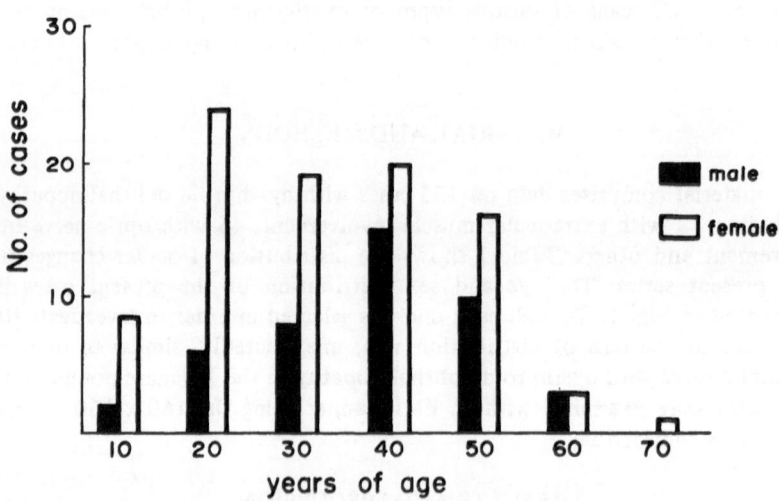

Fig. 1

The inferior section (B in Fig. 2) of the CT scan is positive, showing marked bilateral enlargement of the inferior rectus muscle. This corresponded to the clinical findings.

According to our previous study (Inoue et al., 1971), disturbances of elevation characterized about 60% of the cases with extraocular muscle involvement in dysthyroid ophthalmopathy.

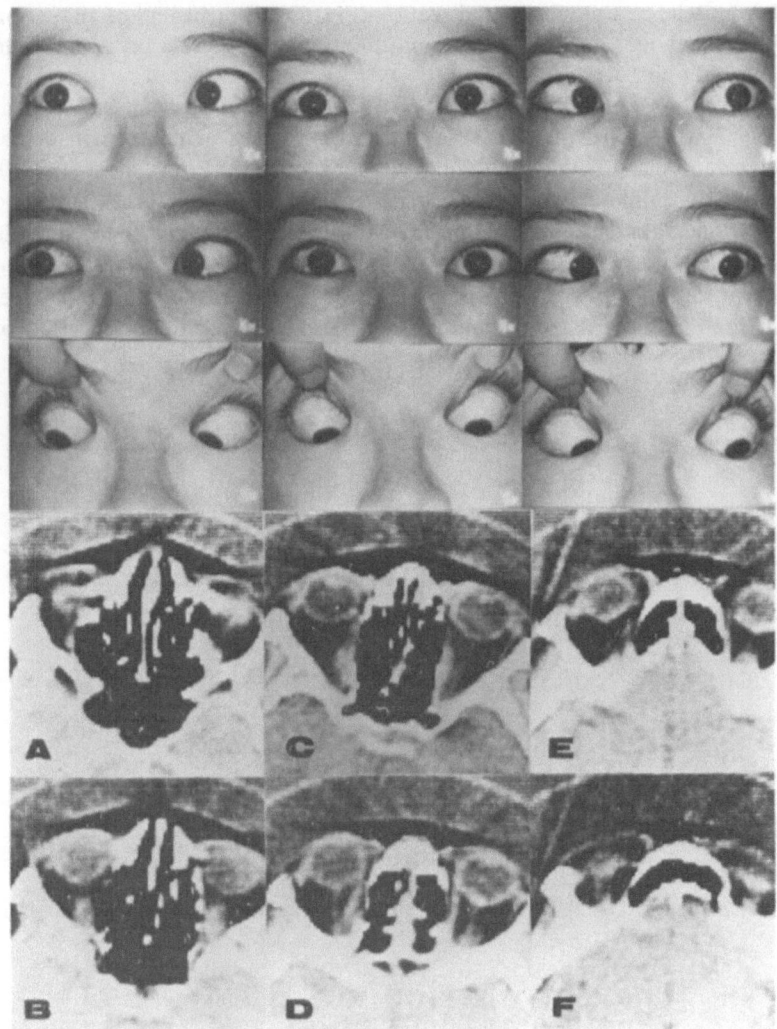

Fig. 2. Top: Female, 37 years. Grade of exophthalmos R – 17 mm, R – 18 mm. Esotropia, advanced and aged stages of disturbance of abduction due to myopathy of the medial rectus muscle, accompanied by the limitation of elevation. Bottom: CT-scan reveals enlargement of inferior rectus muscle. Changes of medial rectus muscle are seen also in the mid-orbital sections (C, D). There seems to be pathological enlargement of the superior rectus muscle in the higher orbital sections (E, F).

Disturbances of abduction, caused by changes in medial rectus muscle, exert traction on the eyeball medially, resulting in esotropia at an advanced stage.

In most cases, disturbances of abduction are accompanied by limitation of elevation in various degrees. Therefore, positive scan is frequently encountered in inferior rectus muscle on the inferior section as well as in medial rectus muscle on the mid-orbital section (Fig. 3). Disturbances of abduction accords in about 20% of the cases with extraocular muscle involvement in dysthyroid ophthalmopathy.

Table 2 represents the incidence of correlations between extraocular muscle involvement and CT scan. It shows degrees of changes in ocular involvement classified by modified Werner's criteria (Inoue et al., 1976). Where only minimal changes are observed, 7 out of 26 cases show no correlation. It is notable that in 82% of cases with extraocular muscle involvement, ocular changes correspond to the results of CT-scan.

Present results show clearly that in cases of extraocular muscle involvement the clinically affected muscles are closely related to the location of

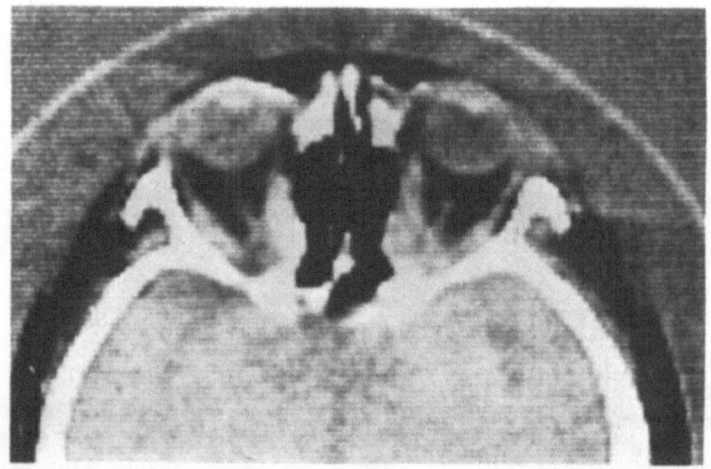

Fig. 3. Changes are characteristic in the orbital apex, filled with enlarged muscles.

Table 2

The correlation of EOM involvement with CT scan

Degree of changes	No. of cases	Correlation with CT scan
minimal	26	19
moderate	15	12
marked	31	28
total	72	59 (82%)

the changes shown by CT scan. However, the reverse is not always true. Positive scan of enlargement of extraocular muscles is not always associated with clinical disturbance of eye movement limited to the affected muscle shown by CT-scan. In cases with ocular myasthenia, negative scan of the orbital space is observed, as expected.

Optic nerve involvement

Regarding optic nerve involvement, a positive scan characterized by abnormally high-density tissue filling the orbital apex (a pathologic feature of muscle cone) was shown in every case, as reported earlier (Enzmann et al., 1976; Inoue et al., 1977). A few of them show the characteristic chorioretinal fold and papilloedema caused by the increased pressure of orbital soft tissue. Positive scans of all muscles are usually seen in some of the orbital sections. A markedly positive scan of the orbital space is observed, especially at the orbital apex (Fig. 3).

Table 3 shows the correlation between 45 cases with optic nerve involvement and their CT-scans. The incidence of correlation in the present cases is 76%. In these cases, enlargement of the medial rectus muscle is not consistently associated with the clinical severity of dysthyroid ophthalmopathy, in contradiction to what has been reported by Enzmann (1976). Changes in the medial rectus muscle are easily detected by CT-scan, and positive scan is obtained in all cases with abduction deficiency.

Eyelid retraction and eyelid swelling

In dysthyroid ophthalmopathy, numerous cases show exophthalmos unaccompanied by extraocular muscle changes determined clinically. Some of them involve upper-eyelid retraction or swelling of the eyelids.

Table 3

The correlation of optic nerve involvement with CT scan

Degree of changes	No. of cases	Correlation with CT scan
minimal	32	24
moderate	10	7
marked	3	3
total	45	34 (76 %)

In our clinical experience, extraocular muscle changes show a tendency to occur most frequently in middle-aged patients. As extraocular muscle changes seem to be related to age, we have divided these common cases into two groups, one under 40 years and one over that age.

In cases of upper eyelid retraction, positive scans of enlarged muscle are seldom obtained in the under-40 group, but in the over-40 group positive scans in inferior rectus muscle are observed in 20% of the cases (Table 4).

On the other hand, in cases with puffy eyelids, positive scans of enlarged muscles are observed more frequently than in the lid retraction group and show the same tendency in cases over 40 years (Table 5).

Concerning changes of inferior and medial rectus muscles, the differences between patients over and under 40 was considered to be more significant in the lid-swelling group.

Table 4

Relation of age to CT scan in cases with upper eyelid retraction (10 cases in each group)

Age (yrs.)	Degree of Exophthalmos (mm)	CT scan			
		inf.	med.	lat.	sup.
< 40	13 ~ 23	0	0	0	0
40 ≦	13 ~ 20	4	2	0	0

No. of eyes with positive scan
of enlarged muscles

Table 5

Relation of age to CT scan in cases with swelling of eyelids (10 cases in each group)

Age (yrs.)	Degree of Exophthalmos (mm)	CT scan			
		inf.	med.	lat.	sup.
< 40	15 ~ 22	4	2	0	4
40 ≦	14 ~ 23	9	11	5	6

No. of eyes with positive scan
of enlarged muscles

CONCLUSION

As from old, endocrine exophthalmos was attributed to a unitary cause, such as changes in soft tissue including fatty tissue in the orbital space. However, clinically extraocular muscle changes are also considered to play a significant part in the development of endocrine exophthalmos. From the results obtained by CT-scan in cases with various types of dysthyroid ophthalmopathy we formed the view that the development of endocrine ophthalmopathy depends on a dual mechanism involving changes of ophthalmopathy extraocular muscles as well as soft fatty tissues.

From these results we have learned that the concept of a dual mechanism represents another step forward in the study of endocrine exophthalmos.

REFERENCES

Coleman, D.J., et al. High resolution B-scan ultrasonography of the orbit. V. Changes of Graves' disease. *Arch. Ophthal.* 88: *465* (1972).

Enzmann, D., et al. Computed tomography in Graves' disease. *Radiology* 118: *615* (1976).

Inoue, Y., et al. Clinical study on dysthyroid ophthalmopathy in Japanese. Report I. Clinical approach to dysthyroid ophthalmopathy and definition. *Acta Soc. Ophthal. Japan* 75: *929* (1971)

Inoue, Y., et al. Problems of extraocular muscle involvement in dysthyroid ophthalmopathy. *Folia Ophthal. Japan* 27: *954* (1976).

Inoue, Y., et al. Dysthyroid ophthalmopathy and computed orbtial tomography. *Japan J. Ophthal.* 21 (in press, 1977).

Kroll, A.J., et al. Dysthyroid ocular myopathy. Anatomy, histology and electron microscopy. *Arch. Ophthal.* 76: *244* (1966).

Authors' address:
Eye Division
Olympia Medical Clinic
6-35-3 Jingumae, Shibuya-ku
Japan

MANAGEMENT OF VERTICAL SQUINT IN
ENDOCRINE ORBITOPATHY

H. KRUSE & W. RÜSSMANN

(Cologne, W. Germany)

The pathogenesis of dysthyroid orbitopathy is largely unknown. Immunological disease has been discussed recently. No correlations have been found between the dysthyroid state and the development of endocrine orbitopathy. It occurs even in patients with euthyroidism or hypothyroidism. Often the eye symptoms appear with a latency of several years after the onset of endocrine disturbance and in other cases they are the first sign of this disease.

Histological examination of orbital tissues reveals mainly lymphocytic infiltration of muscles, fat and connective tissues. Oedema and, later on, fibrosis of the orbital fat and the external eye muscles occur (Fells, 1976). Secondary to these findings proptosis and oculomotor imbalance develop.

Sometimes the intraocular pressure is found to be increased, especially in upgaze. This increase may be caused by compression of the globe or by increased resistance of the orbital veins. This opinion is supported by Veirs (1972).

In most cases the inferior rectus muscle is involved, followed by the medial rectus muscle (Fells, 1976). The patient seems to suffer from superior rectus muscle palsy with hypotropia and restriction of elevation to the midline or just beyond it. The differential diagnosis can be very difficult if there are only few signs of endocrine orbitopathy and/or monolateral manifestation or no obvious signs of dysthyroid disease. Lid lag should be especially looked for. The forced duction test and electromyography can be helpful.

From the orthoptic point of view the therapeutic aim is to enable the patient comfortable binocular single vision by prisms or by surgery, if prescribing prisms fails. Recently we performed an inferior rectus recession in four patients because of hypotropia.

CASE REPORTS

A 59 year old woman, suffering from endocrine orbitopathy for seven years, was admitted in our clinic for extraocular muscle surgery. No binocular single vision was obtained with prisms, and headaches continued. On the first examination gaze up of the left eye was nearly impossible. The left hypotropia measured up to 30 p dpt. A 4.5 mm recession of the left inferior rectus muscle was done with a satisfying result. Binocular single vision was recovered except for upgaze (Fig. 1a, b, 2a, b).

Another woman, 67 years old, suffered from the same disease for 2.5 years; after X-ray radiation of the orbital tissue the intraocular pressure increased, and electrotonography revealed a decreased outflow facility of the left eye. After 4.5 mm recession of the left inferior rectus, diplopia had dis-

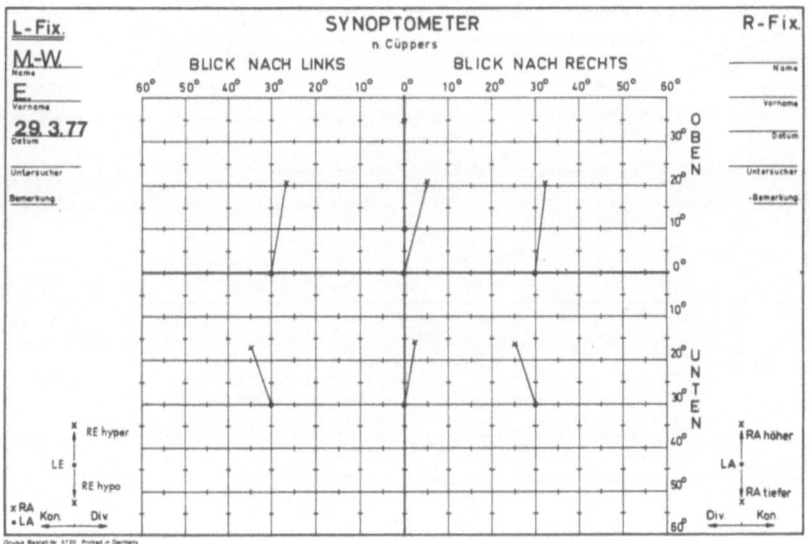

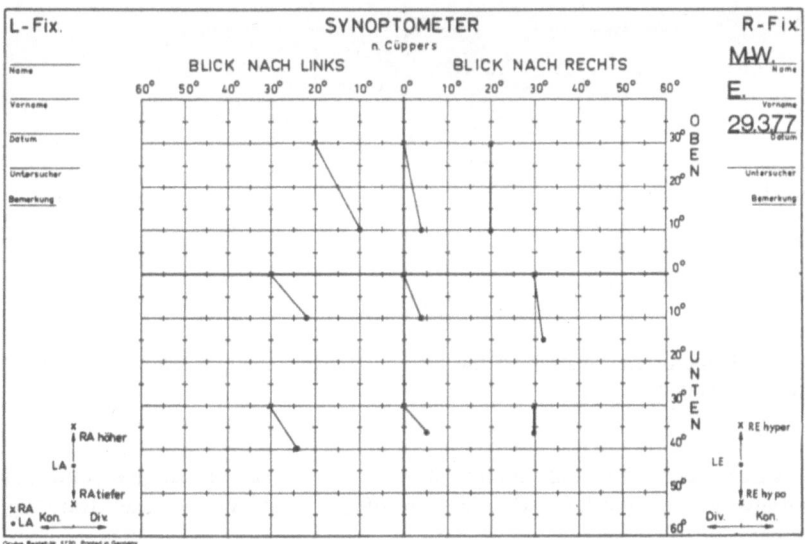

Fig. 1. Synoptometer analysis of case 1 before treatment; a) left eye fixation, b) right eye fixation.

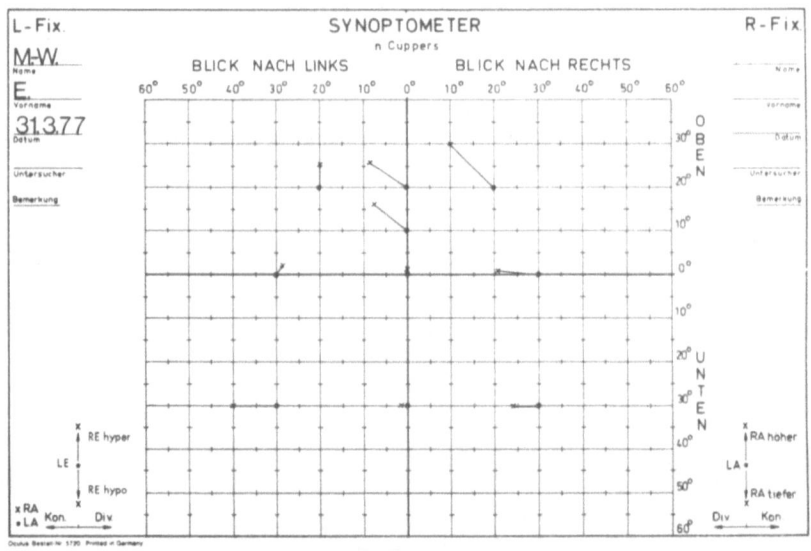

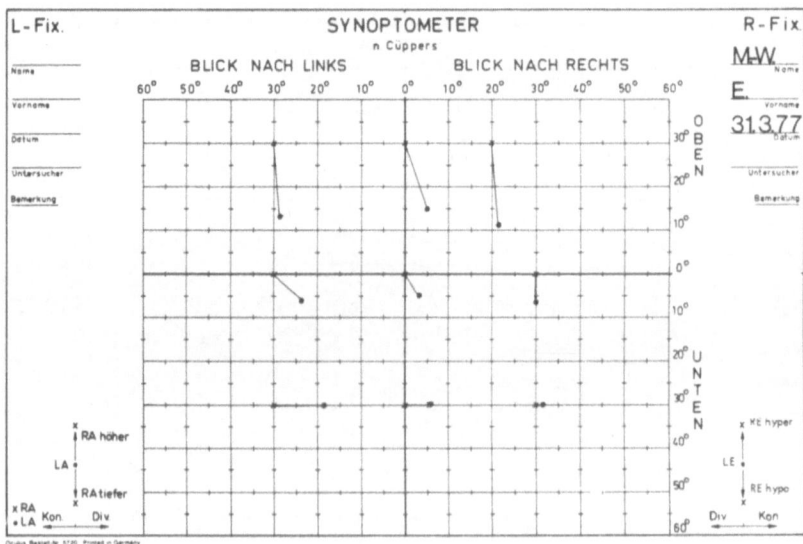

Fig. 2. Synoptometer analysis of the case 1 after treatment; a) left eye fixation, b) right eye fixation.

appeared, but the still increased pressure required antiglaucomatous therapy. Some time later, the pressure of the right eye increased too (Fig. 3a, b).

A third woman, 52 years old, complained of diplopia for about four months, inudced by endocrine orbitopathy. In addition, the intraocular pressure was increased, right more than left. After a 4.5 mm recession of

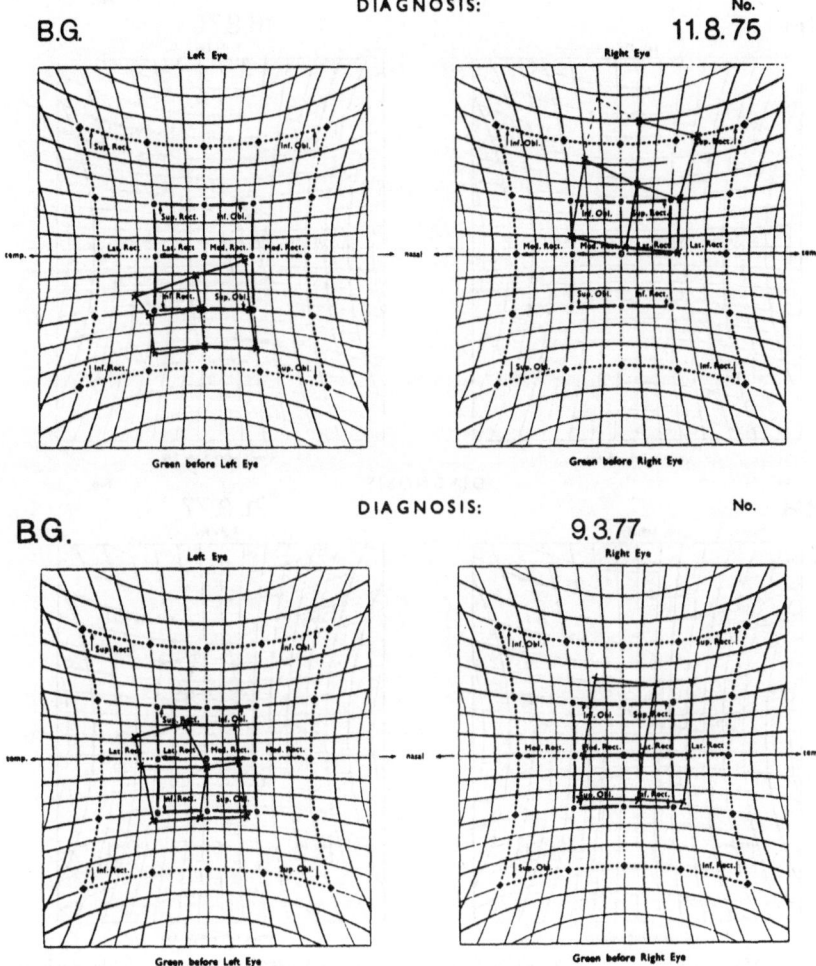

Fig. 3. Hess-screen of case 2; a) before treatment, b) after treatment.

the right inferior rectus muscle electrotonography revealed borderline values of outflow facility only of the left eye, while the intraocular pressure was now the same in both eyes (Fig. 4a, b).

A fourth case (a 51 year old woman, suffering from thyroid disorder for one year) did not show any changes of intraocular pressure. A 4.5 mm recession of the right inferior rectus removed hypotropia (Fig. 5a, b).

The results of electrotonography, performed on some of our patients, may demonstrate that changes in the behaviour of orbital tissues may be also responsible for secondary glaucoma in endocrine orbitopathy. The compression theory is supported by the fact that the intraocular pressure increases if the patient looks to the side opposite to the involved muscle. Often both mechanisms will be found together; i.e. a restricted venous drainage as well as strangulation of the globe. Therefore some decrease of intraocular press-

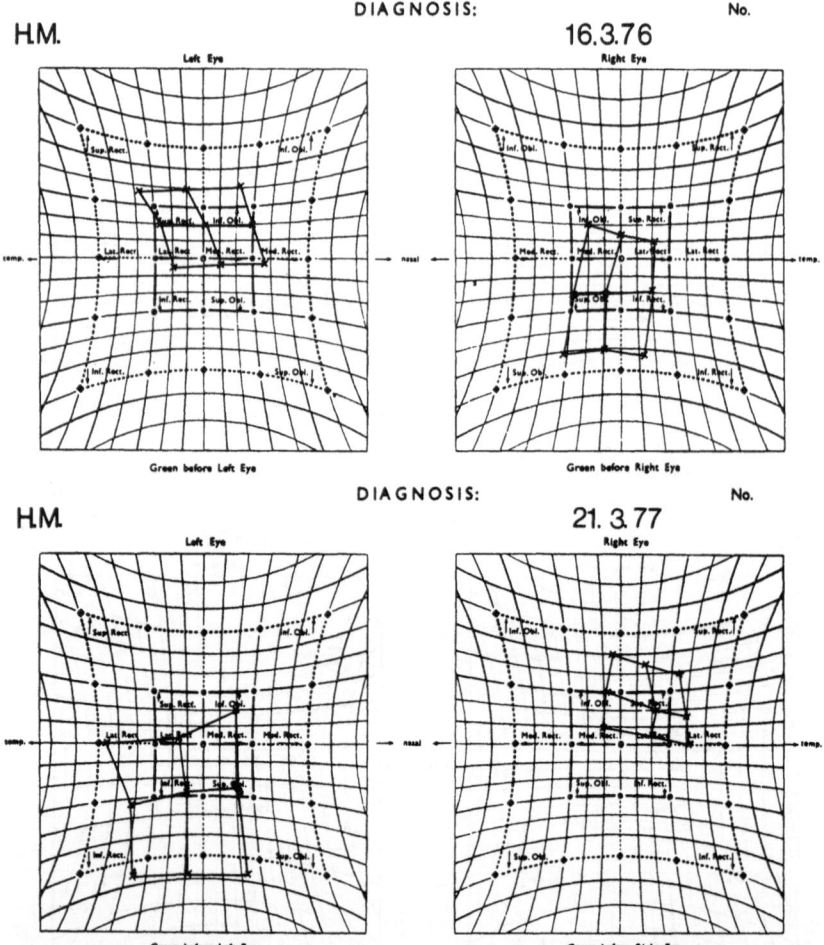

Fig. 4. Hess-screen of case 3; a) before treatment, b) after treatment. This patient overcame the postoperative right eye hypertropia by a large fusional amplitude in vertical direction.

ure may be obtained by recessing fibrotic extraocular muscles. To get a fair correction of deviation and sufficient effects on the intraocular pressure Tenon's capsule should be carefully dissected and relaxed.

We do not agree with Zauberman (1969), who recommends resection of the ipsilateral antagonist. In our opinion, this method does not respect pathophysiological mechanisms. The ocular motility could get worse, and the intraocular pressure could be increased, even if hypotropia is actually decreased.

Any therapeutic procedure should respect the whole pathophysiological situation, as far as it is known, as well as the possible secondary effects. Under these preconditions the recession procedure in cases with squint, caused by endocrine orbitopathy, seems to be the more logical principle and to have a better effect from both points of view.

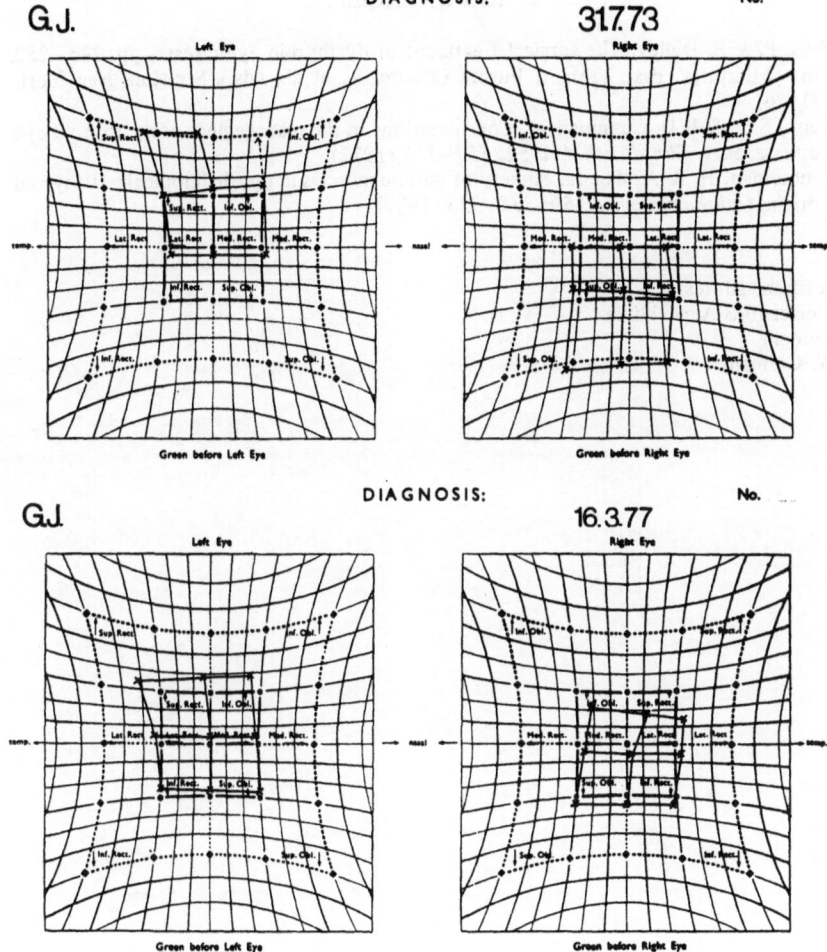

Fig. 5. Hess-screen of case 4; a) before treatment, b) after treatment.

SUMMARY

Four cases of endocrine orbitopathy which suffered from diplopia caused by vertical deviation of one eye are reported. Two of them also had an increased intraocular pressure especially in gaze up. In both cases electrotonography proved decreased outflow facility. In all patients the inferior rectus muscle was recessed with satisfying results (binocular single vision in primary position). It is concluded that this method seems to be the logical therapy concerning the fibrosis of extraocular muscles as a cause of the deviation as well as a cause of the increased intraocular pressure.

REFERENCES

Fells, P. & B. Dulley. The surgical treatment of dysthyroid eye disease. pp. 245–252 in: Orthoptics: Past, Present, Future (Moore, S., et al., eds.). Stratton, New York (1976).

Veirs, E.R. & R.D. Cunningham. Considerations in the management of dysthyroid eye disease. *Surg. Clin. North Am.* 52: *353–358* (1972).

Zauberman, H. & A. Magora. Surgery of paretic muscles in ophthalmoplegia of thyroid origin. *Ophthalmologica* 159: *333–338* (1969).

Authors' address:
Universitäts Augenklinik
Cologne
W. Germany

Proc. 3rd Int. Symp. on Orbital Disorders, Amsterdam 1977

A CASE REPORT ON A 15 YEAR OLD GIRL WITH HYPERTHYROIDISM AND MYASTHENIA GRAVIS. DISCUSSION OF DIAGNOSIS AND ETIOLOGY ON THE RELATION BETWEEN THESE DISEASES

R.J.W. DE KEIZER

(Amsterdam, The Netherlands)

CASE REPORT

A 14 year old girl was seen in our outpatient department for the first time with headache-dizziness-diplopia, ptosis and proptosis of the left eye. She had also a bad rhinitis with lymph nodes of the neck, so we gave her antibiotics. One week of this therapy had no results, so we took her to the hospital for observation.

General examination revealed the typical diagnostic features of hyperthyroidism (nervousness, weight loss, decrease tolerance to heat, pulse rate up to 160 p/min., frequent loose bowel movements, excessive perspiration).

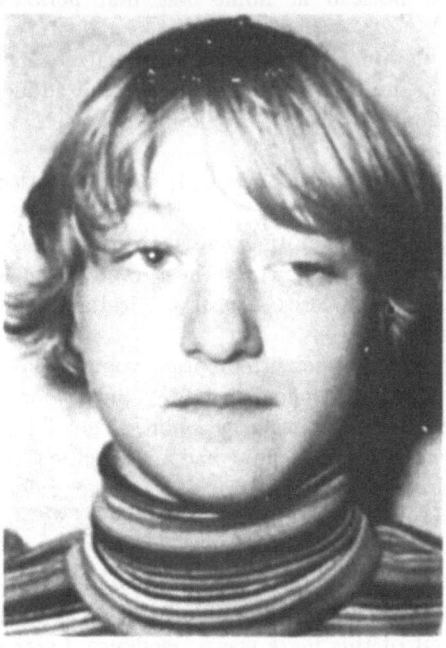

Fig. 1. A 14 year old girl with thyrotoxicosis and myasthenia gravis when referred to our outpatient department. Ptosis left eye.

363

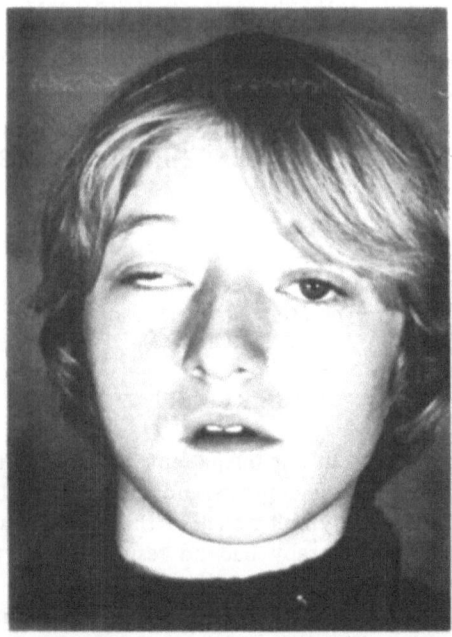

Fig. 2. The same patient on the day of hospitalisation. Ptosis right eye.

The only symptom noticed at home was that perhaps her neck had broadened.

Ophthalmic examination: R ptosis, strabismus divergens with diplopia in all directions (due to limitation of upward gaze and adduction gaze of the left eye), normal vision.

Medical diagnosis (clinical and laboratory): Graves' disease and thyrotoxic myopathy.

Neurologic examination was normal and gave the same diagnosis. But does this diagnosis cover the girl's illness? The symptoms seemed more severe than we had seen in other cases. Was it a pituitary gland disease or an orbital complication?

But all examinations: perimetry, computer tomography, chest and skull films, phlebography, electroencephalography, ultrasound, were normal. Only the visually evoked response gave a hint of possible chiasma trouble. The electro-myogram with neostigmine had an aspecific result.

The therapy consisted of 40 mg carbimazol 4 times daily. After one week there was a little improvement, ptosis and diplopia were decreased. After three weeks there was total ophthamoplegia and keratitis lagophthalmo, the physical symptoms were the same. Propanolol 4 x 40 mg daily was added to the carbimazol. From the clinical view the girl had to be also a myasthenia gravis but of this there was no evidence. Later a second electro-myogram of the eye muscles with neostigmine was done which was positive for the diagnosis myasthenic syndrome.

364

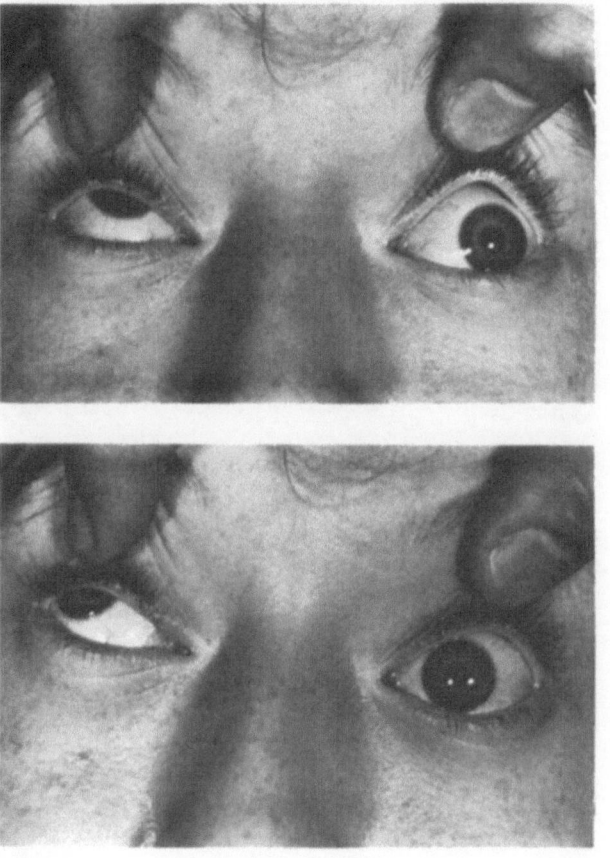

Figs 3, 4. The same patient, with upward gaxe and to the right direction.

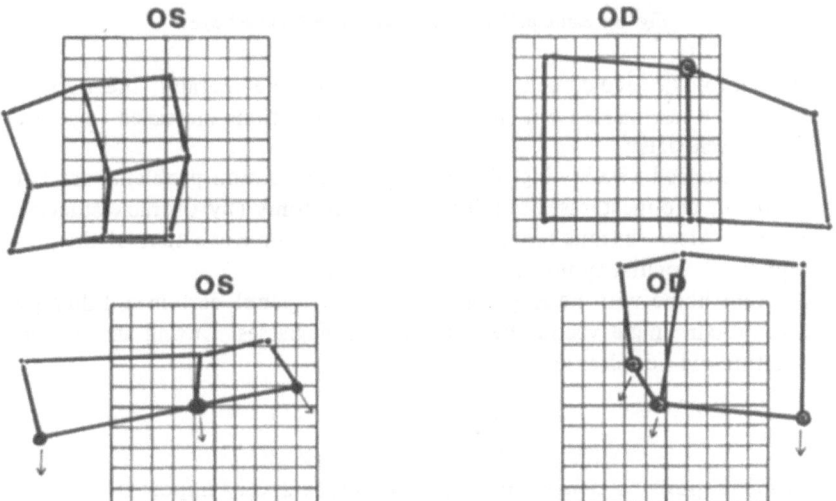

Fig. 5. Orthoptic examination when patient was in hospital for the first time.
Fig. 6. Orthoptic examination 4 weeks after hospitalisation after carbimazol therapy.

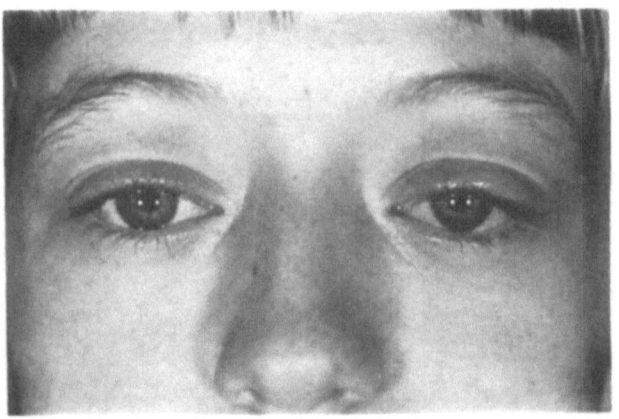

Fig. 7. Same patient after 6 weeks with open eyes.

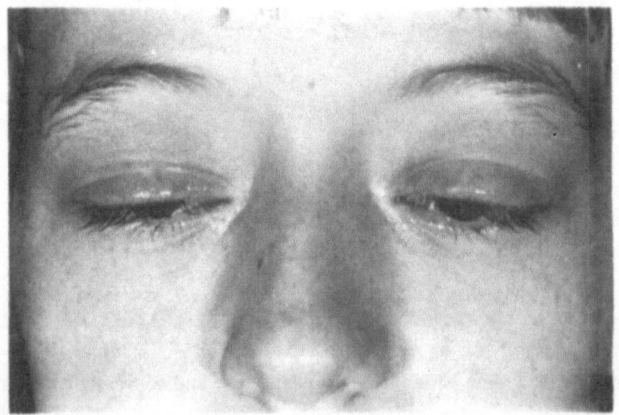

Fig. 8. Same patient after 6 weeks with closed eyes.

The neurologic department took her over for the therapy, the thyroid function had normalised but myasthenic manifestations increased to severe bulbar muscle palsy.

Since disturbed swallowing, dysarthria, and respiration problems did not improve on cholinesterase inhibitors, a thymectomy (by thoracic surgery) was done. After thymus removal we saw a quick improvement of the girl, except for the ocular symptoms.

She went home with neostigmine, atropine, propanol, carbimazol therapy and to obtain single vision she got 18Δ prism glasses. During six months the picture did not alter any more.

DISCUSSION

Myasthenia gravis, a neuro-muscular disorder, is a very important disease; 50% of these patients are first seen by the ophthalmologist. 40% have

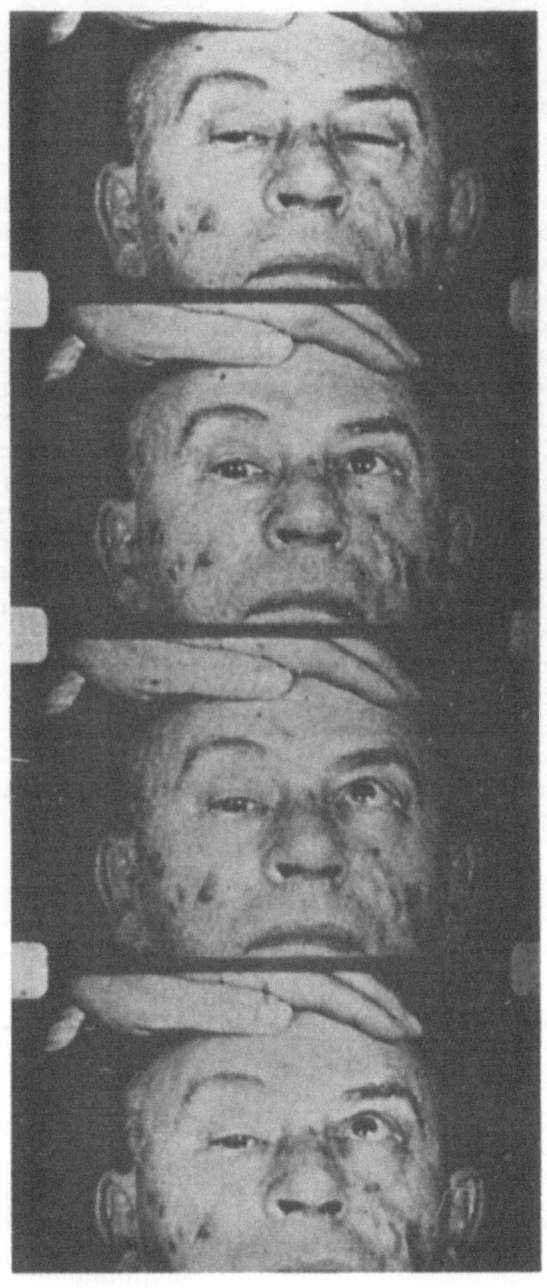

Fig. 9. **Twitch phenomenon**: patient first looks down and then back to primary position. A quarter of a second the palpebral fissure widens more than normal. Pathognomic for myasthenia gravis.

ocular and bulbar symptoms and 15% show ptosis with limited eye movements.

Essential in making a clinical diagnosis and pathognomonic for myasthenia are the following symptoms:

1. Diplopia, the range changes during the day with a maximum in the evening.

2. Ptosis, also varies during the day.

3. Ptosis changes with horizontal eye movements and with optokinetic nystagmus.

4. Twitch phenomenon: when the patient looks first down and after that back again to the primary position, the palpebral fissure widens during a quarter of a second.

5. Rapid eye movements: small amplitude and rapid saccades of a few degrees in association with total ophthalmoplegia. Clinically one sees 'quiver' movements. (Cogan & Yee, 1977).

6. Ptosis which is first localized right and they left, (see our patient).

The diagnosis is made regularly with the edrophoniumchloride or prostigmine test and electromyograms of eye muscle, m. adductor pollicis or hypothenar muscles (Care should be taken of muscle temperature, they have to be at room temperature.) If one cannot perform an electromyogram, one can still do the D-tubocurarine test (with the help of an aneaesthesiologist), myasthenia patients are very sensitive to it; or a test with Decamethonium iodide, myasthenic muscles being more resistant to it than normal muscles.

Clinically the diagnosis is made with edrophonium which gives within seconds a decrease of ptosis and in one of both eyes an increase in intraocular pressure (about 8 mm).

When one of these tests is positive the four types of the masasthenia syndrome have to be differentiated:

a. Lambert Eaton syndrome, a presynaptic myasthenic syndrome with bronchial carcinoma.

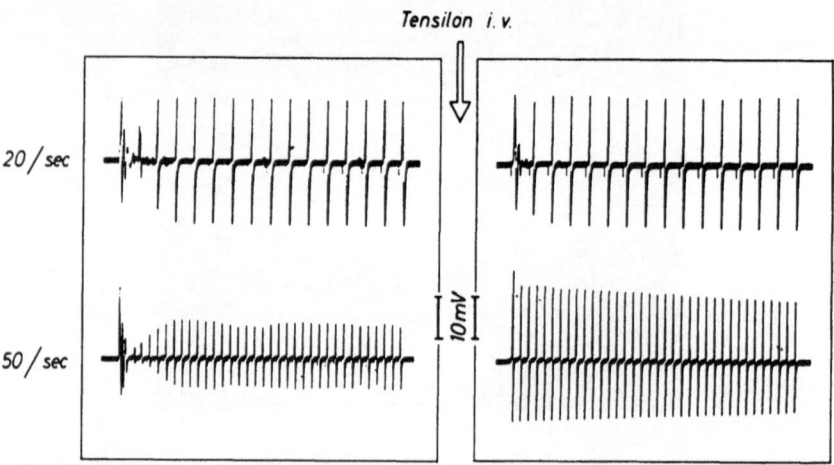

Fig. 10. Electromyogram in myasthenia patients with the reaction on tensilon with low and high frequency, left side normal myasthenic registration, right side after tensilon.

Tables 1+2. Tensilon and neostigmine tests for making the diagnosis mysthenia syndrome

---

Test no. 1

Neostigmine = inhibitor cholinesterase.
Against the central and muscarine activity of this drug first given atropine (this has no effect on the diagnostic signs).
With EMG.

Test no. 2.

- directly neuromuscular activity, anticholinergic
- take 10 mg = 1 cc, give first 2 mg in 15 sec. to patient; when no effect in 30 sec. give the other 8 mg. When after 2 mg a cholinergic reaction after 30 min. give 1 mg.
- it is working in 1–2 min., after 5 min. gone.
. normal muscles no effect
. it acts as antagonist for curare
. sometimes positive when neoastigmine negative
- if dosage too high → more weakness
Atropine also given before action or ready for injection.

---

b. Myasthenia induced by the antirheumatic drug D-Penicillamide.
c. Antibiotic induced myasthenia, sometimes by the combination of antibiotic-narcotic drugs; also presynaptic localised. A good response to calcium given parenterally (Tables 3, 4, 5).

As a reminder all prohibited drugs in myasthenia are given in Table 6.
d. The autoimmune disease myasthenia gravis pseudoparalytica.. For a good understanding of the autoimmunologic disorders the fundamentals of the immunology are important, see Table 7.

Table 3. Symptoms of the Antibiotic-induced myasthenia

Clinical manifestation:

---

outer eye
oropharyngeal ⟩ muscle weakness
intercostal

proximal arm-and legsmuscles weakness reflexes low or zero.

Table 4. The combination of the special antibiotics and other kinds of drugs in antibiotic-induced myasthenia

---

Exacerbation of symptoms

---

1. after anaesthesia   ether
                         tubocurarine
                         succinylcholine
                         flaxedil
2. by hypocalciaemia
3. by kidney diseases

Table 5. The kind of antibiotics which induce the myasthenia syndrome

Neomycin
Streptomycin
Kanamycin
Polymyxin
Bacitracin
Colistin

Table 6. General contra-indications in myasthenia

– minor and major tranquillizers
– morphine
– kinine
– kinidine
– chloroquine
– antibiotics and narcotic drugs who also can give the special myasthenia syndrome
– difantoine
– procainamide

Table 7. The fundamentals of immunology

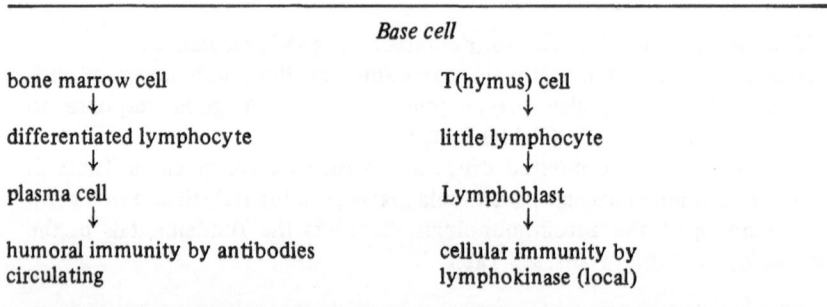

	Base cell
bone marrow cell ↓	T(hymus) cell ↓
differentiated lymphocyte ↓	little lymphocyte ↓
plasma cell ↓	Lymphoblast ↓
humoral immunity by antibodies circulating	cellular immunity by lymphokinase (local)

T System: biochemistry unknown. Delayed sensitisation (tuberculine).
B System: – all antibodies have the same basic structure 2 light and 2 heavy chains = immunoglobulins.
– one antibody molecule has reaction with one antigen molecule.

In the last four years the study of myasthenia gravis has thoroughly changed our knowledge about the etiology. The original conception was that malfunction of the presynaptic region of the nicotine acetyl choline receptor (ACHR) produces the disease. Recent investigations (see below) have demonstrated that the disorder of the neuromuscular junction is localised in the post-synaptic region and is of auto-immune origin.

A short survey on the actual knowledge of the pathogenesis shows that:
1. 75% of myasthenia gravis (M.G.) patients had IgG in the serum which blocks partially or totally the relation bungarotoxin-acetylcholine receptor in the neuromuscular junction (Bender, 1975).
2. Electron-microscopic examinations of muscles shows a lower rate of receptors in M.G. without any allergic base. There must be a functional and structural damage of the ACHR (Drachman, 1973).

3. When ACHR is injected into rappits, they get myasthenia gravis (Patrick, 1973).
4. Lymphocytes, specially transformed, give a special cellular sensitisation which decreases with haemodialysis or prednisone (Almon, 1974. Aahronov, 1975).
5. Lymphocytes from lymph nodes injected into rabbits also produce M.G. but they do not develop it when thymectomy is performed (previously T-cell dependent) (Grobb, 1976).
6. When human M.G. IgG is injected into mice they get M.G. which is dependent on C_3 complement (Toyka, 1977).
7. Normally when prednisone is given to rats they get total lysis of the thymus gland but when the rate have had experimental M.G., lymphoid tissue persists in the thymus after 50 days. If thymectomy was done before inoculation of experimental M.G. the rats still get M.G. but in a low grade (Sanders, 1977).
8. Extracts of thymus tissue contain acetylcholine receptors suggesting that an autoimmune reaction against ACHR might be initiated in the thymus gland itself (Kao & Drachman, 1977).
9. Clinical and laboratory investigations show us that there is a difference between young and old myasthenic patients. Old people react very well to corticosteroid therapy and less to acetylcholinesterase inhibitor medication or operation. Young women, if operated within three years after the first symptoms, respond favourably to thymectomy. They have also a good response to inhibitors of cholinesterase. Especially in the young women this relation with thymus can be shown in the laboratory (Patrick & Richardson, 1976).

Contraty to these investigations, Douglas (1976) was unable to find any difference in age-sex, except in mild and severe disorders. All his patients got high doses of prednisone followed by exacerbations of myasthenia gravis. (Be careful with this corticosteroid therapy. It can precipitate a myasthenic crisis in the first days.)
10. At this very time the registration of a specific antibody against the neuromuscular junction itself of myasthenia gravis patients is under research in the laboratory of Feltkamp (personal communication).

Summary

Myasthenia gravis is an autoimmune disorder of ACHR with antigen-antibody reaction, humoral and thymus cell dependent lymphocytes, and dependent on a serum complement factor. Perhaps the muscle cell junctions in the thymus itself are the source of the antibodies.

Myasthenia and thyroid disease

The frequency of M.G. in thyrotoxic patients is about 1%; thyrotoxicosis occurs in patients with myasthenia gravis in 9% and hypothyroidism in 6% (non-toxic goitre 2.1%). The combination is very rare in children (under 15 years of age). Up to 1968 only 4 cases were described and our case is perhaps the fifth.

371

Sometimes the two diseases can influence each other by increasing or decreasing their symptoms. For a proper diagnosis it is necessary to regulate the thyroid function. In hypothyroid subjects the electromyogram can give positive results for M.G. while after regulation there is a normal one. Aspecific or normal electromyograms in hyperthyroid cases can give evidence of myasthenia after normalising the thyroid function.

What is the direct relation between these two diseases?

1. Phosphorylation is disturbed in hyperthyroidism by high doses of thyroid hormones, by which the transfer of potential energy to muscle activity is decreased. But phosphorylation is also an essential factor in the production of acetylcholine.

2. In both disorders antibodies against thyroid and/or muscle tissue are demonstrable without, however, identifying either disease. The proportion of antibodies in the different diseases are shown in Table 8. It is very remarkable that 6–30% of normal persons have these antibodies. An explanation is given by Feltkamp (1976). He claims that inhibition and/or stimulation of T- and B-systems is disturbed by check of suppression of the formation of antibodies as in normal situations. More information on the nature of the diseases can be obtained from the qualitative level of antibody titres. The highest are found in Hashimoto thyroiditis.

Table 8. Quantities of antibodies in blood samples against thyroid tissue of served diseases

Hashimoto disease	99.9%
Hypothyroidism	90 %
Hyperthyroidism	75 %
Pernicious anaemia	50 %
Non toxic goiter	50 %
Thyroid carcinoma	10 %
Normal persons	1-30%

What kind of hyperthyroidism has our patient? Graves' disease of Hashimoto thyroiditis? Clinical manifestations indicate the diagnosis Graves' disease. However, histological evidence of autoimmune thyroiditis can be found in all kinds of these disorders, even in thyroid carcinoma. All of these autoimmune disorders have to be differentiated; they have their own symptoms but sometimes in a commonly predisposed population there is overlapping: Brown (1974) shows this hypothesis in the Venn diagram, a very good method of interpretation of the relation between the Hashimoto thyroiditis and Graves' hyperthyroidism, and Graves' ophthalmopathy (Fig. 11).

SUMMARY

Thyroid disease and myasthenia gravis both have relations with the thymus gland and its antigen-antibody formation. In the autoimmune disorder group they play a related, but not identical role and proper determination is very difficult. The function of the thyroid gland should be normalised in any case.

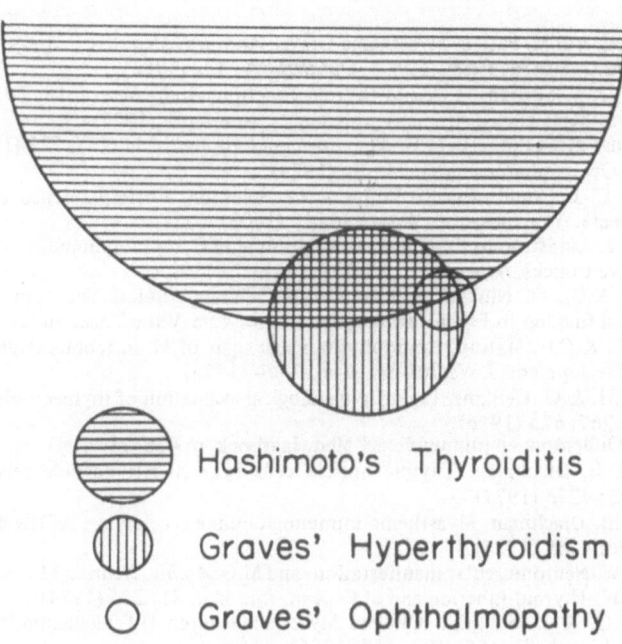

Hashimoto's Thyroiditis

Graves' Hyperthyroidism

Graves' Ophthalmopathy

Fig. 11. Venn's diagram. Relative frequency of Hashimoto/s thyroiditis, Graves' hyperthyroidism and Graves' ophthalmopathy.

REFERENCES

Aahronov, A. & O. Abransky. Humoral antibodies to acetylcholine receptors in patients with myasthenia gravis. *Lancet* II: *340–342* (1975).

Aalmon, R.R. Serum globuline in M.G. inhibition of bungarotoxin. Binding to acetylcholine receptors. *Science* 186: *55–72* (1974).

Bender, A.N. & W. King Engel. A serum factor blocking acetylcholine receptors of the human neuromuscular junction. *Lancet* I: *7907* (1975).

Borenstein, S. & J.E. Desmedt. Temperature and weather correlates of myasthenia fatigue. *Lancet* II: *63* (1974).

Brown, J. Thyroid physiology in health and disease. *Ann. Int. Med.* 81: *68-81* (1974).

Cecil, Loeb. Textbook of medicine, Saunders Company (1973).

Cogan, D.G. Myasthenia gravis. *Arch. Ophthal.* 74: *217* (1965).

Cogan, D.G. & R.D. Yee. Rapid eye movements in M.G. I, II, *Arch. Ophthal.* 94: *1083, 1465* (1976).

Cohan, S.L., K.L. Dretchen & A. Neal. Malabsorption of pyridostigmin in patients with myasthenia gravis. *Neurology* 27: *299* (1977).

Neurology 294(13): *722* (1976).

Crone, R.A. Diplopia, Excerpta Medica (1973).

Douglas Mann, J. & T.R. Johns. Long-term administration of corticosteroids in M.G. *Neurology* 26: *729* (1976).

Elmquist, D. & C. Matson. Acetylcholine receptor protein. *Arch. Neurol.* 34: *7* (1977).

Feltkamp, T.E.W. Het nut van de bepaling van autoantistoffen. Med. Jaarboek, p. 435 (1976).

Feltkamp, T.E.W. HLA typering en autoantistoffen bij patienten met M.G. *N.T.v.G.* 118: *895* (1974).

Finn, R. & P.M. Coates. Plasma exchange (R. Pinching). *Lancet* 22/I: *190*; 19/2: *428* (1977).
Festhoff, B.W. & B.M. Patten. Myasthenia Gravis. *Ann. Int. Med.* 81: *225–246* (1974).
Frenkel, M. M.G. current trends. *Am. J. Ophthal.* 61: *522* (1966).
Gaelen, L.H. & S. Levitan. M.G. and thyroid function. *Arch. Neurol.* 18: *107* (1968).
Grob, D. Myasthenia gravis. Academy of Sciences, New York (1976).
Grob, D. Cause of weakness in M.G. *New England J. of Med.* 294 (13): *722* (1976).
Havener, W. Ocular pharmacology. Mosby (1974).
Hamburger, J., G. Zandman, R. Volpé & D. Solomon. Correspondence euthyroid Graves' disease. *New Engl. J. of Med.* 296: *17* (1003).
Hill, P.K. & J. Lindstroom. Experience autoimmune M.G. no morphometric abnormalities of nerve truncks. *Neurol.* 2: *27, 200* (1977).
Hendrikson, K.G., O. Nilsson, J. Rosen & H. Schiller. Clinical Neurophysiological, morphological findings in Eaton Lambert syndrome. *Acta Neurol. Sca.* 56: *117* (1977).
Heilbronn, E. & C.H. Matson. Neurophysiological signs of M. in rabbits after receptor antibody development. *J. Neurol. Sci.* 24: *59–64* (1975).
Horowitz, S.H. & G. Genkins. Elextrophysiological evaluation of thymectomy in M.G. *Neurology* 267: *615* (1976).
Hymans, W.Ouderdom en immunologie. Med. Jaarboek, p. 425 (1976).
Kao, I. & D.B. Drachman. Thymic muscle cells bear ACHR possible relation M.G. *Science* 195: *4273* (1977).
Kao, I. & D.B. Drachman. Myasthenic immunoglobuline acceleratest ACHR degraditive. *Science* 196: *4289* (1977).
King Engel, W. Neuromuscular manifestations and M.G.*Archiv. Neurol.* 114: *663* (1961).
King Engel, W. Thyroid function and M.G.*Ann. Int. Med.* 81: *225* (1974).
Kommerell, G. & D. Schmidt. Okuläre Myasthenie durch D-Penicillamin-Behandlung. *Klin. Mbl. Augenheilk.* 168: *409–413* (1976).
Lefvert, A.K. & G. Matella. Antibodies against human cholinerg receptor protein in patients with M.G. Studies during immunosuppresive treatment. *Acta Med. Sca.* 201 (3): *181* (1977).
Mittag, T. (K. Nakao). Antiacetylcholine receptor IgG in neonatal M.G. *New. Engl. J. of Med.* 297 (3): *196* (1977).
Oosterhuis, H.J.G.H. Het histologisch beeld van de thymus in verband met resultaat van de thymectomie bij M.G. *N.T.v.G.* 118: *238, 96* (1974).
Oosterhuis, H.J.G.H. Studies in M.G. Clinical study. *J. Neurol. Sci.* 1: *512* (1964).
Oosterhuis, H.J.G.H. & T.E.W. Feltkamp. Studies in M.G. Part II. Relations with immunology. *J. Neurol. Sci.* 4: *417* (1967).
Osher, R.H. & J.L. Smith. Ocular myasthenia gravis and Hashimoto's thyroiditis. *Am. J. Ophthal.* 79: *6* (1975).
Ramsey, I. Thyroid disease and muscle dysfunction. W. Heineman Med. Books Ltd. (1974).
Patrick, J. & J. Lindstrom. Autoimmune response to ACHR serum gobuline in M.G. inhibition of -bungarotoxin. *Science* 180: *871* (1973).
McQuitten, P. & H.E. Caton. Myasthenic syndrome associated with antibiotics. *Arch. Neurol.* 18: *402* (1968).
Rahi, A.H.S. & A. Garner. Immunopathology of the eye. Blackwell, p. 245 (1976).
Rosenberg, J.N. Euthyroid disease. *New. Engl. J. of Med.* 296 (4): *223* (1977).
Richardson, D.P. & I. Patrick. Cellular immunity in M.G. response to purified ACHR and autologons thymocytes. *New. Engl. J. of Med.* 294 (13): *722* (1976).
Rosman, N.P. Neuologic and muscular aspects of thyroid dysfunction in childhood. *Ped. Cl. N.A.* 238: *575* (1976).
Sambrook, M.A. & H. Reid. M.G. clinical and histologic features in relation to thymectomy. *J. Neurol., Neurosurgery, Psych.* 39: *38-43* (1976).
Schlezinger, N.S. & M. S. Corin. M.G. associated with hyperthyroidism in childhood. *Neurology* 18 (1968).
Sanders, D.B., T.R. John, E. Cobb & M. Eldefraim. Experimental autoimmune M.G. in rats. *Arch. Neurol.* 34: *75* (1977).
Toyka, K.V. & D. Drechman. M.G. Study of humoral immune mechanism by passive transfer to mice. *New Engl. J. of Med.* 286 (3): *125* (1977).

Walsh, F.B. & W.F. Hoyt. Clinical neuro-ophthalmology, pp. 1277–1297. Williams-
Wilkins, Baltimore (1969).

Author's address:
Koopvaardijstraat 52
Zaandam
The Netherlands

SPONTANEOUS CAROTID-CAVERNOUS FISTULAS AND ASEPTIC CAVERNOUS SINUS THROMBOSIS – TWO RELATED DISORDERS

JAN BRISMAR & GUDRUN BRISMAR

(Lund, Sweden)

Spontaneous carotid-cavernous fistulas were earlier considered rare but have been diagnosed with increased frequency following the use of selective external and internal carotid artery injections in the angiographic evaluation of orbital disorders. These fistulas are typically supplied by branches from both the external and internal carotid arteries, and often have bilateral feeders. They usually have an insidious onset, and the symptomatology may give rise to suspicion of intraorbital tumour.

We have had the opportunity to examine with both carotid arteriography and orbital phlebography seven patients who were later proved to be suffering from a spontaneous carotid-cavernous fistula. These patients form the basis of this report. The ophthalmological and roentgenological findings in six of these patients have earlier been presented elsewhere (Brismar & Brismar, 1976a,b).

METHODS

Standard angiographic techniques were used; in most cases bilateral selective external and internal injections were made. For orbital phlebography 10 cc of contrast medium was injected during 1 second, following percutaneous cannulation of a frontal vein (Brismar 1974).

RESULTS

In all seven patients a carotid-cavernous fistula was demonstrated at carotid angiography. In one patient the fistula was probably caused by rupture of a demonstrable intracavernous internal carotid artery aneurysm; in the remaining six cases no etiologic factor could be suggested. In one of these cases the fistula was supplied solely by the ipsilateral accessory meningeal artery; in the remaining cases both internal and external carotid feeders were observed. In three cases bilateral arterial supply was found.

At phlebography countercurrent filling of the fistula was achieved in six cases. The cavernous sinus in all these cases had an amputated, deformed appearance, with all its posterior and lateral outlets partly or completely occluded (Fig. 1). In one of these six cases a thrombus was also demonstrated in the superior ophthalmic vein that drained the fistula (Fig. 2); in

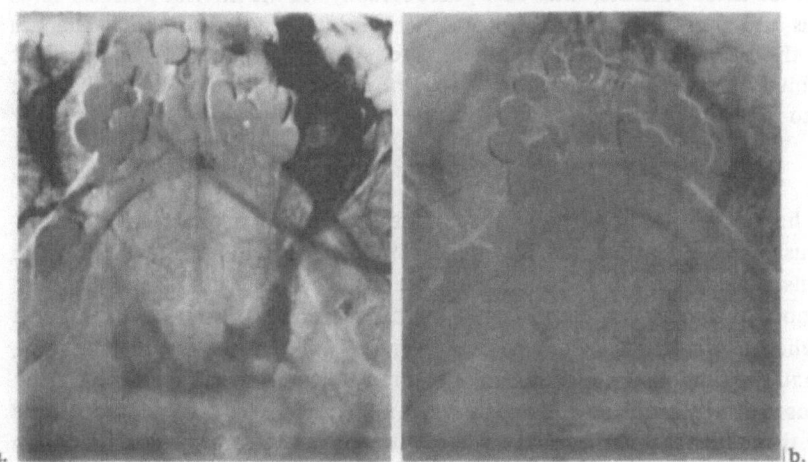

Fig. 1. Spontaneous carotis-cavernous fistula draining through both superior ophthalmic veins. Basal views, a) orbital phlebography, b) right external carotid angiography. Cavernous sinus is deformed with posterior and lateral outlets occluded.

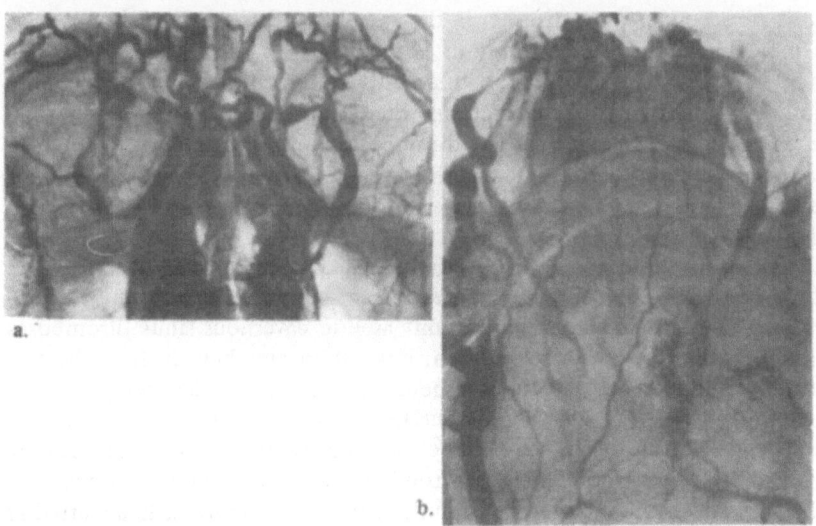

Fig. 2. Spontaneous carotid-cavernous fistula. Orbital phlebography, a) a.p., b) basal projections. Cavernous sinus has an irregular post-thrombotic appearance. Thrombus in right superior ophthalmic vein (←).

another patient, who had earlier had symptoms and signs indicating that the fistula drained also through the contralateral superior ophthalmic vein, an occlusion of that vein developed between two phlebographic examinations. In the seventh case, phlebography disclosed total occlusion of a superior ophthalmic vein which had at a previous angiography drained the fistula. In two of these patients, skull base phlebography via the inferior petrosal sinus was also performed and demonstrated widespread postthrombotic changes in the basal sinuses of the skull. In three of the cases, contrast material at orbital phlebography passed in retrograde direction through the fistula back into the feeding arteries.

DISCUSSION

It has earlier been reported that carotid-cavernous fistulas may spontaneously close (Sattler, 1920; Locke, 1924; Taniguchi et al., 1971). The constant correlation between spontaneous carotid-cavernous fistulas and venous thromboses, demonstrated in this material, has not been observed earlier, however, and could be demonstrated only thanks to phlebography. That the demonstrated deformity of the cavernous sinus is not an illusion caused by insufficient filling is proved not only by its sharp contours and by the fact that the injection was effective enough to force contrast medium back into the feeding arteries in three cases, but also by the fact that it could be observed, though less obviously, also at angiography. The etiology of spontaneous carotid-cavernous fistulas is obscure and, among other causes, primary disorders of the vascular wall have been mentioned (Walsh & Hoyt, 1969). It is possible of course that both the fistula and the thrombosis are secondary to a disorder in the vascular wall. We believe, however, it is more likely that the thrombosis is secondary to the fistula – whatever may be the etiology of the fistula. This statement is supported by the findings in three cases in this material where thrombosis developed or propagated between examinations. The thrombosis could then be caused either by vascular wall injury due to the high intravenous pressure, or by stagnation or reversal of flow in some veins caused by the fistula, according to the principle of the water aspirator.

It is obvious that if a carotid-cavernous fistula spontaneously heals through thrombosis, the end result will appear as an aseptic cavernous sinus thrombosis. This leads to another question: aseptic cavernous sinus thromboses are also disorders of obscure origin; how often are they, in fact, the end result of spontaneous carotid-cavernous fistulas? The clinical symptomatology will not help to answer this question with any certainty as the symptoms and signs are often the same for both disorders. In one patient of ours with an aseptic cavernous sinus thrombosis, however, the symptoms indicated that a fistula might have been the cause: the symptoms had started as a period with a bubbling sound in one ear.

SUMMARY

Seven consecutive patients with spontaneous carotid-cavernous fistulas were examined with both carotid angiography and orbital phlebography. Phlebography gave countercurrent filling of the fistula and in all seven cases disclosed extensive thromboses in the skull base sinuses. This remarkable correlation between fistulas and thromboses has not earlier been observed, and raises the question: How often are 'aseptic cavernous sinus thromboses' secondary to healed fistulas?

378

REFERENCES

Brismar, G. & J. Brismar. Spontaneous carotid-cavernous fistulas. Clinical symptomatology. *Acta Ophthal. Kbh.* 54: *542* (1976).

Brismar, G. & J. Brismar. Spontaneous carotid-cavernous fistulas. Phlebographic appearance and relation to thrombosis. *Acta Radiol. (Diagn.)* 17: *180* (1976).

Brismar, J. Orbital phlebography. I. Technique. *Acta Radiol. (Diagn.)* 15: *369* (1974).

Locke, C.E., Jr. Intracranial arteriovenous aneurysms of pulsating exophthalmos. *Ann. Surg.* 80: *1* (1924).

Sattler, Ch. In: Handbuch der gesamten Augenheilkunde, Vol. 9 (A. Graefe & T. Saemische, eds.). Engelmann, Leipzig (1920).

Taniguchi, R.M., J.A. Goree & G.L. Odom. Spontaneous carotid-cavernous shunts presenting diagnositc problems. *J. Neurosurg.* 35: *384* (1971).

Walsh, F.B. & W.F. Hoyt. Clinical neuro-ophthalmology, Volume 2, p. 1714. Williams & Wilkins Comp., Baltimore (1969).

Authors' address:
Departments of Diagnostic Radiology & Ophthalmology
University Hospital
S-221 85 Lund
Sweden

Proc. 3rd Int. Symp. on Orbital Disorders, Amsterdam 1977

THE TOLOSA HUNT SYNDROME

P. DWYER JONES, P. EUSTACE & J. TOLAND

(Dublin, Ireland)

This rather rare clinical condition was first clearly defined by Hunt et al. (1961) who also re-described the pathology of Tolosa's case (1954). The condition is best described as retro-orbital pseudotumour producing, because of its different location, a different set of signs and symptoms to orbital pseudotumour, namely painful ophthalmoplegia in a white eye. Neurological involvement is not confined necessarily to the third cranial nerve, the fourth, fifth and sixth as well as the optic nerve and the oculo sympathetic fibres may be involved. Investigations suggest only involvement of the cavernous sinus. Spontaneous resolution and occasional recurrences are usual.

In our experience three clinical features strengthen the diagnosis, negative angiography, suggestive orbital phlebography and dramatic response to steroids exhibited systematically.

The aetiology of the condition is quite unknow but undoubtedly it represents a similar pathological process to orbital pseudotumour, the site of the inflammation being more posteriorly sited (Levy et al., 1975).

This paper reports three cases and emphasises the salient features of the condition, in particular the abnormality of orbital phlebography and the extensive differential diagnosis.

CASE REPORTS

Case 1

Mrs. E.R. aged 65

Presented on 29/12/'74 complaining of severe pain in the right temple and radiating into the right eye which had been present for two days. Horizontal and vertical diplopia had also been present for two days. Her family had noticed slight drooping of the right upper lid for four days. She was referred to the National Neurosurgical Unit with a presumptive diagnosis of carotid aneurysm possibly sited at the posterior communicating artery junction. On examination she was found to have vision of 6/24 with two m.ms of proptosis; the pupil was sluggish in reaction and slightly dilated. There was slight ptosis and limitation of all eye movements in particular adduction.

Investigations included a normal glucose tolerance test: E.S.R. 8 mm/hour and negative carotid angiography. Orbital phlebography showed poor filling of the superior ophthalmic vein and the apex of the cavernous sinus. Systemic steroid were commenced, the dose being prednisolone 60 mgms daily.

Within forty-eight hours there had been complete relief of pain and also dramatic improvement in the range of eye movements. Systemic steroids were continued for the next two months in reducing dosage. There was complete resolution of all clinical signs and during a two year observation period there has been no recurrence.

Case 2

Mr. S.A. aged 35

There was a history of severe pain in the right temple and right eye spreading back to the occiput for one week. For four days there had been drooping of the upper lid and diplopia when the lid was elevated. He was referred to the National Neurosurgical Unit on 15/2/'77. On examination visual acuity was 6/6 in either eye, there was partial ptosis with moderate levator action. There was 2 mm of reducible proptosis; pupillary reflexes and corneal sensation were normal. The eye was white. Eye movements were limited vertically and medially. Glucose tolerance test was normal. E.S.R. was 11 mm/hour, carotid angiography was normal but orbital phlebography showed failure of opacification of the superior ophthalmic vein and the cavernous sinus. Systemic steroid in a dose of prednisolone 60 mgms produced complete relief of pain in 24 hours with marked improvement in range of movement. Steroids were stopped after 2 months. There has been no recurrence to date.

Case 3

Mr. J.K. aged 45

Had had dull pain behind the left eye with slight vertical diplopia. He was referred to the National Neurosurgical Unit on 14/4/'77. On examination visual acuity was 6/6 in both eyes; there was slight ptosis. The eye was white and pupillary reflexes were normal. There was slight limitation of vertical movement and some limitation also of adduction. Carotid angiography, E.S.R. and glucose tolerance test were normal. After 24 hours treatment with systemic steroid there was almost complete resolution of all clinical signs. Treatment was continued for six weeks. There has been no recurrence to date.

DISCUSSION

The diagnostic problem of painful ophthalmoplegia is not uncommon. It is common knowledge that carotid aneurysm particularly at the junction with the posterior communicating artery is often signalled by painful ophthalmoplegia with pupillary involvement, the so-called surgical third. Since the aneurysm is potentially treatable at this time, carotid angiography is mandatory in all cases of painful ophthalmoplegia. Perhaps not so widely recognised is the frequency with which diabetes or pre-diabetes may produce painful ophthalmoplegia usually with sparing of the pupil, the medical third. Giant cell arteritis is a much rarer cause of medical third but should always be considered in the older age group. In children by far the commonest cause of painful ophthalmoplegia is ophthalmolegic migraine. There is an unfortunate tendency for recurrence and later attacks may fail to resolve totally.

Pituitary apoplexy must also be considered as a cause of painful ophthalmoplegia although often bilateral in these cases. There are other rare causes, Herpes Zoster, tenosynovitis of the superior oblique tendon, neoplasm, etc.

It is our policy to combine orbital phlebography with carotid angiography in these patients who are also screened with a glucose tolerance test and an E.S.R.

In the cases described in this paper a dramatic response to systemic steroids greatly assisted the clinical diagnosis. Orbital phlebography was extremely helpful in the two cases in which it was carried out.

A further case of interest has been seen in which systemic steroids were commenced after negative investigations. There was no clinical improvement within 48 hours and the patient now developed a diabetic glucose tolerance curve and subsequently developed clinical diabetes.

As to aetiology this is quite unknown but there is little clinical doubt that the process is identical to orbital pseudotumour. Both Tolosa-Hunt Syndrome and orbital pseudotumour have been associated with Reidels thyroiditis, mediastinal and retro-peritoneal fibrosis as well as Dupytrens contracture and sclerosing cholangitis. All these conditions, it is felt, may have a similar pathology (Levy et al., 1975).

SUMMARY

The important clinical features of the Tolosa-Hunt Syndrome are presented as demonstrated in three clinical cases. The differential diagnosis is outlined and value of orbital phlebography in pinpointing the cavernous sinus is confirmed. The dramatic response of these cases to systemic steroids is re-emphasised.

REFERENCES

Hunt, W.E., J.N. Meagher, H.E. Lefever & W. Freman. Painful ophthalmoplegia, its relationship to indolent inflammation of the cavernous sinus. *Neurology* 11: *56–62* (1961).
Levy, T.S., J.E. Wright & G.A.S. Lloyd. Orbital and retro-orbital pseudotumors. pp. 364–367, in: Modern Problems in Ophthalmology, Vol. 14 (1975).
Tolosa, E. Periarteritic lesion of the cavernous sinus with clinical features of carotid infraclinoid aneurysm. *J. Neurol. Neurosurg. Psychiat.* 17:*300–302* (1954).

Authors' address:
The Mater Misericordiae Hospital and the
National Neurosurgical Unit
The Richmond Hospital
Dublin
Ireland

THE TOLOSA HUNT SYNDROME

DANIELE ARON-ROSA & DOMINIQUE DOYON

(Paris, France)

Arising from lesions of the orpital apex, the Tolosa Hunt syndrome has received increasing attention in recent years. This syndrome is characterised by recurrent, unilateral painful acute ophthalmoplegia (involvement of the ophthalmic division of the trigeminal nerve) usually without involvement of the optic nerve, and responds dramatically to steroid therapy within 48/72 hours.

In 1954, Tolosa described a 47-year-old man with self-limited left orbital pain. The pain recurred after several months and became associated with ptosis and subsequently total ophthalmoplegia. The patient died two days after exploratory craniotomy and an autopsy revealed that the intracavernous portion of the left carotid was wrapped in granulomatous tissue and that the lumen of the cavernous sinus was partially replaced by a similar process.

In 1961, Hunt et al. reported 6 similar cases and reviewed the cases of Tolosa's patient. They concluded that the process was not an arteritis but an inflammatory reaction limited to the cavernous sinus and that corticosteroid therapy was beneficial. In 1962, Lakke reviewed the superior orbital fissure syndrome and reported another case. In 1966 Smity & Taxdal were the first to apply the term 'Tolosa-Hunt syndrome' to this entity. They described 5 additional cases and stressed the importance of steroid administration as a diagnostic test because of the dramatic therapeutic response.

Mattew & Chandy (1969) reported 22 cases and in one case found an irregular stenosis of the intracavernous portion of the internal carotid artery. Lesser & Jampol (1972) reported one case who had a positive anti-nuclear factor associated with exacerbations of the disease.

Spindler (1975), reporting one case, described the possible angiographic findings which provided evidence of isolated periarteritis disease of the intra-cavernous carotid-artery. Sondheimer & Knapp (1973) reported a complete angiographic study in 3 cases all with phlebographic abnormalities and reviewed 14 cases. Lapresle & Said (1975), on the other hand, reporting 3 cases found all angiographic studies to be normals.

The purpose of this report is to review 10 personal cases in which the follow-up was between two and five years, and an attempt has been made to isolate the most constant clinical, radiological and CAT's features and the signs which may help to avoid the confusion with other pathological conditions in the same region such as space occupying lesions, aneurism, nasopharyngeal growths, meningitis, diabetes, multiple sclerosis, temporal arteritis, sphenoid sinus infections, mucocele or ophthalmoplegic migraines.

MATERIAL AND METHODS

This paper includes 10 cases of recurrent painful ophthalmoplegia. Besides a complete clinical investigation in all 10 cases, neurological examination, routine laboratory investigations of blood, urine, stools and cerebrospinal fluid were done, complete thyroid investigation was demanded for the 8 adults, special rhumathoid tests, sedimentation rate and research of anti-nuclear factors. L.C.R. cells were done in all cases. Temporal artery biopsy was performed in all adults; all patients had standard radiological investigations including study of the sphenoidal fissure and sinuses, complete repeated angiographic study (arteriography and phlebography), 8 patients were explored with C.T. and all patients had an isotopic scanning of the orbit.

Three patients who had alternating Tolosa Hunt syndrome and attacks of orbital psuedo-tumour, were excluded from this paper as discutable in the nature of the process.

RESULTS

Clinical features

Age and sex incidence is shown in Table 1:

Age group, years	No. of patients
10–19	2
20–29	1
30–39	2
40–49	4
50–59	0
60–69	1

The ages ranged from 10 to 65 years, the most frequent being between 30–49 (6 patients). Of 10 patients, 4 were female, which is in agreement with Sondheimer & Knapp, but differs from Mathew & Chandy who found 15 males and 7 females among 22 patients.

Symptoms and onset

In all 10 cases symptoms started with pain around the orbit, in the retro and/or periorbital region, and it preceded the ophthalmoplegia; the pain is most commonly retro-orbital (6 cases) but presently extends (9 cases) to the temporal and frontal regions (Table 2).

Table 1. Clinical findings (I); Tolosa Hunt, 10 cases

	Present	Absent
Pain around the orbit	10	0
Ophthalmoplegia	10	0
III nerve	8	2
IV nerve	2	8
VI nerve	4	4
Pupils paresis	2	7
Horner's syndrome	1	
Response to steroid therapy	10	0

Table 2. Clinical findings (II). Tolosa Hunt, 10 cases.

	Present	Absent
Chemosis	3	7
Proptosis	4	6
Optic nerve involvement	0	10
Unilat. low opthalmic blood pressure	2	8
Recurrences	9	1

The ophthalmoplegia may be manifested by isolated third or sixth nerve palsy, more rarely it can be total. Initial involvement of the 3rd nerve (especially SR) is more frequent (8 cases) than of the 6th nerve (4 cases) the IV nerve was only twice involved and this involvement accompanied a complete ophthalmoplegia.

The pupils are said to be usually spared but 3 patients had a positive response to the cocaine test, two patients had a totally irresponsive pupil for 2 days – and one patient presented a Horner syndrome besides the orbital pain which belongs to the Vth disfunction. Involvement of the 5th cranial nerve is not uncommon and observed in 8 cases, the first division of the 5th nerve was the most frequently involved (7 cases) resulting in 6 peri-orbital painful hypesthesia and depression of corneal reflex in 2 cases. Disfunction of the mandibular nerve was never observed. This involvement is of importance to distinguish Tolosa Hunt syndrome from pseudo-tumor of the orbit, in which painful ophthalmoplegia may be present, but the 5th nerve is spared and there may be signs of orbital inflammations.

Although noticed in some cases, by Mathew & Chandy (1970) and Sond-heimer (1973), we never observed real involvement of the optic nerve, nor abnormalities of the fundus in any case, but one patient complained for a few days of a blurred vision. Other features were observed inconstantly, such as a mild chemosis in 3 cases for a few days during the onset of the

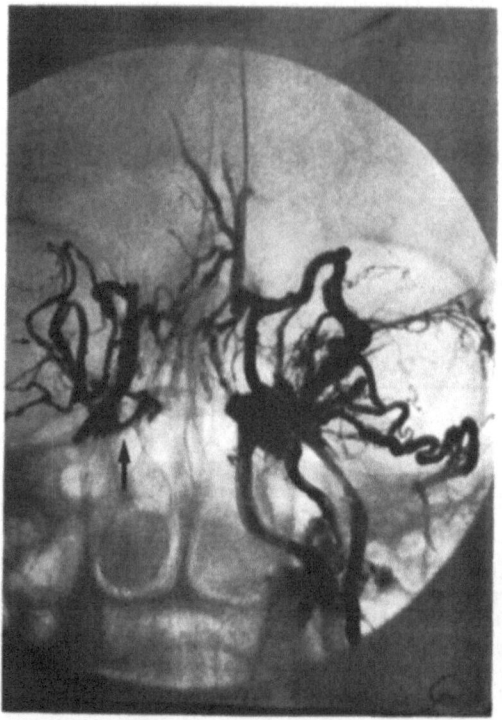

Fig. 1. C.H., 43 years old. Tolosa Hunt syndrome on the right side. Phlebography. This case responded well to the corticosteroid treatment.

Aspect before treatment was started. Note the narrowing of the superior ophthalmic vein. Compared with the left side, the vascularisation is only impaired on the right side.

affection. Real proptosis was discutable and always less than 2 mm and observed in 4 cases.

We observed 4 times a significant difference in the ophthalmic blood pressure which was unilaterally lowered on the side of the syndrome. A slight unilateral elevation of eye pressure was noted in 2 cases.

Remissions and recurrences

Spontaneous remission with partial and complete recovery of ophthalmoplegia is, together with the recurrence, one of the main features of the disease; recurrences were observed in all cases:

— 2 patients had 5 episodes
— 4 patients had 3 episodes
— 3 patients had 2 episodes
— 1 patient had 1 episode (in this case the follow-up is in less than 18 months). It should be pointed out that in one patient (5 episodes) alternatively the right and the left side were involved (Table 3).

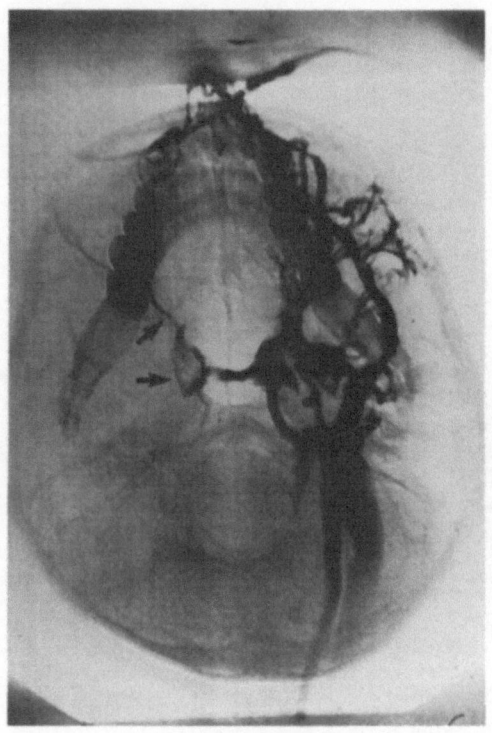

Fig. 2. C.H., **43 years old. Tolosa Hunt syndrome on the right side. Phlebography.**
The irregular aspect and the reduced circulation of the right cavernous sinus is even more conspicuous on this figure (Hirtz). It indicates a narrowing of the terminal portion of the superior ophthalmic vein, as the vein on the other side in the same region is at least twice as large.

Table 3. Radiological findings. Tolosa Hunt, 10 cases.

	Normal	Abnormal	Not done
Optic canal sphen. cleft	10	0	0
CAT's examin.	8	0	2
Isotop. scanning	6	4	0

Steroid response

All patients were given 60 mg Prednisone daily, in 9 cases the pain disappeared after 2 days, and after 8 days in 9 cases ophthalmoplegia regressed. Only one of the cases, who had received surgery, improved more slowly and partially.

387

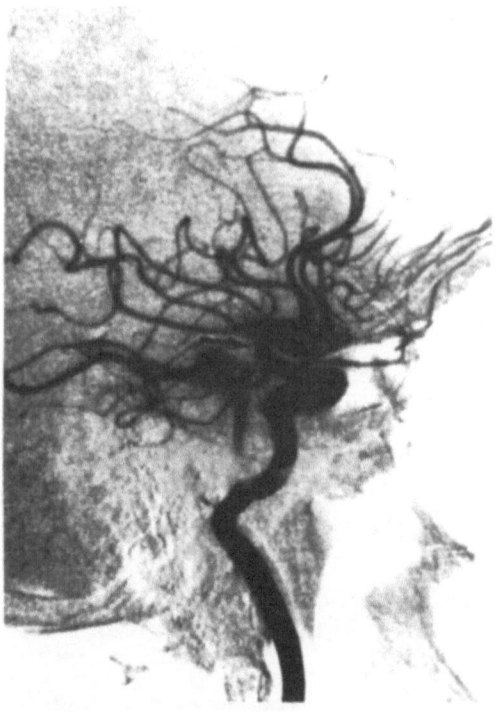

Fig. 3. C.H., 43 years old. Tolosa Hunt syndrome on the right side. Right carotid angiography.
Irregularity and stenosis of the carotid siphon in the cavernous sinus.

Biological findings

The erythrocyte sedimentation rate was moderately elevated in 6 patients, never exceeded 40 mm during the first hour, and normalised in one week after steroid treatment; only in 4 cases was it noticed to be elevated during recurrences.

All other laboratory examinations were negative including cerebrospinal fluid analysis, glucose tolerance test, thyroid dysfunction tests, rheumathoids test (Waller-rose latex, research of the HLAW 27).

Only one patient had a positive response to research of antinuclear factor and to our knowledge it has only been reported once by Lesser & Jampol (1974), and it is interesting to point out that the antinuclear factor is also positive in a good proportion of patients with rheumathoid arthrites, scleroderma; some medications (INH hydralazine etc.) and sometimes in dermato myositis, polyarteritis, Hashimoto thyroiditis, pulomonary fibrosis, ulcerative colitis and in some malignant neoplasm.

Temporal artery biopsy was done for 8 adults and revealed to be negative. The thyroid tests were all negative.

Routine examination of the skull sphenoidal fissure optic canal, sinus, were normal in all the cases, as well as in the other real cases previously reported (Table 4).

Carotid angiography showed a narrowing of the cavernous portion of the internal carotid artery in 5 cases, but was normal in the 5 others – the possibility of arteriosclerotic lesions may be excluded, 2 patients were less than 15 years old and the 3 others less than 45 years old and had an opposite normal carotid artery – it should be emphasized that all these 5 patients had a lowered ophthalmic pressure on this side.

Table 4. Angiography. Tolosa Hunt, 10 cases.

	Normal	Abnormal
Intern. carotid	5	5 (stenosis of syphon)
Phlebography	5	5
Repeated phlebo: 4 cases abnormal		4

Orbital venography showed abnormalities in 7 cases, 5 were not discutable and slightly different to these described by Sondheimer & Knapp (1973).

Only in 2 cases was a stenosis of the end of the superior ophthalmic vein observed, the ipsilateral cavernous sinus was partially occluded in 5 cases, 2 other cases presented a finer cavernous sinus compared to the same opposite side.

Orbital venography was repeated in 4 of our patients, 3 months and 2 years after the onset and outsides from a recurrence, no change was observed. This suggested, as said by Sondheimer & Knapp (1973), that in some cases the inflammatory process progress as to fibrosis. It must also be pointed out that the angiography was completely normal in the other cases.

CAT's examination (computerised tomography) was possible in 8 cases, and was repeated twice 4 weeks and 3 months after the onset – we obtained no positive response.

Echography was negative in all 10 cases.

Gammagraphic scannign showed a limited positive response in 4 cases (using marked Technecium), which disappeared after clinical improvement.

Surgical explorations of the lateral aspect of the cavernous sinus with biopsy was done in the previous case (one of the 2 children) and showed a thickening of the dura and a granulamatous inflammation of the dura on the border of the orbital fissure, which, according to Tolosa Hunt, respond to this disease which is due to an indolent non-specific inflammation within the cavernous sinus and the orbital sphenoidal cleft. In this case the carotid was noted to be thick and rigid although it was a child's arteriography. It appears that the clinical findings are more constant and typical than radiological images.

DISCUSSION

The Tolosa Hunt painful ophthalmoplegia has to be distinguished from other causes of painful ophthalmoplegia with or without trigeminal dysfunction, which included sphenoid fissure syndrome, cavernous sinus syndrome, parasellar syndrome, trauma, pansinusites, intracavernous carotid aneurism, nasopharyngeal tumors, pseudo tumors of the orbit, ophthalmic migraine: clinical features, especially pain recurrence and dramatic response to steroid therapy remain the best argument for the Tolosa Hunt syndrome.

Patients with temporal arteritis may have painful ophthalmoplegia and elevated sedimentation rates, and also respond to steroid therapy, but this condition reveals some evident differences. The average age in patients with temporal arteritis is 10 years older than in Tolosa Hunt syndrome and the ratio of female to male is about 4 to 1, the majority of these patients have general symptoms and the sedimentation rate is superior and usually more than 80 mm/h. Neuorpapillitis with blindness is never encounteren in Tolosa Hunt but frequent and frequently bilateral in Horton's disease, third and sixth nerve palsy are far more frequent in Tolosa syndrome. Mainly, temporal artery biopsy are positive in 85% of Horton's disease and negative in all patients with Tolosa Hunt syndrome.

Finally, response to steroid is more dramatic in the Tolosa Hunt syndrome than in the real pseudo tumors of the orbit.

CONCLUSIONS AND SUMMARY

10 cases of painful ophthalmoplegia are reported — in all cases pain marked the onset of the disease and the condition was mostly unilateral. Recurrence and dramatic response to steroid therapy were more constant features than angiographic findings which may be completely normal.

CAT permitted elimination of a tumor of the cavernous sinus in 7 cases, but in one case which was operated an aggravation followed surgery. In spite of complete investigations of all patients some questions remained unanswered:

− Is it an inflammatory or an allergic inflammatory process? (The presence of antinuclear factor in a single case does not enable us to answer this question.)

− Why is the process confined to the superior orbital fissure? Mathew & Chandy tried to find a similarity between this syndrome and Bell's palsy although the two syndromes have not been shown to coexist.

− Is the Tolosa Hunt syndrome comparable to the pseudo-tumor of the orbit? Although the dura mater is inserted on the border of the sphenoidal cleft, some patients may alternate the two syndromes.

REFERENCES

Di Chiro, G. Carotid angiography in eight cases of unilateral ophthalmoplegia. *Acta Radiol.* 50: *132–136* (1958).
Hunt, W.E. Tolosa-Hunt syndrome: one case of painful ophthalmoplegia. *J. Neur. Surg.* 44: *544* (1976).

Hunt, W.E., J.N. Meagher, H.E. Lefever et al. Painful ophthalmoplegia. Its relation to indolent inflammation of the cavernous sinus. *Neurology* (Minn.) 11: *56–62* (1961).

Lakke, J.P. Superior orbital fissure syndrome. Report of a case caused by local pachymeningitis. *Arch. Neurol.* (Chicago) 7: *289–300* (1962).

Lapresle, J. & G. Said. Ophtalmoplégie douloureuse alternante et récidivante, contribution à l'étude du syndrome de Tolosa Hunt. Serv. de Neur. du Centre Hospitalier de Bicêtre (0000).

Lesser, R. & L.M. Jampol. Tolosa Hunt syndrome and antinuclear factor. *Am. J. Ophthal.* 71: *732–733* (1974).

Mathew,   & J. Chandy. Painful ophthalmoplegia. *J. Neurol. Sci.* 11: *243–256 (1970)*.

Smith, J.L. & D.S (1970).

Smith, J.L. & D.S.R. Taxdal. Painful ophthalmoplegia. The Tolosa Hunt Syndrome. *Am. J. Ophthal.* 61: *1466–1472* (1966).

Sondheimer, F.K. Angiographic findings in the Tolosa Hunt syndrome: Painful ophthalmoplegia. pp. 105–106, 112–113 in: Kanpp: Neuroradiology (1973).

Spindler, H. Painful ophthalmoplegia: the Tolosa Hunt syndrome. *Med. J. Austr.* 213: *645–646* (1973).

Tolosa, E.J. Perioteritic lesions of the carotid siphon with the clinical features of a carotid infraclinioidal aneurysm. *J. Neurol. Neuorsurg. Psychiatr.* 17: *300–302* (1954).

Authors' address:
Hôpital Trousseau
24 Av. du Dr. Arnold-Netter
Paris 12
France

ASEPTIC VENOUS THROMBOSIS OR TOLOSA-HUNT SYNDROME: DISCUSSION OF DIAGNOSTIC CRITERIA WITH REFERENCE TO 12 PERSONAL CASES

GUDRUN BRISMAR & JAN BRISMAR

(Lund, Sweden)

Painful ophthalmoplegia, i.e. affection of the ocular motor nerves as well as the trigeminal nerve, may be caused by a variety of lesions affecting the superior orbital fissure or the cavernous sinus. It has thus been described in association with neoplasms (especially nasopharyngeal carcinoma growing along the skull base), intracavernous carotid aneurysms, carotid cavernous fistulas and inflammatory conditions (specific, such as tuberculosis and syphilis, as well as unspecific). Sometimes, however, no underlying disorder is found in spite of extensive evaluations. Hunt et al. (1961) noticed that such cases often responded dramatically to steroid therapy, and suggested that cases exhibiting such a response might constitute a diagnostic entity, probably caused by some low-grade nonspecific inflammatory condition. Several similar cases have since been presented by different authors and the condition is now known as the Tolosa-Hunt syndrome. In a few cases surgery has been performed, disclosing granulomatous changes in the region of the superior orbital fissure – cavernous sinus (Tolosa, 1954; Lakke, 1962; Schatz & Farmer, 1972; Levy et al. 1975). Singular cases have been subjected to orbital phlebography demonstrating occlusion of the superior ophthalmic vein (Sondheimer & Knapp, 1970; Milstein & Morretin, 1971; Hunt, 1976).

Rad et al. (1970) presented 10 cases with similar symptomatology, all but one examined with orbital phlebography, that disclosed occlusion or defective filling of the superior ophthalmic vein or the cavernous sinus. These cases were interpreted as aseptic thrombosis and heparine therapy was successfully employed in 8. The authors suggested that several cases earlier published as Tolosa-Hunt syndromes might in fact have been thromboses.

The aim of this study is to discuss the differential diagnosis in cases with unexplained painful ophthalmoplegia, with reference to a personal patient material.

MATERIAL

The material consists of 10 patients with: 1. symptoms and signs that indicate a lesion in the cavernous sinus or the superior orbital fissure, 2. phlebographic findings of occlusion or defective filling of the superior ophthalmic vein and/or the cavernous sinus, 3. no underlying disorder disclosed in spite of extensive investigations. Two additional patients with similar clinical findings will also be discussed. Seven of the patients in this material have been presented earlier (Brismar & Brismar, 1977a,b).

RESULTS

The clinical findings are summarized in Table 1.

Case 8

49-year-old woman, tired for a couple of months. Acute onset of moderate left frontotemporal headache and diplopia. Examination discloses left N III paresis with ptosis and dilated retinal veins. Orbital phlebography (Fig. 1):

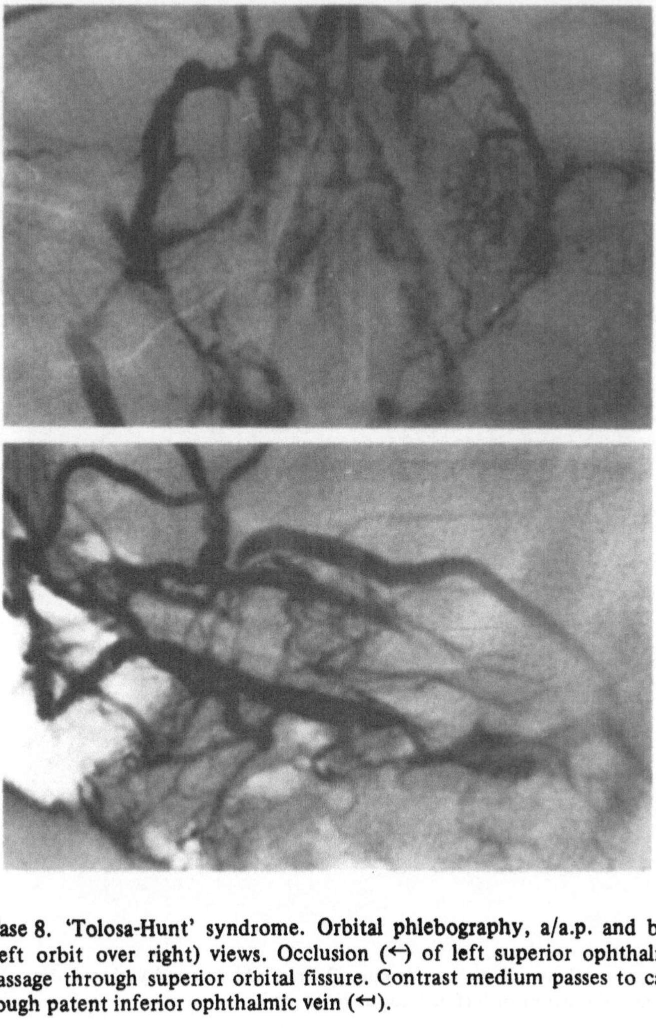

a

b

Fig. 1. Case 8. 'Tolosa-Hunt' syndrome. Orbital phlebography, a/a.p. and b/oblique lateral (left orbit over right) views. Occlusion (↤) of left superior ophthalmic vein during passage through superior orbital fissure. Contrast medium passes to cavernous sinus through patent inferior ophthalmic vein (↤).

Left superior ophthalmic vein occluded at passage through superior orbital fissure. Collateral circulation through inferior ophthalmic vein. Steroids were followed by immediate improvement. In half a year symptoms and signs of cerebral ischemia indicating a more disseminated vascular disorder.

Case 9

27-year-old woman, earlier healthy. Acute onset of leftsided retro- and intraorbital pains. After 14 days also paresis of left N VI, 5 days later affection of the second trigeminal branch and another three days later also leftsided ptosis. Orbital phlebography (Fig. 2): Defective filling of lateral portion of left cavernous sinus. Steroids followed by prompt disappearance of symptoms and signs. One month later, after reducing dosage of steroids, rightsided symptoms and signs. Once more prompt response to steroids. Thereafter free from symptoms on low dose of steroids.

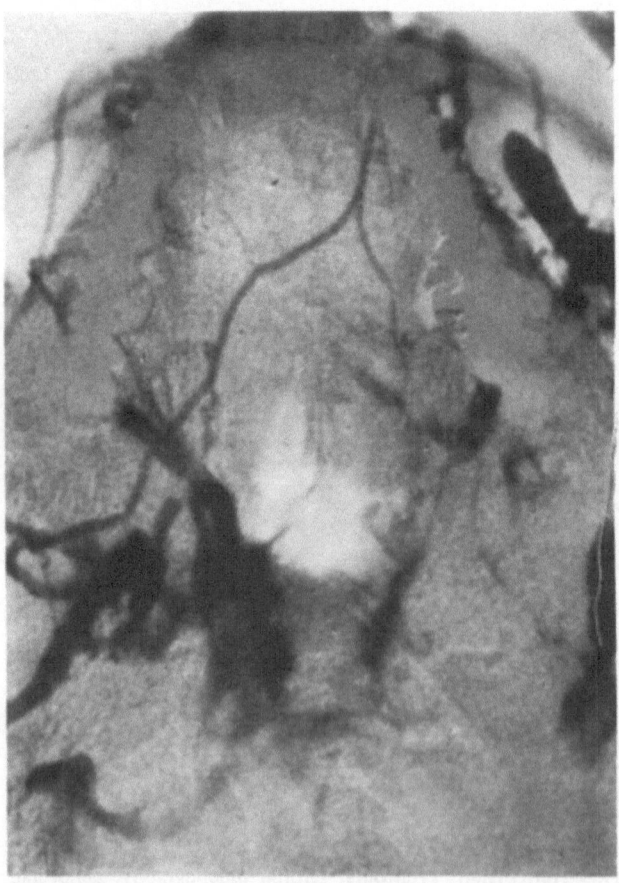

Fig. 2. Case 9. 'Tolosa-Hunt' syndrome. Orbital phlebography, basal view. Defective filling of lateral portion of left cavernous sinus (←).

DISCUSSION

A comparison between the clinical findings in previously presented 'Tolosa-Hunt' materiats (57 patients) and in the material with 'aseptic cavernous sinus thrombosis' of Rad et al. (10 patients) shows certain differences (Brismar & Brismar, 1977a). While pains and ocular palsies are constant findings in both materials, trigeminal involvement as well as signs of external and internal venous congestion were much more frequent in the material of Rad et al. These differences are not pronounced enough, however, to permit a differentiation between the two diagnoses in the single patient.

A dramatic response to steroid therapy has been used as an important criterion in the diagnosis of a Tolosa-Hunt syndrome. Such a response, however, may be encountered in many different disorders, including parasellar tumours (Thomas & Yoss, 1970) and is therefore of limited diagnostic value. Neither does a positive response to heparine therapy with necessity indicate the presence of a thrombosis – spontaneous remissions are characteristic of the Tolosa-Hunt syndrome. The clinical findings, in the single case, not only fail to differentiate between the Tolosa-Hunt syndrome and an aseptic thrombosis – they also fail to exclude an underlying disorder.

Case 12

74-year-old woman with 30-year history of arterial hypertension. For a couple of years episodes with redness and pain in left eye. Acute onset of severe intermittent leftsided retro-orbital pains, nausea. In one week also left proptosis, paresis of left N III and N VI as well as involvement of the first trigeminal branch. Steroids were of no effect. Orbital phlebography: Sharply demarcated occlusion of left cavernous sinus. Carotid angiography discloses a leftsided intracavernous carotid aneurysm.

We consider the diagnoses 'Tolosa-Hunt syndrome' and 'aseptic cavernous sinus thrombosis' as exclusion diagnoses – they must not be used until alternative diagnoses are excluded with reasonable security. Skull base tomography, nasopharyngoscopy with biopsies and carotid angiography are therefore required in the evaluation of painful ophthalmoplegia.

The findings at orbital phlebography sometimes aid in the differential diagnosis – a displacement of the venous structures indicates a tumour, a filling defect may indicate thrombosis. In most cases, however, phlebography only demonstrates occlusion of the superior ophthalmic vein without any displacement, a finding confirming the presence of a lesion but not aiding in the differential diagnosis. There are also cases with a clinical history, typical for a Tolosa-Hunt syndrome, but with normal phlebography.

Case 11

60-year-old woman, earlier healthy. Consulted with a 14-day history of pains behind right eye and right abducent nerve palsy. Orbital phlebography: normal. Prompt response to steroid therapy. No recurrence during six months follow up.

One case in our material, presented in greater detail elsewhere (Brismar et al., 1976), originally behaved as a typical 'Tolosa-Hunt' case with a dramatic improvement following steroid therapy. The disorder had a recurrent and progressive course, however, and ended with exitus in a few years in a clinical picture of generalized cerebral arteritis. Our patient, No. 8 (presented above), shows some similarities with progressive symptomatology. These cases, though fulfilling all suggested diagnostic criteria, markedly differ from most cases published as Tolosa-Hunt syndromes.

Evidently the diagnostic criteria generally used permit a wide variety of disorders to be classified as Tolosa-Hunt syndromes. Still the criteria may be too narrow in some respects, as the required steroid response may exclude closely related cases.

We think it better to use the designation: 'retroorbital pseudotumour', introduced by Levy et al. (1975), and to use it for all cases with painful ophthalmoplegia in which no underlying disorder can be demonstrated, i.e. both for the 'Tolosa-Hunt cases and for the 'aseptic thromboses'. The name 'retro-orbital pseudotumour' has two advantages: 1. it constantly reminds us that the symptoms and signs do in fact indicate the possibility of a tumour,

Table 1. Symptoms and signs in 12 patients with painful ophthalmoplegia.

Case nr	1	2	3	4	5	6	7	8	9	10	11	12
Sex, age	F,56	F,63	M,58	M,72	F,53	M,72	F,44	F,49	F,27	F,62	F,60	F,74
Pains	O	O	O	O	O	O	O	O	O	O	O	O
Palsy N III	O	O	O	O		O	O	O	O			O
N IV	O	O	O	O			O		O			O
N VI	O	O	O	O	O	O	O		O		O	O
Affection of N V$_1$	O	O										O
N V$_2$		O								O		
Proptosis	O			O			O					
Lid swelling												
Dil. conjunct. veins				O		O						O
retinal veins								O				
Disc blurring							O					
Red. visual acuity	O	O			O	O	O					O
Def. visual fields						O	O	O				O
Recurrences	O		O		O	O	O		O			O
Pathol. phlebogr.	O	O	O	O	O	O	O	O	O	O		O

Cases 1–10 demonstrated occlusion or defect filling of cavernous sinus and/or superior ophthalmic vein raising the differential diagnostic problem: 'Tolosa-Hunt syndrome'? 'Aseptic cavernous sinus thrombosis'? In case 11 phlebography was negative. In case 12 the symptoms and signs were caused by an intracavernous carotid aneurysm; in the remaining cases no underlying disorder was found.

although no tumour has been disclosed; 2. it is vague enough to reveal our lack of knowledge of the underlying disorder.

SUMMARY

Twelve patients with painful ophthalmoplegia were examined with orbital phlebography. In eleven cases occlusion or defective filling of the superior ophthalmic vein or the cavernous sinus was found; in one case phlebography was negative. In one of the cases an intracavernous carotid aneurysm was found; in the remaining cases no underlying disorder could be disclosed in spite of extensive evaluation. Possible diagnoses are 'Tolosa-Hunt syndrome' and 'aseptic cavernous sinus thrombosis'. An analysis of the diagnostic criteria for these two disorders reveals that a valid differentiation is in many cases impossible.

REFERENCES

Brismar, G. & J. Brismar. Aseptic thrombosis of orbital veins and cavernous sinus. *Acta ophthal.* (Kbh.) 55: *9* (1977).

Brismar, G. & J. Brismar. Thrombosis of the intraorbital veins and cavernous sinus. *Acta radiol. (Diagn.)* 18: *145* (1977).

Brismar, G., J. Brismar & S. Cronqvist. Complications of orbital and skull base phlebography. *Acta radiol. (Diagn)* 17: *274* (1976).

Hunt, W.E. Tolosa-Hunt syndrome: one case of painful ophthalmoplegia. *J. Neurosurg.* 44: *544* (1976).

Hunt, W.E., J.N. Meagher, H.E. Lefever & W. Zeman. Painful ophthalmoplegia. Its relation to indolent inflammation of the cavernous sinus. *Neurology* (Minneap.) 11: *56* (1961).

Lakke, J.P. Superior orbital fissure syndrome. Report of a case caused by local pachymeningitis. *Arch. Neurol.* (Chicago) 7: *289* (1962).

Levy, I.S., J.E. Wright & G.A.S. Lloyd. Orbital and retro-orbital pseudotumours. *Med. Probl. Ophthal.* 14: *364* (1975).

Milstein, B.A. & L.B. Morretin. Report of a case of sphenoidal fissure syndrome studied by orbital venography. *Amer. J. Ophthal.* 72: *600* (1971).

Rad, M. v., P. Wolf & K. Tornow. Die blande Thrombose des Sinus cavernosus. *Dtsch. med. Wsch.* 96: *457* (1971).

Schatz, N.J. & P. Farmer. Tolosa-Hunt syndrome: the pathology of painful ophthalmoplegia. In: Symposium of the University of Miami and the Bascom Palmer Eye Institute. Neuro-ophthalmology, vol. 6, p. 102. C.V. Mosby, St. Louis (1972).

Sondheimer, F.K. & J. Knapp. Angiographic findings in the Tolosa Hunt syndrome: Painful ophthalmoplegia. *Radiology* 106: *105* (1973).

Thomas, J.E. & R.E. Yoss. The parasellar syndrome: problems in determining etiology. *Mayo Clin. Proc.* 45: *617* (1970).

Tolosa, E.J. Periarteritic lesions of the carotid siphon with the clinical features of a carotid infraclinoidal aneurysm. *J. Neurol. Neurosurg. Psychiat.* 17: *300* (1954).

Authors' address:
Departments of Ophthalmology and
Diagnostic Radiology
University Hospital
S-221 85 Lund
Sweden

Proc. 3rd Int. Symp. on Orbital Disorders, Amsterdam 1977

BLINDNESS ASSOCIATED WITH RETROBULBAR HEMORRHAGE

TED T. HUANG & S.R. LEWIS

(Galveston, Texas)

The exact sequence of events leading to blindness in patients with retrobulbar hemorrhage remains unclear. However, it is believed that an abnormally high pressure developed within the bony orbit can play an important role in the pathogenesis of this complication. This concept is supported by the clinical finding of blindness coinciding with the onset of intraocular hypertension, lid edema, chemosis and proptosis, clinical features considered characteristic of intraorbital hypertension caused by an expansile mass in the retrobulbar compartment. This entity has attracted much attention in recent years because such complications occurred in individuals who had the cosmetic procedure of blepharoplasty (Hartley et al., 1973). While some have advocated decompression of the globe by perforating the anterior chamber of the eye as the treatment for this complication (Hartley et al., 1973; Hueston & Heinze, 1974), our clinical experience indicated that a more conservative approach in management is preferred (Huang et al., 1977). This includes an immediate control of factors such as systemic hypertension or coagulation abnormality. To further support this method of management, an experimental study was designed to investigate the effects of an abnormally high pressure within the bony orbit upon the ocular structures. The information accumulated from this study forms the basis of this report.

MATERIAL AND METHODS

In 24 rabbits, autogenous blood obtained by cardiac puncture was injected into the retrobulbar space in one eye and as a control, 0.9 percent saline solution was injected into the opposite eye. No anesthesia was used. The injection created a situation closely resembling the clinical entity of retrobulbar hemorrhage (Figure 1). The intraocular pressure was then measured with the Schioetz tonometer in both eyes immediately, and then 10, 15, 30, 45 and 60 minutes, two, three, 24 and 48 hours after injection. Simultaneously, the visual status was qualitatively measured by observing the size of the pupil and by noting the eyelid movements in reaction to bright light stimulation.

The orbital contents were also removed at the same time intervals for histological studies to ascertain whether any changes had taken place in the optic nerve, retina, retinal and periocular vessels.

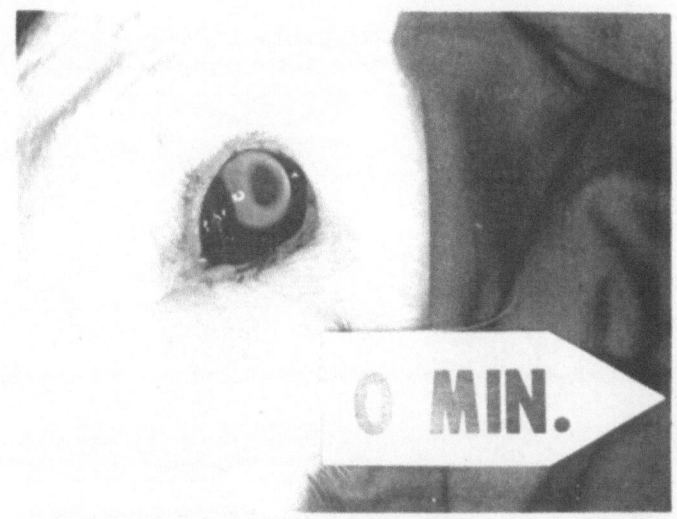

Fig. 1. The onset of chemosis, lid edema and proptosis were immediate after injections. The appearance resembles the clinical entity of retrobulbar hemorrhage.

RESULTS

The intraocular pressure measured in the unanesthetised rappits, prior to retrobulbar injection of whole blood and of 0.9 percent saline solution ranged from 6.5 mmHg to 12.2 mmHg with a mean pressure reading of 9.2 mmHg. An intraocular pressure of 40 to 40 mmHg was achieved by injecting either the whole blood or 0.9 percent saline solution into the retrobulbar space. However, the pressure had never exceeded 55 mmHg. A loss of pupilary reactivity to bright light stimulation was usually accompanied by absent light-eyelid reflexes (Table 1). In most instances, the pressure began to decrease within minutes following the injection and came down to normal limits within two to three hours (Figure 2). The light perception remained absent for at least another three to four hours and frequently remained somewhat sluggish for the first 24 to 36 hours. A full recovery of these reflexes and a resolution of proptosis were observed in all animals by 48

Table 1.

Light-pupillary reflex	−	−	−	±	±	+	+++	+++
Light-eyelid reflex	−	−	−	±	+	++	++++	++++
		¼ hr	½ hr					
Time elapsed after injection	0 hr			1 hr	2 hrs	3 hrs	24 hrs	48 hrs

(−) to (++++): Denote the magnitude of reaction to light stimulation.

399

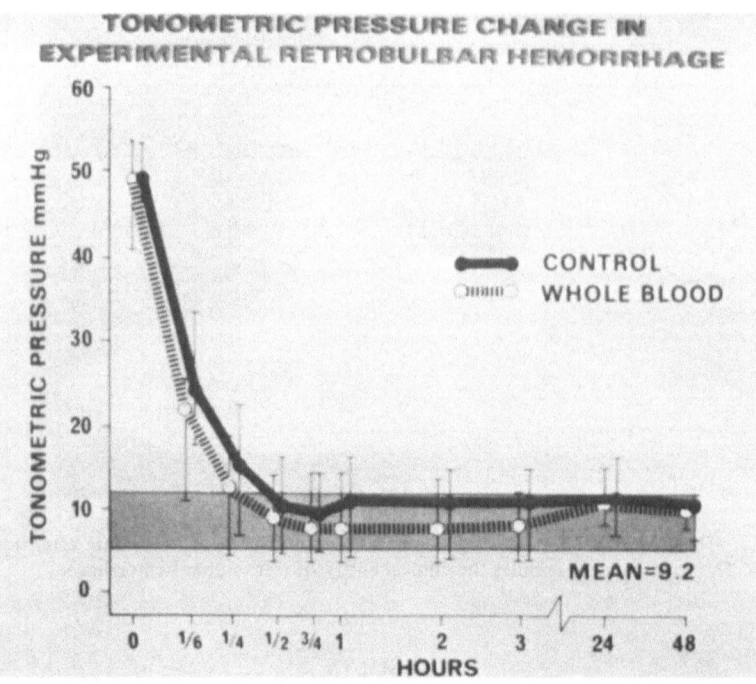

Fig. 2. The highest intraocular pressure achieved from injections of an autogenous blood and of 0.9% saline solution varied between 42 and 55 mmHg. This began to decrease within minutes following the injection and returned to the normal level within two to three hours. (Reproduced with permission from the Journal of Plastic and Reconstructive Surgery.)

hours following the injection (Fig. 3). The histologic sections of the eyes obtained at the same time interval revealed surprisingly little. The retinal vessels were found to be free of obstruction in all specimens examined. Furthermore, neither the retina nor the optic nerve showed any effect from the high pressure within the bony orbit and within the globe (Fig. 4).

DISCUSSION

Although an elevated pressure within the bony orbit caused by an expansile mass in the retrobulbar space is said to be the responsible factor for blindness, the exact sequence of events leading to this catastrophic complication remains undefined. While Fry postulated from his observations in Cynomolgus monkeys that the visual disturbance is probably caused by a venous collapse which leads to retinal hypoxia form stagnation (Fry, 1969), an occlusion of the central retinal artery was thought to be the responsible factor in many clinical encounters (Goldsmith, 1967; Kransbar et al., 1974).

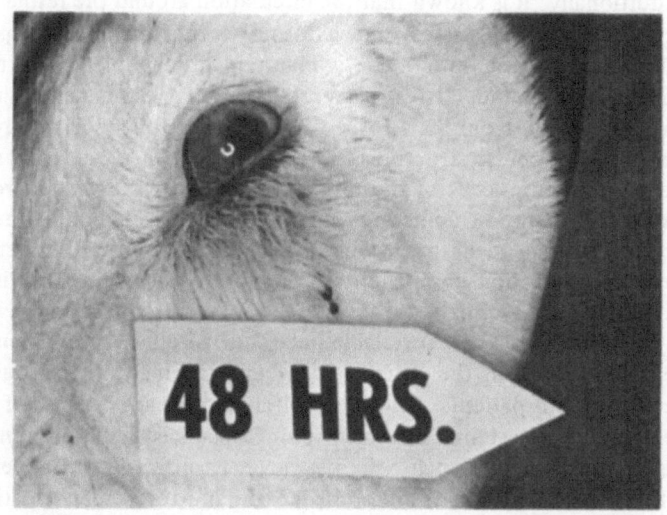

Fig. 3. Proptosis usually subsided by the end of 48 hours. Full recovery of vision occurred also.

These findings, however, were not observed in this study. Differences in anatomical configurations of the orbit, histological architectures of the periorbital and periocular tissues, and the lack of rigid anatomical boundaries anteriorly around the orbit may account for the discrepancies in manifesta-

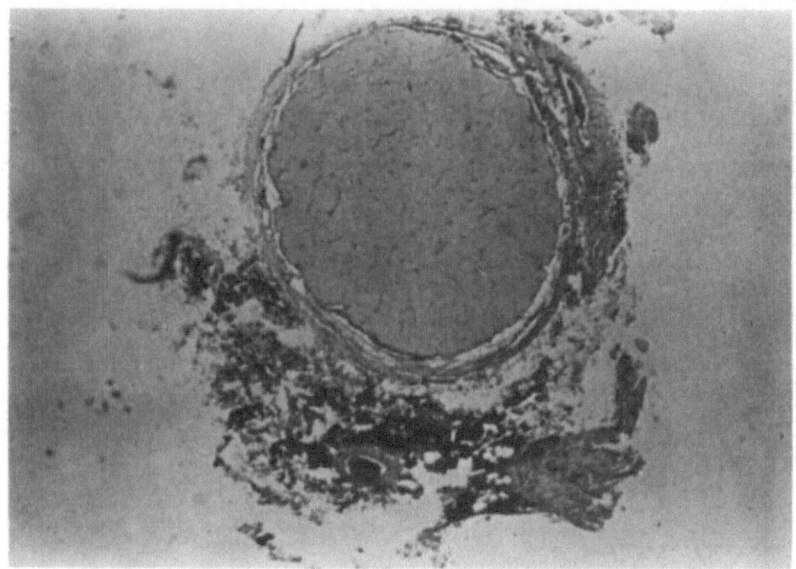

Fig. 4. The histologic section of the optic nerve from animals sacrificed at the end of 24 hours showed no evidence of permanent damages.

401

tions. Additionally, it is known that the circulation around the retina is protected by various compensatory mechanisms so that the blood supply to both the retina and the optic nerve is maintained adequately even though the entire system is under stress (Hayreh, 1971). A permanent injury to these structures occurs only if a force of great magnitude persistently compresses against the ocular structures. In spite of such adequate blood supply to the eye, the neural cells of the retina and the optic nerve are probably quite vulnerable to the ischemic injury. Any disturbance in circulation may, therefore, cause these cells to become unresponsive to usual light stimulation. Mechanical traction upon the optic nerve caused by anterior displacement of the globe may further aggravate the injury. These changes, in contrast to vascular injuries, are reversible once the causative factor is removed.

Unlike those found in the animal study, an extremely high intraorbital pressure is found in patients suffering orbital hemorrhage because of persistent bleeding from systemic hypertension or occult coagulation abnormality. The treatment under such circumstances, as shown in our experience, should firstly aim to lower the blood pressure and to correct clotting defects (Krauser et al., 1974). If the intraorbital pressure remains elevated, an orbital decompression must be carried out by detaching the lateral canthal ligament from its bony origin.

SUMMARY

Visual disturbance caused by hemorrhage in the retrobulbar space is probably related to an abnormally high pressure within the bony orbit. The treatment should aim to correct the causes of bleeding and to reduce the intraorbital pressure in order to avoid a permanent damage upon ocular structures.

REFERENCES

Fry, H.J. Reversible visual loss after proptosis from retrobulbar hemorrhage. Reproduction of the syndrom in Cynomolgus monkey. *Plast. & Recon. Surg.* 44: *480* (1969).
Goldsmith, M.O. Occlusion of the central retinal artery following retrobulbar hemorrhage. *Ophthalmologica* 153: *191* (1967).
Hartley, J.H., J.C. Lester & W.E. Schatten. Acute retrobulbar hemorrhage during elective blepharoplasty. *Plast. & Recon. Surg.* 52: *8* (1973).
Hayreh, S.S. Pathogenesis of occlusion of the central retinal vessels. *Am. J. Ophthal.* 72: *998* (1971).
Huang, T.T., B. Horwitz & S.R. Lewis. Retrobulbar hemorrhage. *Plast. & Recon. Surg.* 59: *39* (1977).
Hueston, J.T. & J.B. Heinze. Successful early relief of blindness occurring after blepharoplasty. *Plast. & Recon. Surg.* 53: *588* (1974).
Kraushar, M.F., M.H. Seelenfreund & D.B. Freilich. Central retinal artery closure during orbital hemorrhage from retrobulbar injection. *Ar. Am. Acad. Ophthal.* 78: *66* (1974).

Authors' address:
Division of Plastic & Reconstructive Surgery
The University of Texas Medical Branch
Galveston, Texas
USA

Proc. 3rd Int. Symp. on Orbital Disorders, Amsterdam 1977

ASPECTS ON THE DIAGNOSIS OF VENOUS MALFORMATION OF THE ORBIT

F. OSMERS, H. BUSSE & H.-P. SCHIFFER

(Münster, W. Germany)

On the basis of recent collective data a vascular tumor or vascular dysplasia is the cause of about 14 to 25% of cases of unilateral exophthalmos (Table 1). Special attention ought to be paid to venous malformations in the group of vascular neoplasms of the orbit. From a pathological-anatomical view-point these are classified as: cavernous haemangioma, venous aneurysm or varicosity, capillary angioma, plexiform angioma and some rare vascular tumors. Histology reveals mostly polymorphic mixed types, rarely a pure type.

Venous malformations are among the vascular tumors of the orbit especially common. From the literature over 50% of all intraorbital haemangiomas are cavernous (Housepian & Trokel, 1973). We describe here the x-ray diagnosis of 20 cases of venous malformation of the orbit from the common cases of the radiological clinic and the eye clinic of the University of Münster.

In the roentgen-native technique applied to the orbit, orbit excavation is a nonspecific sign of intraorbital space occupation — we have 2 cases of this type in our 20 cases. The x-ray proof of intraorbital phleboliths (Fig. 1) is, on the contrary, evidence for a soft tissue haemangioma — often a varix or a cavernoma, whether the orbit is excavated or not (Tänzer, 1972).

Further invasive radiological methods of examination such as angiography must be regarded critically. In our opinion orbitaphlebography is the examination of choice for the direct proof of intraorbital venous malformations, also if the vessel tumor is separated from the main venous circulation in a siding as is often the case. Carotid angiography, however, gives only

Table 1. Frequency of intraorbital vascular disease as a cause of 'intraorbital space-occupying lesion'.

	Orbital tumor/ unilateral exophthalmos	intraorbital vascular disease
Palmer (1965)	2073	319 (= 15%)
Mennig (1970)	883	119 (= 14%)
Aron-Rosa & Doyon (1972)	257	62 (= 24%)
Vignaud et al. (1974)	197	49 (= 25%)

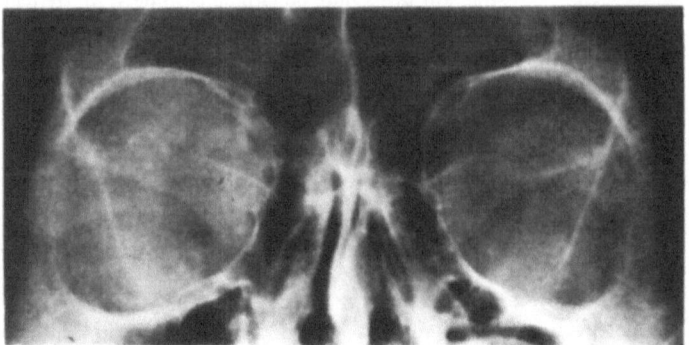

Fig. 1. Phleboliths in the right orbit.

rarely useful results, because in cases of intraorbital space occupation changes in the course of the ophthalmic artery are rare and are usually not diagnostic. In addition, a sufficient contrast filling of the orbit veins almost never occurs during a carotid angiography with the usual technique (Krayenbühl & Yasargil, 1965).

From the 59 orbit phlebographies carried out up till now we could prove a venous malformation in 20 cases; in 10 of these cases an operation was performed (Table 2).

For a technique of examination we used the percutaneous catheterisation of the frontal vein – and if this was not successful we laid bare the facial vein at the border of the lower jaw and catheterised it up to the angular vein.

Table 2. Phlebography of the orbit (n = 59). Radiological Clinic, Münster/W.Germany.

Phlebography – findings	n	Histology	n
vascular disease	20	varicosis	5
		venous aneurysm/cavernom	4
		art.-venous angioma	1
space-occupying lesions	12	metastatic carcinoma of breast	2
		metastatic bronchial carcinoma	1
		plasmocytoma	1
		lympho-sarcoma	1
		haemangiopericytoma	1
		haemangioendothelioma	1
		meningeoma	1
		fat herniation through dehiscence of orbital fascia	1
		pyomucocele orbital roof	1
		histiocytosis	1
		lipoma	1
no findings	27		

The normal result of an orbital phlebogram (Fig. 2) makes visible several vein areas of the orbital and face regions. Especially notable the superior ophthalmic vein filled well with contrast and showed a constant course in the a-p view as a typical rhombus form open in a medio-basal direction.

The phlebographic x-ray diagnosis offers, besides the topographical result, often a pointer to the real diagnosis:

1. Calibre enlargement and irregularities of the superior ophthalmic vein and its smaller branches (varicosis, Fig. 3).

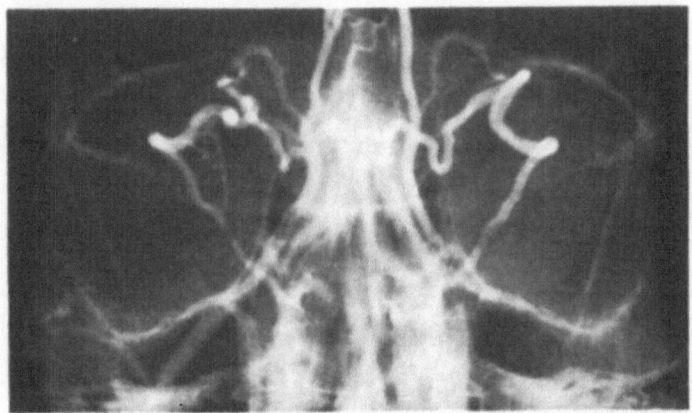

Fig. 2. Phlebography of the orbits: both superior ophthalmic veins, show regular course.

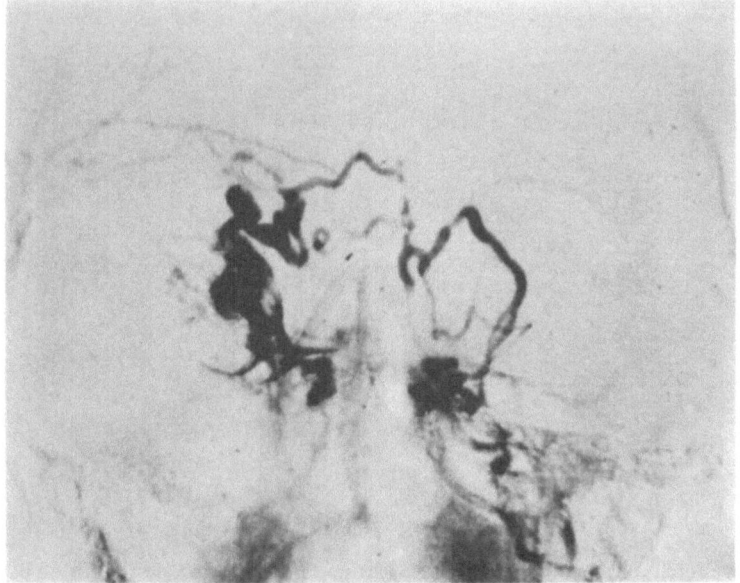

Fig. 3. Varicose enlargement of the right superior ophthalmic vein.

405

2. Homogenous contrast filling of larger chambered blood spaces, which are usually not completely filled with contrast medium, and showing horizontal fluid levels (cavernoma and venous aneurysm).

3. After injection the very late filling with contrast of a venous angioma, with long persistence of contrast medium.

4. Contrast escape into the orbit as evidence of bleeding or also thrombosis of larger orbital veins, which occur as complications of a venous angioma, but are rare, however.

Because the angioma is often filled with thrombotic material and lies on a siding, the blood circulation in the vascular tumor is extremely reduced.

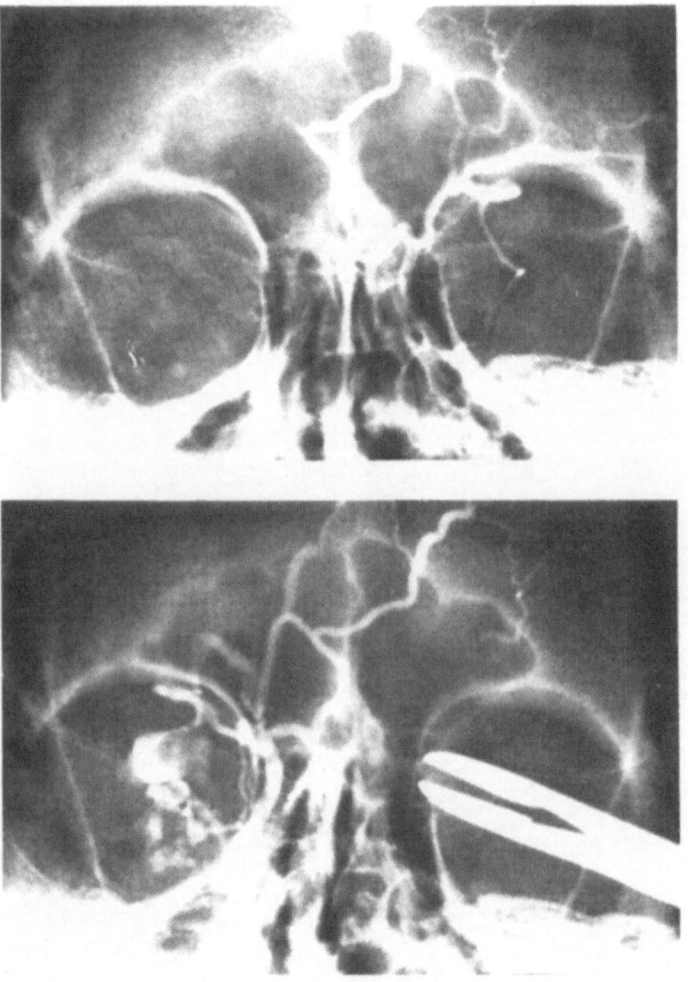

Fig. 4. Orbital phlebography: a) on the right no filling of veins, on the left no pathologic findings; b) compression at the inner canthus: now the right demonstrates a cavernous angioma.

This must be thought of during the investigation, otherwise false negative results will occur. The necessary condition is a series angiography, and as a preliminary emptying the vessel tumor as much as possible by pressure on the yee, and with intermittent exophthalmos the investigation should be performed in the symptom-free interval. Especially important is the compression of the facial and fronto-temporal drainage in order to obtain better contrast of the orbital veins. Sometimes it is only through compression of the superior ophthalmic vein of the healthy side that the filling of a vessel tumor on the other side succeeds (Fig. 4a,b).

Besides the primary congenital often multilocular malformations, venous malformations develop following intracranial or orbital arteriovenous abnormalities with shunt-effect (Lloyd et al., 1971). On the basis of arterial pressure venous dilatation, hypertrophy or varicosis occurs.

The cause of this can be arteriovenous angioma (Fig. 5a,b) which leads to orbital varicosis or carotid-cavernous-sinus-fistula. In both cases the investigation of choice is a carotid angiography and not phlebography, because the veins cannot usually be retrogradely filled with contrast media against the arterial pressure.

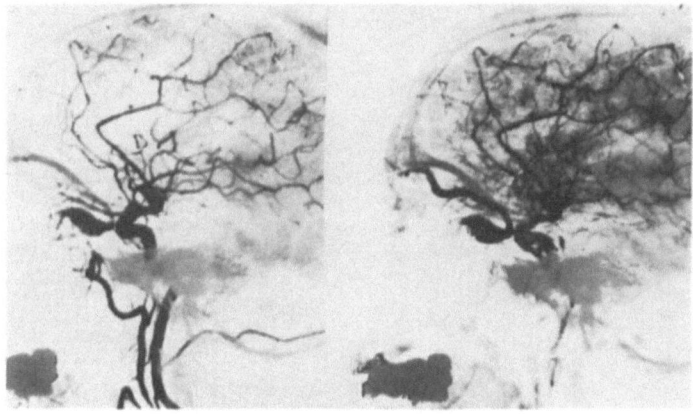

Fig. 5. Carotid angiography: a) opacification via ophthalmic artery of a retrobulbar angioma; b) contrast-medium-outflow via hypertrophic superior ophthalmic vein.

We have tried to show the value of various radiological methods of investigation for the diagnosis of venous malformations of the orbit. It can be accepted that other procedures also, such as computer tomography are able to show the presence of small intraorbital venous malformations, but that the delineation of the topography and the important vessels of supply will remain the domain of the phlebographical investigation.

REFERENCES

Aron-Rosa, D.S. & D.L. Doyon. Malformations vascularies orbitaires. *Ann. d'Occulist.* (Paris) 205: *667* (1972).

Housepian, E.M. & S. Trokel. Tumors of the orbit. In: Neurological Surgery, Vol. III. Saunders, Philadelphia (1973).

Krayenbühl, H. & M.G. Yasargil. Die cerebrale Angiographie. Thieme Verlag, Stuttgart (1965).

Lloyd, G.A., J.E. Wright & G. Morgan. Venous malformation in the orbit. *Br. J. Ophthal.* 55: *505* (1971).

Mennig, H. Geschwülste der Augenhöhle und ihre operative Behandlung. Thieme Verlag, Leipzig (1970).

Palmer, B.W. Unilateral exophthalmos. *Arch. Otolaryng.* 82: *416* (1965).

Tänzer, A. Die Röntgendiagnostik der Orbita im Nativbild. *Radiologe* 12: *397* (1972).

Vignaud, J., C. Clay & L.T. Bilaniuk. Venography of the orbit. *Radiology* 110: *373* (1974).

Authors' addresses:
F. Osmers
Radiological University-Clinic
Jungeblodplatz 1
D-44 Münster
W. Germany

H. Busse & P. Schiffer
Universitäts-Eye Clinic
Westring 15
D-44 Münster
W. Germany

Proc. 3rd Int. Symp. on Orbital Disorders, Amsterdam 1977

THE TOLOSA-HUNT SYNDROME
(painful ophthalmoplegia)

J.T.W. VAN DALEN

(Amsterdam, The Netherlands)

ABSTRACT*

The Tolosa-Hunt syndrome is characterized by recurrent unilateral retro-orbital pain with extra-ocular palsies, and by a dramatic response to steroids. The cause of the syndrome is an inflammatory reaction of the cavernous sinus.

Orbital phlebography usually shows stenosis in the superior ophthalmic vein together with non-opacification of the cavernous sinus on that side, and is said to be characteristic.

A case-history is reviewed and the differential diagnosis is discussed.

Author's address:
Eye Department
Ophthalmological Clinic of the University of Amsterdam
Wilhelmina Gasthuis
104, 1e Helmerstraat
Amsterdam
The Netherlands

* The complete paper has been published in the Proceedings of the Joint meeting of the Netherlands Ophthalmological Society (171st meeting) and the Irish Ophthalmological Society (Amsterdam — March 30-April 1, 1977), pp. 167–172. Junk, The Hague. 1977.

HERNIATED LACRIMAL GLANDS AND THE
TECHNIQUE OF SUSPENSION

BYRON SMITH

(New York, N.Y., USA)

ABSTRACT

Herniation of the lacrimal gland is a condition that occurs unilaterally or bilaterally. Either or both lobes of the lacrimal gland may prolapse, Orbital lobe prolapse may be associated with blepharochalasis, a disease of puberty. A surgical technique for the repair of prolapsed lacrimal glands is outlined. The importance of adequate hemostasis and closure of the orbital septum is stressed.

The lacrimal gland occupies the lacrimal fossa in the upper temporal quadrant of the bony orbit. It is divided into the orbital and palpebral lobes by the lateral horn of the levator aponeurosis (Whitnall, 1932). Relaxation of the suspensory ligaments may result in the conjunctival prolapse of the palpebral lobe. Eversion of the upper lid especially in older individuals will reveal the typical pinkish grey mass bulging from the lateral aspect of the everted tarsal plate.

Herniation of the orbital lobe posterior to the orbital septum is a less common condition which presents more often as a bilateral symmetrical bulge beneath the skin of the temporal one-half of the upper lids. Palpation of the displaced gland is accomplished by gentle manipulation of the mass between the examiner's thumb and index finger. With gentle external pressure in the direction of the lacrimal fossa, the orbital lobe may be reduced and replaced. One may feel its disappearance as it slides under the orbital rim.

Herniation of the orbital lobe of the lacrimal gland may be associated with blepharochalasis, a disease which is manifest at puberty (Duke-Elder, 1975). The attenuated, vascular skin of the upper lids has a baggy appearance and overhangs the eyelashes. The lid fold is often obliterated. This disorder is more common among blacks and more highly pigmented individuals. The patients with blepharochalasis often reported increased lid swelling with emotional bouts of crying and lacrimation or with menstruation (Smith & Petrelli, 1977). The treatment of herniated lacrimal gland is surgical.

TECHNIQUE

An incision is made through the skin in alignment with the supratarsal fold (Figure 1-A). The upper lip of the incision is undermined deep to the orbicularis muscle. This dissection is carried upward to the temporal two-thirds of the superior orbital rim (Figure 1-B). At this point, the attachment of the orbital septum to the periorbita is exposed and incised two millimeters below the bony rim (Figure 1-C). This two millimeter apron of tissue attached to the periosteum is important because it is needed in the proper closure of the wound. The periosteum should not be disturbed.

Pressure upon the globe is accompanied by protrusion of the lacrimal gland through the incision (Figure 1-D). It is recognized by its pinkish grey color and its firm consistency in contrast to the orbital fat which is yellow and soft. If excessive orbital fat is present, it should be removed. Hemostasis is mandatory. A biopsy of the anterior margin of the lacrimal gland is performed. The biopsy defect is closed with a secure absorbable suture.

Suspension of the gland into its normal position is accomplished by passing a double-armed suture through the anterior margin of the gland. This is done by means of a whip stitch so that the suture will not pull out of the glandular tissues when the suture is tied. The two needles of the four-zero chromic catgut are then passed from behind, forward through the periosteum of the anterior portion of the lacrimal fossa (Figure 2-E, F, G, H). We use a nasal speculum as a means of exposing the fossa and recipient area into which the suture is passed. As this suture is pulled up and tied securely, the lacrimal gland is mobilized and fixed back into the lacrimal fossa.

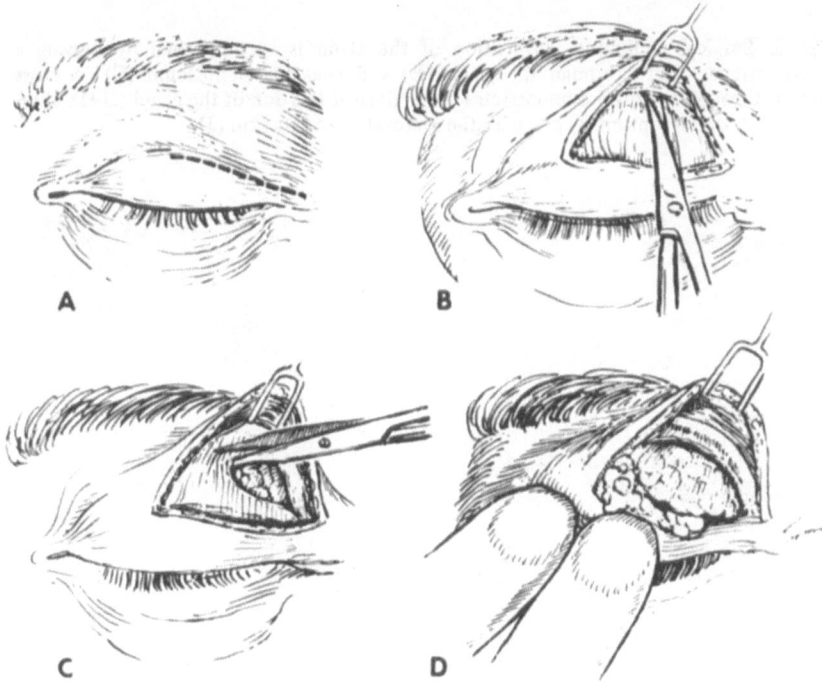

Fig. 1. Surgical technique. After the skin incision is made in the supratarsal fold. (A), the upper lip of the incision is undermined deep to the orbicularis muscle (B). The orbital septum is incised, (C), and the lacrimal gland is prolapsed by gentle digital pressure (D).

411

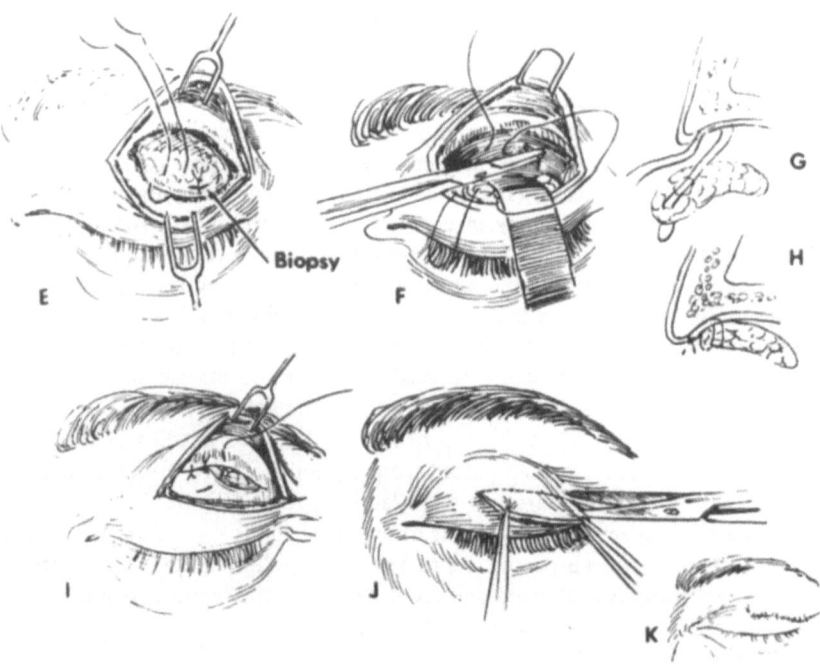

Fig. 2. Surgical technique. Suspension of the gland is accomplished by passing a double-armed suture through the gland (E) and engaging periosteum (F). A cross section through the orbit demonstrates the periosteal fixation of the gland (G-H). Closure of the orbital septum (I) precedes the removal of excess skin (J).

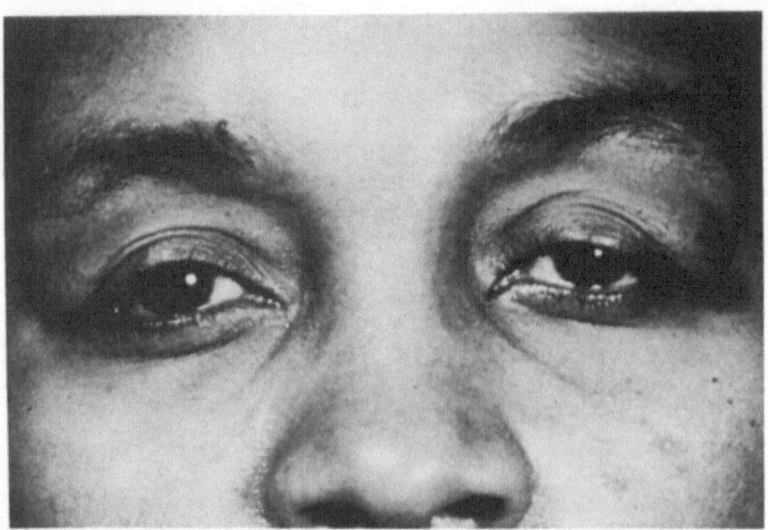

Fig. 3. A forty-two year old black female demonstrates the typical appearance of bilateral prolapsed lacrimal glands.

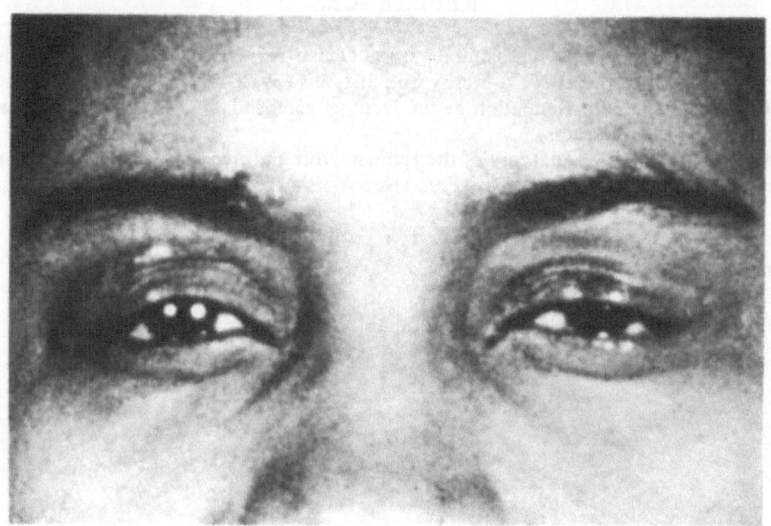

Fig. 4. Postoperative photograph of patient illustrated in Figure 3.

The orbital septum is closed by interrupted four-zero catgut sutures (Figure 2-I). Any excessive skin and redundant orbicularis muscle is excised (Figure 2-J). The skin wound is closed with a continuous suture of five-zero nylon. A light pressure dressing is applied. The skin suture is removed in five or six days.

The lady illustrated in Figure 3 is a forty-two year old black who presented with the typical findings of bilateral symmetrical herniation of the lacrimal glands. Surgical repair was performed as described above, and the postoperative result is shown in Figure 4. Observed for more than ten years, she remains asymptomatic.

DISCUSSION

Four salient features of this procedure deserve comment. First, hemostasis is mandatory since the vascular lacrimal gland will tend to bleed and may cause a hematoma with wound disruption. Secondly, the biopsy of the gland should be done routinely to rule out an orbital neoplasm. Thirdly, the suture through the lacrimal gland should be tied before passing the double arms through the periosteum in order to prevent slippage. Fourthly, care should be taken to close the orbital septum securely along the line of surgical entry two millimeters below the orbital rim. This will provide insurance against a future prolapse of the gland.

Of the three patients treated surgically, none has developed complications or recurrent prolapse during the follow-up period ranging from five to ten years. However, the recurrent prolapse of the lacrimal gland is possible if care is not taken to secure the gland to the periosteum and to close the orbital septum.

413

REFERENCES

Duke-Elder, S. System of Ophthalmology, the Ocular Adnexa. Part I: Diseases of the Eyelids. Vol. XIII, p. 350. C.V. Mosby Co., St Louis (1975).

Smith, B. & R. Petrelli. Herniation of the lacrimal glands. Trans. Am. Acad. Ophthal. Otolaryng. (1977, in press).

Whitnall, S. Ernest. The Anatomy of the Human Orbit and Accessory Organs of Vision, 2nd ed., p. 144. Oxford University Press, New York (1932).

Author's address:
32 East 64th Street
New York, N.Y. 10021
USA

Proc. 3rd Int. Symp. on Orbital Disorders, Amsterdam 1977

LATERAL ORBITAL DECOMPRESSION

IRA SNOW JONES

(New York, N.Y., USA)

When a volume of fluid or tissue is greater than the space available to contain it, it may overflow the space, lead to increased pressure of the contents of the space, or enlarge the space. Increased pressure of the contents within the space may not be sufficient in the case of a resistant capsule to enlarge the structures, and the pressure may rebound upon the tissue itself, leading to ischemia, fibrosis and atrophy. If the boundaries of space are rigid, as in the skull, help from outside must be obtained to enlarge the space, since the pressure of the tissue within it will not avail. If the encapsulating structures are elastic, as is the case with the scrotum, the space can enlarge with no discernible increase in pressure. The bony orbit will enlarge in response to an increased volume in the early years of life, but after age seven the strength of the bony orbit becomes increasingly greater and less likely to be deformed by intraorbital pressure. Only the base of the orbit or the anterior opening is closed by tissues which have greater elasticity and which may respond to the demand for greater orbital volume. The soft tissues of the orbit offer a site of predilection for the accumulation of fluid, for round cell infiltration, and for diffuse enlargement containing elements of these two mechanisms, as well as chemical changes in the fluid-binding properties of the tissues. At various stages, this increased volume of orbital contents leads to stretching of the elastic tissues at the front of the orbit to increase the volume, followed by increased intraorbital pressure, followed by ischemia of some of the structures which have been subjected to this pressure and which cannot resist it. For these reasons, it is many times desirable to use outside factors to enlarge the orbit to a greater extent than could be brought about by the internal demands of the volume of tissue offered to be contained within the orbit.

INDICATIONS

Slow-growing, benign tumors which are incompletely removed occupy space and, in some instances, it will be helpful to enlarge the orbit by fenestrating or removing one of the bony walls. Sometimes, decompression is done as a measure of convenience to make a later surgical procedure easier. The majority of decompressions, however, are done for diffuse infiltrations of

415

the orbit of the kind seen in inflammatory pseudotumor of the orbit and in Grave's disease.

In choosing cases of diffuse infiltration of the orbit for decompression, it is generally better to delay during the active and increasing infiltration stage. If possible, stabilize the process by medical, anti-inflammatory, endocrine, or radiation modes. The concept that surgery during the active stage causes an exacerbation may have validity, but the efficacy of anti-inflammatory drugs is sufficient so that in extreme cases where surgery cannot be delayed it may be done even in the active phase. The stable cases may be exophthalmic but with relatively soft retrobulbar tissues, and these can be identified by the easy replaceability of the globe with the fingers. They may be quite firmly exophthalmic, with difficult replaceability of the globe, and the greater the degree of firmness and resistance to replaceability, the poorer the effect of decompression will be. There is an unproved theory that many cases which are easily replaceable at first gradually become lardaceous due to ischemic factors and poor circulation in the crowded orbit. By extrapolation, it is then thought that decompression early may prevent the development of the fibrotic and lardaceous type of infiltration which responds poorly.

CHOICE OF PROCEDURE

Various kinds or orbital decompression have been suggested, including roof, lateral wall, inferior wall, medial wall, and optic canal. The base of the orbital pyramid is someqhat slanted laterally — i.e., the distance between the apex of the orbit and the lateral rim is shorter than that for any other wall. Accordingly, removing bone laterally opens the orbit more than any other ablation of bone if it is understood that unroofing the orbit is not going to remove the superior rim. The lateral wall is also more easily attacked, since there are fewer important structures to traverse, and the field which one traverses is clean. If additional decompression is required, it is easy to add an inferior and even a medial decompression. The chief difficulty with a superior decompression, aside from the surgical technique problem, is the fact that a large superior decompression allows sagging of the dura and frontal lobe into the orbit, so that what otherwise might be good relief of orbital volume and pressure requirements is compromised by this encroachment.

SECONDARY FACTORS TO BE CONSIDERED IN PLANNING ORBITAL DECOMPRESSION

The diffuse infiltration patients often have difficulties in closing the lids because of the curve of the globe on which the lids are forced by the protrusion of the globe; they sometimes have problems of excess sympathetic tone resulting in retraction of the lids; and they often have extraocular muscle imbalance, usually with the globe looking down instead of assuming the primary position, and usually with the globe failing in elevation more and earlier than in other directions of gaze. A good deal of the muscle problem is due to fibrosis and loss of elasticity, especially with inferior muscles. For this reason, it is often found desirable to combine other procedures with the lateral decompression. Forced duction tests should be performed under anesthesia, and, if the inferior rectus is inelastic, it can either be cut free or receded. If lagophthalmos is a problem, even after the decompression, a lateral tarsorrhaphy of 3—6 mm can be instituted. It will usually be found better not to attempt to alleviate unusual upper lid retraction at the same time as the surgery for decompression. One wishes to see the stabilized condition after decompression before deciding on scleral tarsal grafts and other lid-lengthening procedures. It is usually better surgical judgement to do the decompression on only one side at a time, first because the amount of exophthalmos is asymmetric, second because the amount of improvement can only be guessed at, and one wishes to see what the first side does before trying the second, and third because there is always the risk of functional damage from the surgery, and one does not wish to jeopardize both eyes at the same time. A prediction about the amount of globe recession which can be obtained can be made from the replaceability of the globe before surgery. Little or no effect may be obtained if the posterior structures are lardaceous, and 3—5 mm of recession of the globe can be obtained in the more favorable case. Oftentimes, the globe does not immediately go back after decompression has been done, but one will find that the replaceability has improved so that it is softer and easier to push the globe back with the fingers. In these cases, as the natural tissue elasticity asserts itself, the amount of improvement will increase.

MENSURATION

Exophthalmometry by both the Hertel and the Much method should be done beforehand. Photographs in profile and full face should be taken. Endocrine evaluation, in the case of Grave's disease, is necessary, and advice on the use of suppressive corticosteroid therapy in the post-operative period should be in hand. Visual fields and visual acuity are necessary. Sometimes, the proposal is made to open the optic nerve sheath and attempt to decompress the optic nerve if there have been field changes. I doubt the efficacy of this, and I advise that one avoid the extra risk of trying to decompress the optic nerve or the optic canal, since sometimes this results in worsening of the field or complete loss of vision.

TECHNIQUE

For reasons already discussed, I prefer the Kronlein type of lateral orbitotomy, using the Berke modification and leaving out the bone segments which are removed. I have made a number of modifications over the hears to give greater relief of orbital contents. The first has to do with bone cuts: instead of the Keystone arrangement suggested by earlier authors, I prefer to make the cuts in the bone parallel and as far superior and inferior as can be done and still have bone break free. It is most important to rongeur the broken edge of bone as far back as the bites can be conveniently made. The muscle on the outside of the bone flap can be dissected free and used as a point of re-attachment for the lateral canthus, but the periosteum on the outside of the bone should be removed with the bone. It does not seem necessary to remove the periosteum or periorbita on the inside of the bone, since this is a thin membrane and retracts when it is opened. I prefer not to open the periorbita immediately overlying the lateral rectus muscle, but to open above and below in order to protect the lateral rectus muscle as much as possible from post-operative adhesions. In most instances, the lower pole of the lacrimal gland will offer in the wound, and this can be taken as one of the biopsy specimens. If muscle is to be taken, the inferior rectus or the inferior oblique is less likely to suffer from excision of a small portion. If the orbital fat appears normal, it need not be biopsied, but it it is firmer than normal some of this material should also be taken for microscopic study. It should not be overlooked that a good digital exploration of the orbit should be carried out, even though one is confident of the diagnosis of Grave's disease. Digital exploration also gives information about the amount of thickening of the extraocular muscles, and, in conjunction with the forced duction test carried out before beginning the surgery, this is quite helpful. If the inferior rectus is not elastic and is enlarged, it can be receded or subjected to free tenotomy by enlarging the incision along the inferior conjunctival fornix. There are even some cases in which the mass of the inferior rectus muscle is so great that the anterior half of it may be excised. Pulling out and excising any considerably amount or orbital fat poses dangers, since blood vessels may be drawn out with the fat, and excessive bleeding may occur. Careful hemostasis is important because the reduction in tamponade action which is brought about by the decompression makes losing of blood more likely to occur. The lateral tarsorrhaphy is most easily accomplished while the canthus remains divided from the Kronlein procedure. This can be done in any acceptable fashion, but I prefer splitting the lid into anterior and posterior leaves, denuding the epithelium from the margin of both leaves, and closing both leaves separately. The soft tissues can be closed in the same manner in which they were opened, but care should be taken not to re-attach the lateral canthal ligament too firmly far back; this makes the lids too tight against the globe and hinders easy opening and closing. The firm dressing and headroll usually advocated have given way in my hands to a somewhat softer, less constrictive dressing without a headroll. The constrictive dressing and headroll, in the presence of hemorrhage and swelling, can lead to an undesirable pressure upon the globe. Postoperatively, if the general medical man or endocrinologist agrees, suppressive corticosteroid therapy should be employed.

COMPLICATIONS

The early complications of lateral decompression include hematomas, diffuse bleeding, inflammatory swelling, and double vision. If a hematoma collects under the temporal flap and is appreciated early, the blood can be drained by opening the incision and gentle pressure. At a later date, when the blood has coagulated, this does not produce drainage, and one must wait until liquefaction begins to occur. Exacerbation of swelling and kindling of inflammatory swelling are best handled by suppressive agents, such as cortisone, but if for any reason cortisone cannot be used, butazolidin is a helpful second choice. Transitory double vision is best handled by covering one or the other eye, with periods of both eyes being uncovered to help this to disappear more quickly. Late complications include decrease in the visual field, reconstitution of the lateral wall with firm, fibrous tissue or with bony exostoses, and limitation of lateral rectus action by adhesions. A decrease of the visual field often responds to intensive corticosteroid therapy in consultation with the endocrinologist, especially if it due to post-operative swelling. There are, unfortunately, cases in which the decrease in field cannot be categorized and in which it does not improve.

Reconstitution of the lateral wall, if it has a bony component, is most likely encountered in younger patients, and it it is of a dense connective tissue and fibrous nature can be encountered in any age group. In some of those cases, re-operation is efficacious.

Limitation of lateral rectus action is best left alone if it is of a tolerable degree. Further surgery to remove adhesions often results in even more adhesions forming. If it is decided that something has to be done, the smallest amount of lysis of adhesions, which is effective, can be carried out, and at the most lateral point away from the lateral rectus which can be identified. If one pulls on the lateral rectus and feels with the scissor point, oftentimes a single band can be identified and snipped.

ADDITIONAL SURGERY

Although the lateral decompression may offer the best improvement of any single procedure, it is apparent in many patients that a much greater amount of decompression room is needed. My colleague, Dr. William C. Cooper, has been experimenting with three-compartment decompression — that is, in addition to the lateral compression, the floor and the medial wall are also removed. This effectively doubles the amount of room for prolapse of orbital tissues, and it appears to offer greater retroplacement of the globe than has previously been achieved.

RESULTS

The 34 orbits presented here showed a range of difference in exophthalmometer measurements between the before- and after-surgery observations of −5 to +14. That is, one patient at last observation was 5 mm more proptatic and one 14 mm less so after decompression. Obviously, the patient who became more so was still in the active phase or orbital infiltration and was poorly chosen. The patient with the sensational 14 mm improvement was

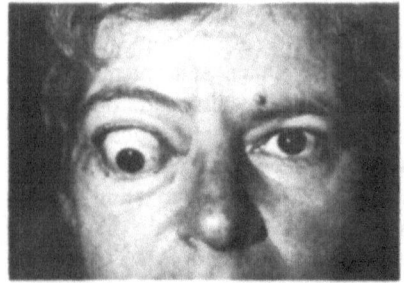
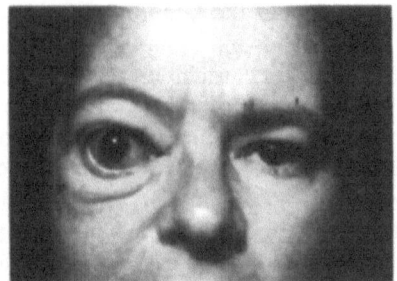

Fig. 1. E.L. *Left:* Before surgery R; *Right:* One year later.

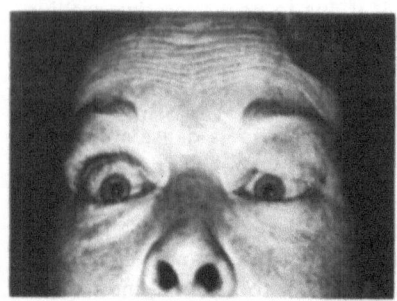
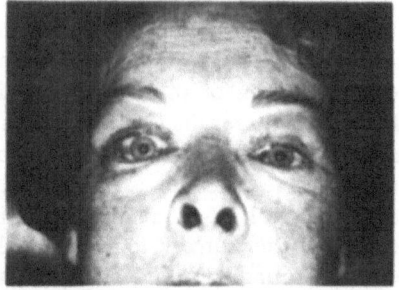

Fig. 2. M.M. *Left:* Before surgery; *Right:* Three weeks later.

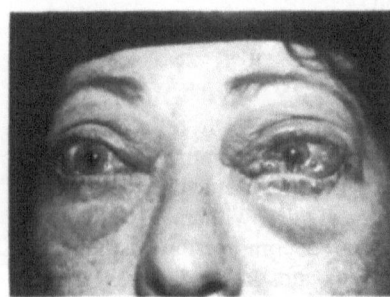
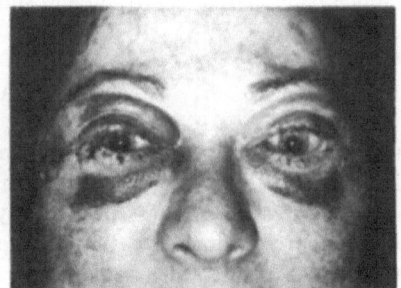
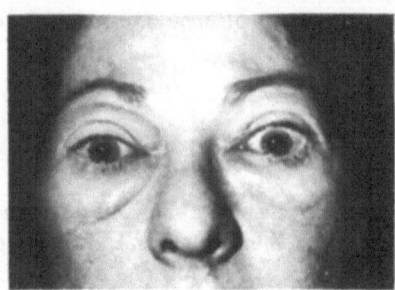

Fig. 3. S.R. Top: *Left* — Before surgery R and L; *Right* — Two weeks later; Bottom: One year later.

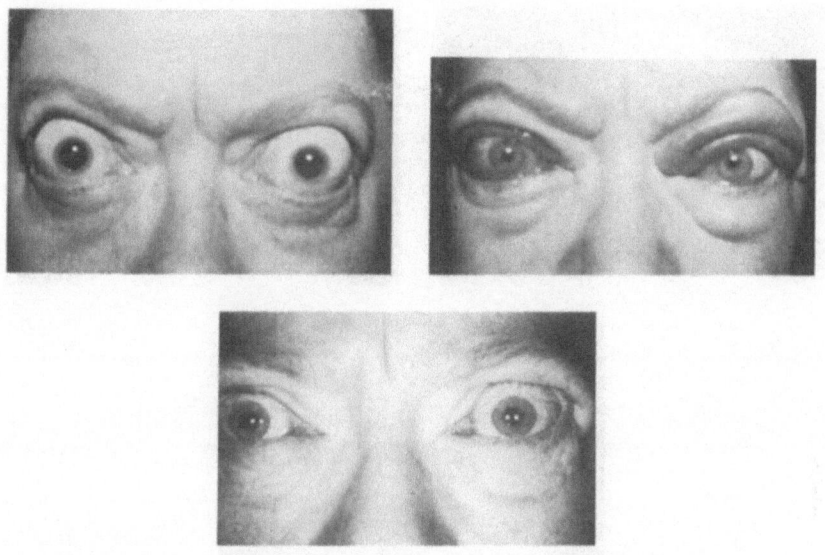

Fig. 4. M.H. Top: *Left* – Before Surgery o.u.; *Right* – Three weeks later; Bottom: Five years later.

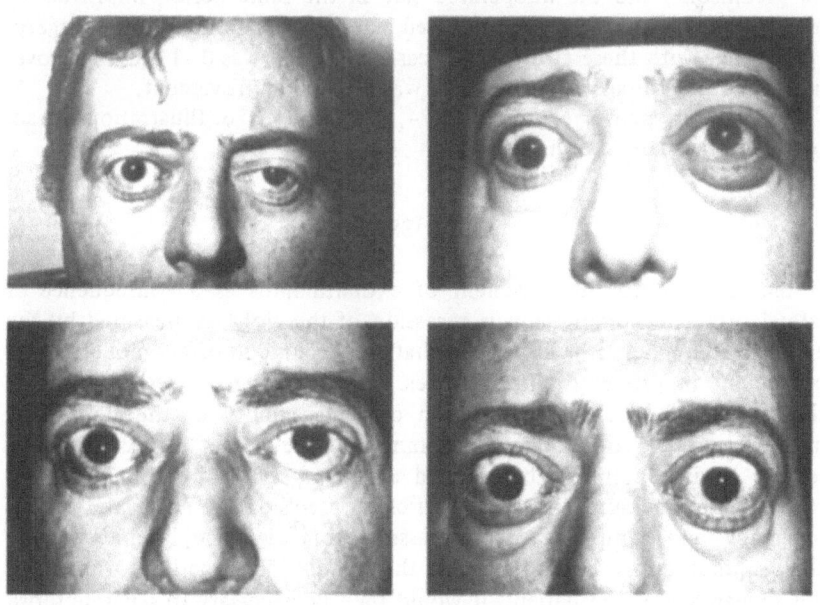

Fig. 5. H.M. Top: *left* – Before surgery L; *Right* – Two months later; Bottom: *Left* – One year later; *Right* – Five years later.

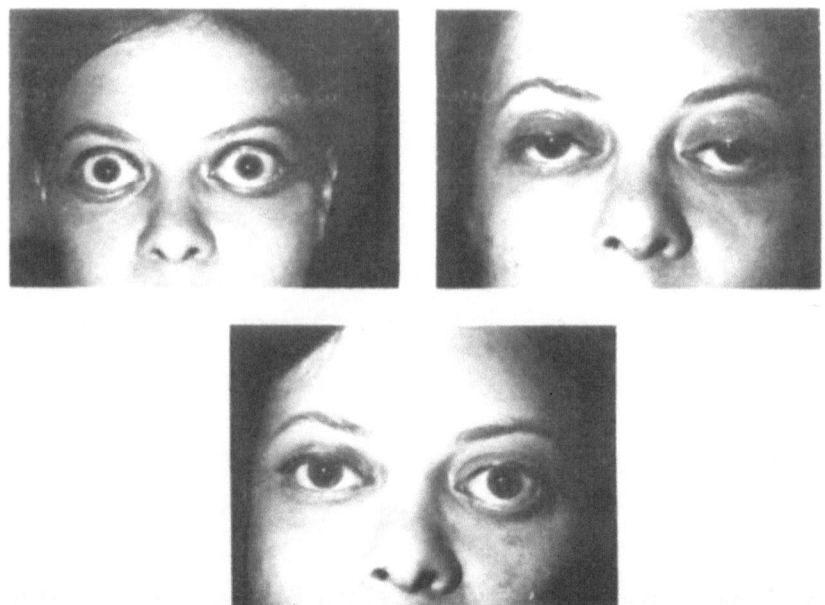

Fig. 6. L.H. Top: *Left* – Before surgery o.u.; *Right* – Four months later; *Bottom* –Six months later.

on prednisone, and the unoperated side in the same period improved 11 mm. Perhaps 3 mm on the unoperated side may be ascribed to the surgery.

The range with these two unusual cases excluded was 0–11 mm improvement, and the average of all the cases was 3.5 mm improvement.

The cases are active records of 1974, 1975 and 1976. Illustrations of six representative cases are shown.

DISCUSSION

If the standard for improvement of exophthalmos as a consequence of lateral orbital decompression is recession of the globe as measured by the exophthalmometer, it will be seen that this technique offers moderate improvement in properly selected cases. If one adds to this standard, as I think should be done, the question of replaceability of the globe after decompression, a firm statement cannot yet be made, because this will require orbitotonometry before and after surgery, and I am only now beginning to measure this with sufficient precision to make the results repeatable and significant. My impression from digital replacement of the globe is that the technique helps. If the standard is to be improvement in the appearance of the patient, it would then be necessary to separate those cases who have no lateral tarsorrhaphy from those who do, and this seems unfair to the patient, since a lateral tarsorrhaphy is such a helpful adjunct

Table of cases

Patient	Orbit	Exophthalmo- meter	Post-op measurements
R.M.	Right	31	27
E.L.	Right	30	28
M.M.	Left	22	27
J.W.	Left	31	24
S.R.	Right	31	30
S.R.	Left	31	30
M.H.	Right	25	25
M.H.	Left	33	28
H.M.	Left	32	30
L.H.	Right	28	26
L.H.	Left	31	28
B.A.	Right	20	27
B.A.	Left	32	26
A.B.	Right	31	17
N.F.	Right	30	25
N.F.	Left	29	24
T.O.	Left	31	25
M.T.	Right	27	23
J.W.	Right	33	22
M.K.	Right	22	22
E.K.	Left	26	24
H.A.	Left	24	22
J.C.	Right	23	23
L.T.	Right	25	24
L.T.	Left	30	24
S.S.	Right	32	34
S.S.	Left	36	32
V.H.	Left	24	20
C.D.	Left	28	26
L.C.	Right	34	30
L.C.	Left	32	29
M.B.	Right	30	26
M.B.	Left	30	26
G.P.	Right	28	23

at the time of the lateral decompression. There exist, of course, a number of cases in whom lateral tarsorrhaphy alone has been done, and, if these could be compared with those in whom lateral decompression alone has been done, it might give the answer. As to the question of whether a helpful prophylactic effect against fibrosis and permanent changes in the orbit can be secured in those decompressions done early, it is obvious that a long study with many patients will be necessary, and even then, because of the variable natural course of the disease, it might not be possible to make an accurate statement.

SUMMARY

Lateral orbital decompression often gives improvement, sometimes is unavailing, and occasionally may be harmful. When combined with inferior rectus and lid surgery, it offers a positive improvement in many exophthalmos cases.

Author's address:
73 East 71st Street
New York, N.Y. 10021
USA

THE SURGICAL TREATMENT OF ENDOCRINE EXOPHTHALMOS

ANDRE CASTERMANS, GASTON LAVERGNE
& ALAIN VAN GARRSE-LYSENS

(Liège, Belgium)

The surgical treatment of endocrine exophthalmos has long been a challenge. The proof lies in the multiplicity of the proposed techniques (see for example Lanier, 1975). The first of these techniques, originated by Dollinger (1911), was a mere application of the temporal approach described by Krönlein (1888). The technique was then used repeatedly (Guyton, 1946; Moran, 1956; Smith, 1965; Long & Ellis, 1966). The upper, extradural approach of the orbit was proposed by Naffziger first in 1931 and then again in 1938. Poppen in 1934 and Hamby in 1970 used it with certain modifications. Orbit decompression through the inferomedian wall was used for the first time by Sewall in 1936. This method was taken over and modified by Ogura & Walsh (1957), Hirsch (1950), Spira, Gerow & Hardy (1974).

All these procedures attempt to decompress the orbit, the accepted hypothesis being that proptosis is the consequence of an increase in intraorbital pressure. Certain observations suggest that this explanation is perhaps too simple. Lavergne & Winand (1973), for example, showed through biochemical and histological studies that the orbital fat and the oculomotor muscles were greatly modified in endocrine exophthalmos.

During attempts to correct exophthalmos using Krönlein's method the authors made observations which confirmed the latter views. External orbitomy does not provoke any bulging of the orbital tissues, even after incision of the periorbit. Moreover, a large lipectomy effected through this approach does not induce retraction of the eyeball, because orbital fat is infiltrated and indurated; the extrinsic muscles are pale and distended. Nor can it be excluded that the muscular involvement was in certain cases worsened by the steroid treatment which the patients received.

In view of this situation we have attempted to perfect a surgical technique whose principle is to advance the orbital frame, since the eyeball seems not to be able to be retracted. It should be mentioned that Tessier (1969) and Rougier et al. (1977) explored this possibility.

SURGICAL PROCEDURE

We propose a technique which moves the whole of the external and inferior walls of the orbit, since it is the relation of the globe to these structures

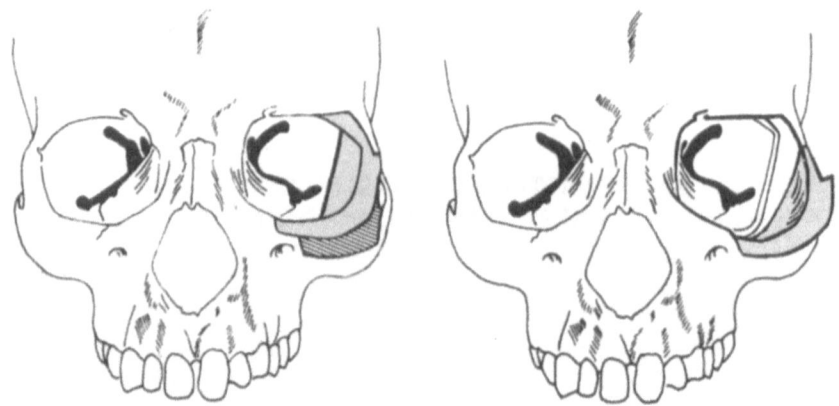

Fig. 1a-b. Step osteotomy of external and inferior walls of the orbit.

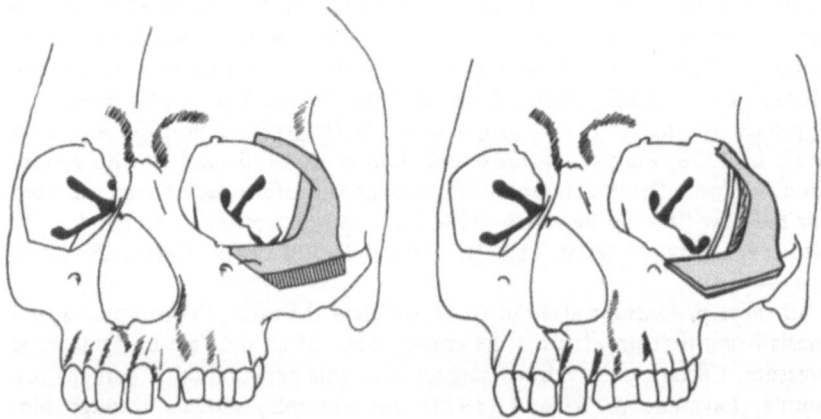

Fig. 2a-b. Curvilinear osteotomy of external and inferior walls of the orbit.

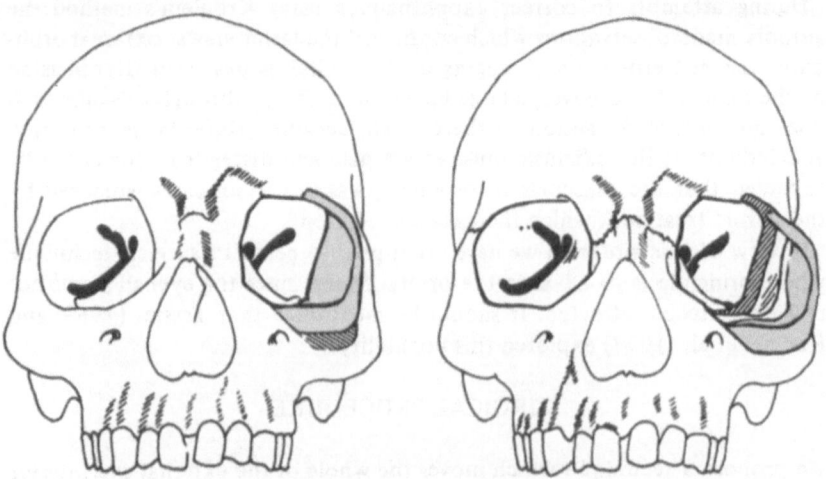

Fig. 3a-b. Sagittal osteotomy of the outer process of the orbit.

426

which determines the existence of exophthalmos. A double approach is used: at the level of the tail of the eyebrow and the lower eyelid at its junction with the cheek, or even through the conjunctiva. Through adequate osteotomies, the free part of the external wall and the floor up to the sphenomaxillary fissure are detached in one block. Upwards the section is extended up to the level of the external quarter of the superior orbital rim. Below, it stops at the level of the infraorbital foramen. We experimented with three types of mobilisation and we finally chose the third one which appears to be the most effective:

– a step osteotomy at the level of the upper and lower sections (Fig. 1a,b) with a horizontal osteotomy of the anterior wall of the sinus.

– a curvilinear osteotomy at the upper section and an oblique osteotomy at the lower section (Fig. 2a,b). This procedure provides movements of greater amplitude than the former. Like the former, it requires a bone graft, which is generally obtained from the osteotomy segment of the anterior antral wall.

– a sagittal osteotomy of the ecternal orbital rim without altering the procedure for the osteotomy of the anterior wall of the sinus. The block composed of the external and inferior walls is raised and after trimming of the distal edge it is fixed in external luxation with respect to the thin remaining external orbital process (Fig. 3a,b). One obtains by this method a considerable projection of the orbital frame which thus blocks itself; there is no need of osteosynthesis, except at the fronto-orbital junction. The forward movement may be adjusted by reducing the depth of the overhanging orbital wall.

Table 1. Ophthalmologic status before and after operation

Patients Age in years	Exophthalmos in mm pre-op	post-op	Lagophthalmos in mm pre-op	post-op	Follow-up in years
DE lo 69	r.e.24 l.e.24	22 22	0	0	6
DI gi 36	r.e.26 l.e.22	22 22	1–2	0	6
QU ma 27	r.e.29 l.e.28	29 26	2 2	2 0	3
LA gi 27	r.e.21 l.e.23	22 23	0	0	3
SC da 35	r.e.26 l.e.26	21 20	3 3	0 0	3
DE an 65	r.e.27 l.e.24	24 21	6 3	2 0	2½
LI ch 33	r.e.22 l.e.22	18 18	0	0	1
VA ja 20	r.e.25 l.e.21 (unoper.)	21 21	0	0	3 months

OPERATIVE OBSERVATIONS

These methods, mainly the third one, offer the possibility of a controlled and significant mobilization of the orbital frame in the three directions of space. They provoke a considerable expansion of the orbital cavity.

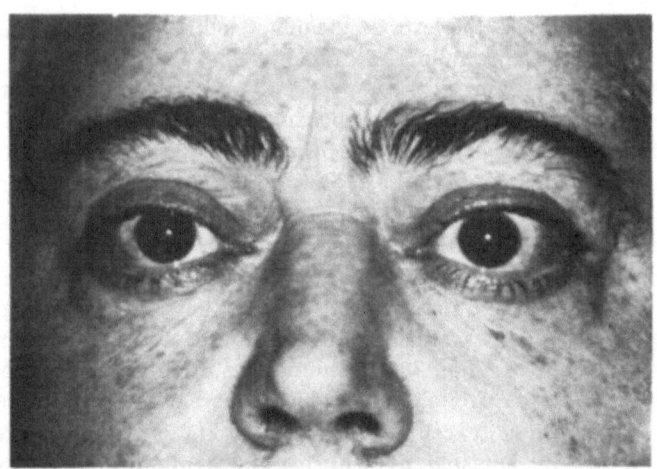

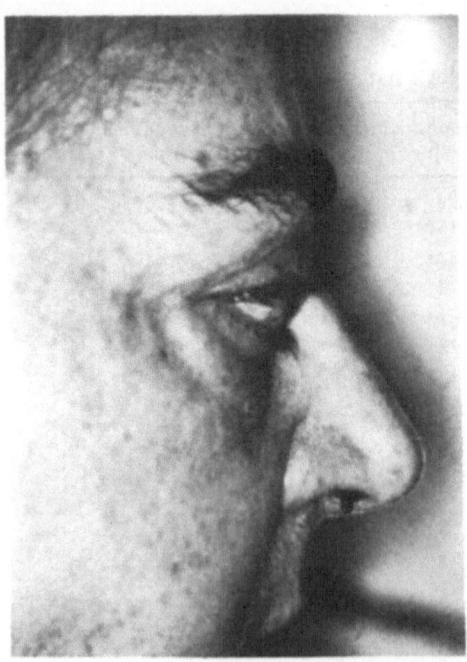

Fig. 4a-b. Patient MA: preoperative views.

They also increase the tension of the external palpebral ligament which may constitute an adjuvant to the treatment by increasing the pressure of the palpebral apparatus on the eyeball.

RESULTS

The best control in this case is that of the ophthalmologist who can objec-

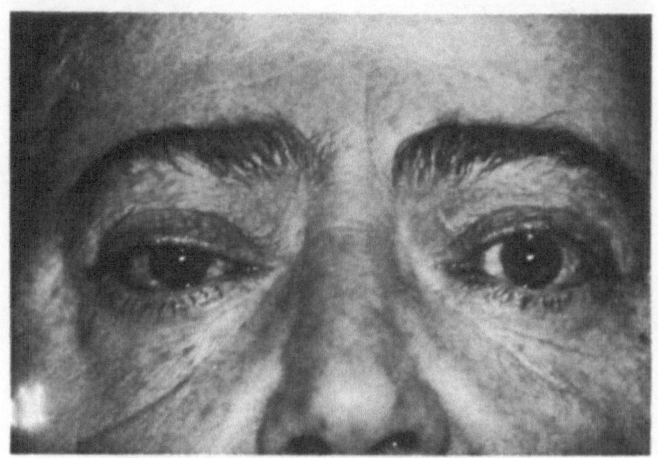

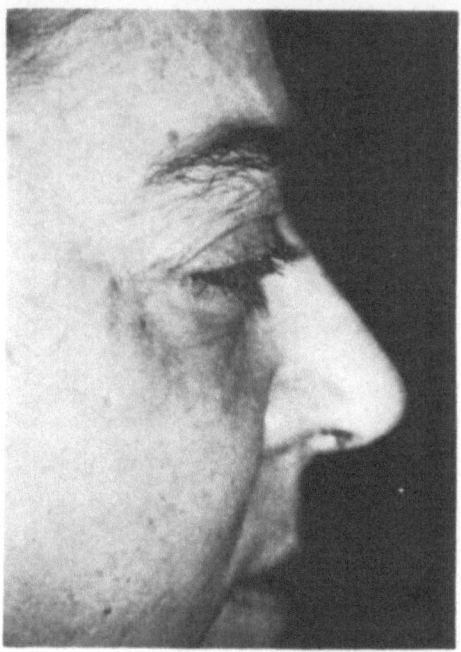

Fig. 5a-b. Patient MA: postoperative views.

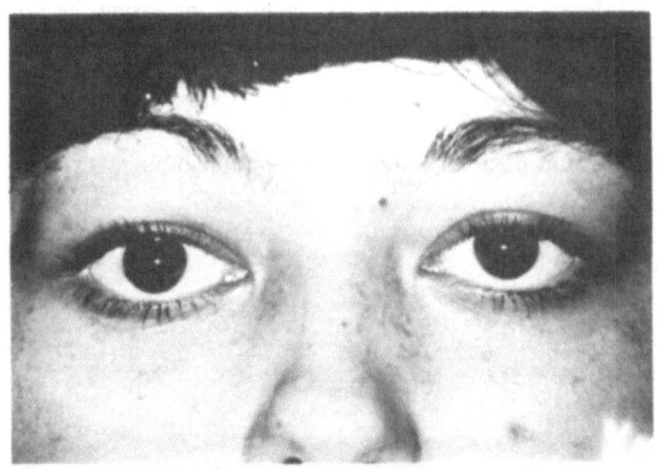

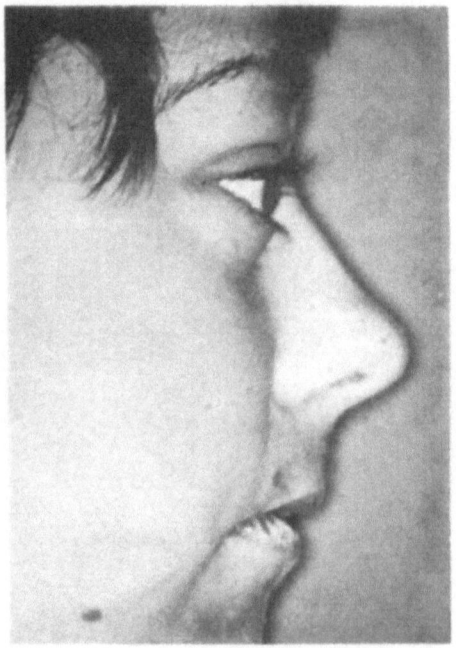

Fig. 6a-b. Patient VA: preoperative views.

tively measure the difference between the pre- and post-operative state (Table 1).

The main benefit of the operation has been the reduction of the exophthalmos (10 eyes out of 13) (Fig. 4a,b 5a,b, 6a,b, 7a,b). Exophthalmos is more than a cosmetic trouble. It is responsible for lagophthalmos exposing the anterior segment of the eye and leading to a serious risk of

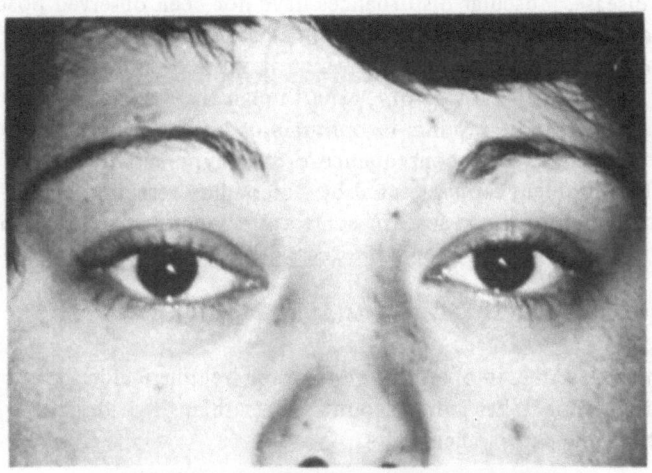

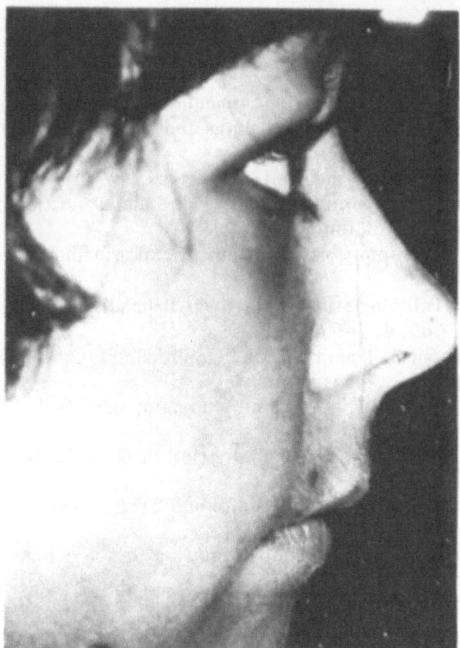

Fig. 7a-b. Patient VA: postoperative views.

infection of the conjunctiva and ulceration of the cornea. In 7 out of 8 eyes exposed to that complication, lagophthalmos was suppressed and it was improved in one further eye. So one eye only did not get any benefit of the operation.

Surgery was without any effect on the other symptoms of thyrotoxic exophthalmos such as chemosis, troubles of eye movements or of ocular pressure, oedema of the optic disc, all symptoms related to the auto-immune disease. Muscular disturbances have not been observed post-operatively and have not been aggravated when existing before.

From a purely cosmetic point of view, it must be noted that all results have not been totally satisfactory, even though the eyeball could be retracted in most cases. The residual lagophthalmos occasionally observed seems, at least in part, to be a consequence of the hyperactivity of the Müller muscle. This problem can be treated by a secondary resection of this muscle by the conjunctival approach. In some cases secondary corrections were made on the eyelids mainly for skin excess.

SUMMARY

The authors describe an operative method for treating endocrine exophthalmos. This method takes into account, better than those described before, the reality of the pathological facts.

REFERENCES

Dollinger, J. Die Druckentlasting der Augenhöhle durch Entfernung der äusseren Orbita und bei hochgradigem Exophthalmus und Konsekutiver Hornhauterkrankung. *Dtsch. Med. Wschr.* 37: *188* (1911).

Guyton, J.S. Decompression of the orbit. *Surgery* 19: *190* (1946).

Hamby, W.B. Orbital decompression for exophthalmos, in: Clinical Neurosurgery. Williams and Wilkins Co., Baltimore, USA (1970).

Hirsch, O. Surgical decompression of malignant exophthalmos. *Arch. Otolaryng.* 51: *325* (1950).

Krönlein, R.U. Zur Pathologie und operativen Behandlung der Dermoid-Cysten der Orbita. *Beitr. Klin. Chir.* 4: *149* (1888).

Lanier, V.C. The Surgical Treatment of Exophthalmos. A review. *Plast. Reconstr. Surg.* 55: *56* (1975).

Lavergne, G. & R. Winand. Exophtalmie endocrinienne. *Bull. Soc. Belge d'Ophtal.* 163: *170* (1973).

Long, J.C. & G.D. Ellis. Temporal decompression of the orbit for thyroid exophthalmos. *Am. J. Ophthal.* 62: *1089* (1966).

Moran, R.E. The correction of exophthalmos and levator spasm. *Plast. Reconstr. Surg.* 18: *411* (1956).

Naffziger, H.C. Progressive exophthalmos following thyroidectomy. Its pathology and treatment. *Ann. Surg.* 94: *582* (1931).

Naffziger, H.C. Progressive exophthalmos associated with disorders of the thyroid gland. *Ann. Surg.* 108: *529* (1938).

Ogura, J.H. & T.E. Walsch. The transantral orbital decompression operation for progressive exophthalmos. *Laryngoscope* 72: *1078* (1962).

Poppen, J.L. Exophthalmos: diagnosis and surgical treatment of intractable cases. *Am. J. Surg.* 64: *64* (1944).

Rougier, J., P. Tessier, F. Hervouet, M. Woillez, M. Lekieffre & P. Derome. Chirurgie plastique orbito-palpébrale, 498 pp. Masson éd. Paris (1977).

Sewal, E.C. Operative control of progressive exophthalmos. *Arch Otolaryng.* 24: *621* (1936).

Smith, J.P. Progressive exophthalmos: cure presentations: preliminary report of new surgical techniques used in treatment. *Laryngoscope* 75: *1160* (1965).

Spira, M., F.J. Gerow & B.S. Hardy. Surgical decompression of the orbit for endocrine exophthalmos. *Fort. Kief. Ges. Chir.* 18: *35* (1974).

Tessier, P. Expansion chirurgicale de l'orbite. *Ann. Chirurgie Plastique*, 14: *207* (1969).

Authors' address:
Departments of Maxillo-facial Surgery and Ophtalmology
66 bvd de la Constitution
4020 Liège
Belgium

Proc. 3rd Int. Symp on Orbital Disorders, Amsterdam 1977

EXPERIENCES WITH MEDIAL DECOMPRESSION OF THE ORBIT

VERNON H. SMITH

(Birmingham, England)

Decompression of the orbit by a medial approach was first suggested by Sewall (1936) but only isolated cases in which the technique had been used for the relief of endocrine exophthalmos were reported (Kistmer, 1939; Schall & Reagan, 1945; Spencer Harrison, 1956; Boyden, 1956) until Smith (1972, 1975) reported the results in 15 cases. The present paper relates further experience with the operation. For the first time some degree of statistical analysis of the results is possible.

MATERIAL

Patients suffering from endocrine exophthalmos were referred from a wide area to the author. In most cases there had already been attempts to treat the condition with systemic steroids and in the few where this was not the case, a trial was given, so that no patient was operated on in which general medical measures had not been tried and proved unsuccessful. The majority of the patients were euthyroid at the time of surgery although eight out of twenty-four were taking carbimazole. In all, 45 orbital decompressions were performed on twenty-four patients, of which eight were men. The ages of the patients ranged from 27 to 68 years and the exophthalmos had been present from one to ten years prior to surgery. Most patients had been exophthalmic for 3 to 4 years.

INDICATIONS FOR SURGERY

There was no common indication for surgery present in all patients (Table 1). Gross and incapacitating diplopia, particularly vertical diplopia was the

Table 1. Indications for surgery in 24 patients

	Case No.
Diplopia	21 (87.5%)
Exposure keratitis	17 (71%)
Poor cosmetic appearance	11 (46%)
Pain	9 (37.5%)
Visual loss	7 (29%)

commonest, and of the 3 patients who did not complain of double vision, 2 had gross visual impairment in one eye and the third in both. Exposure keratitis was present in a high proportion but was only accepted as a true indication for surgery if it had been demonstrated that local supportive measures were not controlling it. In those patients in whom pain was considered an indication, the pain was a severe retrobulbar aching and was considered as a separate entity from the pain associated with exposure keratitis. The cosmetic appearance of all 24 patients naturally fell short of perfect, but in 11 it was considered to be sufficiently distressing to amount to an indication for surgery in itself. Finally in only 7 patients was loss of visual field and acuity the main indication for surgery. This may seem strange when compared with the attitude to orbital decompression held only a few years ago (Friedman & Jones, 1967) but medial decompression has proved such a successful procedure in the hands of the author that some broadening of the indication for operation seemed justifiable.

Technique

The technique has been described previously (Smith 1975) and in essence consists of an exenteration of the ethmoid air sinuses and a decompression of the orbit medially by incising the orbital fascia and allowing the orbital contents to bulge into the dead space so created. The only addition to the technique as described has been to wire the medial palpebral ligaments together in bilateral cases, which were the vast majority, to prevent sagging of the inner canthi which sometimes occurred tending to mar the cosmetic result.

RESULTS

In 45 decompressions carried out on 24 patients, the overall average decompression was 4.8 mm. The immediate pre-operative exophthalmometry reading was taken as the first point of comparison and the exophthalmometry reading at the last post-operative visit as the second. The type of exophthalmometer varied but was standard for any one case. The period of post-operative follow-up has varied from over 5 years to 7 months. In practice there has been little variation in the decompression achieved after 3 months from surgery. Perhaps unexpectedly the decompression achieved in men (14 cases in 8 men) has been less (average 4.5 mm) than in women (31 cases in 16 women) in which it averaged at 4.9 mm. The range of decompression however, has been considerable (Table 2) varying from 2 mm to 11 mm.

There were, however, certain features common to all cases. In no case was post-operative infection a problem, and no case sustained any damage to the optic nerve. Indeed all 7 patients who complained of visual impairment before surgery were able to report improvement, in some cases dramatically so, such as 5/60 to 6/9 in 7 days. The numbers here, however, are too small to permit any statistical analysis, and many other factors have to be considered. One patient had been known to have bilateral papilloedema for 5

Table 2. Decompression achieved

number of patients	milimetres of decompression
3	2
15	3
5	4
6	5
9	6
1	7
2	8
2	9
1	10
1	11
45	Total

months before surgery and her vision only improved to 6/18 and 6/24, which unfortunately was just enough to give her diplopia, associated in part with a pre-existing convergent squint.

Diplopia, if the patient complained of it before the operation, was another symptom that improved considerably. Of the 21 patients with diplopia before surgery, 2 subsequently required squint surgery and 4 others still found this diplopia troublesome although less so than before this operation. There were 2 others who also had squint surgery but they did not have diplopia pre-operatively (see below).

Complications

An interesting feature of this operation was that while it could be relied on to produce an adequate decompression of the orbit, in the majority of cases a significant degree of retraction of the upper lids remained, and for this, Henderson's procedure was performed on 39 out of 45 decompressions. Only 4 patients (6 orbits) did not require it. At the same time as the Henderson's procedure a lateral tarsorrhaphy was also performed to restore the stretched palpebral aperture to a more normal length. Residual exposure keratitis was seen in 4 patients, all of whom had decompressions of 4 mm or over and this was easily controlled by medical means.

Table 3. Complications of medial decompression

Residual lid retraction requiring Henderson's procedure	20 (83%)
Residual exposure keratitis	4
Diplopia requiring squint surgery	4
Trichiasis	2
Poor cosmetic appearance	2
Lacrimal obstruction	1
Recurrent exophthalmos	1

As mentioned above, 4 patients required horizontal squint surgery. Two of these had not complained of diplopia prior to surgery but had been suffering from significant visual impairment. With the recovery in their vision diplopia became troublesome.

Two patients had, and still have some degree of trichiasis and in 2 who were operated on prior to the introduction of canthal wiring, the cosmetic appearance at the medial canthus was poor. Of the remainder one patient developed lacrimal obstruction which was cleared surprisingly easily by probing, but the most instructive complication was that of the patient who had a recurrence of his endocrine exophthalmos. A decompression of 4 mm in the right eye and 3 mm in the left had been achieved by surgery and his diplopia and appearance was much improved. However, one year after his operation his exophthalmos recurred to its original degree. Prior to surgery, intensive systemic steroids had failed to reduce the exophthalmos but when the recurrent proptosis was treated with 60 mgm Prednisolone daily the condition regressed in one week to the post-operative state and has remained so for 12 months after tailing off his steroids.

DISCUSSION

Decompression of the orbit by the medial route allows the orbital contents to expand into an actual rather than a potential space as with the lateral (Krönlein, 1889) and supra-orbital approaches (Naffziger, 1931). The transantral approach of Walsh & Ogura (1957) also allows the orbital contents to expand into an acutal space but through this approach it is difficult to exenterate all the ethmoid sinuses and removal of the floor of the orbit is frequently followed by serious problems with the vertically acting recti (Friedman & Jones, 1967; Young, 1971). While medial decompression cannot be said completely to cure the diplopia seen so frequently before surgery it has a much better record in this respect than other operations. Finally and most important, it seems to be safe. In spite of the close relation of the optic nerve to the site of dissection at the apex of the orbit, no case reported has sustained any optic nerve damage, and all those who had visual impairment before surgery reported improvement. The other potential danger is infection and all cases receive systemic antibiotics because of the risk of infection spreading from the nasal mucosa to the orbital tissues. While all cases complain of nasal obstruction in the post-operative period, which normally lasts about 10 days, there has been no case of orbital cellulitis.

REFERENCES

Boyden, G.L. *Laryngoscope* 66: *633* (1956).
Friedmann, A. & B.R. Jones, *Trans. Ophthal. Soc. U.K.* 87: *431* (1967).
Harrison, M.S. *Lancet* 1: *508* (1956).
Kistner, F.B. *J. Am. Med. Assn.* 112: *37* (1939).
Kronlein, R.U. *Beitr. Klin. Chir.* 4: *149* (1889).
Naffziger, H.C. *Ann. Surg.* 94:   *582* (1931).
Schall, L.A. & D.J. Reagan. *Ann. Otolaryng.* 54: *37* (1954).

Sewall, E.C. *Arch. Otolaryng.* 24: *621* (1936).
Smith, Vernon H. *Trans. Ophthal. Soc. U.K.* 92: *485* (1972).
Smith, Vernon H. *Mod. Probl. Ophthal.* 14: *446* (1975).
Walsh, T.E. & J.H. Ogura. *Laryngoscope* 65: *544* (1957).
Young, J.H.D. *Proc. Roy. Soc Med.* 64: *929* (1971).

Author's address:
Birmingham & Midland Eye Hospital Church Street
Birmingham B3 2NS
England

Proc. 3rd Int. Symp. on Orbital Disorders, Amsterdam 1977

LACRIMAL PROTHESES
(EL ASWAD PROTHESIS)

MOHAMED A.H. EL ASWAD

(Cairo, Egypt)

INTRODUCTION

Since in 1970 Waller first installed a metallic naso-lacrimal tube (called a lacrimal style by C. Callahan), intubation of lacrimal passages has been tried frequently.

Probing of the lacrimal passage by increasing diameter gives generally poor results with a high ratio of recurrence of obstruction. A surgical fistula between the lacrimal sac and the nose, which was done first by Totti, gives good results, especially the mucosa-lined fistula, but if there is a recurrence no hopeful alternative is available.

Successful results of artificial intubation-drainage of minute body cavoties by synthetic tubes in the inner ear and the ventricles of the brain made me think of making a synthetic prothesis in the shape of the lacrimal passages which can be left there permanently to drain tears, especially when the lacrimal sac is about. Many materials have been tried, but polythelene proved to fit the purpose.

HISTORICAL NOTES

In 1713 Anel recommended probing the naso-lacrimal duct followed by irrigation. About 1724 Woolhouse seems to have been the first to try a short circuit from the lacrimal sac to the nose by excising the sac, piercing the lacrimal bone with a trocar, and inserting a drain through this opening. For some months after operation the passages were kept open by tubes of either gold, silver or lead. In 1735 Monro exposed the lacrimal sac and passed shoemaker's awl down the naso-acrimal duct followed by a seton which was left in its place.

If the naso-lacrimal duct had beeen obstructed the lacrimal bone was pierced by a special pin and a drain was left in position.

In 1851 Bowman was the first to show that the puncta and canaliculi could be dilated with probes of graduated sizes which bear his name to this day. In 1868 Berlin excised the lacrimal sac. In 1891 de Wecker performed partial dacryo-adenectomy (the palpebral lobe) for epiphora.

Until the beginning of the twentieth century probing and dacryocystectomy were the accepted therapy for obstruction of the tear passages and

439

consequent dacryo-cystitis. In 1893, Caldwell passed a probe down the naso-lacrimal duct and cut down to this with a bur applied within the nose. This was a precessor of the West-Polyak operation.

In 1904 Toti described this method of dacryocystorhinostomy in which he excised the medial wall of the lacrimal sac, removed the lacrimal fossa and the anterior lacrimal crest. He spared the nasal mucosa except for an opening which corresponded in size and shape to the remaining lateral wall of the sac. Any intervening ethmoidal cells were removed and the anterior tip of the middle turbinate was excised. No sutures were used to unite the edges of the nasal and sac mucosa, but the nose was bandaged in order to press the mucosae against each other.

In 1910 West improved Caldwell's operation by making a larger opening in the naso-lacrimal duct and enlarging this upwards in the lacrimal fossa. The mucous membrane of the duct and lower part of the sac were resected. Later West removed most of the sac. Polyak claimed that he had done this in 1908. In 1912 Blascovics excised the sac, removed the bone of the lacrimal fossa, and implanted the canaliculi into the nose. In 1914 Kuhnt turned the nasal mucosa round the anterior edge of the bony opening and sutured it to the periosteum. The sutures were brought through the skin medially to the skin incision.

In 1920 Ohn was the first to suture the nasal mucosa to the sac, posteriorly and anteriorly, and in 1921 Dupuy-Dutemps and Bourget improved on this by mobilizing the anterior and posterior flaps by short horizontal incisions at each end of the vertical incisions in the sac and nasal mucosa, which facilitated the suturing of these panel-like flaps. Equally in 1921 Mosher described a combined intranasal and external approach.

In 1935 Tikhomorow advised injection of alcohol into the palpebral lobe of the lacrimal gland; in 1937 Jameson described subconjunctival division of lacrimal ductules; and in 1958 Whitwell wrote about denervation of the lacrimal gland for intractable epiphora.

Chronological scheme of other methods:

1958	Moran	Retrograde entubation
1960	Barrie Jones	Canaliculi dissection on nylon thread
1960	Summerskill	Acrylic N.L. tube
1963	Stallard	Conjunctivo-rhinostomy
1963	Dalgleish	Retrograde threading
1970	Lester Jones & Callahan	Pyrex tubes
1974	M. El Aswad e.a.	Lacrimal prothesis (Original)
1977	M. El Aswad	Lacrimal prothesis (Open closed type)

MATERIAL AND METHODS

After many trials I have made two types of lacrimal protheses: the open cavity and closed cavity types (Figs. 1 and 2).

The main line of the prothesis is a bulb 4 mm in diameter, coinciding with the lacrimal sac where a naso-lacrimal tube emerges from its lower border and one or more canaliculi tubes emerge from its lateral border.

440

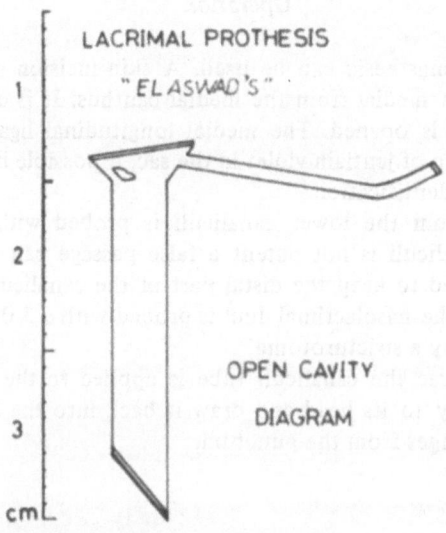

Fig. 1. Lacrimal prothesis. Closed cavity type (diagram).

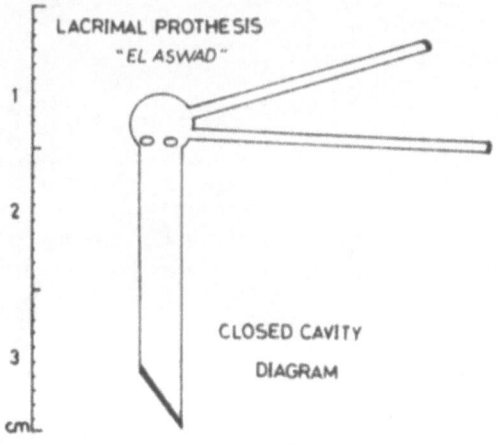

Fig. 2. Lacrimal prothesis. Open cavity type (diagram).

The naso-lacrimal tube is 20 mm long and 3 mm in diameter with a wide draining opening.

The canaliculi tubes are 30 mm long, 1.0 mm in diameter, with a tapering narrow lateral end to facilitate its admission through the canaliculi. The closed cavity type is a prothesis with a closed bulb cavity. In the open cavity type the bulb is represented by a rim of 2 mm height over the naso-lacrimal tube just to give insertion for the canaliculi tube, and one lower canaliculi is usually enough.

Radio-opaque 'Vygon' polyethylene tubes are used for easy identification during and after the operation.

Operation

Local or general anasthesia can be used. A skin incision is made over the lacrimal sac 4 mm medial from the medial canthus. It is deepened till the sac or the cavity is opened. The medial longitudinal ligament has to be spared. An injection of jentiain violet in the sac, if possible before the operation, helps in the identification.

From the punctum the lower canaliculi is probed with a 1 mm blunt probe. If the canaliculi is not patent a false passage can be made by the probe but it is tried to keep the distal part of the canaliculi and the punctum area intact. The nasolacrimal duct is probed with a 3.0 mm probe. Any adhesions are cut by a stricturotome.

From the open sac the canaliculi tube is applied to the tip of the small probe to fit firmly to its head and draw it back into the lacrimal caniculi until the tube emerges from the punctum.

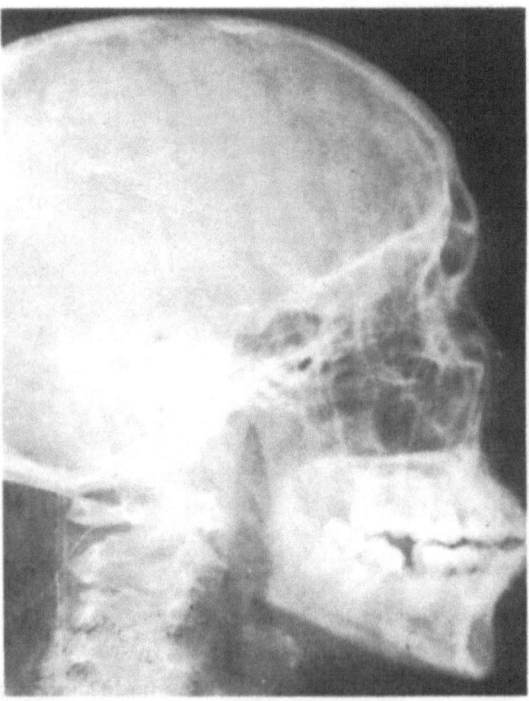

Fig. 3. X-ray picture showing radio opaque lacrimal prothesis in the naso-lacrimal duct.

The naso-lacrimal tube is introduced with the large probe inside. The bevelled surface should look medially and proceed until it is felt that the lower end rests on the inferior conchae. If the nasal tube is too long, it can be cut short until the rim of the bulb rests on the bone of the lacrimal fossa. The sac, the lacrimal facia and the subcutaneous muscles are closed with catgut in separate layers, and then the skin is closed.

The canaliculi tube is left emerging from the punctum to enable syringing through it. Syringing is done daily with antibiotic for 5 days, then the tube is cut with mild pressure on the punctum so the cut end retracts about 3 mm inside the punctum.

The prothesis is X-ray screened before closing the wound to be sure of its position in the bony naso-lacrimal duct (no false passage). If the punctum is closed by adhesions from the start or if multiple traumatic wounds are present, reconstruction is done with the tube inside and the tube is left in its place, emerging from the lid margin, for about one moth to be sure of re-epithelialisation of the canaliculi.

DISCUSSION

The practice of tubing the lacrimal passages by synthetic tubes that are removed afterwards is generally liable to restenosis or obstruction.

Mucosa-lined dacrio-cysto-rhinostomy is a good promising operation, but it is also a difficult bleeding operation and many surgeons report contra-indications if the nasal mucosa is unhealthy. Even if this operation is indicated, what is the treatment if it fails?

This operation is easy, can be done in the out-patient clinic, even with local anaesthesia.

Indications

A. Absolute indications

1. Trauma to the lacrimal passages with avulsion of the canaliculi or the sac especially if accompanied with fractures of the maxillary bone.
2. Recurrence after imperfect dacrio-cystectomy, the prothesis can be put into the cavity replacing the lacrimal sac.
3. Recurrence after closure of the dacriocystorhinostomy fistula.
4. Diseases of the nasal mucosa, e.g. atrophic rhinitis.

B. Relative indications

5. Lacrimal fistula (congenital and post-inflammatory).
6. Symblepharon with closure of the punctum.
7. Chronic decriocystitis in unfit patients.
8. Infants, after failure of probing to relieve lacrimal obstruction.
9. To replace dacryo-cystectomy in small hospitals, in the absence of a skilled surgeon or with poor equipment.
10. Old age.

The prothesis has been tried in 32 different cases of naso-lacrimal duct obstruction and trauma of the lacrimal canalculi. It was well tolerated, not a single case of rejection was observed.

At first, small diameters of 1 and 2 mm were made of the naso-lacrimal tube. These were usually obstructed but increasing the lumen to 3 mm kept them open. Introduction throught the bony naso-lacrimal duct, especially in young females, became difficult.

The question of epiphora has to be discussed more extensively in the following cases. In our series four cases (11%) still have epiphora after installing the prothesis.

The dynamics of lacrimal circulation or drainage and the forces controlling it are not well understood. Most of the early authors, including Ploman, believe that the tear transport system is not a mere passive process but depends on contraction of orbicularis oculi muscle. Some think that the lacrimal sac was compressed during lid closure, resulting in a flow from the sac to the nasal cavity. Frieberg believes that canaliculi have the major role in pushing tears to the lacrimal sac by their propelling contraction and on the suction of tears from the conjunctival sac. He supports his view by the fact that transport of tears continues after surgical dacryocysto-rhinostomy which prevents the lacrimal sac from sucking tears towards it as it is no longer a closed cavity.

This idea is supported by me, for results indicate that cases with healthy canaliculi give better results.

Ploman demonstrated that volumetric changes occur during blinking by radiographic measures. These changes were present mainly in the canaliculi and to a lesser extent in the lacrimal sac. Jones gave the concept of what he called 'the lacrimal pump', and he claimed that on closing the lid the puncti are closed, canaliculi become shorter and the lacrimal sac distends. The shortening of the canaliculi gives a positive pumping effect, pushing the tears medially, helped by the distention of the sac and the closure of the puncti. When opening the eye, the distention of the sac ends and tears run to the nose. This push-pull mechanism forms the lacrimal pump.

Rosengren & Maurice recorded pressure variations in the canaliculi and sac during blinking. Brienen & Snell believed that the pressure rise within the conjunctival sac at the moment of lid closure is the sole propelling force of tear flow.

The expansion and contraction of the lacrimal sac are felt to be the results of pressure fluctuation within the conjunctival sac. In my opinion a chronically inflamed lacrimal sac loses its role in the lacrimal pump; if it has had a role from the start, and so the canaliculi may be the sole part which shares in this mechanisms, e.g. in cases of chronic dacryocystitis or in cases of trauma to the lacrimal sac. We got benefit from the punctum function and part of the canaliculi in lacrimal prothesis application by leaving the punctum and the distal third or half of the canaliculi fee.

The polyethylene tube does not interfere with shortening and elongation of the canaliculi when blinking, as stated by previous authors, and the closure and opening of the punctum is also left free. I recommend using a canaliculi tube of a softer consistency than polyethylene (e.g. silicon), and I am arranging to try this out in the future, using different grades of hardness. In cases of trauma of the canaliculi it is important to keep the lateral parts of the canaliculi and punctum intact, but the medial parts can be replaced by a false passage for the tube if the normal canaliculi cannot be identified. Probing begins from the punctum and can continue through a false passage to open in the lacrimal fossa joining the prothesis with no harm at all as the tube is left in permanently.

If the lacrimal sac or its remnant cavity are not sufficient to co-apt the ampulla of the prothesis, the lacrimal fascia is sutured over the ampulla covered by muscle and skin. Not a single case of lacrimal fistula occurred after such a manoeuvre as the naso-lacrimal duct is patent.

Some patients claim that on sneezing they have a gurgling sensation at the medial angle of the eye. Symptomatic relief of epiphora and a clinical absence of regurge was observed in 25 patients (78%).

Conjunctivo-rhinostomy with a polyethylene or silicon tube, described earlier, to be introduced directly in the nose from the medial canthus usually moves from its place due to the lack of good fixation and may be extruded. Our prothesis takes the shape of and coincides with the normal passages and even if it is removed (which has occurred once on request of the patient after 6 months from its application) it leaves patent normal passages.

In one case the tube was cut flush with the punctum. After two weeks the patient developed a corneal ulcer at the nasal side of the cornea which appeared to be traumatic (i.e. from the tip of the tube); especially polyethylene hardens after this time. The ulcer healed after medical treatment and shortening of the tube in the canalculi.

Faulty introduction of the naso-lacrimal tube in the maxillary sinus may occur, but X-ray screening of the area before closing the wound will avoid this. The tube has to be replaced correctly later with no significant harm.

Swelling of the sac area with signs of acute dacriocystitis occurred once and was relieved by antiobiotics and syringing. More work and experience with this prothesis is needed to estimate its advantages.

SUMMARY

A new polyethylene lacrimal prothesis having the shape of the lacrimal passages and which is left in place permanently is described. Its indications and a comparison with older methods of draining the lacrimal sac are discussed.

REFERENCES

Beard. Plastic and reconstructive surgery of the eye and adnexa. Mosby, St. Louis, p. 171 (1967).

Brienen, J.Q. & C.Q.R.D. Snell. The mechanism of the lacrimal flow. *Ophthalmologica* 159: *223* (1969).

Duje-Elder, S. System of ophthalmology, Volume XIV, p. 434. Kimpton (1972).

Fasanella. Complications in eye surgery phils, p. 133 (1965).

Jones, L.T. Epiphora. II. Its relation to the anatomic structures and surgery of the medial canthal region. *Am. J. Ophthal.* 43: *203* (1957).

Maurice, D. dynamics and drainage of tears. *Int. Ophthal. Clinics* 13: *1* (1973).

Mustarde. Repair and reconstruction in orbital regions, p. 228. Edinburgh (1966).

Ploman, K.G., A. Engel & F. Knutssun. Experimental studies of the lacrymal passageways. *Acta Ophthal.* 6: *55* (1928).

Rosengren, B. On lacrimal drainage. *Ophthalmologica* 164: *409* (1972).
Stallard. Eye surgery, 4th ed. Bristol (1965).
Veirs. Symposium on surgery of the ocular adnexa, p. 113. Mosby, St. Louis (1966).

Author's address:
Department of Ophthalmology
Tanta University
Cairo
Egypt

Proc. 3rd Int. Symp. on Orbital Disorders, Amsterdam 1977

ORBITAL RECESSION IN CRANIOFACIAL SURGERY

J.C.H. VAN DER MEULEN

(Rotterdam, The Netherlands)

ABSTRACT

In the past years orbital osteotomies have been used to correct major cranio-facial deformities in an increasing number of cases. While in general the results are extremely gratifying, complications may, however, occur, e.g. the creation of intra- and extra-orbital 'dead space' and the occurrence of tele-canthus and enophthalmos. A technique has been developed to eliminate these complications, or at least to reduce their severity.

Author's address:
Lambertweg 40
Rotterdam
The Netherlands

SURGICAL APPROACH TO THE ORBITAL CONNECTIVE TISSUE IN CASES OF TRAUMATIC DIPLOPIA

T.H. OEI

(Amsterdam, The Netherlands)

Diplopia after trauma may be due to a defect of the orbital walls in combination with a change in the structure of the connective tissue system in the orbit. Up to now it has been generally accepted that in cases of blow-out fractures the muscle-fibres are incarcerated in the fracture.

In cases of fracture of the orbital floor, the vertical eye movements will be diminished. Formerly, these cases were considered as an acute situation in which operation should be performed within a certain time, to prevent — as we assumed — a necrosis of the muscle fibres during the incarceration.

In the many cases on which we have operated, we found only fatty and connective tissue in the prolapsing tissue. An effort to find muscle fibres during the operation was not successful. Even with the aid of faradic stimulation we were not able to demonstrate contractile tissues in the prolapsing tissues. At present we are inclined to postpone the acute treatment. The majority of the motility disturbances in blow-out fractures may be due to haematoma in the orbit.

Nowadays we wait a few days and order the patient to practise vertical eye movements. This has proved to be beneficial. If no improvement of the motility occurs, a surgical restoration of the blow-out will be necessary. We perform this operation by sub-periostal approach, free the prolapse from the fracture hole and cover this hole by a thin teflon plate.

But the generally accepted treatment does not always solve the problem of diplopia. In our opinion the functional anatomical mechanism of blow-out fractures is more complex than has hitherto been assumed. We can ask ourselves the following questions:

1. Why is it that vertical motility disturbances by incarceration of muscle in cases of blow-out fractures of the orbital floor never have the characteristics of the most exposed muscle, lying nearest to the orbital floor: the inferior oblique muscle?

2. Why have we not invariably found muscle fibres in the prolapse during operation?

3. Why does diplopia occur and persist in cases where the fracture of the orbital floor is not severe?

4. Why does the diplopia not improve in many cases after adequate restoration of the orbital floor?

These questions may be answered by the study of Koornneef (1977). In his paper he showed us the connective tissue septa lying between the eye-ball, the muscles and the orbital walls. Up to now little attention has been paid to the importance of the connective tissue in relation to the motility of the eyeball. This can be illustrated by a number of patients.

The first patient had a neuro-fibroma of the infra-orbital nerve. She was operated on; the tumour was removed, together with a large part of the orbital floor. No restoration of the floor by teflon plate was done. She had diplopia for a few days postoperatively. After one week diplopia had disappeared. This case clearly illustrates that the orbital floor is not indis-pensible for eye movements. It is probable that the connective tissue system in the orbit keeps the eyeball in its place and makes normal eye movements possible, even without an orbital floor.

The second patient got a wooden stick into the left orbit during skating. He sustained a blow-out fracture; he had hypertropia of the left eye and severe motility disturbances, especially when looking downwards, causing diplopia. X-ray pictures showed a cloudy maxillary sinus and displacement of the orbital floor. Two days after the accident an orbitotomy was performed. The forced duction test was done, the eyeball appeared to be completely stuck. The prolaps into the maxillary sinus was freed, little pieces of wood were removed and the fracture was covered with teflon. Two months later the motility had not improved much and the patient still had diplopia.

Again X-ray pictures were taken and these showed that the teflon plate was still in its place. Nevertheless, a large shadow could be seen around the orbital floor. The motility chart looked like a paralysis of the inferior rectus muscle. Electromyography was performed and it revealed a perfectly normal and functioning inferior rectus muscle. The shadow around the orbital floor, the contradictory results of the orthoptic and EMG findings gave support to the assumption that abnormal scar-connective tissue could probably be held responsible. Eight months after the first operation the teflon plate was removed via conjunctival approach and the inferior rectus muscle was freed as far as possible from the adherent connective tissue lump. Immediately post-operatively, a slight motility improvement was obtained. The patient was told to practise eye movements frequently. Again a few months later motility was even better with the result that the patient could look straight ahead without having diplopia.

It is probable that a rather 'normal' connective tissue system had de-veloped around the freed inferior rectus muscle, influenced by his practising eye movements, and permitting better eye movement. Today, one year post-operatively, eye movements have improved even more and the diplopia has been reduced. This fact supports our theory that changes in the connective tissue in the orbit can influence eye movement.

449

REFERENCE

Koornneef, L. Spatial aspects of orbital musculo-fibrous tissue in man. Swets & Zeit-linger, Amsterdam (1977).

Author's address:
University Eye Clinic
Wilhelmina Gasthuis
104, 1e Helmerstraat
Amsterdam
The Netherlands

Proc. 3rd Int. Symp. on Orbital Disorders, Amsterdam 1977

FOREIGN BODY REACTION AFTER ORBITAL
TEFLON IMPLANTATION

K. MÜLLER-JENSEN

(Karlsruhe, W. Germany)

The early operative management of blow-out fractures of the orbit has become a routine procedure in well-organized hospitals and orbital centers for the past 20 years (Smith & Regan, 1957). One of the best known orbital surgery facilities in Europe is the Orbital Center Amsterdam, formed and guided by Bleeker (Bleeker & Lyle, 1970; Bleeker & Ommen, 1959).

The literature of the past 20 years is replete with positive reports and statistics on the early management of orbital blow-out fractures. (Converse et al., 1967; Lerman, 1970). For several years it has been questioned whether principal and early surgery in blow-out fractures was always appropriate. The specific indications deferring immediate surgical repair and using medical observation are less precise than those for initial intervention. For example, on follow-up of patients who were operated on immediately 15 to 38% had unstaisfactory cosmetic results and 10 to 15% had symptomatic diplopia. These percentages varied with the particular speciality of the managing physician (Emery & v. Noorven, 1971, 1972). It has been proven that posttraumatic diplopia cleared spontaneously in 50% of nonsurgical patients within two weeks.

Motility sometimes recovers not because of, but in spite of surgical management (Müller-Jensen & Schneider, 1975). It was emphasized, that retrobulbar and intramuscular hemorrhage can produce typical signs of blow-out fracture: inability to elevate the globe, vertical diplopia, and hypesthesia over the distribution of the infra-orbital nerve, Submucosal hematoma and mucosal swelling localized to the roof of the maxillary sinus can look like a 'hanging-drop' opacity caused by herniated orbital contents.

In a series of 63 patients operated upon within the last 8 years both at the University Clinic Munich, and in the Municipal Hospital Karlsruhe, severe postoperative complications with unsatisfactory results were observed in only four cases. In addition, 33 patients (50%) kept a minor degree of persistent diplopia. All patients were treated by the trans-eyelid approach or a combined Caldwell-Luc approach (32%). The fractured orbital floor was reinforced by a sheet of teflon in all cases. None of these plates were attached to the orbital floor.

Fifty-nine patients showed good wound healing and marked reduction of the diplopia within the first postoperative week. The four patients with severe postoperative complications will be discussed:

1. This 40-year old man suffered a complex crushing injury with zygomatico-maxillary fracture and marked diplopia resulting from incarceration of the inferior rectus muscle. A combined Caldwell-Luc and trans-eyelid operation was performed with interosseous wiring of the zygomatico-maxillary lines of separation. Bony fragments were partly removed, partly restored to their original position. Because of the marked defect, the teflon implant had to be very large (Fig. 1). Diplopia cleared within 2 weeks, but wound-healing was not adequate. After three months, the teflon plate had to be removed because of anterior migration (Fig. 2).

2. A similar case of zygomatic fracture with extrusion of the implant was observed in a 33-year old man in which the teflon plate was not anchored to the underlying bone.

Normally, this procedure is not necessary, but in large defects with interosseous wiring, the plate should be fixed to the orbit by wire or with a 'tongue' of the implant inserted into the anterior aspect of the fracture following the technique of Smith & Putterman, (1970).

These methods − either to drill a hole in the orbital rim to secure the implant (Browning & Walker, 1965) or to anchor the implant by a bent flap placed into the anterior aspect of the fracture − can prevent anterior migration and extrusion.

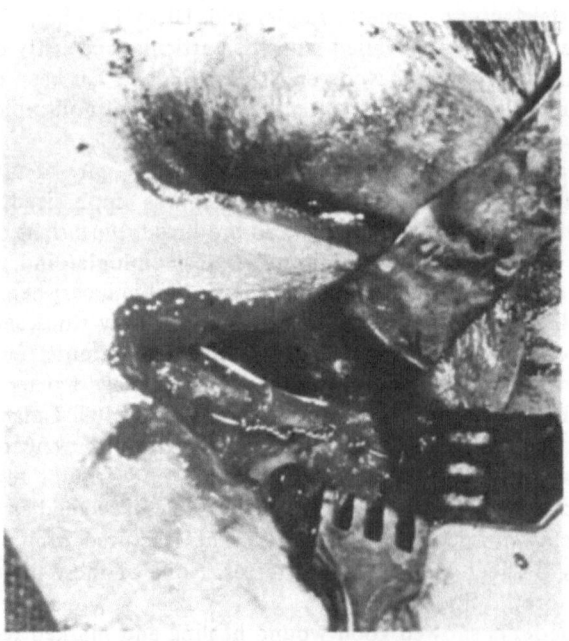

Fig. 1. Zygomatico-macillary fracture in a 40-year old man. Operative situation after interosseous wiring and teflon implantation without anchoring of the implant.

452

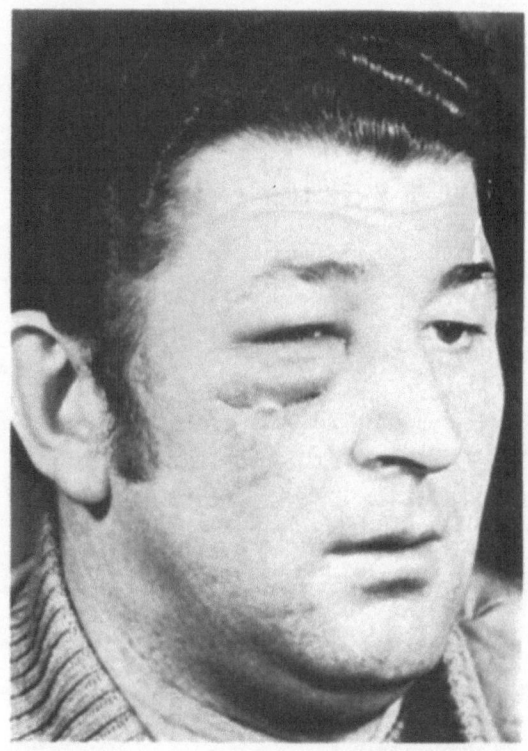

Fig. 2. Same patient as in Fig. 1, 6 weeks after surgical repair. Extrusion is present due to anterior migration of the teflon implant.

3. Another problem is demonstrated in the case of a 60-year old man who suffered a pure blow-out fracture by the traumatizing force of a human fist. The x-ray shows herniation or orbital contents. A large curved eyelid incision provoked disturbance of the lateral lymphatic passages with persistent lid edema (Fig. 3).

This complication can easily be avoided by a straight incision, diverging slightly downwards laterally, as emphasized by Converse (1962) and Hoette (1970).

4. There are probably different etiologic factors responsible for hyperplastic scarring without extrusion or migration of the alloplastic implant. This 48-year old man with a typical orbital floor fracture which resulted from a car accident was treated by a transeyelid approach with subperiosteal teflon implantation. The cosmetic result was unsatisfactory.

We felt that a chronic infection of the maxillary sinus was one factor for the inflammatory irritation of the lowerr lid. I also think that difficulties in adaptation of the periosteum, which occasionally is damaged during the operative procedure, can lead to extrusion of the plate and to irregular scarring.

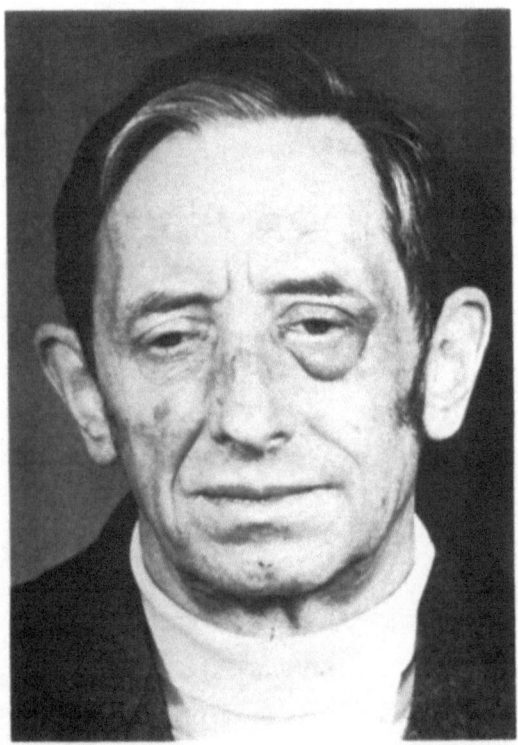

Fig. 3. 60-year old patient with blow-out fracture. 3 months postoperative. Persistent lid edema due to disruption of the lateral lymphatic passages.

SUMMARY

The percentage of postoperative complications can be diminished by adequate fixation of the implants, careful adaptation of the different layers of periosteum, orbicularis muscle and skin, as well as postoperative care of the sinuses by antibiotics snd good drainage.

Because good spontaneous reconstitution occurs in 50% of patients treated medically, the indication for operative management or blow-out fracture should be strictly limited to cases in which the initial or follow-up examinations within the first 2 weeks show typical extraocular muscle imbalance with persistent diplopia in addition to roentgenographic evidence.

REFERENCES

Bleeker, G.H. & B. van Ommen. Early treatment of orbital fractures. *Ophthalmologica* (Basel) 138: *40–53* (1959).
Bleeker, G.H. & T.K. Lyle. Fractures of the orbit. Excerpta Medica, Amsterdam (1970).

Browning, C. & R. Walker. The use of alloplastics. *Am. J. Ophthal.* 60: *684–698* (1965).

Converse, J.M. Blow-out fracture of the orbit. *Plast. Reconstr. Surg.* 29: *408* (1962).

Converse, J.M., B. Smith, M.F. Obear & D. Wood-Smith. Orbital blow-out fractures. A ten-year survey. *Plast. Reconstr. Surg.* 39: *20* (1967).

Emery, J.H., G.K. von Noorden & D.A. Schlernitzauer. Orbital floor fractures: long-term follow-up of cases with and without surgical repair. *Trans. Am. Acad. Ophthal. Otolaryng.* 75: *802* (1971).

Emery, J.M., G.K. von Noorden & D.A. Schlernitzauer. Management of orbital floor fractures. *Am. J. Ophthal.* 74: *299–306* (1972).

Hoette, H.H. Orbital fractures. Van Gorcum & Comp., Amsterdam (1970).

Lerman, S. Blow-out fractures of the orbit. *Br. J. Ophthal.* 54: *90–98* (1970).

Müller-Jensen, K. & J.U. Schneider. Besondere Verläufe bei Orbitaboden fraktur. *Klin. Mbl. Augenheilk.* 167: *596–600* (1975).

Smith, B. & A.M. Putterman. Fixation of orbital floor implants. *Arch. Ophthal.* 83: *598* (1970).

Smith, B. & W.F. Regan. Blow-out fracture of the orbit. *Am. J. Ophthal.* 44: *733* (1957).

Author's address:
Augenklinik der Städt. Krankenanstalten
18 Moltkestrasse
7500 Karlsruhe
W. Germany

CORRECTING THE DEFICIENCY OF THE SUPRA-ORBITAL RIM IN CRANIOSTENOSIS BY RADICAL OSTEOTOMIES. ABOUT 28 CASES

DANIEL MARCHAC, JEAN COPHIGNON, JEAN-FRANCOIS HIRSCH & DOMINIQUE RENIER

(Paris, France)

ABSTRACT

In 1972 we first started to treat the cosmetic sequellae of craniostenosis, especially of the oxycephalic type, with retrusion of the forehead and supra-orbital rim, and often with exophthalmic appearance.

We designed a procedure with radical mobilization of the skeleton of the anterior cranial vault by osteotomies and rocking and advancement of the supra-orbital rim. A kind of bony Z plastic allows an easy contention without bone-grafts.

This procedure having proved very effective and the cranial vault remodelling being quite well tolerated by the patients, we were encouraged to treat younger children, even babies, in order to solve at the same time the functional (intra-cranial hypertension) and the cosmetic problem.

Facial craniostenosis — Crouzon and Apert diseases — are of special interest in this respect, and we have started to operate on them very early, during the first 2 or 3 months of life, to make a radical frontal advancement including the upper part of the orbit.

In 5 cases the result is so far very gratifying, and this has encouraged us to continue and to try also the liberation of the lower part of the orbit.

Authors' addresses:
Hôpital St. Louis,
Hôpital Lariboisière, and
Hôpital des Enfants-Malades
Paris
France

Proc. 3rd Int. Symp. on Orbital Disorders, Amsterdam 1977

THE SURGICAL MANAGEMENT OF ORBITAL TUMOURS

J. WRIGHT

(London, England)

ABSTRACT

The routine use of all new investigative techniques has substantially altered the surgical management of orbital disease. The author describes the basic technique of orbital surgery and shows methods of dealing with extensive orbital tumours, particularly those which require exenteration combined with resection of all the orbital walls.

Author's address:
Moorfields Eye Hospital
City Road
London EC1V 2PD
England

Proc. 3rd Int. Symp. on Orbital Disorders, Amsterdam 1977

MUCOCOELE OF MAXILLARY SINUS
(A film)

ALSTON CALLAHAN

(Birmingham, Ala, USA)

Although mucocoeles of the frontal and ethmoid sinuses are relatively common, they rarely develop in the maxillary sinus.

A 10 year old girl had noticed blurred left vision and diplopia in upward and downward gaze for several weeks. The left eye was 3 mm higher and 3 mm anterior to the right eye. The visual fields were normal. Pressure against the left globe and pressure inside the inferior orbital rim met with firm resistance. There was pain in and tenderness over the left maxillary sinus.

Ultrasonography and x-ray studies revealed a globular cystic mass about 3 cm in diameter in the left maxillary sinus. It extended through the orbital floor in a large bony dehiscence.

The film shows the operative technique of obtaining a minimal scar through a subciliary incision in the lower lid, the removal of 100 cc of brownish fluid from the cavity, the removal of the cavity walls and flushing of the remaining tissues with potassium chloride solution, and the insertion of a curved strip of supramyd sheeting 0.3 mm thick, large enough to serve as the floor. This sheet was fixed in place with sutures through the inferior orbital rim. During the operation and especially during the insertion of the plate, the optic nerve head was observed for possible interference with the blood flow.

The patient has been observed postoperatively for two years with no recurrence.

Author's address:
Eye Foundation Hospital
Birmingham, Alabama
USA

MEDICAL TREATMENT OF MALIGNANT ORBITAL TUMOURS IN CHILDREN

P.A. VOÛTE & J. DE KRAKER

(Amsterdam, The Netherlands)

Orbital swellings in childhood can be either benign or malignant. Benign swellings are haemangiomas, lymphangiomas, neurofibromas, orbital cellulitis, cysts and many others. Although many of them can give rise to alarming clinical symptoms resembling malignant tumours, a conservative though adequate treatment should be given. This is especially necessary in orbital haemangiomas in siblings. These haemangiomas will nearly always regress spontaneously, resulting in complete disappearance.

Malignant tumours of the orbit are to be divided in primary and metastatic tumours. The metastatic and systemic are represented by neuroblastomas, myeloid leukemia and histiocytosis X. The primary tumours are the rare Ewing-sarcomas and osteosarcomas of the orbital bones, and the rhabodomyosarcomas. The rhabdomyosarcomas are the most frequent malignant orbital tumours. Mostly they are localised in the orbit as well as in the nasofaryngeal sinusses. They occur most frequently in the first ten years of life, chiefly in children under five years old.

Rhabdomyosarcomas have the reputation of spreading at an early stage to lymphnodes and by the bloodstream to the lungs. This is not common in orbital rhabdomyosarcomas, probably because they are recognised early. Spreading to and through the meninges is more often.

The clinical presentation is mostly:
1. Visible tumour.
2. Proptosis with displacement.
3. Diplopia.
4. Signs suggestive of acute inflammation as oedema and rapidly developing hyperaemia of the orbital tissues.

A multidisciplinary approach is necessary for all childhood tumours and orbital rhabdomyosarcomas are not different in this aspect.

Radiotherapy, surgery and chemotherapy are the three modalities of treatment. It has to be borne in mind that all three *can* be used, but that they do not *have to* be used. In treatment one has to decide on twe points:
1. Cure with mutilation, or
2. Cure with minimal or no mutilation, but taking the risk that no cure will be obtained.

Nowadays it is possible to take into consideration that a cure with minimal or no mutilation is possible due to chemotherapy. Cure rate is high and with chemotherapy mutilating treatment with radiotherapy and surgery can be prevented or diminished. Chemotherapy has serious systemic side effects, but used before surgery and radiotherapy it can diminish the extend of surgical or radiotherapeutical procedures. And it can prevent the development of distant metastasis.

From October 1971 ot November 1975, 40 patients were seen by us with a rhabdomyosarocma in all sites of the body. Nine were localised in the orbit or nasofaryngeal sinus with extension in the orbit. Three patients died despite treatment and 6 seem to be cured. All were treated with chemotherapy following a treatment schedule of Vincristine, Actinomycine D and Cyclofosfamide and adjuvant radiotherapy if necessary. Exenteration of the orbit was not necessary in these patients. This treatment regime was instituted after having good treatment results in rhabdomyosarcomas of the urogenital tract and nasofaryngeal region where surgery and radiotherapy has to be very mutilating.

In childhood cancers one has to consider:
1. That the patient never decides for himself.
2. That the patient has to be treated and cured to have a normal live expectancy for his age group.
3. That one is treating a child that has to lead a normal social live, and treatment can interfere with the normal development of the body or parts of the body.

In summary one could say that quality of suvival is just as important as survival as such.

Authors' address:
Working Group on Childhood Tumours
Antoni van Leeuwenhoek Ziekenhuis and Emma Kinder Ziekenhuis
Amsterdam
The Netherlands

Proc. 3rd Int. Symp. on Orbital Disorders, Amsterdam 1977

AN ACCURATE AND SIMPLE TECHNIQUE FOR MEGAVOLTAGE THERAPY OF INTRA-ORBITAL TUMOURS

J. SCHIPPER & K.E.W.P. TAN

(Utrecht, The Netherlands)

INTRODUCTION

Malignant intra-orbital tumours, other than basal cell and squamous cell carcinoma on or near the eyelids, are very rare and, even in large centres, seldom seen by the radiotherapist. The commonest, treated by radiotherapy at the university hospital in Utrecht, are:
— retinoblastoma in infants, and
— intra-orbital metastases of primary tumours elsewhere in the body.

The first aim of radiotherapy for these patients is adequate treatment of the whole tumour area. The second is the preservation of some degree of useful vision if there is a potential chance to do so. This can lead to conflicting requirements with regard to the radiation technique as for instance in the treatment of retinoblastoma. One has to protect as much as possible the anterior segment of the eye with, as the most sensitive component, the lens. Even with low doses cataract can be induced (Merriam et al., 1972). But, on the other hand, the entire retina has to be treated with a high and uniform radiation dose because of the high incidence (84%, Reese, 1963) of multifocal tumours in the same eye and, as we and other authors (Thompson et al., 1972; Ellsworth, 1969) have experienced, new lesions can develop in the anterior retina if that region was not included in the treated volume.

In most centres for radiotherapy retinoblastoma is treated by a single lateral high-energy X-ray beam. The temporal field of 3 x 3 cm up to 5 x 5 cm is arranged as accurately as possible to cover the entire retina and to exclude the lens. After the installation of our 6 MeV linear accelerator in 1968, we started to treat retinoblastoma and intra-orbital metastases with this technique. We found however this method not accurate and reproducible enough, especially in the treatment of retinoblastoma with tumour foci anterior to the equator of the eye. The description of the improved radiation technique, which is in use from 1971, will be given in relation to the treatment of the most interesting and difficult tumour, retinoblastoma in infants.

TREATMENT TECHNIQUE

A first improvement was made by the introduction of sharply collimated D-shaped fields, after the technique as Bagshaw & Kaplan (1966) described in 1966. In our system these D-shaped fields, especially contoured to guard the lens and to irradiate only the tumour and tumour at-risk area (Fig. 1), are achieved by precision machined 11 cm thick lead collimators. With help of a specially designed collimatorholder the collimators are placed in the beam at 83 cm from the focus. The tumourous eye is located exactly in the isocentre of the accelerator, at 100 cm from the focus.

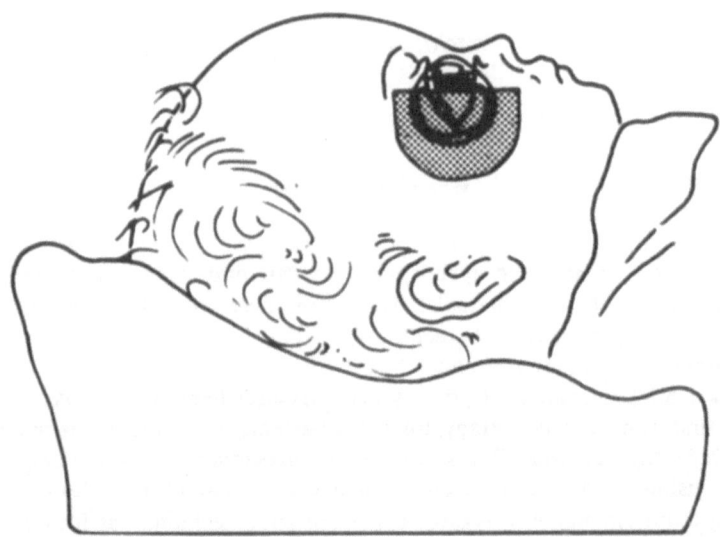

Fig. 1. A lateral, sharply collimated, D-shaped treatment field covering the entire retina and excluding the lens.

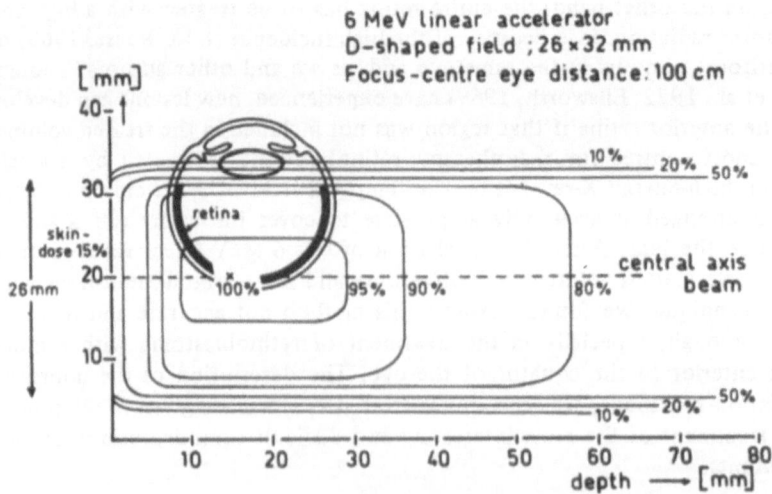

Fig. 2. The isodose-distribution of a D-shaped field of 26 x 32 mm, in a plane through the central axis of the eye and the central axis of the beam, using a 6 MeV linear accelerator. The lateral beam is positioned with the anterior 50%-isodose line against the back of the lens.

462

a plane through the central axis of the beam and the central axis of the eye, shows some of the specific advantages of the high-energy X-ray beam of a 6 MeV linear accelerator. The irradiation dose at the surface of the skin is only 15% of the maximum dose that, at a depth of 1.5 cm, is located nearly in the middle of the eye. The knife-edged character of the collimated beam is illustrated in Figure 3 by the cross-plot of the relative dose distribution along the central axis of the eye. The penumbra-width between the 20% and 80% dose-points is only 2 mm. If the tumour is confined to the posterior segment of the eye, behind the equator, the beam is set up with the 50% dose-point against the back of the lens, as is shown in Figure 3. If there is an extensive seeding in the anterior vitreous, the beam is moved forward over 2 mm with an increased risk on cataract formation because a larger portion of the lens is irradiated. If only the posterior segment of the lens is located in the beam we experienced up to now only a very mild form of cataract. Probably this is caused by the fact that most of the epithelial lens cells are in a narrow band just anterior to the equator of the lens and only a few at the posterior segment.

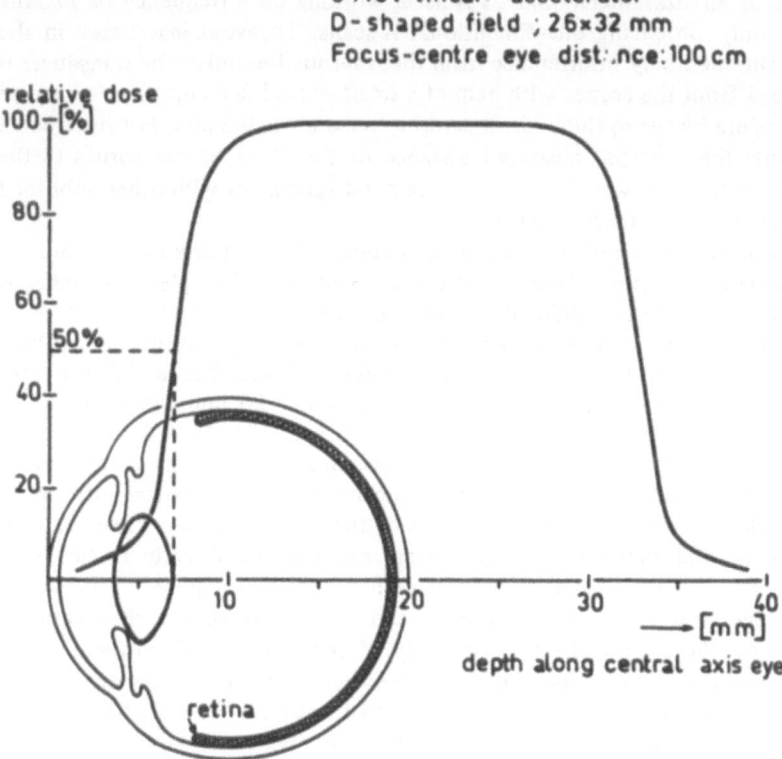

Fig. 3. Dose profile of a lateral D-shaped field of 26 x 32 mm along the central axis of the eye. The beam is positioned with the anterior 50% dosepoint against the back of the lens.

463

Accurate and reproducible treatment of the eye with a sharp-edged beam, excluding the lens or with only the posterior segment of the lens in the beam, is only possible if:

(a) the very young patients are sedated during treatment,

(b) the position of the eye and of the lens are exactly known,

(c) the head and the eye are fixed during the treatment and

(d) the setting-up of the beam is based on the position of the eye during the treatment and not, as is generally done, on the position of the lateral bony canthus or, after an accurate localisation of the eye and the lens, on marks on the skin.

Nevertheless the irradiation technique has to be simple, because with a small number of patients it is difficult to maintain experience in complicated techniques.

The very young patients are sedated by a slow-induction inhalation anesthesia consisting of a mixture of nitrous oxide and oxygen with 1% of halothane given by intubation. The patients are fully awake in approximately 10 minutes after finishing of the treatment and can be managed easily as out-patients. At the first treatment the position of the lens with reference to the cornea is determined ultrasonically. An inexpensive industrial ultrasonic unit of Krautkrämer (USM 2) is used, working on a frequency of 12 Mhz and only procucing one-dimensional A-scans. To avoid inaccuracy in the measurements by interference from the transmission pulse, the transducer is spaced from the cornea with help of a small water filled cup, that is fixed to the sclera by the eyelids. The measuring accuracy is 0.2 mm. For the treated infants the averaged measured distance of the front of the cornea to the back of the lens was 7 mm. This is in good agreement with other published data (Charles J. Brown, 1975).

For positioning and fixation of the patient's head during the treatment a thin-walled, highly pliable, plastic bag filled with fine plastic granules is used, which becomes rigid after evacuation with a vacuum pump.

For positioning and fixation of the eye we use X-ray localisation contact-lenses, made by Medical Workshop, Groningen. These lenses with different diameters of respectively 10.5 mm, 17 mm and 20 mm, are modified by extending the steel capillair with a soft iron rod (Fig. 4). A contact-lens of suitable diameter is fixed to the eye by creating a low vacuum in the corneal chamber of the lens. The lens automatically adjusts in a central position, so that the iron pin and the central axis of the eye are in line. Then the contact-lens and thereby also the eye are magnetically directly fixated to a perspex millimeter scale, as as shown schematically in Figure 5. The desired distance between the lens of the eye and the anterior edge of the treatment field can be set up directly with help of the mm-scale if (a) the distance between the front of the cornea and the back of the lens of the eye, (b) the distance between the millimeter scale and the edge of the irradiation beam and (c) the total length of the contact-lens, are measured.

Positioning of the beam is simple and easy with an overall accuracy of 0.5 mm. Because the centre of the eye is located in the isocentre of the accelerator, treatment can be done under any desired angle as is schematically illustrated in Figure 6. In the case that the left eye has to be treated and the

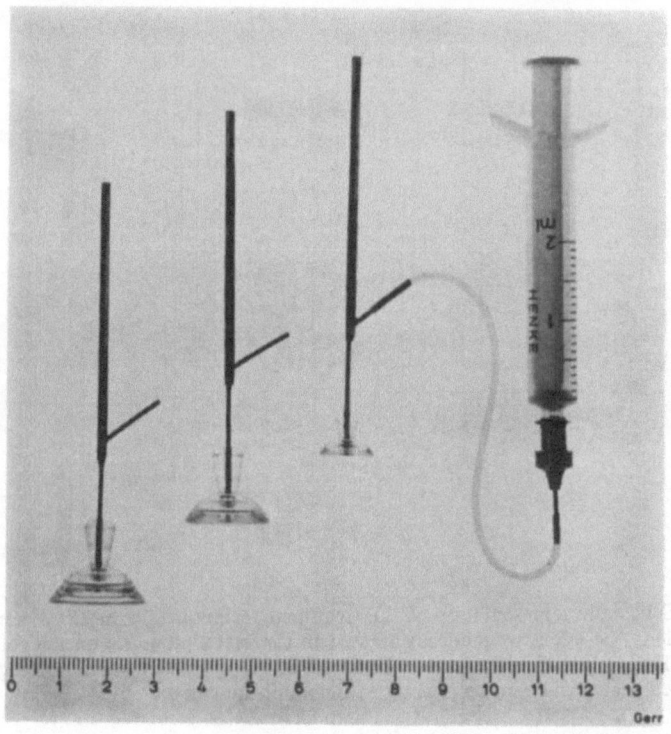

Fig. 4. Contact-lenses used for positioning and fixation of the eye. The lenses are modified by extending the steel capillair with a soft iron rod, to allow magnetic fixation of the lens to the collimatorholder.

contralateral eye has to be spared treatment can be done with the oblique lateral field 2a. If afterwards the right eye is affected with tumour, treatment can be done with field 2b. Figure 7 shows a practical example of a unilateral treatment of retinoblastoma. Radiation therapy of bilateral tumours in or behind the eyes is possible just as easy and with the same accuracy by fixation of both eyes with contact-lenses and giving alternately the fields 1a and 1b of Figure 6. A practical example of bilateral treatment of both eyes is given in Figure 8. This patient was treated for intra-orbital metastases from a primary breast carcinoma.

Verification of the correct position of the irradiation beam can be done by (a) making a portal film on the linear accelerator or by (b) direct measurment of the radiation dose on various places on the eye with help of small thermoluminescent dosemeters placed in a little perspex holder fixed to the contact-lens. We found that, if the whole treatment system is measured and calibrated correctly, verification of the beam position is not strictly necessary.

In the period from 1971 uptil now 20 eyes in 17 patients with retinoblastoma and 6 intra-orbital metastases in 5 patients have been treated with

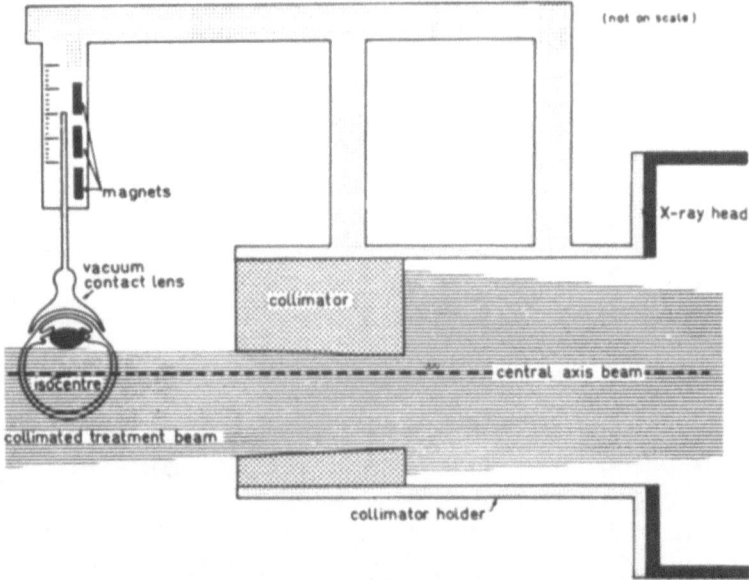

Fig. 5. Schematic representation of the treatment technique. By means of a modified contact-lens the eye is magnetically fixated to a perspex mm-scale on the collimator-holder. The desired distance between the lens of the eye and the anterior edge of the collimated beam can be set up directly with help of the mm-scale.

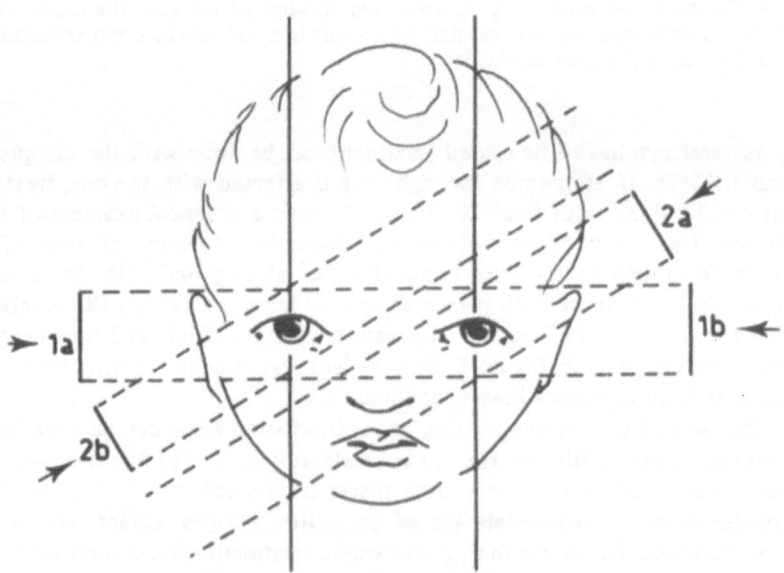

Fig. 6. Schematic representation of the treatment of unilateral and bilateral retino-blastoma or intra-orbital metastases. If the left eye is affected and the contralateral eye has to be spared, treatment can be carried out with the oblique field 2a. If afterwards the right eye is affected, treatment can be done with field 2b. If both eyes are tumo-rous simultaneously, treatment can be carried out by giving alternately the fields 1a and 1b.

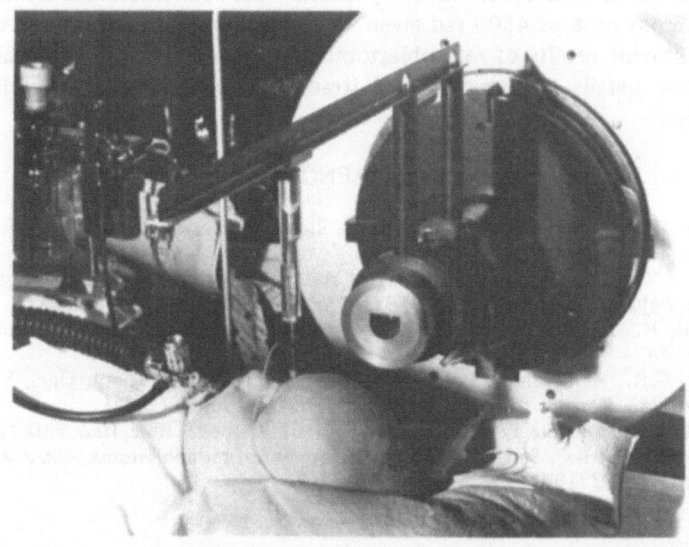

Fig. 7. Unilateral treatment of retinoblastoma. By means of the contact-lens the eye is magnetically fixated to the perspex mm-scale on the collimatorholder. Because the left eye has been enucleated before, the right eye is treated with a lateral field like field 1a in Figure 6. The head of the anesthetized patient is immobilized with an evacuated plastic pillow.

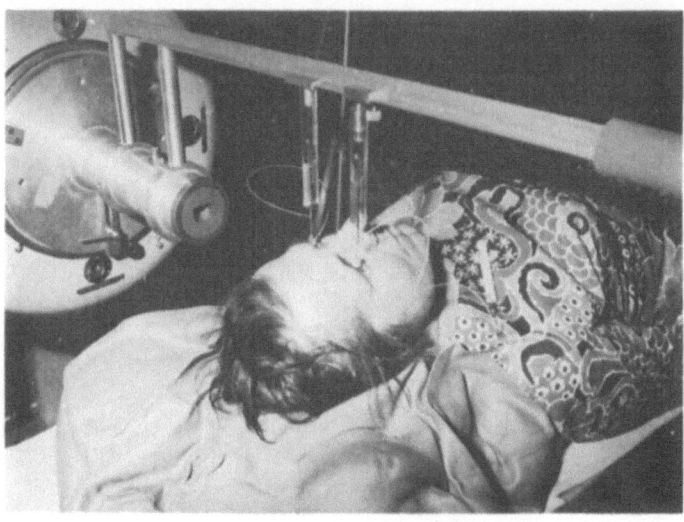

Fig. 8. Treatment of a patient with bilateral intra-orbital metastases from a primary breast carcinoma. Both eyes are fixated. The eye most near the focus of the accelerator is always placed in the isocentre. The eyes are anesthetized locally.

this irradiation technique. All the patients with retinoblastoma received a total tumour dose of 4500 rad given in 15 fractions, 3 fractions per week. The treatment results of retinoblastoma and, separately, the technical and dosimetric details of the described irradiation method will be published elsewhere.

REFERENCES

Bagshaw, M.A. & H.S. Kaplan. Supervoltage linear accelerator therapy. VIII. Retinoblastoma. *Radiology* 86: *242–246* (1966).
Charles, M.W. & N. Brown. Dimensions of the human eye relevant to radiation protection. *Phys. Med. Biol.* 20: *202–218* (1975).
Ellsworth, R.M. The practical management of retinoblastoma. *Trans. Am. Ophthal. soc.* 67: *462–534* (1969).
Merriam, G.R., A. Szechter & E.F. Focht. Front. Radiation Therp. Onc., Vol. 6, pp. 346–385. Kargerl. Basel/University Park Press, Baltimore (1972).
Reese, A. Tumors of the eye. 2nd ed., pp. 84–161. Harper & Row, New York (1963).
Thompson, R.W., R.C. Small & J.J. Stein. Treatment of retinoblastoma. *Am. J. Roentgen.* 114: *16–23* (1972).

Authors' address:
Dept of Radiotherapy
University Hospital
101 Catharijnesingel
Utrecht
The Netherlands

Proc. 3rd Int. Symp. on Orbital Disorders, Amsterdam 1977

RADIATION THERAPY OF ORBITAL TUMORS

P. LOMMATZSCH & S. MAU

(Berlin, E. Germany)

This paper presents a brief survey on the controversial field of radio-ophthalmology, based on work done at the University Eye and Tumor Clinic in Berlin. The essential problems of this field have already been discussed in the fundamental work by Lederman (1956).

RADIOTHERAPY OF PRIMARY ORBITAL TUMORS

The diagnosis of all primary orbital tumors has to be confirmed by histological examination. If the surgeon considers the tumor unsuitable for complete removal, the patient is sent to the radiotherapist. A postoperative radiation therapy is also indicated after incomplete excision of the malignant tumor.

In most of our cases, we are dealing with sarcomas of the lymphatic tissue, sometimes bilateral, rapidly growing sarcomas — especially in children — malignant tumors of the lacrimal gland, and metastatic tumors.

Radiation technique

If the eye has been removed and the tumor has not been excised completely, irradiation of the empty orbit is no problem. The application of high energy electrons has the advantage of less damage to the brain and the other eye as compared with X-rays or gamma-rays.

In some special cases, e.g. in patients with only one seeing eye, the sound eye of the orbit involved must be preserved, and the tumor around or behind the eyeball should be destroyed by irradiation. Such patients always present great problems, because on the one hand the tumor cells should be given a high dosage and, on the other hand, the eye has to be kept outside the radiation field.

The eye is radiosensitive and the following thresholds should not be exceeded in order to avoid severe radiogenic damage:

cornea	2000 rd
lens	200 rd
retina	3000 rd

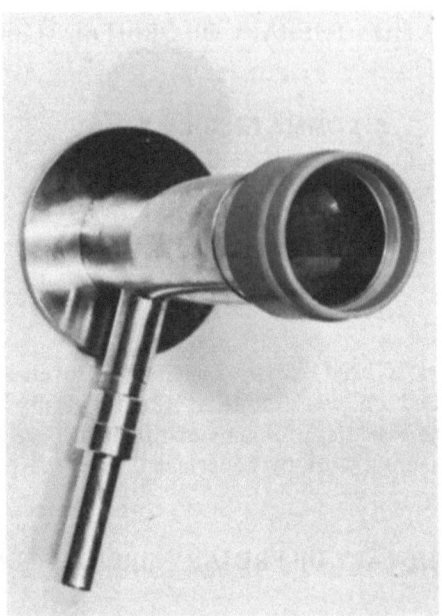

Fig. 1. Special eye tube for orbital irradiation with the betatron.

Lederman (1956) introduced the high and super voltage radiation with a frontal and temporal field. By direct or indirect eye protection the anterior part of the eyeball can be kept out of the area of damaging effects. Halnan (1962) described super voltage irradiation (4 MeV) with two angular frontal

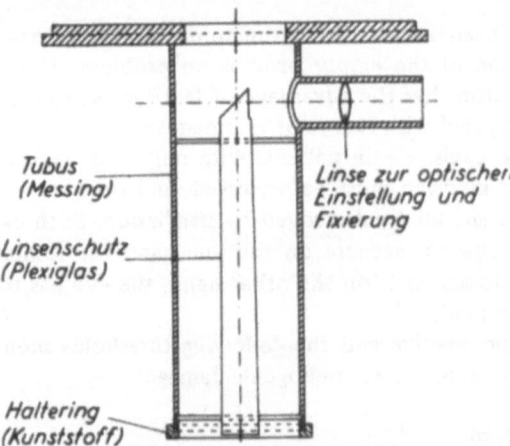

Tubus
(Messing)

Linsenschutz
(Plexiglas)

Haltering
(Kunststoff)

Linse zur optischer
Einstellung und
Fixierung

Fig. 2. Schematic view of this tube showing the central plexiglass stick to protect the eye.

470

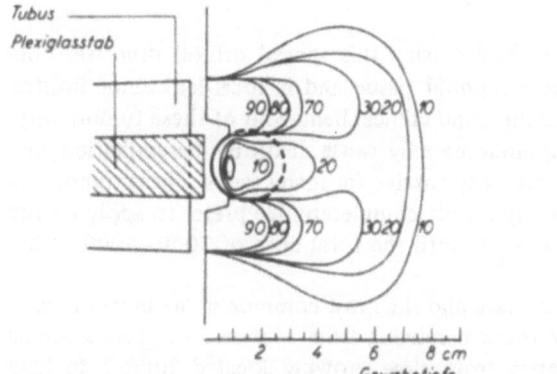
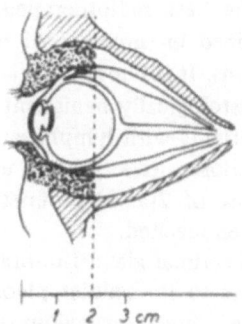

Tubus
Plexiglasstab

90 80 70 30 20 10

10 20

90 80 70 30 20 10

2 4 6 8 cm
Gewebetiefe

1 2 3 cm

Fig. 3. Isodose curves of the betatron eye tube.

fields and two absorbing wedges, but lens protection achieved in this way seems imperfect. Hohl (1972) recommended rotating high voltage radiation of the socket. The anterior part of the eye receives about 60% of the tumor dose behind the eye. This percentage is higher than that which can be attained by using Lederman's technique.

We recommend high energy electrons for the treatment of patients suffering from orbital tumors involving only the anterior part of the socket. In such cases the eye can be protected either by a direct shield of lead or tungsten or by the indirect method, using a 'plexiglass' stick fixed in the centre of the irradiation tube. For this reason we constructed a special tube for the 15 MeV betatron. Thus the irradiation field can be adjusted under optical control (Figs. 1–4). The lens remains outside the 10% isodose.

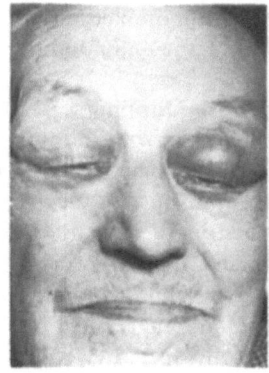
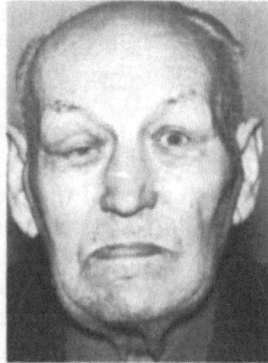
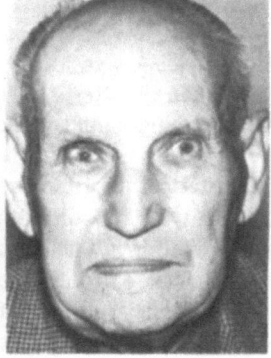

Fig. 4a. Bilateral lymphosarcoma of the anterior part of orbita.
Fig. 4b. 1 day after treatment with high energy electrons using the special eye tube and 3000 rd.
Fig. 4c. After 4 months the tumor was completely destroyed.

471

The best radiotherapeutic results using this special orbital tube were obtained in sarcomas of the lymphoid tissue and in local leukaemic infiltrations. It is known that structure and clinical behaviour of these tumors vary. Histologically benignant lymphoma may cause death by dissemination, and patients with lymphosarcoma may survive for many years. These tumors are radiosensitive and will usually recede completely. We prefer to apply a daily dose of 200 rd 5 times a week until the total dose of 3000–4000 rd has been reached.

Lacrimal gland tumors are rare and the most common is the mixed tumor. Due to its cellular pleomorphism ranging from adenoma to adenosarcoma the clinical behaviour varies from slow growing located tumors to high malignancy with generalized metastases.

As Lederman pointed out, lacrimal gland tumors are best treated by a combination of surgery and postoperative radiotherapy. The removal of the sound eye must be avoided. The postoperative super voltage or telecobalt irradiation with 5 times 200 rd a week up to a total dose of 6000 rd has to include the lacrimal fossa and large parts of the frontal bone to prevent the tumor cells from spreading through the orbital roof into the neighbouring bone. As a rule, in most patients the sound eye can be protected by a suitable shield.

The rhabdomyosarcoma of the orbit is a rare tumor and occurs mainly in children. In our experience this tumor is highly radiosensitive, but there is hardly any chance of curing it by radiotherapy, for this tumor will soon recur. Neither can recurrences be prevented by primary orbital surgery, not even by exenteratio. Therefore, we recommend a combined therapy though it will hardly succeed in saving the eye.

Lederman (1972) published his experience with 17 orbital rhabdomyosarcomas (1941–1961), and he concluded that this tumor can rarely be cured by primary radiation therapy, as recurrences after a period of impressive shrinkage are the rule and the result is only transitory. Irradiation before surgical treatment may facilitate the procedure of tumor excision or exenteratio. We irradiated these with a dose of 4000 rd before and 2000 rd after surgical operations.

Sagerman, Tretter & Ellsworth (1972) published good results in 7 cases out of 15 patients treated by using primary telecobalt beams without any eye protection. Radiation cataract, as the lesser evil, occurred in every case.

Metastatic tumors, mostly from cancer of the breast, prostata, bronchus or from sympathicoblastoma, should be treated by radiation therapy under eye protection, because the patients may survive for many months. In such cases we use a frontal field of high energy electrons, the sound eye being shielded, and a temporal field from telecobalt. This second field is tilted by $10°$ to dorsal for keeping the other eye out of the radiation zone.

RADIOTHERAPY AFTER ENUCLEATION OF
PATIENTS SUFFERING FROM CHOROID MELANOMA

We observed that postoperative radiation therapy of the socket after enucleation caused a higher survival rate of patients suffering from choroidal melanoma. This has been confirmed by statistical comparison. The reason for this effect is not quite clear, and it is an open question how local irradiation can have an influence on the growth on metastases in other organs (Lommatzsch & Dietrich, 1976).

We prefere radiation therapy with high energy electrons (15.5 MeV) and a circular frontal field. As can be seen from the isodose curves it is possible to protect the cerebral tissue behind the orbit. We apply 200 rd per day 5 times a week until 6000 rd are reached with a month's break after 4000 rd.

It should be made quite clear that the possibilities of radiation therapy of primary malignant orbital tumors are limited. Only in some cases, especially with lymphatic tumors, can we succeed in destroying the tumor and saving a seeing eye. Close cooperation between orbital surgeons and radiotherapists should be a good basis for favourable therapeutic results.

REFERENCES

Halnan, K.E. Tumors of the eye treated by radiotherapy. *Radiol. Clin.* 13: *19–28 (1962)*.

Hohl, K. Augenmalignome. Handbuch der medizinischen Radiologie, Bd. XIX, pp. 258–297, Springer-Verlag (1972).

Lederman, M. Radiotherapy in the treatment of orbital tumors. *Br. J. Ophthal.* 40: *592–610* (1956).

Lommatzsch, P., W. Seidel & G. Fürst. Spezielle Bestrahlungstechniken bei der Anwendung hochenergetischer Elektronen in der Augenheilkunde. *Klin. Mbl. Augenheilk.* *150: 45–50* (1967).

Lommatzsch, P. & B. Dietrich. The effect of orbital irradiation on the survival rate of patients with choroidal melanoma. *Ophthalmologica* (Basel) 173: *49–52* (1976).

Sagerman, R.H., P. Tretter & R.M. Ellsworth. The treatment of orbital rhabdomyosarcoma of children with primary radiation therapy. *Am. J. Roentgenol., Radium Ther. & Nucl. Med.* 114: *31–34* (1972).

Authors' addresses:
P. Lommatzsch
Augenklinik Städtisches Klinikum Berlin-Buch
Karower Strasse 11
1115 Berlin
East Germany

S. Mau
Geschwulstklinik des Bereiches Medizin der
Humboldt-Universität (Charité) Berlin
Schumannstrasse 20
104 Berlin
East Germany

Proc. 3rd Int. Symp. on Orbital Disorders, Amsterdam 1977

THE VISUAL EVOKED RESPONSE AS A SIMPLE DIAGNOSTIC PROCEDURE IN CASES OF OPTIC NERVE AND CHIASMAL LESIONS

J.T.W. VAN DALEN, A.M. FRENS & G.P.M. HORSTEN

(Amsterdam, The Netherlands)

ABSTRACT

The visual evoked response may be used as a diagnostic method for optic nerve and chiasmal lesions. We discuss a number of patients, in which the VER was the only indication for the existence of lesions in the visual system (including optic nerve and chiasmal lesions).

In several cases the diagnosis was confirmed by means of computer-assisted tomography.

The visual evoked response (VER) is a simple and quick method to test the integrity of the visual system. The VER is a gross electrical signal which reaches its maximum over the occipital cortex in response to visual stimuli.

There are two types of visual stimuli which may be used to elicit the VER:
a) Diffuse unpatterned light flashes.
b) Pattern stimulation, e.g. the checker-board patterns.

The reaction to conventional flashing is a combination of luminance response and contrast. The visual response to checker-board stimulation can be regarded as a more specific contrast response. Possibly the best method of VER-recording is the use of both methods, light-flashing and checker-board stimulation.

In the literature we found many disagreements among the various authors about the nature and significance of the deflections in the evoked response. Moreover, there usually is a great deal of variation in the results between subjects and, although to a lesser extent, in the same subject at different times of recording, even when the stimulation conditions are kept constant. This variability can be ascribed to a great number of factors, such as visual attention, habituation, electrode positioning, flash intensity, etc.

As already mentioned, the interpretation and coding of the obtained response varies from author to author. One of the well-known contemporary workers on the VER is Cijanek (1961, 1964, 1969). He subdivided the VER into eight deflections (Fig. 1). He demonstrated that the time between the administration of the flash and the appearance of peaks I, II and III is relatively constant. The conduction time between starting the flash and the occurrence of peak II seems quite reliable (Cijanek, 1969), and is used in our electrophysiological unit as an important parameter. (Many other criteria are used by other investigators.)

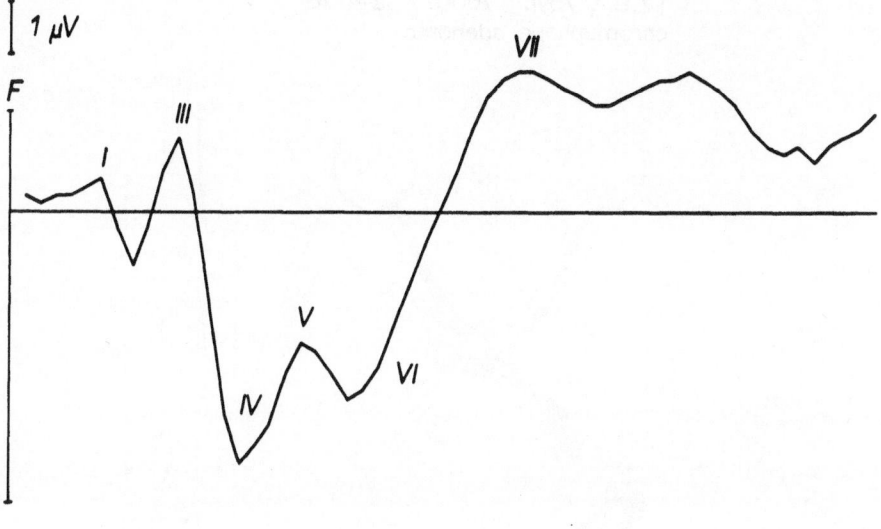

Fig. 1. The VER is subdivided into eight deflections (Cijanek).

The VER results in a number of patients, obtained by means of conventional flashing, will be discussed here.

Flashing of one eye gives rise to potentials along the optic nerve and, due to the semi-decussation in the optic-chiasm, to potentials along both optic tracts. In this way flashing of one eye will activate both occipital lobes.* It seems highly probable that a process affecting the optic nerve, the chiasmal and retro-chiasmal pathways may cause a delay in this latency time, together with an alteration of the whole VERcomplex. Chiasmal lesions, e.g., a chromofobe adenoma, may affect the crossing fibers and, more or less, spare the uncrossed fibers, as was the case in the first patient we want to discuss.

The patient was a seventy-five year old lady with a visual acuity of 2/60 in the right eye and 3/4 in the left eye. In the skull-X-ray an enlargement of the sella turcica was visible and a pituitary abnormality was suspected. The VER shows a markedly poor differentiation over the right occipital lobe indicating more damage on the right side of the optic chiasm (Fig. 2). On operating, a chromofobe adenoma was found, which indeed exerted more pressure on the right than on the left side of the chiasm.

The next patient to be discussed was a now four year old boy, who presented a retrobulbar tumor of the left orbit which was found to be an optic glioma, with extension into the cerebral cavity through the optic foramen. During the operation the left eye was enucleated together with a great deal of the intra-cerebral part of the tumor (Fig. 3). The VER from the right eye

* In normal subjects, the peak II latency time will show the same value (about 40 msec).

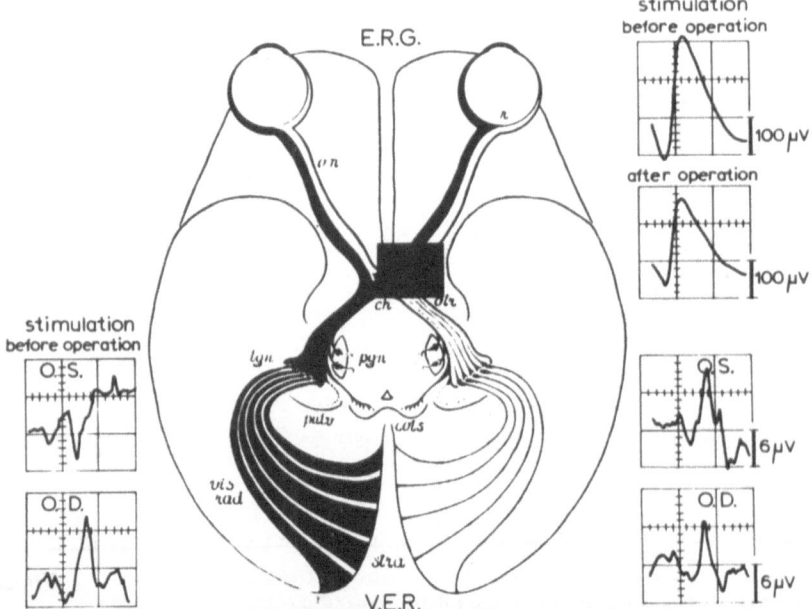

T.Z.B. ♀ 75yr.   760077   2-4-76
chromophobe adenoma

Fig. 2. The VER obtained from the right occipital region is definitely abnormal. The VER from the left occipital region is abnormal when the right eye is stimulated, but when the left eye is stimulated a normal latency time is found.

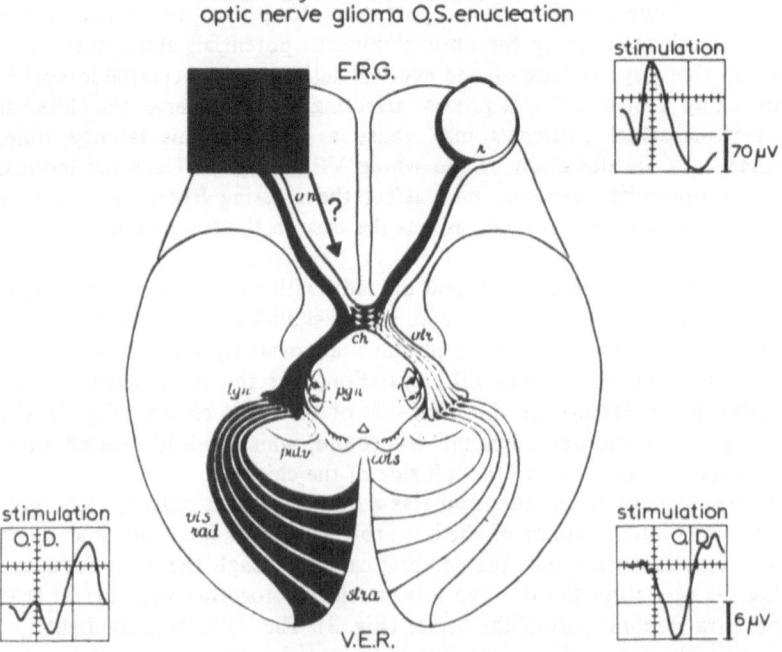

M.K.♂ 2yr.   750155   2-9-75
optic nerve glioma O.S. enucleation

Fig. 3. An abnormal VER is found after stimulation of the right eye; an extension from the tumor should be considered.

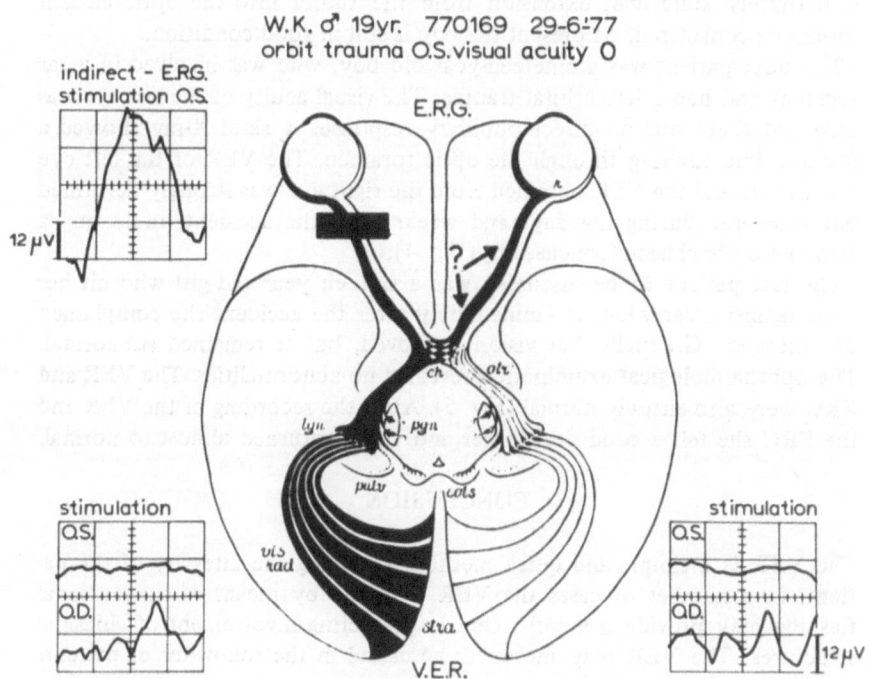

W.K. ♂ 19yr. 770169 29-6-77
orbit trauma O.S. visual acuity O

indirect – E.R.G.
stimulation O.S.

E.R.G.

12 μV

stimulation
O.S.

stimulation
O.S.
O.D.

O.D.

12 μV

V.E.R.

Fig. 4. The VER from·the left eye is absent; no VER latency time can be measured when the right eye is stimulated.

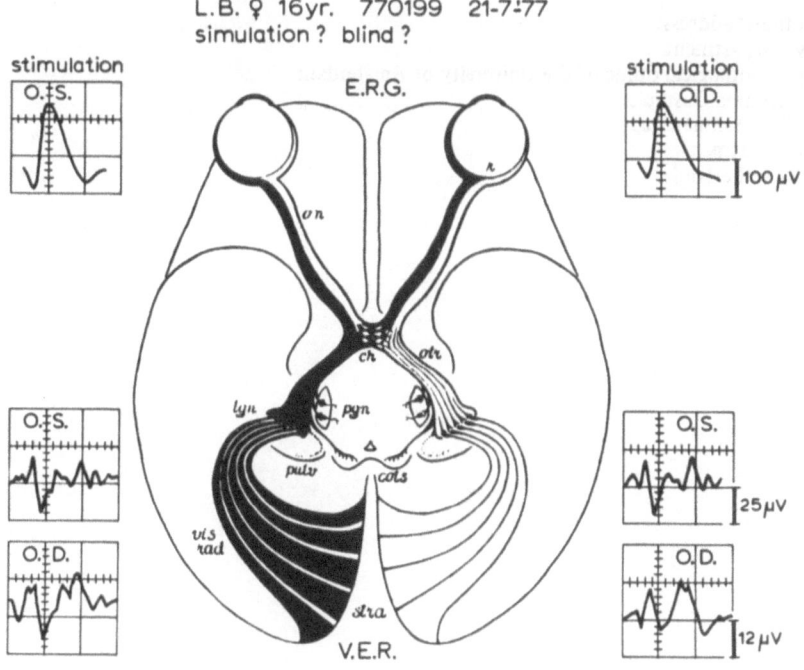

L.B. ♀ 16yr. 770199 21-7-77
simulation ? blind ?

stimulation
O.S.

E.R.G.

stimulation
O.D.

100 μV

O.S.

O.S.

25 μV

O.D.

O.D.

12 μV

V.E.R.

Fig. 5. The ERG and VER obtained from the left and right eye are entirely normal.

is definitely abnormal; extension from the tumor into the optic chiasm should be considered. At present the boy is still in good condition.

The next patient was a nineteen-year old boy, who was involved in a car accident and had a left orbital trauma. The visual acuity of the left eye was zero and there was no direct pupillary response. A skull X-ray showed a fracture line running through the optic foramen. The VER of the left eye was absent and the VER obtained from the right eye was strongly deformed but recovered during the days and weeks after the accident, indicating a damaged optic chiasm (concussion) (Fig. 4).

The last patient to be discussed was a sixteen year old girl who hit her head against a car window. Immediately after the accident she complained of blindness. Gradually her vision improved, but it remained subnormal. The ophthalmological examination revealed no abnormalities. The VER and ERG were also entirely normal (Fig. 5). After the recording of the VER and the ERG she felt a good deal better and vision returned almost to normal.

CONCLUSION

The VER is a simple and quick method of testing the integrity of the patient. In a number of cases the VER obtained by means of conventional flashing may provide a helpful clue in predicting involvement of chiasmal structures. The VER may moreover be useful in the follow-up of patients operated on for an orbital or retro-orbital lesion.

Comparison of responses from the left and right occipital lobe may provide further information concerning the nature of a possible disease.

Authors' address:
Eye Department
Opthalmological Clinic of the University of Amsterdam
Wilhelmina Gasthuis
104, 1e Helmerstraat
Amsterdam
The Netherlands

Proc. 3rd Int. Symp. on Orbital Disorders, Amsterdam 1977

FOLDS IN THE POSTERIOR POLE OF THE EYE IN ORBITAL DISORDERS

R. WIJNGAARDE & G. BLAAUW

(Rotterdam, The Netherlands)

The routine examination of patients with orbital diseases includes funduscopy. Although papilloedema and optic atrophy are frequently seen, changes outside the optic disc occur less often. These changes include scleral indentation by tumors, which lie against and impress the eye, and which are often surrounded by circular folds. In this paper we want to discuss a second phenomenon, which is much less understood. This is the occurrence of linear and curved folds, which are found remote from the tumor, and which usually occur between the optic disc and the macula.

SUBJECTS

From a series of approximately 200 patients with orbital diseases 12 cases were found where folds were present upon funduscopy. Table 1 shows some data of these cases. The total series includes miscellaneous tumors, cases with inflammatory pseudotumors, thyroid dysfunctions, vascular abnormalities, and cases with orbital trauma. In this series a cavernous haemangioma was found in 10 patients, seven of whom had folds in the posterior pole. Of the three patients without folds, one had a large tumor which lay outside the muscle cone, in the two others the haemangioma was present inside the muscle cone.

Table 1. Some data concerning 12 cases with folds in the posterior pole.

	no. of patients	age years
cavernous haemangioma	7	3–60 (mean 41)
benign lacrimal gland tumor	1	57
neurinoma	1	20
mucocele	1	23
metastasis	1	61
thyroid dysfunction	1	47

DISCUSSION

Choroidal folds are lines or grooves of the posterior pole of the eye, which appear as approximately parallel alternating light and dark lines usually radiating from the disc across the macula. Since their description by Nettleship in 1884 they have been noticed in ocular, orbital and intracranial diseases. The introduction of fluorescein angiography has greatly aided in their diagnosis. Norton (1969) described them as alternating hypo- and hyperfluorescent lines. Until the use of fluorescein angiography, a clinical distinction between retinal and choroidal folds was difficult.

Retinal and choroidal folds have been described incidentally. Table 2 presents a summary of these cases from the literature. From a total of 83 reported cases with retinal and choroidal folds, which were observed during funduscopy, an orbital disorder was present in 36 cases.

The pathogenesis of folding is still not clear. Bullock & Egbert (1974a, b) demonstrated the ability of Bruch's membrane in fresh cadaver eyes to form parallel folds. Choroidal folds were produced in vivo in cat's eyes by traction on the optic nerve or by hypotony after paracentesis. Traction caused the folds to assume a parallel alignment opposite to the direction of traction. They thought that choroidal folds are produced by any mechanism that forces Bruch's membrane to fold, and that traction on the optic nerve plays a role in the characteristic orientation of choroidal folds. Von Winning

Table 2.

		orbital disorders	intraocular disorders	intracranial disorders	congenital
Nettleship	1884	–	–	1	–
Birsch & Hirschfeld	1930	1	–	–	–
Kugelberg	'32	1	–	–	–
Blegvad	'44	1	–	–	–
Della Porta	1954–'55	–	5	–	–
Hedges	'59	2	–	–	–
Vedel-Jensen	'59	1	–	–	–
Wolter	'62	3	–	–	–
Norton	'68	3	7	–	–
Rosen	'67	2	4	–	–
Scott	'67	–	–	1	–
Shikano	'68	1	1	–	–
Almaric	1968–'70	–	–	–	4
Hyvärinen	'70	3	–	–	–
Krill	'70	2	1	–	–
Gass	'71	–	1	–	–
Velzeboer	'71	1	–	–	–
de Laey	'71	–	1	–	–
Newell	'73	8	8	–	–
Bird	'73	–	–	8	–
Wolter	'74	1	–	–	–
Bullock	'74	6	4	1	–
		36	32	11	4

Table 3. Folds in 36 patients with an orbital disorder reported in the literature.

1915–1968	cavernous haemangioma	1
	other causes	6
1968–1974	cavernous haemangioma	5
	other causes	24

(1972) suggested, that edema of the posterior pole may play a role as well. Edema of the retina causes the retina to fold over the pigment epithelium, which may then show edematous changes due to the formation of subretinal fluid, thus causing the pigment epithelium to fold as well.

From our series a marked preference for an occurrence of folds in patients with a cavernous haemangioma seems to be present. The tumor is usually situated in close relation to the optic nerve. It may be that traction on the optic nerve is a main factor in the production of folds in these cases. Blood circulation factors may play a role as well, causing hyperaemia and congestion of the choriocapillaris.

We performed fluorescein angiography only in those cases where folds were noticed during funduscopy. More cases might, however, be discovered when angiography had been performed routinely. We have grouped the cases with folds from the literature in relation to the time of the development of fluorescein angiography (Table 3). It is evident from this table, that the frequency of occurrence of folds in patients with a cavernous haemangioma was not greatly altered after the introduction of fluorescein angiography.

SUMMARY

From a series of 200 patients who visited an orbital clinic, 12 cases are reported in whom folding in the posterior pole was noticed. Seven of these patients proved to have a cavernous haemangioma. In three more cases with the same tumor folding was not present. The close relation of these tumors to the optic nerve was thought to be a main factor in the production of retinal and choroidal folds.

REFERENCES

Bullock, J.D. & P.R. Egbert. Experimental choroidal folds. *Am. J. Ophthal.* 78: *618– 623* (1974a).

Bullock, J.D. & P.R. Egbert. The origin of choroidal folds, a clinical, histopathological and experimental study. *Docum. Ophthal.* 37: *261–293* (1974b).

Nettleship, E. Peculiar lines in the choroid in a case of papillitic atrophy. *Trans. Ophthal. Soc. U.K.* 4: *167* (1884).

Norton, E.W.D. A characteristic fluorescein angiographic pattern in choroidal folds. *Proc. Roy. Soc. Med.* 62: 1–10 (1969).

Winning, C.H.O.M. Von. Fluorgraphy of choroidal folds. *Docum. Ophthal.* 31: *209– 249* (1972).

Authors' address:
Eye Hospital Rotterdam and
Department of Neurosurgery
Erasmus University
Rotterdam
The Netherlands

Proc. 3rd Int. Symp. on Orbital Disorders, Amsterdam 1977

CHOROIDAL FOLDING IN ORBITAL DISEASE

JOHN D. BULLOCK & ROBERT R. WALLER

(Dayton, Ohio / Rochester, Minn.)

Choroidal folds are lines or grooves of the posterior pole of the eye which appear as approximately parallel alternating light and dark lines, usually radiating from the disc across the macula. These folds are seen in a variety of orbital and ocular conditions, including orbital inflammation and tumors, hyperopia, scleritis, choroidal tumors, hypotony, retinal or choroidal detachments, papilledema, or after retinal detachment surgery (Bullock & Egbert, 1974).

Norton (1969) further elucidated the nature of these folds by describing alternating hypo- and hyper- fluorescent lines seen on fluorescein angiography. This fluorescein angiographic pattern is said to result from a folding of the retinal pigment epithelium with thinning of the pigment epithelium at the crest of the fold and a compression of pigment in the trough of the fold. In 1962, J. Reimer Wolter described three pathological changes associated with choroidal folds. He described these changes in the eyes of patients whose orbits were exenterated for malignant tumors. He noted internal limiting membrane folds, Bruch's membrane folds, as well as 'brain-like' corrugations of the retina (Wolter, 1962). Reese (1976) attributed the choroidal folds to indentation of the globe by an orbital tumor. Reese makes the following statement: 'Indentation of the sclera is indicated by retinal striae. This is an accurate localizing sign, and it justifies proceeding with the Krönlein operation for removal of a tumor localized in the orbit at the site indicated by the area of retinal striae.' Numerous clinical observations, however, have gone against Reese's theory. Newell (1973) has observed that in exophthalmos due to orbital tumors, the position of the folds is of no value in localizing the tumor.

In 1974, Bullock & Egbert published two papers describing the mechanisms involved in choroidal folding and performed a number of experimental studies to further elucidate their nature. One experiment involved placing a Fogarty embolectomy catheter behind the eyes of cats and inflating the catheters. This caused a marked proptosis of the eye. In no instance were choroidal folds produced by the Fogarty catheter. In addition, they described a series of patients in whom they had observed choroidal folding. One patient had bilateral orbital pseudotumor with unilateral choroidal folds. They speculated that the folding was due to the greater proptosis on the side with the folds and theorized that a backward traction force on the optic nerve (which emanates from the nasal side of the globe) would be responsible for the choroidal folds radiating from the optic nerve head temporally across the macular area.

They also produced an animal model of choroidal folds in cats by placing polyethylene tubes around the optic nerve and applying traction to the optic nerve. Folds were created in a direction opposite to the applied traction force. Histologic sections were then prepared from the experimental globes and folding of the retinal pigment epithelium was demonstrated. In addition, 'brain-like' corrugations of the retina were also produced, similar to those noted by Wolter (1962).

The above observations led these authors to speculate that one mechanism of choroidal folding may relate to traction on the optic nerve. The following case reports substantiate this new theory of choroidal folding.

Case 1

A forty-five-year-old white female was noted to have a mucocele of the ethmoid sinus. This was documented by a computerized transaxial tomo-

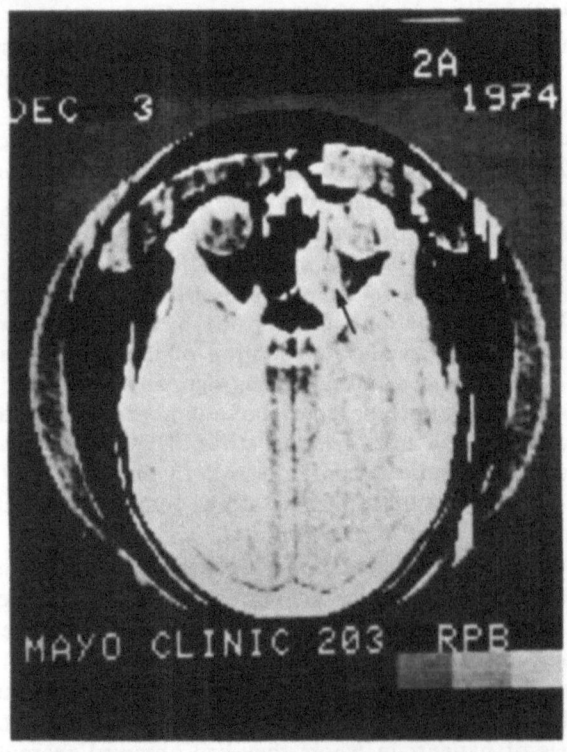

Fig. 1. Computerized transaxial tomographic scan of Case 1 showing prominent right nasal orbital mucocele. Note that the mass does not touch the temporal aspect of the globe.

484

graphic scan (Figure 1). The CT scan shows a mass within the orbit arising from the nasal side of the orbit. The temporal side of the orbit shows no evidence of a tumor touching the sclera. Choroidal folds however, were noted on the temporal side of the right eye (Figure 2). The folding was also demonstrated by fluorescein angiography (Figure 3).

Case 2

A sixty-five-year-old male was seen because of massive proptosis of the left eye. Examination of the left fundus showed prominent choroidal folds radiating from the optic nerve head across the macular area (Figure 4). An EMI scan showed massive proptosis of the left eye with a soft tissue density within the orbital apex. This is thought to represent enlarged extraocular muscles due to Graves' disease. The EMI scan clearly showed no mass lesion contiguous with the sclera at any point, and there is a clear segment of optic nerve observed between the apparent apical lesion and the globe (Figure 5).

DISCUSSION

Previous work (Bullock & Egbert, 1974) has substantiated the observations of Newell (1973) that choroidal folds are of no localizing value in orbital tumors. Their work documented this at the experimental level also. They

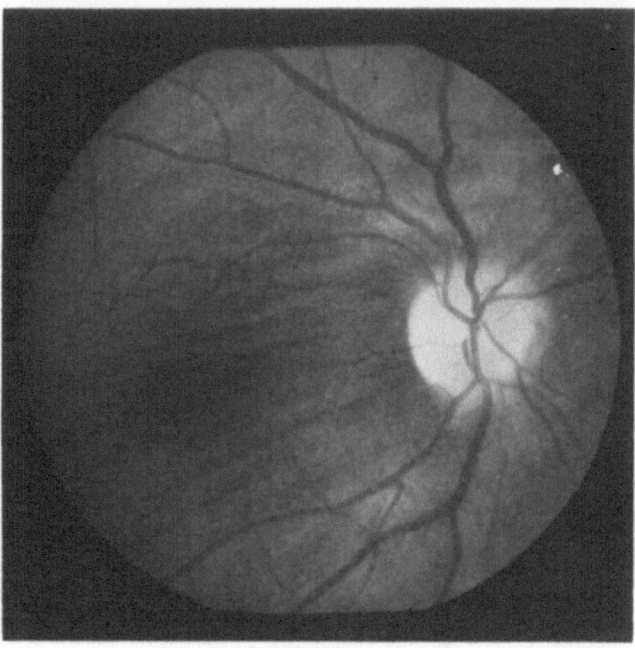

Fig. 2. Fundus photograph, right eye, Case 1, showing prominent choroidal folds radiating from the optic nerve head across the macular area.

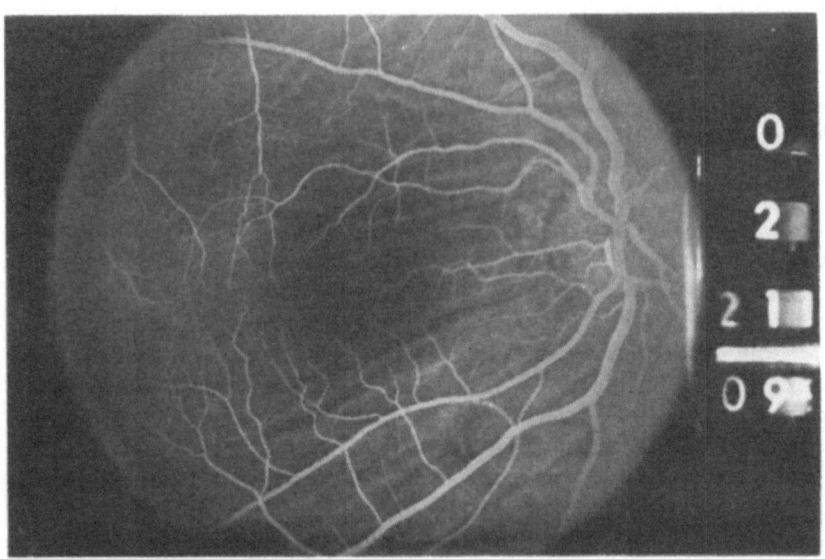

Fig. 3. Fluorescein angiogram, right eye, Case 1, showing typical alternating light and dark retinal lines, in the macular area, indicative of choroidal folds.

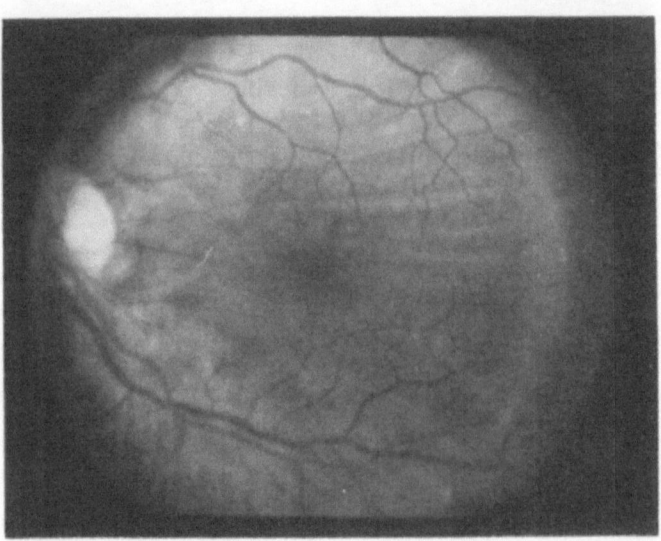

Fig. 4. Fundus photograph, left eye, Case 2, showing prominent choroidal folds radiating across the macular area.

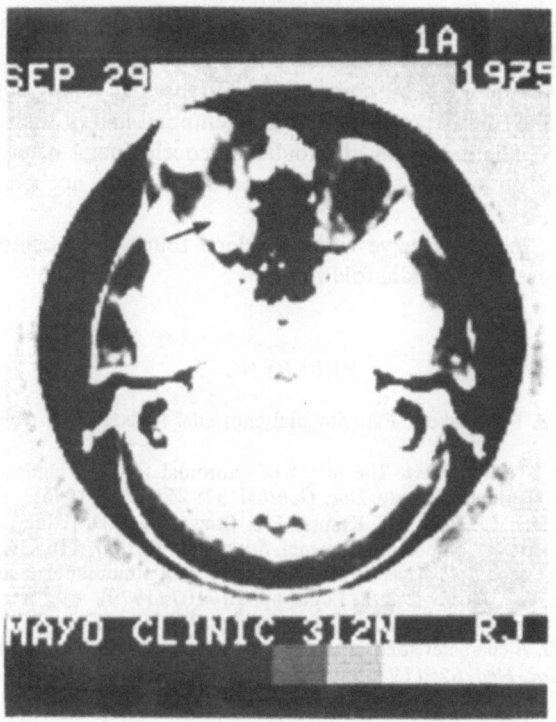

Fig. 5. Computerized tomographic scan, Case 2, showing prominent mass in the apex of the left orbit. Note the absence of scleral touch and the clear segment of the optic nerve between the mass and the globe.

theorized that choroidal folds could be due to traction on the optic nerve in the absence of scleral touch. They created, for the first time, an animal model of choroidal folds based on traction on the optic nerve.

Case 1 documents choroidal folding in a patient with an ethmoid mucocele where the EMI scan shows a tumor on the nasal side of the eye which has not touched the globe temporally, yet the choroidal folds were located temporally. Case 2 shows an apical soft tissue density which does not touch the sclera at any point, and yet choroidal folds were located temporally. These two cases substantiate the newer theory of Bullock & Egbert (1974) and serve to further refute that of Reese (1976).

CONCLUSIONS

1. Choroidal folds are not an accurate localizing sign of an orbital tumor.
2. One mechanism of choroidal folding may relate to traction on the optic nerve in the absence of scleral touch.

487

SUMMARY

Two patients are presented with choroidal folds where the location of the tumor was documented by computerized transaxial tomography. In both cases, choroidal folds were located on the temporal half of the retina. In one instance the patient had an ethmoidal mucocele (nasal orbit) and in the other patient an orbital apex soft tissue density did not even touch the sclera.

Traction on the optic nerve without scleral touch by an orbital tumor is a presumed cause of choroidal folding.

REFERENCES

Bullock, J.D. & P.R. Egbert. Experimental choroidal folds. *Am. J. Ophthal.* 78: *618* (1974).

Bullock, J.D. & P.R. Egbert. The origin of choroidal folds. A clinical, histo-pathological, and experimental study. *Doc. Ophthal.* 37: *261–293* (1974).

Fogarty, T.J., J.J. Cranley, R.J. Krause, E.S. Strasser & C.D. Hafner. A method for extraction of arterial emboli and thrombi. *Surg. Gyn. Obstetr.* 116: *241* (1963).

Gass, J.D.M. Stereoscopic Atlas of Macular Diseases: A funduscopic and angiographic presentation. C.V. Mosby Co., St. Louis, pp. 98–107 (1970).

Newell, F.W., Choroidal folds. *Am. J. Ophthal.* 75: *930* (1973).

Norton, E.W.D. A characteristic fluorescein angiographic pattern in choroidal folds. *Proc. Roy. Soc. Med.* 62: *119* (1969).

Reese, A.B. Tumors of the Eye. Harper & Row, New York. 3rd ed., pp. 434–435 (1976).

Wolter, J.R. Parallel horizontal retinal folding. *Am. J. Ophthal.* 53: *26* (1962).

Authors' addresses:

John D. Bullock
Wright State University
Dayton, Ohio
USA

Robert R. Waller
Mayo Clinic
Rochester, Minn.
USA

Proc. 3rd Int. Symp. on Orbital Disorders, Amsterdam 1977

AN ERG INDICATION OF THE EXISTENCE OF
OPTIC NERVE LESIONS

J.P. WITMER

(Amsterdam, The Netherlands)

The relationship between the amplitude of the b wave and the existence of an optic nerve lesion is still controversial. Experimental observations have shown that a disturbance of impulse propogation through the fibers of the optic nerve can cause changes in the electroretinogram (ERG) (Abe, 1962; Borg & Knave, 1971; Jacobson & Suzuki, 1962).

Clinical observations also show that in patients with section of the optic nerve, optic neuritis, (posttraumatic) optic atrophy and compression of the optic nerve by tumors changes in the ERG, in the sense of supernormal b wave amplitude, are often found (Henkes, 1957; Gills, 1966; Feinsod & Auerbach, 1971, Feinsod et al., 1971).

Feinsod et al. (1971) examined 69 cases of optic nerve atrophy electrophysiologically; 42% displayed a supernormal b wave amplitude. But these workers also described 7 patients with low visual acuity who exhibited an enhanced positive response in the ERG and a reduced or extinct visual evoked response (VER) without signs of optic nerve involvement (Feinsod et al., 1971). The question is, how can the strongly abnormal VER be reconciled with an intact retinal function such as existed in 5 patients?

The existence of centrifugal fibers in the optic nerve leads to the hypothesis of an inhibitory cerebral control on retinal function. Other reports, however, provide histologic and electrophysiologic evidence against the existence of a centrifugal influence on the retina via the optic nerve (Brindley & Hamasaki, 1962, 1966).

These differences in opinion make the enhancement of b wave amplitude in cases of optic nerve affection still controversial. We possess a considerable amount of data on this subject and the positive findings of Feinsod et al. (1971) led us to evaluate our material. From this evaluation we now wish to present a preliminary report, dealing especially with the effect of trauma on the ERG.

In our material, from 1973 till July 1977, we had 315 ERGs requested on suspicion of optic nerve lesions. The ERGs of 151 patients showed an obviously supernormal b wave amplitude.

Of a random sample of 100 patients whose ERG was requested for reasons other than optic nerve lesions, the ERGs of only 11 patients showed an obviously supernormal b wave amplitude. These results point to an evident relationship between optic nerve lesions and amplitude of the b wave.

489

Further, we had the impression that optic neuritis showed a rise of b wave amplitude more often than optic atrophy. It is possible that a relationship exists with the duration of the lesion; this would confirm the findings of Borg & Knave (1971) who studied the long-term changes in the ERG after transection of the optic nerve in rabbits and found a constant increase for the next 8 months, followed by a decrease.

In connection with this symposium we analysed those cases of orbital or cranial trauma which were referred to the electrophysiological unit, most of them from the Orbital Centre of Professor Bleeker. We examined 48 patients with suspected optic nerve lesions due to orbital trauma, including blunt head injury, orbital fracture and orbital stab wound.

Nineteen patients exhibited an obviously supernormal b wave amplitude. 17 of them had a clinically verified optic nerve lesion as evidenced by reduced visual acuity, pallor of the optic disc, visual field defects and an abnormal VER.

Twenty-nine patients exhibited a normal or decreased b wave amplitude, and yet 10 of these had a clinically verified optic nerve lesion. Of these 10 patients, 6 had a lesion of more than 1.5 to 5 years standing before they came to our clinic and 4 showed retinal lesions or impairment of retinal circulation. In the latter 4 cases the generation of the b wave was seriously impaired.

We conclude that an optic nerve lesion can cause an enhancement of the b wave amplitude and that a relationship may exist between the time elapsed after the injury and the amplitude of the b wave. In cases of unilateral orbital trauma a supernormal b wave amplitude could be recorded from both eyes. Probably this bilateral b wave enhancement is caused by concussion of the total optic pathways. This view is supported by the findings in patients with a blunt head injury from our material, whose ERG from both eyes showed a supernormal b wave amplitude.

Additionally we should like to present the case of a 74-year-old woman. For seven months she had been suffering from reduced visual acuity. At admission her visual acuity was: OD 2/60 and OS 2/3. The visual field showed a bitemporal upper quadrantanopia. Electrophysiologically a supernormal b wave was recorded from OD and a normal ERG from OS. The VER on both sides was poorly differentiated and showed a lengthened latency. She was found to have a chromphobe pituitary adenoma. One week after operation the ERG of the right eye had a normal b wave.

SUMMARY

On the basis of the results of this preliminary study of 315 cases of suspected optic nerve lesions, and especially of 48 cases with suspected optic nerve lesions due to orbital trauma, we argue that an enhancement of the b wave amplitude in the ERG may be an indication of the existence of optic nerve lesions.

The author would like to thank Miss A.M. Frens for the skillful technical assistance.

REFERENCES

Abe, N. Effect of section and compression of the optic nerve on the ERG in the rabbit. *Tohoku J. Exp. Med.* 78: *223–227* (1962).

Borg, E. & B. Knave. Long-term changes in the ERG following transection of the optic nerve in the rabbit. *Acta Physiol. Scand.* 82: *277–281* (1971).

Brindley, G.S. & D.I. Hamasaki. Evidence that cat's electroretinogram is not influenced by impulses passing to the eye along the optic nerve. *J. Physiol.* 163: *558–565* (1962).

Brindley, G.S. & D.I. Hamasaki. Histological evidence against the view that the cat's optic nerve contains centrifugal fibres. *J. Physiol.* 184: *444–449* (1966).

Feinsod, M. & E. Auerbach. The electroretinogram and the visual evoked potential in two patients with tuberculum sellae meningioma before and after decompression of the optic nerve. *Ophthalmologica* 163: *360–368* (1971).

Feinsod, M., H. Rowe & E. Auerbach. Changes in the electroretinogram in patients with optic nerve lesions. *Doc. Ophthal.* 29: *169–200* (1971).

Feinsod, M., H. Rowe & E. Auerbach. Enhanced retinal responses without signs of optic nerve involvement. *Doc. Ophthal.* 29: *201–211* (1971).

Gills, J.P. The electroretinogram after section of the optic nerve in man. *Am. J. Ophthal.* 62: *287–291* (1966).

Henkes, H.E. Electroretinography. *Am. J. Ophthal.* 43: *67–86* (1957).

Jacobson, J.H. & T.A. Suzuki. Effects of optic nerve section on the ERG. *Arch. Ophthal.* 67: *791–801* (1962).

Author's address:
Electrophysiology Unit
University Eye Clinic
Wilhelmina Gasthuis
104, 1e Helmerstraat
Amsterdam
The Netherlands

Proc. 3rd Int. Symp. on Orbital Disorders, Amsterdam 1977

ISOMETRIC CONTRACTION OF THE EXTRAOCULAR MUSCLES

J.L. VROOLAND

(Amsterdam, The Netherlands)

For many years investigators have been trying to get a quantitative impression of the pulling power of eye muscles. Until about 1967 the only methods of assessment were Electromyography (EMG) and the Forced Duction Test (FDT). In particular, EMG is of great value. In neurological disease and in trauma it offers the possibility of differentiating between a normal, paretic, or a wholly paralysed muscle. In addition, it is possible to distinguish a paralysed muscle from one that has been trapped in the orbital floor after a 'blow-out' fracture.

In squint, Electromyography was used by many investigators to identify the cause of deviation of the eye or abnormal eye motility. Strachan et al . (1975), Scott (1971) and Madroszkiewisz (1970) all observed strange phenomena in the EMG of the Duane Syndrome.

Lately, we have used a new technique to measure the contraction force of an eye muscle and to correlate it with the EMG. Esslen (1967) already described his method for estimating this force. However, he had to detach the muscles under local anesthesia during an operation for squint and he had to attach some sutures to the muscles in order to make his measurements. Madroszkiewisz (1970) obtained the same result with an oculodynamometer built by himself. Both investigators were in agreement that a muscle in isometrical contraction ·· able to exert the force of 60 gram.

Scott (1971) went as far as freeing the horizontal muscles from the surrounding tissues over a distance of approximately 2 cm posteriorly to the insertion. The muscle was connected by a 3.0 suture to a strain gauge force transducer that was attached to a warm-drive micromanipulator. Before the measurements, the muscles were stretched to a given length. Then, the patient was requested to fix his gaze on a target and with the sutures still attached to the globe, Scott measured the passive globe rotation. He reached an estimate of a gram/degree ratio of 0.4 or more. At the same time he was able to obtain a record of the rapidity of the saccadic movements and of the muscle forces. Under full anaesthesia he obtained values of 0.25 and 0.33 gram/degree for the tonic elasticity of the passive muscle components of the globe suspensory tissues.

In our experiments we use the device shown in Fig. 1. The apparatus consists of a suction cup with a diameter of 12 mm. This cup is placed on the eye and fixed with a negative pressure by pulling the syringe. The pressure is

492

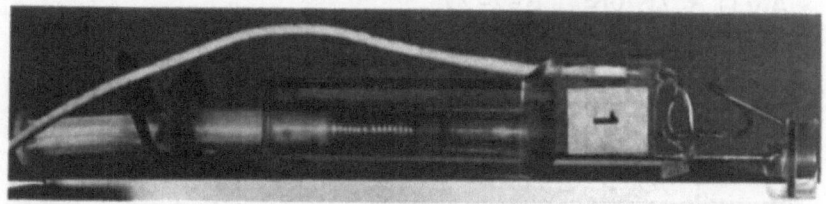

easily-calculated with Boyle's law, PV = C. In our case the volume is in expanded form 0.5 cm³ to 1.5 cm³ and the negative pressure on the eye is approx. 1/3 atmosphere during several minutes. In their experiments, Stephens & Reinecke (1967) used a negative pressure of 70-80 mm, equivalent to 0.1 atmosphere, during the 10 minutes of the experiment. Slight conjunctival irritation was the only complication.

DESCRIPTION OF THE EXPERIMENT

At first, the patient looks straight forward while the cup is fixed on the eye. Then the patient is requested to look 40 degrees to the left or to the right. The electric transducer near the cup gives a signal to the monitor.

In the beginning we had no problems with normal eyes. The experiment was not a burden to the patient as long as we used two harmless anaesthetic eyedrops. Except for an occasional corneal edema of short duration the patients had no ill-effects. We did not experiments on patients operated for glaucoma or on children.

According to these principles, we found that the average horizontal or vertical eye muscle can produce a force of 8-10 grams. But we had problems in cases of passive motility disturbances by adhesion of orbital tissues, as mentioned by Koornneef, for instance, in the case of a trapped muscle.

Figure 2 shows the results of a patient with orbital fracture and diplopia resulting from a trapped inferior rectus muscle. It is evident that the trapped muscle is functioning better than its antagonist, although both muscles showed a normal EMG. Actually, this is not surprising because we have not measured the forces exerted by the muscle itself, but the sum of all mechanical torques.

Here we find:

$$M_O = \Delta_{\omega 1} \cdot Dm$$

where
$\Delta_{\omega 1}$ = rotation force of the eye
D_{ω} = reacting momentum of the apparatus, but when there is a tumor or a fracture with an abnormal rigidity the formula should be:

$$M_O = \Delta_{\omega 2} \cdot (Dm + D_O)$$

D_O = reacting momentum of the eye. It represents here the resistance

493

A.v. D ♂ 46 yrs   6-7-'77

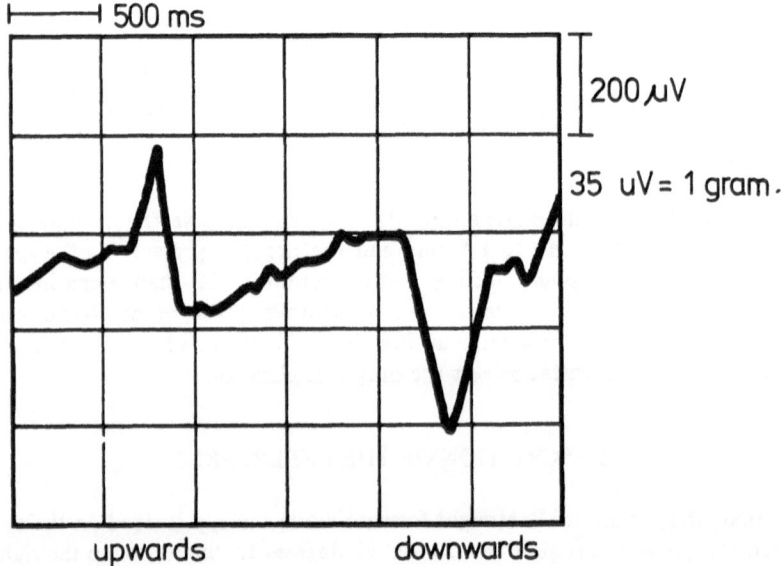

upwards   downwards

and the elasticity of the antagonist and of the orbital tissues. Thus, when D_O becomes greater, $\Delta\omega_2$ has to be smaller.

After combining these formulas, we come to the following comparison

$$\frac{\Delta\omega_2}{\Delta\omega_1} = \frac{D_m}{D+D_m} \leqslant 1$$

Conlusions:
1) D_m has to be as small as possible
2) If D_O increases, we find a smaller value
3) We have to know the relation between D_O and D_m.
This leaves us with two unknown factors to complicate our investigations. Our solution to this problem is that we measure the forces of the eye muscles during activation by the patient. To get information about the elasticity and the resistance we try to move the eye with a known force applied to the suction cup.

For this paper we have limited ourselves to patients suffering from orbital trauma. Future experiments will be devoted to measurements of forces involved in squint or even to the forces involved in convergence movements.

REFERENCES

Collins, C.C., A.B. Scott & D.M. O 'Meara. Elements of the peripheral oculomotor apparatus. *Am. J. Optom.* 46: *510–515* (1969);

Esslen, E. & A. Huber. Electromyografisch Innervationsanalyse des Strabismus Concomitans. Über die beim Strabismus Concomitans wirksamen Muskelkräfte. *Ophthalmologica* 154: *189−200* (1966).

Huber, A. Electromyography of eye muscles. *Trans. Ophthalm. Soc. U.K.* 82: *455− 472* (1962).

Lennerstrand, G. & P. Bachrita. Basic mechanism of ocular motility and their clinical implications. Proc. International Symp. Stockholm, 1974. Pergamon Pres, New York (1975).

Madroszkiewics, M. Oculodynamometry. The strength and work of extra-ocular muscles in squint. *Ophthalmologica* 161: *491−498* (1970);

Metz, H.S., A.B. Scott, D.M. O'meara & H.Za. Stewart. Ocular saccades in lateral rectus palsy. *Arch. Ophthal.* 84: *453−460* (1970).

Metz, H.S. & A.B. Scott. The innervational plasticity of the ocular system. *Arch. Ophthal.* 84: *86−91* (1970).

O'Meara, D.M., H.S. Metz, H.L. Stewart & A.B. Scott. Eye movements pattersn in strabismus. *Invest. Ophthal.* 8: *651* (1969).

Robinson, D.A., D.M. O'Meara, A.B. Scott & C.C. Collins. Mechanical components of human eye movements. *J.Appl. Phys.* 26: *548−553* (1969).

Scott, A.B. Active force tests in lateral rectus paralysis. *Arch. Ophthal.* 85: *397−404* (1971).

Stephens, K.F. & R.D. Reinecke. Quantitative foced dusction. *Trans. Am. Acad. O & O* 71: *324−329* (1967).

Strachan, I.M., B.H. Brown, S.G. Johnson & P. Robinson. New apparatus for measuring forces in strabismus. *Trans. Ophthal. Soc. U.K.* 95: *85−87* (1975).

Author's address:
Nic. Japiksestr. 61
Amsterdam
The Netherlands

Proc. 3rd Int. Symp. on Orbital Disorders, Amsterdam 1977

THE ROLE OF CLINICAL ECHOGRAPHY IN MODERN DIAGNOSIS OF PERIORBITAL AND ORBITAL LESIONS

KARL C. OSSOINIG

(Iowa City, Iowa)

INTRODUCTION

Echography of the orbit has come a long way since it was introduced by Gilbert Baum in 1958 1,2. Baum used a highly sophisticated B-scan unit; although his technique based on very expensive laboratory equipment had no real change of spreading, Baum proved that ultrasonography of the orbit was possible and useful 3. In the early 1960's A-scan methods were developed which helped to detect, measure and localize orbital tumors with a high degree of reliability and accuracy 4-6. At that time, even a limited differential diagnosis of orbital tumors was possible.

During the following years, A-scan equipment was continuously improved; intensive clinical and experimental investigations of the various system parameters were conducted in order to optimize the instrument design for tissue diagnosis in the eye and orbit 7-17. At the same time, relatively inexpensive B-scan equipment was designed, and for the first time both A- and B-scan methods were combined for orbital diagnosis 18-26. In 1971 the first *standardized* A-scan instrument specifically designed for ophthalmic tissue diagnosis was introduced 27-65. Using this instrument and advanced examination techniques, tissue differentiation in the orbit and periorbital region was markedly improved and extended in the early 1970's: more than 25 groups or entities became differentiable with echography. Since 1972, the thickness of the optic nerve and since 1973 the thickness of the straight extraocular muscles have been measured successfully and accurately using standardized A-scan echography 64, 66-68.

B-scan techniques have been applied to the orbit either exclusively 369-72, or combined with nonstandardized A-scan displays 73-80 or in conjunction with standardized A-scan echography 18-22, 64, 68, 81. In the early 1970's it was Jackson Coleman in particular who developed and popularized the B-scan display technique 75-80.

The forte of B-scan echography is the documentation of the topography of orbital lesions. As far as other important information about orbital and periorbital lesions necessary for reliable detection and tissue differentiation is concerned, B-scan echography has always been quite limited and less useful, applicable and reliable than the standardized A-scan method; in orbital diagnosis, B-scan echography rarely adds significant information to the A-

496

scan findings. Even in its main function, i.e. the topographic documentation of lesions, B-scan echography has suffered a setback in recent years with the introduction of improved computerized tomography which produces better pictures from the posterior orbit and the periorbital structures. Nevertheless, B-scan echography is still more effective than CT-scanning in the anterior orbit and often provides finer details of the topography in the retrobulbar space. Therefore, B-scan echography along with Doppler techniques is recommended as a regular supplement to the standardized A-scan method. A detailed discussion of the different roles of the A- and B-scan methods in a combined approach has been published elsewhere 91.

The standardized A-scan method is today the most sensitive and accurate diagnostic tool for evaluating soft orbital tissues. With this method, 99% of orbital lesions can be detected with an accuracy greater than 99% and, in more than 80% of all cases, can be differentiated into 50 different groups or entities with an accuracy better than 80%. In addition, the standardized A-scan method helps to detect pathology in the periorbital sinuses. In the presence of defects in the bony orbital wall such perior retro-orbital lesions can also be differentiated to some degree. All detected lesions, whether intra-, peri- or retro-orbital in location, can be measured with the standardized A-scan method.

EQUIPMENT

Successful orbital diagnosis is based on the use of the standardized A-scan method. So far, the 7200 MA of Kretztechnik is the only A-scan instrument specifically designed (for ophthalmic tissue diagnosis) and also *standardized*. It uses an 8-MHz unfocused probe which produces a parallel beam capable of reaching the orbital apex in the normal orbit (which maximally attenuates the sound waves). Since orbital lesions attenuate ultrasonic waves much less than normal tissues and allow 8-MHz frequencies to penetrate as deep as 15 cm, the orbit can always be examined completely with the standardized A-scan method.

The special design and standardization of the 7200 MA includes all system parameters which influence the appearance and diagnostic value of tissue echograms. A narrow-band amplifier with a maximum response to 8 MHz provides unusually high system sensitivity. Rejection of signals is minimized and just sufficient to avoid disturbing noise. The amplification characteristiscs of the standardized instrument are neither linear nor logarithmic but follow an S-shaped course. This allows for an optimal dynamic range (range of echo intensities which can be displayed simultaneously) and limits the signal height smoothly without cutting off important amplitude information. The high-frequency oscillations of the echo signals are filtered to an optimal degree, thereby simplifying the echograms for visual pattern recognition and, at the same time, avoiding excessive blurring of the information processed. The ratio between horizontal and vertical expansions of the screen display is also optimized and standardized in the 7200 MA.

Figure 1 indicates the flow of information from tissue echoes through signal processing to the displayed echogram. This *signal processing* plays a

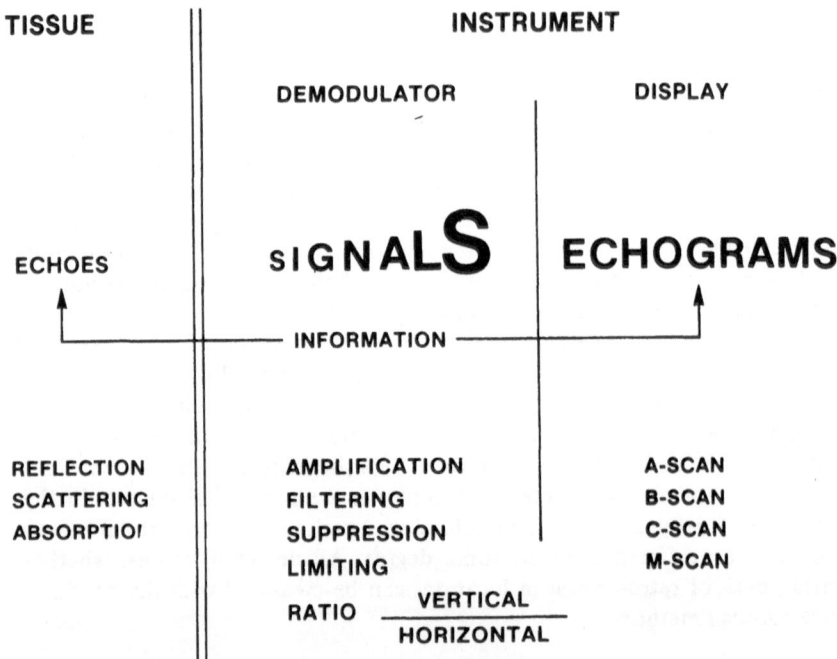

TISSUE		INSTRUMENT	
		DEMODULATOR	DISPLAY
ECHOES		siGNAL**S**	ECHOGRAMS
		INFORMATION	
REFLECTION		AMPLIFICATION	A-SCAN
SCATTERING		FILTERING	B-SCAN
ABSORPTIOI		SUPPRESSION	C-SCAN
		LIMITING	M-SCAN
		RATIO VERTICAL / HORIZONTAL	

Figure 1: Flow of echographic information. The design of echographic instrumentation decisively influences the appearance and diagnostic value of echograms; after echoes are received, it is the signal processing through the demodulator, and there, in particular, it is the mode of signal amplification which is crucial for the clarity and unequivocality of acoustic tissue signatures as displayed on the screen of the echographic instrument.

crucial role in enhancing acoustic differences between various tissues. When processing echo signals, one often must sacrifice some acoustic information to find an optimal compromise between various contradictory requirements. For instance, a very high system sensitivity is required in order to detect fine tissue structures. If system sensitivity is set at too high a level, however, not only noise but also the much stronger echoes from larger tissue structures are enhanced to the point that they mask the weaker echoes from the fine tissue structures; i.e., at toe high a system sensitivity, the resolution of the instrument deteriorates beyond acceptable levels. On the other hand, maximal resolution is also damaging: either system sensitivity is then too low to detect weaker echoes altogether or too many fine, non-characteristic details are over-emphasized and cover up the more characteristic tissue information. The filtering of high-frequency oscillations superimposed on the echo amplitudes is another example. High-frequency oscillations carry information which may be of some value; however, it has to be partially discarded in order to allow the examiner to recognize more important tissue signatures on the screen. On the other hand, filtering of high frequencies must nog exceed certain levels or significant information will be lost.

The design of all system parameters mentioned is equally crucial for obtaining ptimal results in tissue diagnosis. The function of the *S-shaped am-*

plifier characteristics in the design of the standardized 7200 MA will be discussed in more detail to show the radical advantages it offers over the linear or logarithmic amplifiers used in most non-standardized A-scan instruments.

Tissue diagnosis requires both good resolution and sufficient dynamic range (acoustic depth of field). S-shaped amplifiers provide good resolution through the steep central portions of the amplifier curve and sufficient dynamic range through the decreasingly steep slopes of the lower and upper ends of the amplifier curve (*Figure 2*). Neither linear nor logarithmic amplifiers can meet this dual requirement: linear amplifiers (used in most non-standardized A-scan instruments) offer excellent resolution but insufficient dynamic range (often less thand 15 db), while logarithmic amplifiers provide a dynamic range which is often more than 60 db but cannot provide sufficient resolution for tissue diagnosis.

The function of an amplifier can be compared to the function of the eye. In analogy to the normal eye, the S-shaped amplifier curve provides 'acoustic acuity' through its steep central portion and 'acoustic field' through the gradually flattened upper and lower ends of the curve (*Figure 3*). The linear amplifier may be compared to an eye with a hemianopic field defect: it offers excellend acoustic acuity but insufficient acoustic field (*Figure 4*). The logarithmic amplifier is analagous to an otherwise normal eye with central scotoma: it offers abundant acoustic field, but no acoustic acuity (*Figure 5*). A more detailed description of the function of S-shaped amplifiers in acoustic tissue diagnosis has been given elsewhere 89, 91.

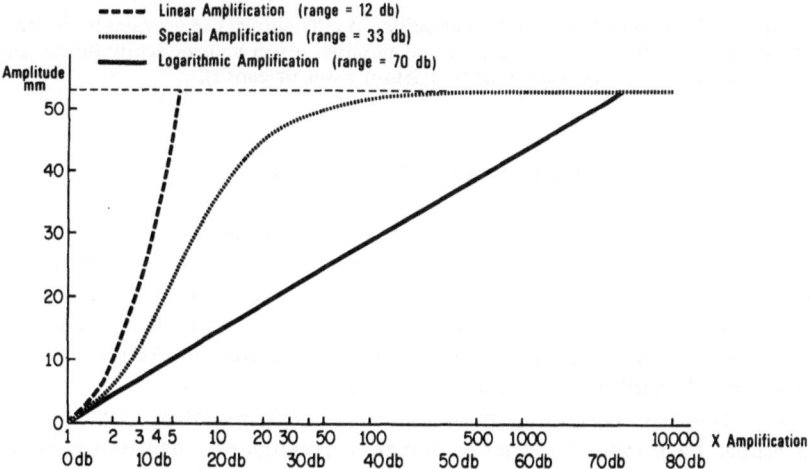

Figure 2: Characteristic curves of linear, logarithmic and special S-shaped amplifiers. These curves indicate· the changes of signal height in response to variation of system sensitivity or echo intensity. With linear amplification signal height doubles when amplification or echo intensity double; . . . with logarithmic amplification the signal height grows by the same constant amount, whereas with the specific S-shaped amplification the response of signal height varies depending orl the initial spike height. Note that in regard to the steepness of the curve and, consequently, its relative sensitivity and dynamic range, the S-shaped amplifier represents a compromise between the two extremes of linear and logarithmic amplification.

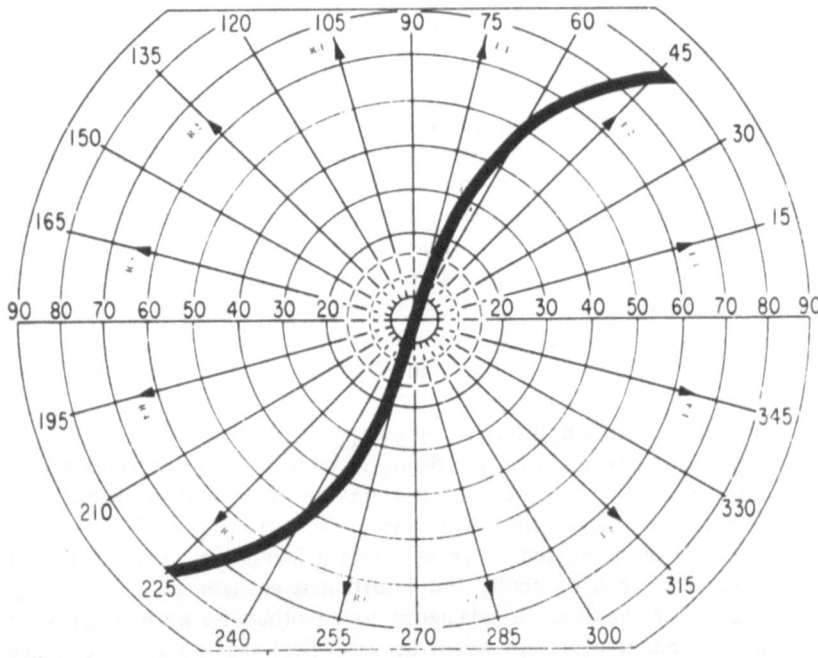

S-Shaped Amplification

Figure 3: Function of the S-shaped amplifier. As the normal eye provides both visual acuity and visual field, the special S-shaped amplifier offers acoustic acuity (important for measurements) and acoustic field (crucial for tissue diagnosis).

EXAMINATION TECHNIQUES

Reliable, accurate and comparable echographic results are assured only if optimized and *standardized* examination techniques are used in conjunction with standardized instrumentation. The *basic examination* is performed first in order to detect or rule out (1) orbital mass lesions, (2) thickening of the optic nerve or extraocular muscles and their sheaths and (3) bony defects or abnormal conditions in the periorbital space.

Next, orbital or periorbital mass lesions are differentiated, localized and measured by means of *special examination techniques* (quantitative, topographic and kinetic echography) and the thickness of the optic nerve and the extraocular muscles and their sheaths are measured accurately. Finally, Doppler techniques are used for a more detailed study of the vascularity of a lesion.

Basic Examination

a) Screening the orbit for a mass lesion: After local anesthetic drops are

500

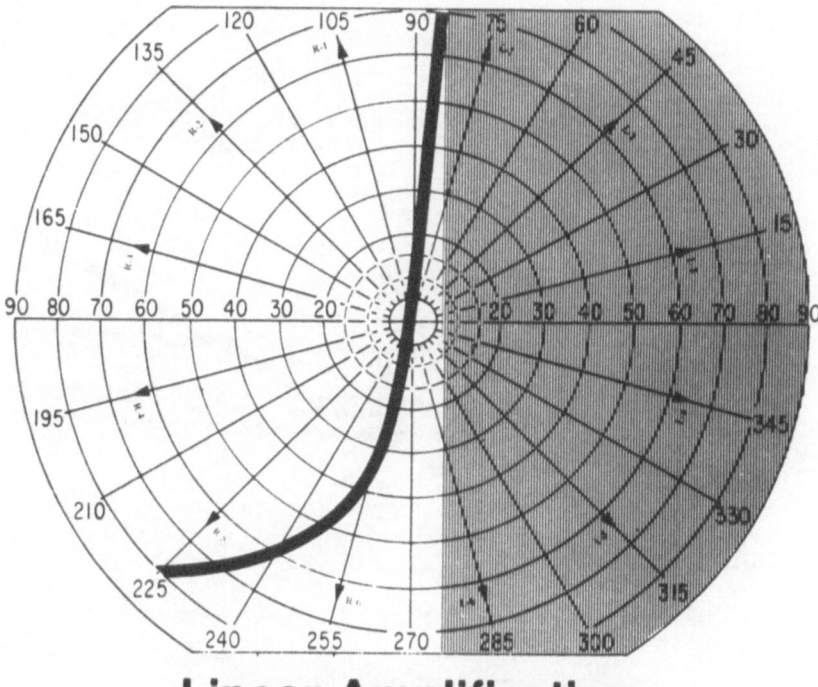

Linear Amplification

Figure 4: Function of linear amplifiers. Comparable to a case of hemianopsia, a linear amplifier may provide acoustic acuity, but it lacks sufficient acoustic ffield.

instilled in both of the patient's eyes and the A-scan instrument is set for orbital examination at tissue sensitivity (a standardized setting), the basic orbital examination is begun with a *transocular approach* (*Figure 6*). The probe is first placed on the conjunctiva next to the limbus at 6:00 and the beam aimed through the center of the globe into the orbital tissues opposite the probe. By shifting the probe toward the fornix and angling it, the anterior and posterior sections of the orbit are scanned along the 12:00 meridian; since most orbital lesions are located in either the upper orbit or the muscle cone, they can thus be detected early during the basic examination. Next, other meridians of the orbit are examined in the same manner. It is usually sufficient to scan 8 meridians.

Using 2% methylcellulose as a coupling agent, the basic examination is continued with a *paraocular approach* (*Figure 7*). The probe is placed directly on the skin of the lids and the beam is directed into the anterior orbit between the globe and bone. Using the paraocular approach, lesions which may escape transocular detection (i.e., small lesions in the most anterior orbit and particularly those behind the orbital rim) are found. Again, several meridians are scanned in this manner.

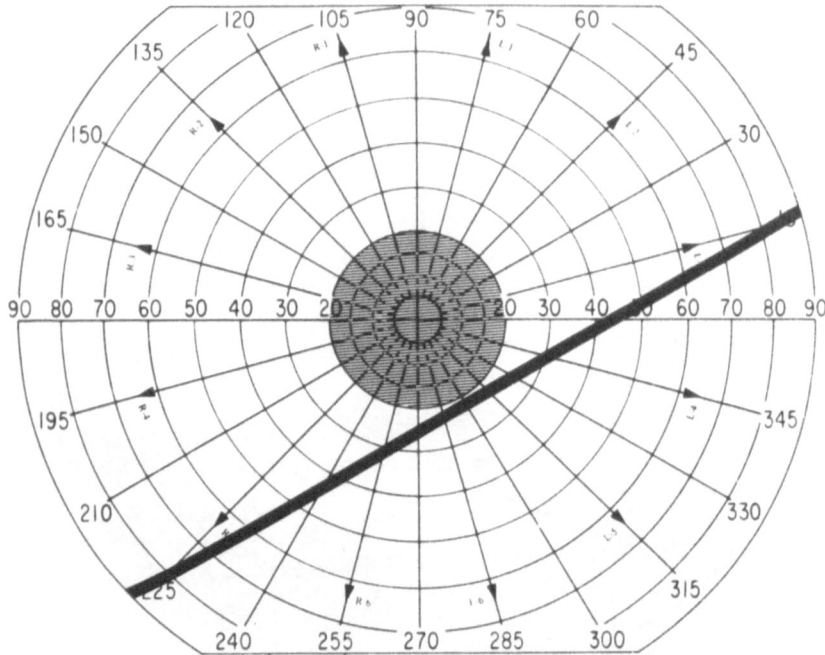

Logarithmic Amplification

Figure 5: Function of logarithmic amplifiers. Comparable to a case of central scotoma, a logarithmic amplifier provides acoustic field but lacks acoustic acuity.

During the basic scanning of the orbit, the examiner carefully monitors the screen display for the appearance of a defect in the orbital pettern.
Normal tissues produce chains of high, overloaded spikes on account of their extremely high reflectivity; most orbital mass lesions are more homogeneous to ultrasound and therefore have a lower reflectivity. Thus, spike heights of mass lesions are less than 100% (*Figure 8*). This 'defect' in the height of the orbital echogram is the most important acoustic criterion of a lesion.

If a lesion is present this *transocular* and *paraocular* scanning of the orbital contents, the bony orbital wall and periorbit requires only a few minutes. Whether or not a lesion is detected, the basic examination is next continued with the display of the optic nerve and extraocular muscles.

b) Display of the extraocular muscles: To display an extraocular muscle, the probe is placed near the equator of the eyeball opposite the muscle to be examined while the patient keeps his eyes in primary gaze position (*Figure 9*). The probe is slightly angled and shifted until a tiny defect next to the scleral spikes is displayed (*Figure 10*). This defect represents the inserting tendon of the muscle. The beam is guided along the course of the muscle posteriorly and the muscle pattern shifts away from the globe towards the

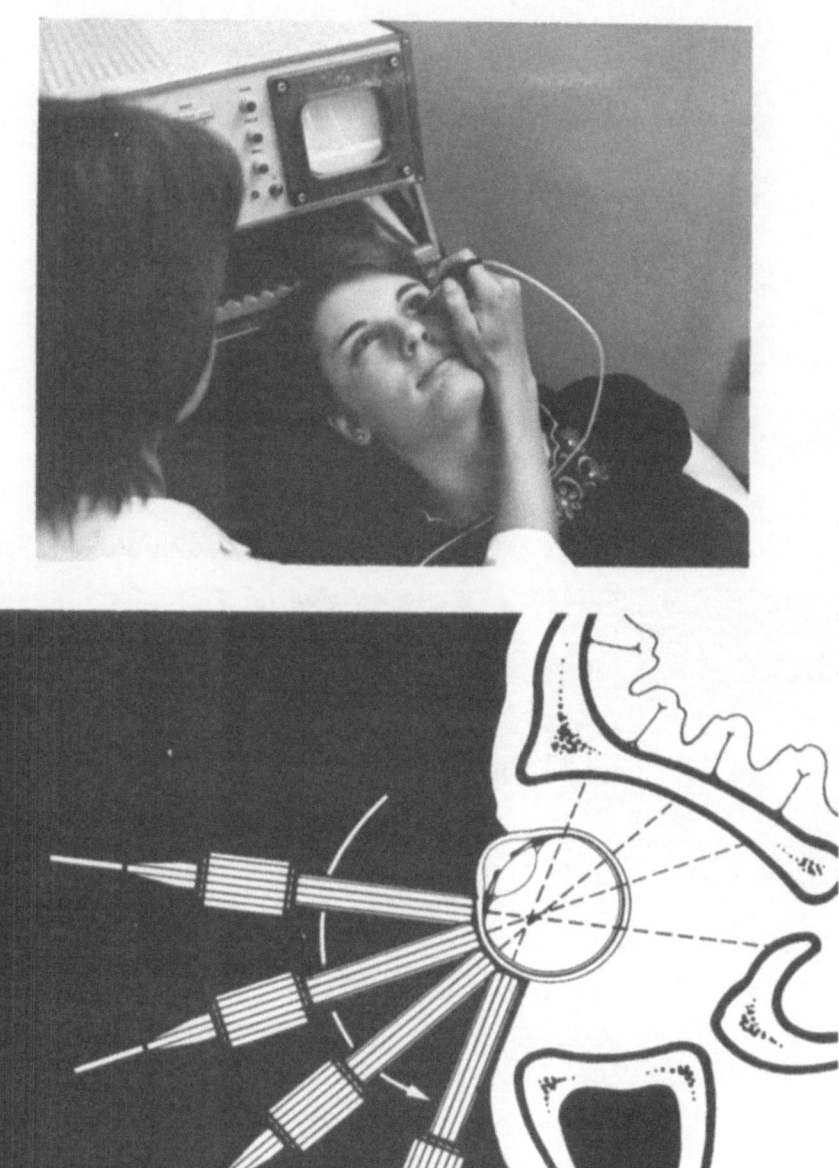

Figure 6: Transocular basic examination of the orbit to detect anterior and posterior lesions. **Above:** first the probe is placed at the limbus in the 6:00 meridian and the sound beam is aimed posteriorly and superiorly in order to examine the posterior orbit at 12:00. **Below:** the probe is shifted from limbus to fornix and angled in order to examine the orbit along the entire 12:00 meridian. Note that the patient is instructed to look toward the meridian examined *(away from the probe)* so that the lens, which would attenuate and refract the beam, does not interfere with the examination. The other meridians are then examined correspondingly.

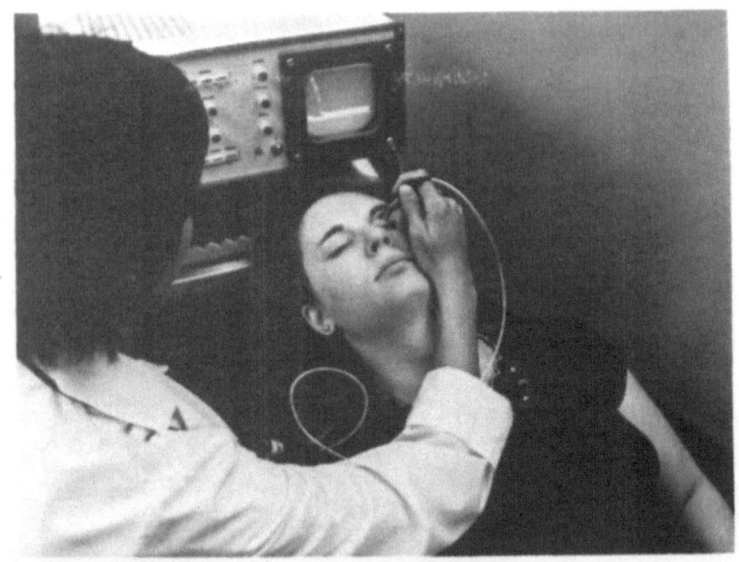

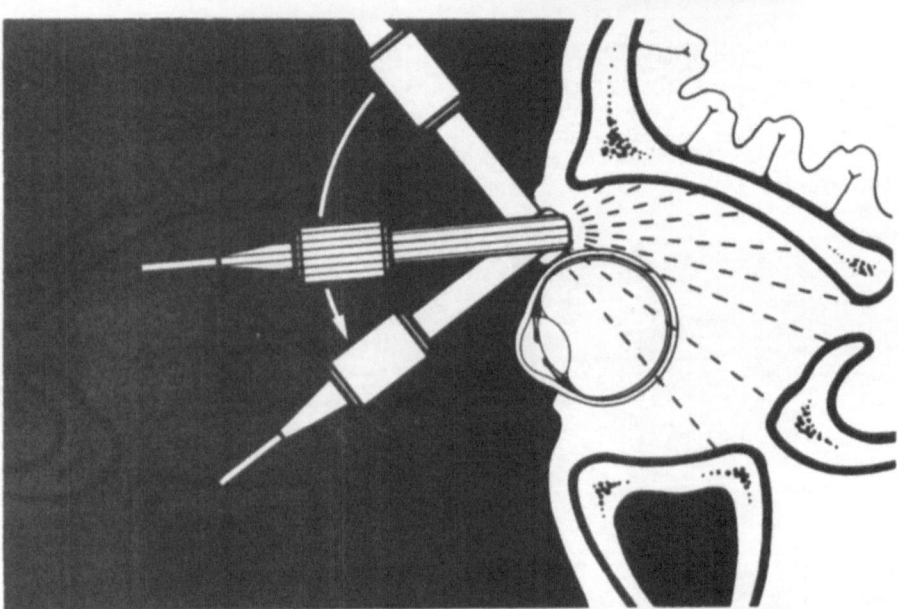

Figure 7: Paraocular basic examination of the orbit to detect lesions in the most anterior orbital sections. **Above:** first the probe is placed on the surface of the upper lid in the 12:00 meridian using methylcellulose as a coupling agent; the sound beam is aimed at the orbital tissues between globe and bone at 12:00. **Below:** by angling the probe along the 12:00 meridian the paraocular tissues alont the entire 12:00 meridian are evaluated (this includes the tissues behind the superior orbital rim). Note tham the sound beam is first directed into the globe and then angled away from the globe in order to more easily identify the paraocular space. The other meridians are then examined in the same fashion.

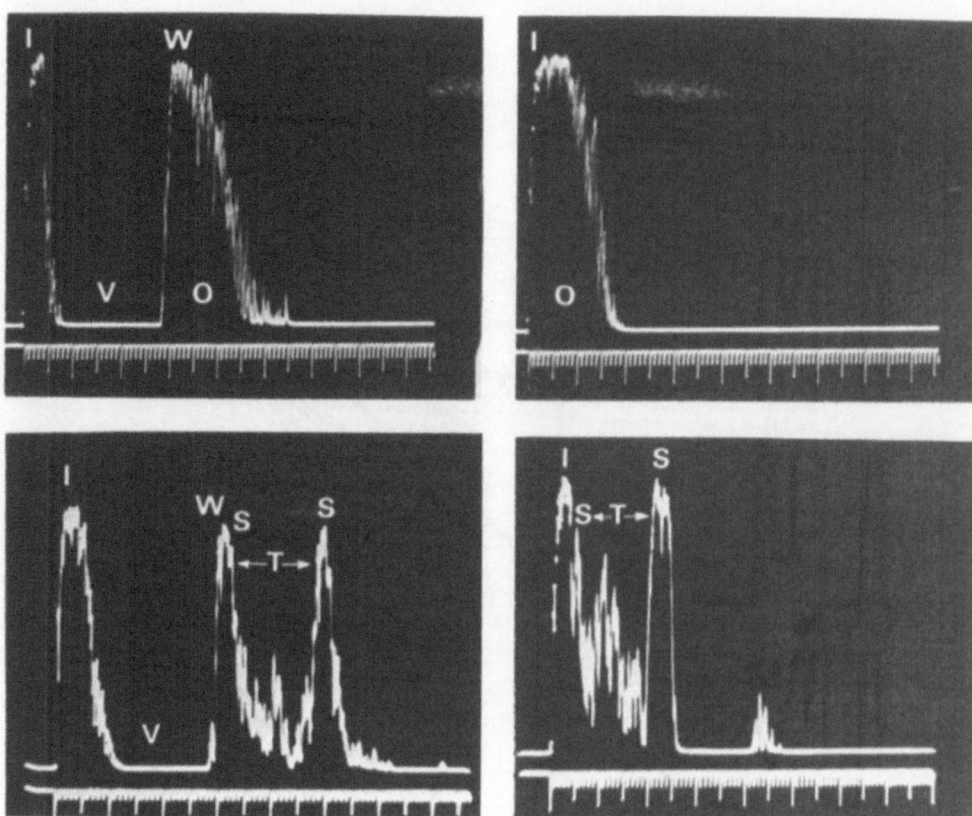

Figure 8: Normal (top) and abnormal (bottom) orbital A-scan echograms. **Left** transocular patterns; **right** paraocular patterns. **I** initial spike representing the tip of the probe or the surface of the tissues examined (anterior) ocular surface, lid surface); **V** normal vitreous (intact baseline); **W** ocular wall opposite the probe (retina, choroid, sclera); **O** normal orbital tissues; **T** orbital tumor; **S** tumor surface. Note that the lesion pattern is not only wider than the normal orbital echogram, but in particular shows a defect in the spike height (lower reflectivity of orbital lesion).

bone signals and at the same time becomes wider and deeper. By slightly angling and shifting the probe the examiner attempts to display the widest possible muscle pattern which still is outlined on each side by maximally high, steeply rising surface spikes. In this way, it is insured that the maximal thickness of the muscle is being displayed by a sound beam perpendicular to the surface of the muscle. To detect thickening of the extraocular muscles, it is sufficient to quickly scan the 4 straight extraocular muscles and observe the width of their defects in the echograms. An exact measurement of the muscle thickness is performed if these defects appear wider than usual: using an electronic measuring scale calibrated in microseconds (which is displayed simultaneously with the orbital echogram), a photographic pic-

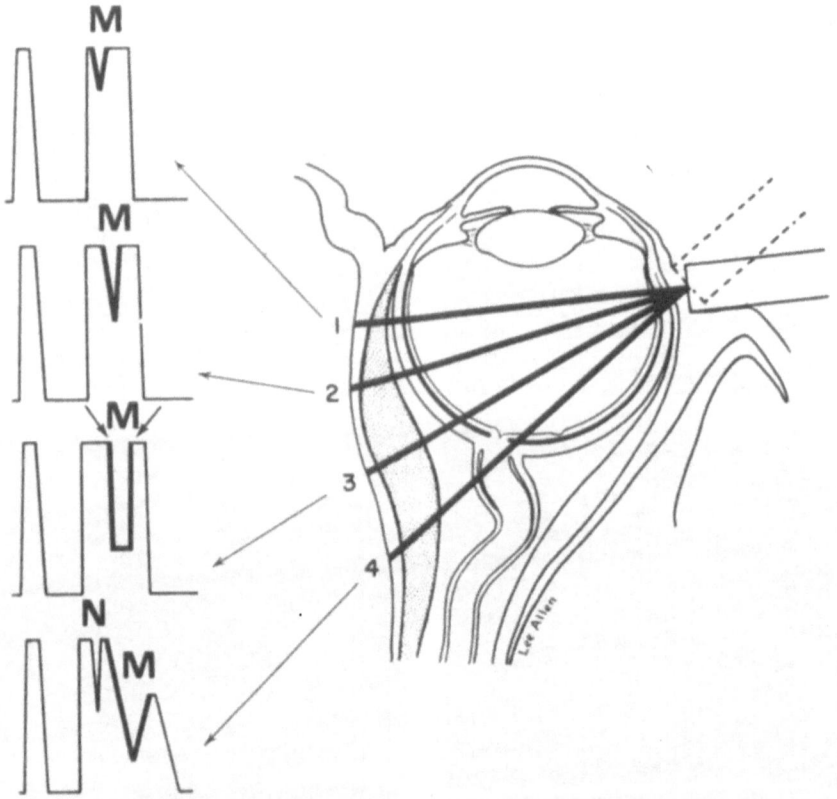

Figure 9: Measurement of thickness of extraocular muscle (right medial rectus muscle in this case). The probe is placed opposite the muscle; first the sound beam is directed perpendicular to the opposite ocular wall reaching the insertion of the muscle **(1)**; then, the sound beam is angled posteriorly in order to display the maximum thickness of the muscle **(3)**. The width of the defect in the orbital pattern representing the muscle indicates the thickness of the muscle, while the steeply rising and falling surface signals on each side of the defect prove perpendicularity of the sound beam to the muscle surface. **M** cross section of muscle (defect in orbital pattern); arrows surface of muscle (steeply rising and falling spikes, if surface reached by perpendicular beam); **N** optic nerve (see *Figure 11*).

ture is taken at a moment when the muscle pattern appears in maximal width outlined by maximally bigh, steeply rising surface spikes. The width of the muscle pattern is then measured on the photograph and the micro-seconds are converted to millimeters using conversion tables.

c) Display of the optic nerve: In order to display and measure optic-nerve thickness, the probe is placed near the temporal equator and the beam is directed toward the medial rectus muscle while the patient maintains primary gaze direction (*Figure 11*). When the beam is aimed more posteriorly

506

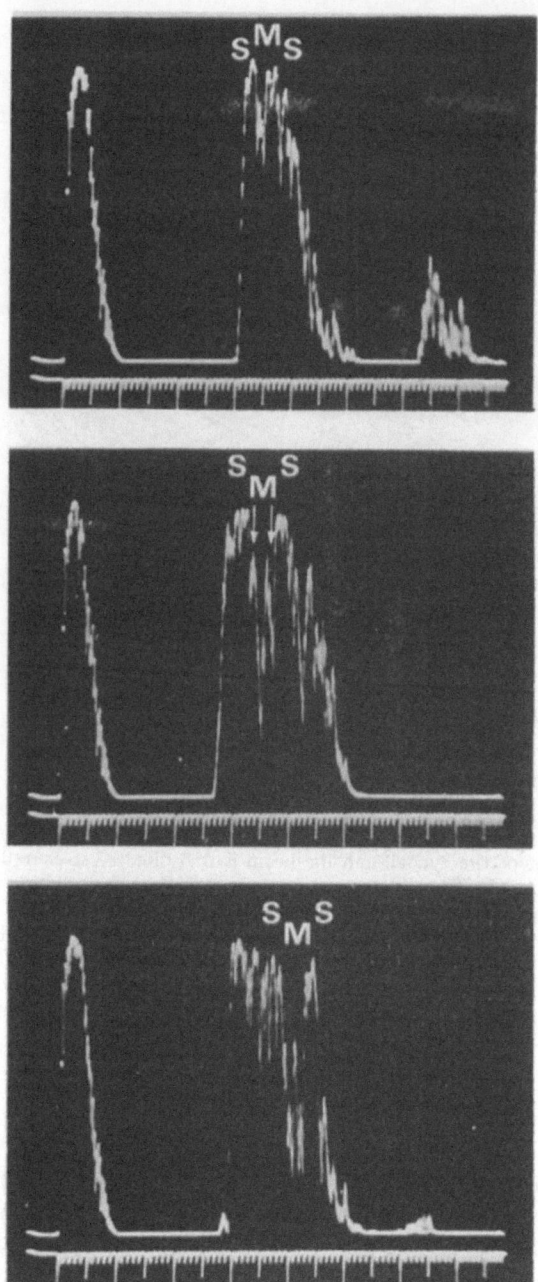

Figure 10: A-scan echograms from normal medial rectus muscle displaying its thickness in its anterior section (**top**: muscle insertion), in the retrobulbar space (**center**) and in the orbital apex **bottem**). **M** defect in the orbital pattern representing a cross section of the extraocular muscle; **S** muscle sheaths; **arrows** surface of muscle bundles.

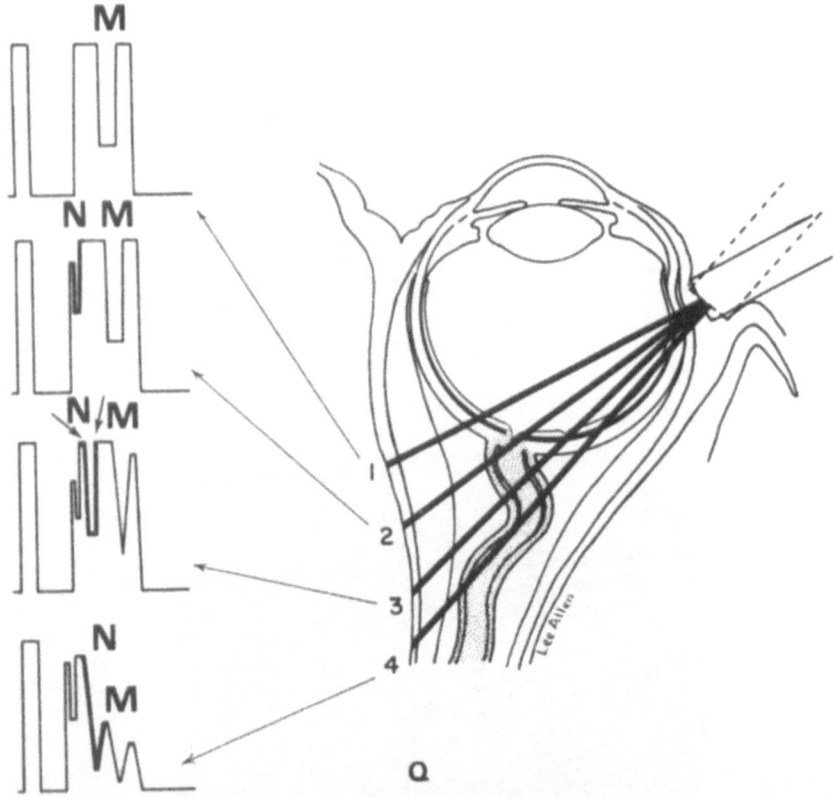

Figure 11: Measurement of optic-nerve thickness. The probe is usually placed near the temporal equator of the eyeball and the beam is first directed so as to display the medial rectus muscle (1). Then the sound beam is angled posteriorly and slightly above the horizontal plane; by angling extensively a further defect appears in the orbital echograms (3 *optic-nerve pattern*). By angling the beam toward the orbital apex and continuously displaying this optic-nerve 'defect', cross sections of the anterior and posterior segments of the orbital optic nerve are displayed. **N** optic nerve (defect in orbital pattern); **arrow** optic-nerve surface (arachnoidal surface); **M** medial rectus muscle (see *Figure 9*).

into the orbit another defect is displayed between the ocular wall and the muscle pattern; this is the optic-nerve 'defect'. The width of this defect is maximized by angling and shifting the beam in order to indicate the maximal thickness of the optic nerve (*Figure 12*). Steeply rising double-peaked surface spikes represent the optic-nerve sheaths; the distance between the two peaks of eacht surface spike reveals the thickness of the optic-nerve sheaths. By shifting the beam more anteriorly or posteriorly, various sections of the optic nerve are displayed along its course through the orbit. Again the thickness is measured from photographic pictures. While most optic nerves are best displayed with the tehcnique described, it is some-

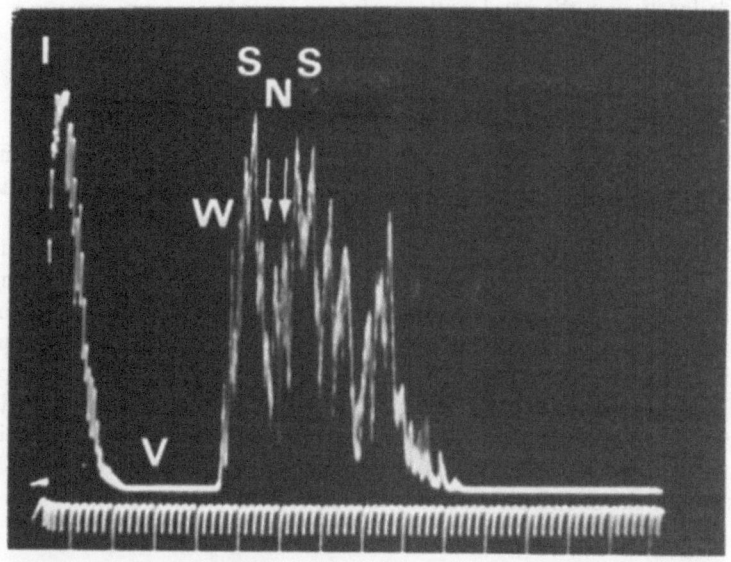

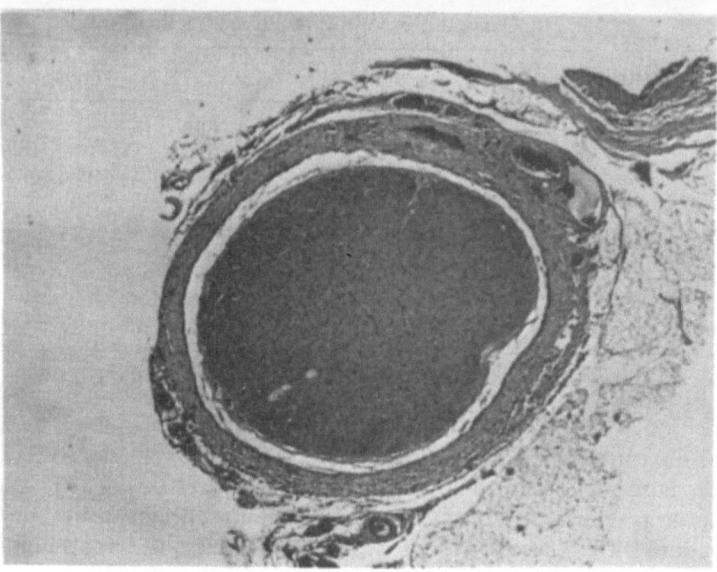

Figure 12: A-scan echogram and histological section representing a *cross section of a normal optic nerve.* I initial spike indicating the surface of the globe where the probe is placed; V normal vitreous; W posterior ocular wall (retina, choroid and sclera; due to oblique sound-beam incidence, the ocular wall signals are weak); N defect representing cross section of the optic nerve; S optic-nerve sheaths (dura and arachnoidea); arrows surface of the nerve itself (surface of pia). Optic-nerve measurements determine maximum distance of the two opposite surfaces of the arachnoidea (two distinct surface spikes).

509

times easier to demonstrate optic-nerve thickness by placing the probe on the inferior or even the nasal ocular surfaces.

2) Special Techniques

a) The first and most important step in the differentiation of orbital mass lesions is to determine the internal structure and reflectivity of a lesion using *quantitative echography*. The instrument is set at tissue sensitivity and the sound beam is aimed through the center of the lesion. If the lesion spikes display a similar height or change their height fromleft to right at a regular pace, the lesion has a regular internal structure. In this case, the lesion is then classified into 1 of 5 groups according to its reflectivity; the spike height within the lesion pattern is expressed as a percentage of the display height (*Table 1*). *Figure 13* illustrates echograms from lesions of various reflectivities displayed at tissue sensitivity. The sound attenuation within a lesion is indicated by the size of the inclination angle 'kappa' (*Figure 14*). The stronger the sound attenuation, the larger is the angle kappa.

Table 1:	Quantitative classification of mass lesions	
Reflectivity	Spike height	Examples
Extremely high	95–100%	Normal tissue
High	60– 95%	Cavernous hemangioma
Medium	40– 60%	Glioma
Low	5– 40%	Pseudotumor
Extremely low	0– 5%	Serous Cyst

b) The next major step in the differentiation of an orbital lesion is to determine its borders. This is done with *topographic A-scan echography*. *Figure 15* shows 4 echograms from low-reflective lesions which differ in their delineation. Diffuse lesions do not display any surface spike; poorly-outlined lesions produce a wide, indistinct surface spike; well-outlined, encapsulated solid lesions produce a distinct and high, steeply rising, single-peaked surface signal, whereas cysts display a very distinct and high, steeply rising and *double-peaked* surface spike.

By measuring the diameter of a mass lesion in different sound-beam directions, the shape and size of the lesion is determined. *B-scan echography* is often helpful in documenting the shape and topographic relationship of orbital lesions with normal ocular structures. In rare instances, B-scan echography adds information not easily obtainable by the use of A-scan echography (*Figure 16*).

510

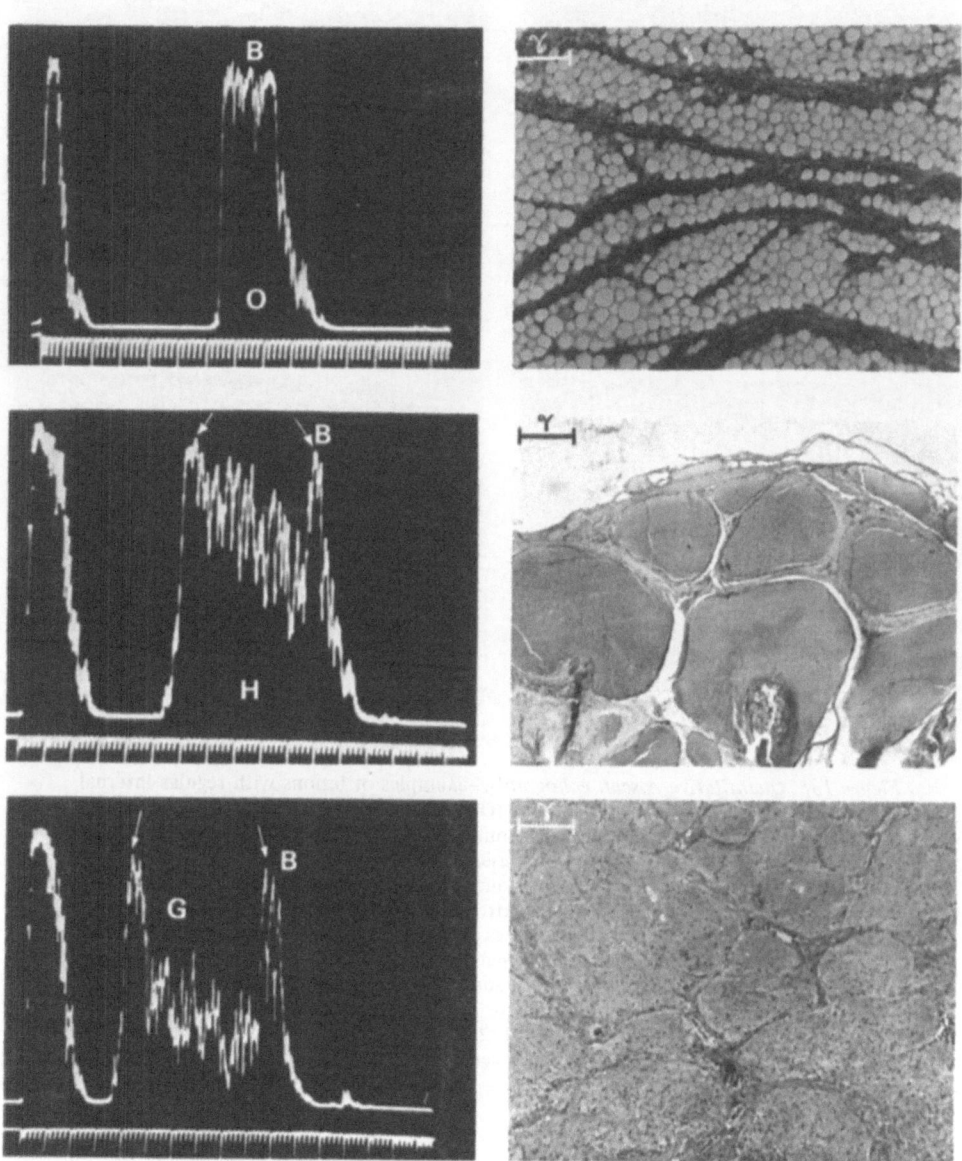

Figure 13: first part. For second part and legend see page 512.

c) The consistency of orbital lesions and their vascularity are determined with kinetic *A-scan echography*. Doppler techniques aid the evaluation of vascularity. As a first step in kinetic echography, the *consistency* of an orbital mass lesion is determined by pushing the globe with the A-scan probe against the lesion in an attempt to squeeze the lesion between the globe and bone. If a lesion is soft, the lesion pattern will decrease markedly in width

511

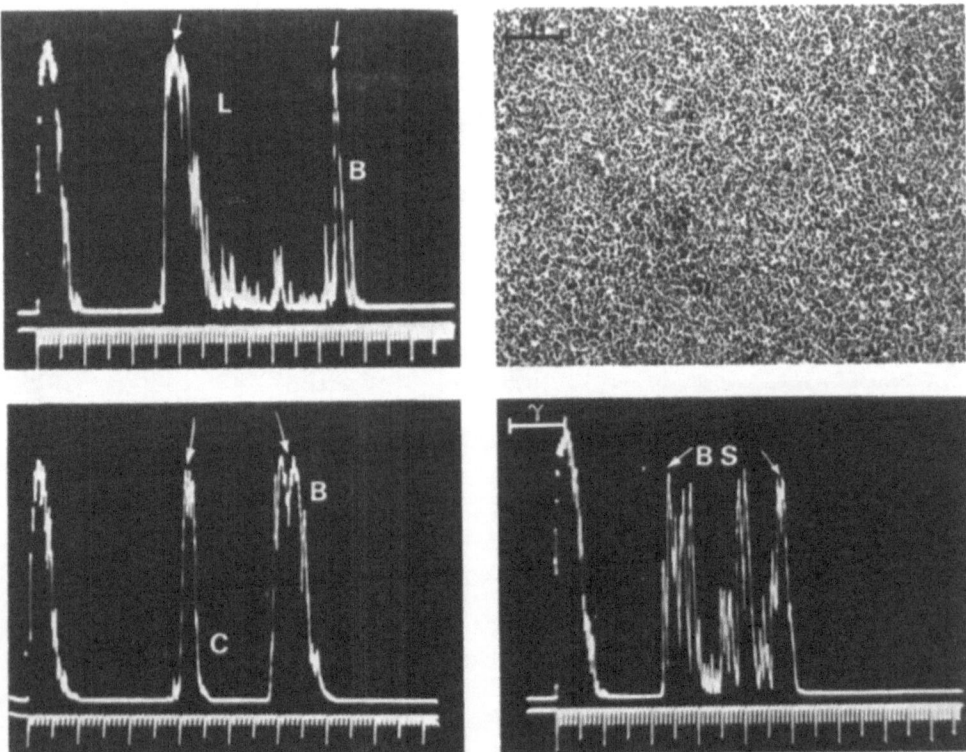

Figure 13: Quantitative A-scan echography--examples of lesions with regular internal structure and extremely high reflectivity (O normal orbital tissues), high (H cavernous hemangioma), medium G optic-nerve glioma), low L lymphoma), and extremely low reflectivity (C epidermoid cyst) and of a lesion with irregular structure (S sinus carcinoma). Histological sections explain the various degrees of reflectivity of each tissue type: very large connectivetissue septa cause extremely strong echoes in normal tissues; large endothelialized surfaces of cavernous spaces produce strong echoes in cavernous hemangiomas; medium-sized trabecular septa creata medium strong echoes in optic-nerve gliomas; and small interfaces between cells and intercellular substance cause weak echoscattering in lymphomas. For quantitative echography a specially designed and standardized A-scan instrument is requiered (7200 Ma Kretztechnik); system sensitivity is set at a standardized level called 'tissue sensitivity'. **Arrows** tumor surface; **B** orbital bone.

during this procedure. If the lesion is hard, however, the width of the lesion pattern will not change.

By holding the A-scan probe still while the beam travels through the lesion, the *vascularity* of a lesion can be shown in the A-scan echogram. Spontaneous and continuous, fast vertical flickering movement of single lesion spikes indicates blood flow within the lesion. If all lesion spikes move in this fashion, the echogram is pathognomonic for an arteriovenous fistula.

Doppler echography can help to evaluate the vascularity of an orbital lesion. If no vacular response is obtained while scanning the lesion with the

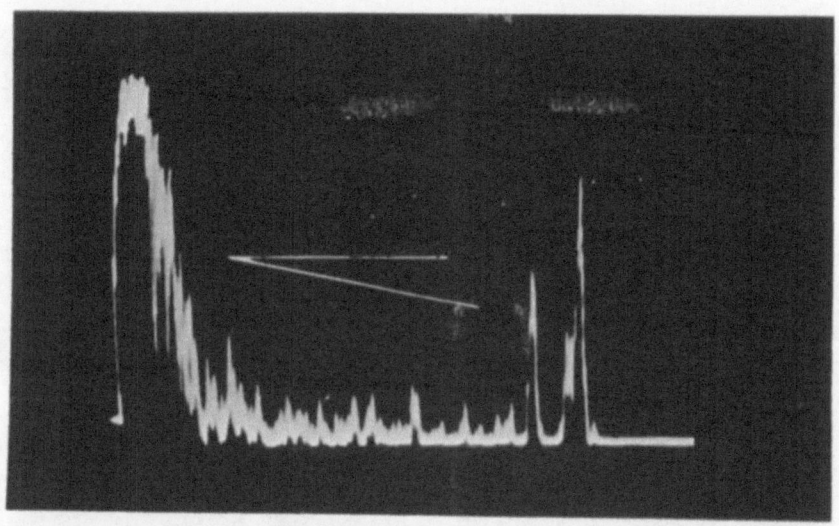

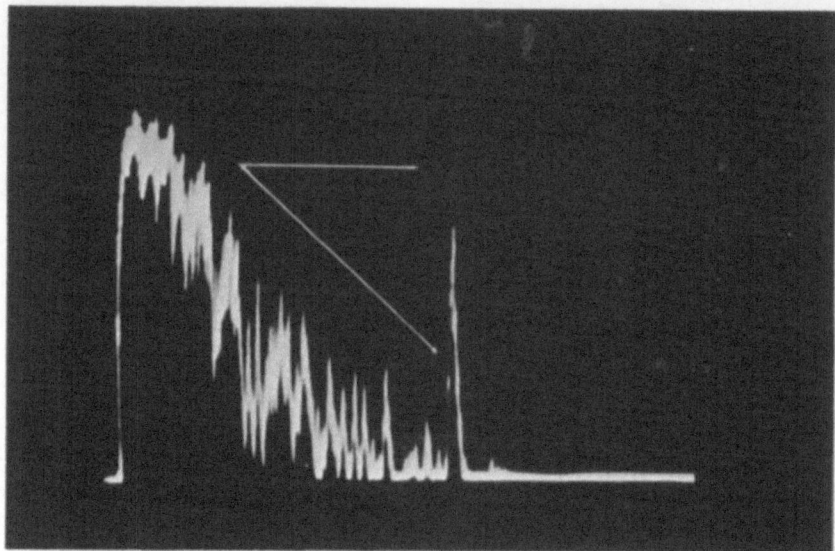

Figure 14: Illustration of the *inclination angle 'kappa'* which is formed by the horizontal baseline and an imaginary line through the centers of the cho spikes. **Top** paraocular echogram from a low-reflective tumor with minor sound attenaution (small angle kappa); **bottom** echogram from tumor with strong sound attenuation (medium angle kappa). Note that the initial spike and the surface and bone signals are excluded from the evaluation of the angle kappa.

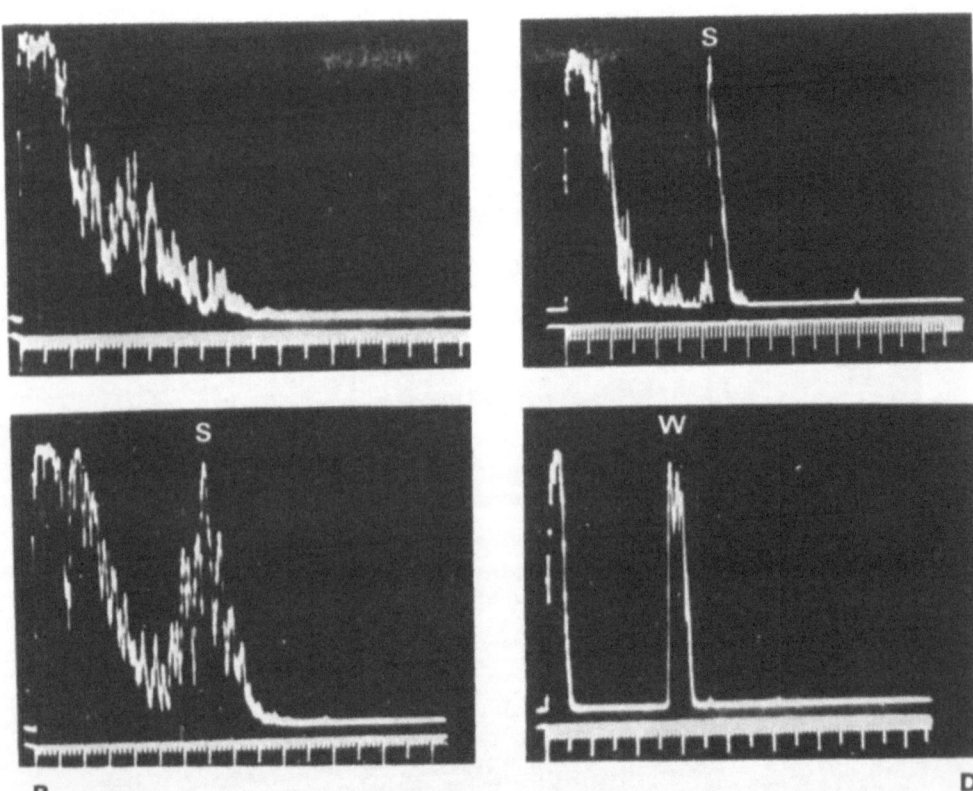

Figure 15: Topographic A-scan echography--examples of low-reflective lesions with different borders. **A** diffuse lesion (no surface signal); **B** poorly outlined tumor (**S** ill-defined multi-peaked surface spike); **C** well outlined lesion (**S** distinct, sharply rising and high, single-peaked surface spike), cyst with thick wall (**W** distinct, steeply-rising, double-peaked wall spike; the two peaks represent the inner and outer surfaces of the cyst wall.

Doppler beam in different directions, the lesion is definitely avascular. When the Doppler examination is positive, it depends on whether the response is directional or diffuse: when the Doppler response is obtained only in one or another direction, the response comes from normal orbital vessels; when the Doppler response is obtained in all sound-beam directions through the lesion, the lesion is proven to be vascularized.

While the beginner is advised to apply the special echographic examination techniques in the order presented, the more experienced examiner will often take shortcuts to save time. He may identify some lesions by type within seconds by simply placing the probe on the eyeball and recognizing the specific pattern. Other lesions may require more time-consuming and meticulous evaluation by even the experienced examiner.

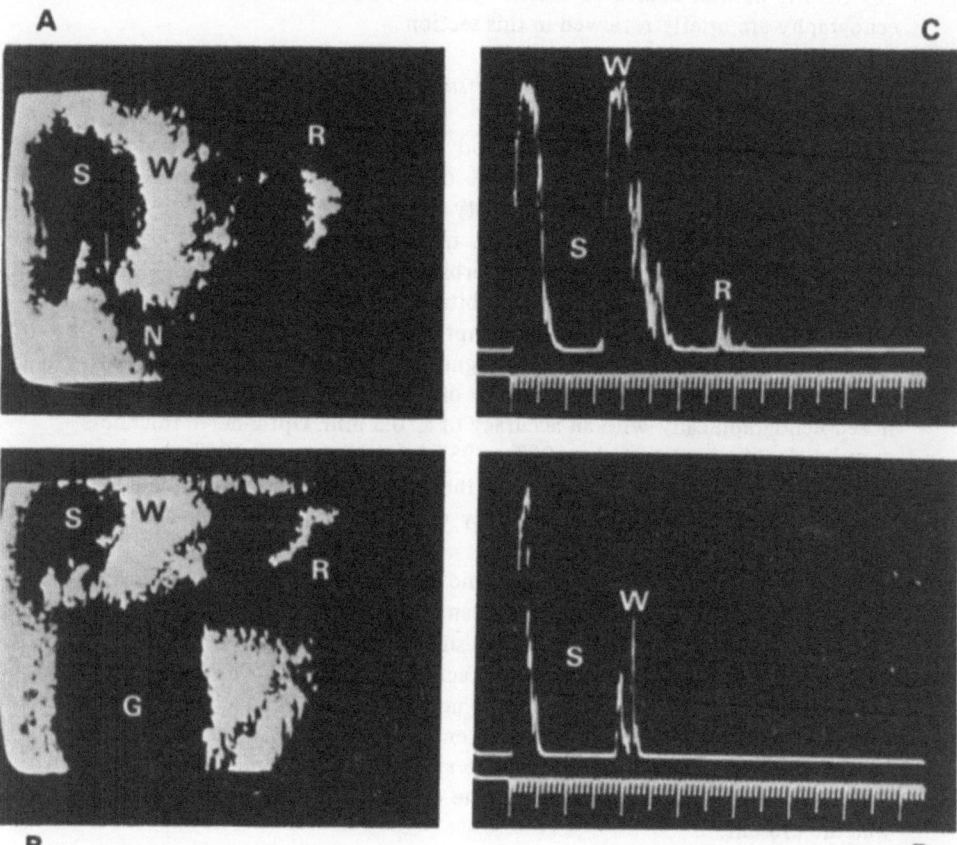

Figure 16: B-scan and A-scan echograms from an enormously *dilated lacrimal sac* in a newborn. **A** B-scan offers unique demonstration of the nasolacrimal duct (**N**) and its ostium in the wall of the lacrimal sac (**arrow**). **B** cross section through both the lacrimal sac and the globe illustrating the topographic relationship between the two. **C** A-scan echogram obtained at tissue sensitivity indicates extremely low reflectivity of the cyst contents (serous fluid) and shows cyst wall. **D** A-scan echogram at reduced system sensitivity clearly demonstrates the two surfaces of the cyst wall. **S** dilated lacrimal sac filled with serous fluid; **G** globe; **W** cyst wall; **R** reverberation signals (duplication of cyst-wall signals).

APPLICATIONS AND RESULTS

There are a variety of useful applications of echography in the evaluation of orbital and periorbital pathology. The uses of echography range from simple axial eye-lenght measurements to disclose pseudoexophthalmos or -enophthalmos to systematic screening of the orbit and periorbit to detect lesions. Echography serves to identify the tissue type and to map the topography of lesions to optimize their treatment, be it surgery, radiation or chemotherapy. Echography is also used to carefully monitor the effects to therapy and to observe the natural course of orbital diseases. There various uses of orbital echography are briefly reviewed in this section.

A) Diagnosis of Soft-Tissue Orbital Lesions

1) Detection:

With the standardized A-scan method (basic examination), 99% of soft tissue lesions can be detected; >99% of the echographic diagnoses are correct. Such a high degree of sensitivity and accuracy holds true for intra-orbital lesions which are larger than 1 mm (when located in the anterior orbit) or 3 mm (when located in the orbital apex). This limitation is of no more than theoretical interest since orbital mass lesions have usually grown to a much larger size before causing symptoms.

Thickening of the optic nerve throughout its orbital course can be diagnosed echographically with an accuracy of *b*
nosed echographically with an accuracy of ± 0.5 mm. Optic-nerve thickness may be classified as normal, as 90% or 95% borderline, or as 100% abnormal as shown in *Table 2*. The thickness of the extraocular muscles can be determined echographically with an accuracy of ± 0.75 mm; it may be classified according to *Table 3*.

Intracranial lesions escape echographic detection with opthalmic instrumentations in the absence of significant bony defects. The presence of significant pathology in the periorbital sinuses can be detected echographically through intact bone. The mere fact that echoes are obtained from a periorbital sinus proves that the sinus is not completely filled with air (which would block the ultrasonic waves from entering the sinus). Echography fails to indicate whether mucous-membrane swelling, fluid, or inflammatory or neoplastic tissues are responsible for the echoes unless defects in the bony wall are present.

The sensitivity and accuracy of orbital echography in detecting soft tissue masses in the orbit and periorbital sinuses is comparable to the roentgenological diagnosis of bony fractures. Just as x-ray techniques are the best means for demonstrating bony lesions, echography is the most reliable and accurate means for diagnosing intraorbital soft tissue lesions.

2) Tissue Differentiation:

More than 80% of detected orbital and periorbital soft-tissue lesions can be differentiated echographically into 50 categories or entities. The accuracy of

Table 2: Thickness of optic nerves (results of the McNutt study of a normal population)

Optic-nerve thickness				Difference between both optic nerves	
90%	95%	100%	*)	90%	95%
4.05	4.30	4.72	mm	0.90	1.10

*) Percentiles of normal population with optic nerves thinner than listed mm-values.

Table 3: Thickness of extraocular muscles (results of the McNutt study of a normal population)

	Individual muscle-thickness			Difference between orbits		
	90%	95%	100%	*)	90%	95%
Medial rectus	5.02	5.20	6.52	mm	1.10	1.36
Lateral rectus	4.88	5.12	5.40	mm	0.90	1.10
Superior rectus	4.32	4.58	5.40	mm	1.15	1.50
Inferior rectus	4.24	4.45	5.32	mm	1.40	1.50

*) Percentiles of normal population with muscles thinner than listed mm-values

this differential diagnosis is more than 80%. Lesions in the periorbital region, however, can only be differentiated if defects in the bony orbital wall allow the ultrasonic pulses to enter those lesions with sufficient energy.

Table 4 lists entities or categories of lesions which may be identified at the present time using the standardized A-scan method aided by B-scan and Doppler techniques. Some lesions, e.g. serous cysts, cavernous hemangiomas of the adult type, arteriovenous fistulas, varices and mucoceles, often produce echograms which are pathognomonic for these conditions. Other lesions, such as dermoid cysts, cannot be diagnosed with this high degree of accuracy; they may be confused with well-encapsulated, roundish, nonvascularized solid lesions of regular structure.

Some lesions, e.g., pseudotumors, lymphomas and sarcomas, often display such similar acoustic properties that they can be identified only as a group; it is rarely possible to differentiate the benign from the malignant entities whithin this group. Other lesions can be identified only through repeated echographic evaluations or with the aid of the clinical picture or medical history. Orbital hematomas, for instance, produce echograms similar to those from pseudotumors. But, unlike pseudotumors, hematomas display a rapid decrease in size and consistency when followed for a few days; also, there is often a history of sudden and most recent onset of proptosis which appears inconsistent with the echographic finding of a large mass. Orbital abscesses cannot be differentiated from pseudotumors either, unless they produce typical pain and signs of inflammation and are echographically proven to have developed within hours or days.

Cavernous hemangiomas (adult type), optic neuropathy and pachymyopathy have been chosen as examples to illustrate the varying potential of standardized echography in differentiating tissues.

a) Cavernous hemangiomas: Cavernous hemangiomas of the adult type,

517

Table 4: Entities and groups of lesions which may be differentiated with the standardized A-scan method aided by the contact B-scan method at the present
time (listed according to location and acoustic properties).

ORBITAL MASS LESIONS

- pseudo-exophthalmus
- pseudo-enophthalmus
- diffuse orbital edema
- orbital cellulitis
- dacryoadenitis
- (epi)scleritis
- abscess/hard infiltrate
- hyperemia/congestion
- plexiform neuroma
- cavernous hemangioma (adult type)
- cavernous hemangioma (infant type)
- lymphangioma
- mixed tumor of the lacrimal gland
- carcinoma metastatic to soft orbital tissues
- arteriovenous fistula (orbital extension of)
- orbital aneurysm/arteriovenous malformation
- varix
- dermoid cyst/hematic cyst
- epidermoid cyst
- Schwannoma A
- Schwannoma B
- lymphoma/pseudotumor/sarcoma
- sclerosing pseudotumor
- neurofibroma
- scirrhous carcinoma
- congenital anophthalmos (with or without cyst)

PERIORBITAL (PSEUDO-) TUMORS

- sinus disease (without bone defect)
- mucocele
- meningocele (encephalocele)
- supraorbital meningioma
- periorbital malignancy (carcinoma)
- fibrous dysplasia
- dacryocystitis

PATHOLOGY OF THE EXTRAOCULAR MUSCLES

- thickened muscles
- endocrine orbitopathy
- acute myositis
- chronic myositis
- hematoma
- metastatic carcinoma
- atrophy

OPTIC-NERVE PATHOLOGY

- swelling
- glioma
- increased fluid/thickening of sheaths
- meningioma
- atrophy

TRAUMA

- foreign body (except in orbital apex)
- blow-out fracture
- bony splinter in orbit
- hematoma
- emphysema

among the more frequently seen orbital tumors, were recognized early as
presenting specific echographic patterns. *Table 5* summarizes the acoustic
differential criteria of these hamartomas. The hallmarks of these round and
often mobile lesions are: (1) honeycomb-like structure, (2) high reflectivity,
(3) marked sound attenuation, (3) well-defined borders (encapsulated) and
(4) firm consistency. Cavernous hemangiomas of the adult type are usually
located within the muscle cone but frequently protrude into the temporal
paraocular space, more often inferiorly than superiorly to the lateral rectus
muscle.

Table 5: Acoustic differential criteria of cavernous hemangioma of the orbit (adult type)

Structure: Honeycomb-like	A
Reflectivity: High (80–95% - spike height)	A
Borders: Well-outline	A (B)
Sound attenuation: Medium	A (B)
Location: Muscle cone	AB
Consistency: Conditionally hard	A
Mobility: Mobile (if not very large)	A
Vascularity: No motion	A
Shape: Rounded	BA

A = A-scan findings
B = B-scan findings
() indicates minor significance

Quantitative A-scan echography often produces patterns pathognomonic for cavernous hemangiomas (*Figure 17*): echograms of these tumors are widened as compared to normal echograms and they exhibit a *shallow defect*. The spike height on the left is between 80 and 95% of the display height. The large amount of blood within the tumor causes the rather strong sound attenuation which is indicated by a medium angle kappa (30° to 60°) of the echogram. *Figure 18* shows histologic sections through a cavernous hemangioma explaining its high reflectivity: the large surfaces of the cavernous spaces are smoothly lined with endothelium and are responsible for strong reflections. Weaker echoes are produced by the blood within and by the connective tissues between the spaces. This honeycomb-like structure often creates a specific echographic pattern: higher and longer spikes (from the large surface of the cavernous spaces) alternate with shorter and lower signals (from the small interfaces of blood and connective tissues).

With *topographic A-scan* or *B-scan echography*, the round to oval shape of a cavernous hemangioma is revealed and its typical location within the muscle cone is established. *Figure 19* presents B-scan echograms from a cavernous hemangioma of the adult type. The B-scan echograms and to an even greater degree the A-scan patterns demonstrate that these tumors are well-outlined.

Kinetic A-scan echography exhibits another typical quality of cavernous hemangiomas of the adult type. When pushing the probe against the globe in order to squeeze the tumor between globe and bone, the first impression is that of a hard lesion: the width of the tumor pattern does not decrease during the initial stage of this procedure. However, prolonged pressure on the tumor will result in a moderate to marked decrease in the width of the

519

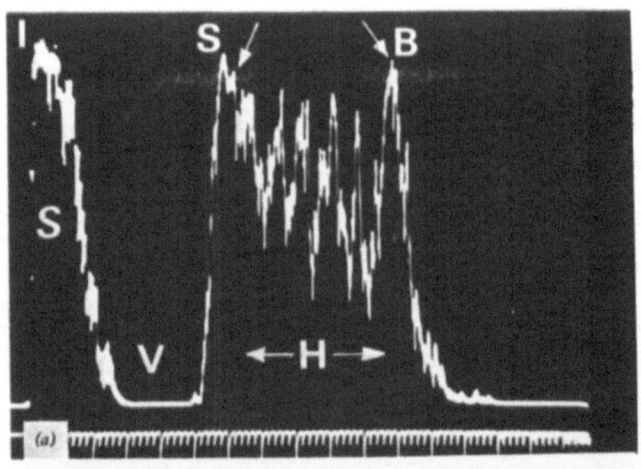

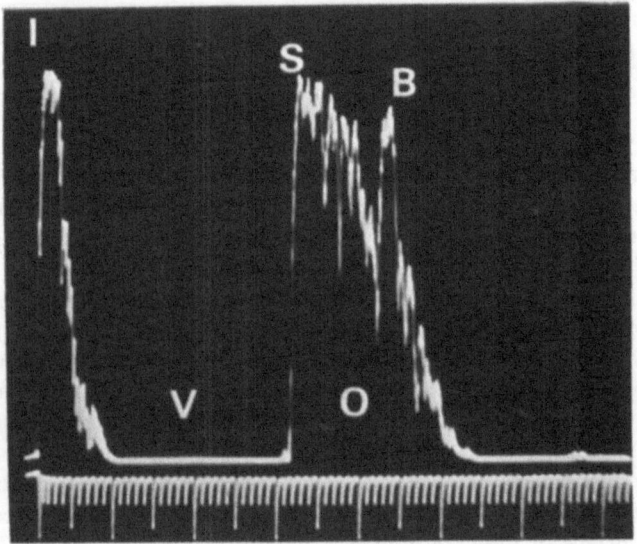

Figure 17: Transocular A-scan echograms from orbital cavernous hemangioma (adult type; (top) and normal orbit (bottom). **I** initial spike representing tip of the probe; **V** clear vitreous; **S** sclera; **H** hemangioma; **B** bony orbital wall; arrows tumor surface; **O** normal orbital tissues. Note the varying height of lesion spikes: longer and higher spikes correspond with the large, smooth, endohelialized surfaces of the cavernous spaces, whereas lower and shorter spikes represent the blood within these spaces (honeycom-like structure). The cho spikes from normal orbital tissues are higher and shorter (more closely spaced); the normal orbital echogram is also narrower and shows a larger angle kappa. Note the shortening of the vitreous line in the abnormal echogram which is caused by indentation of the posterior ocular wall through the tumor.

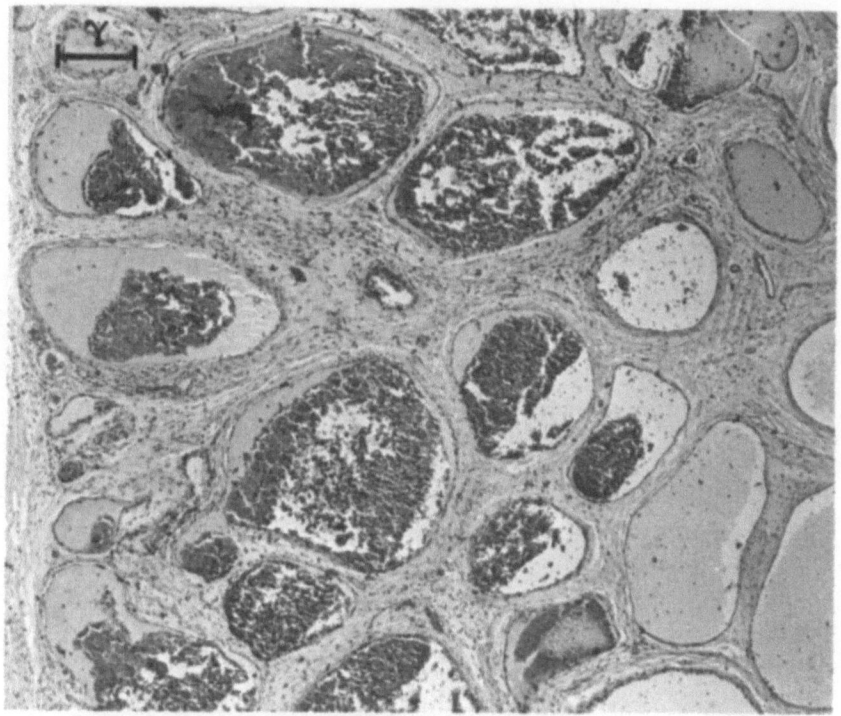

Figure 18: *Histological section from cavernous hemangioma (adult type)* explaining the typical appearance of the echogram (see *Figure 17*). I wave-length (0.19 mm with 8 MHz as used in standardized A-scan echography). The size of the surfaces of the cavernous spaces ranges within or above the wave-length and therefore produces stronger echoes (higher spikes) than the small interfaces formed by blood cells within the spaces (lower spikes). The distances between the longer spikes in the tumor echogram correspond with the width of the cavernous spaces in the hemangioma. The long surface spikes are frequently double-peaked (both surfaces of the septa separating two adjacent cavernous spaces).

echogram (*Figure 20*). This delayed compressibility of cavernous hemangiomas of the adult type is explained by the small calibers of the feeding and draining vessels as compared to the immense overall diameter of the vascular spaces within the lesion. It takes some time to expell sufficient amounts of blood from the lesion to shrink its size. For the same reason, the blood within the tumor is stagnant (like the water in a large swimming pool fed and drained by small pipes) so that no blood flow is detected with either echography or Doppler techniques.

Figures 21, 22 display a histological section and typical A- and B-scan echograms form a *lymphangioma* of the orbit. Note that the honeycomb-like structure is enhanced in these patterns to the point that even the B-scan echogram shows it. This is explained by the extremely low reflectivity of the contents of the vascular spaces in this lesion. Because of the absence of

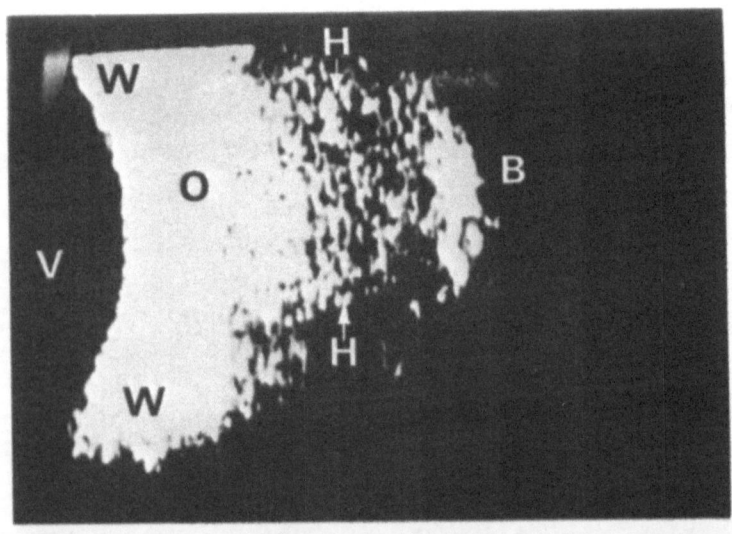

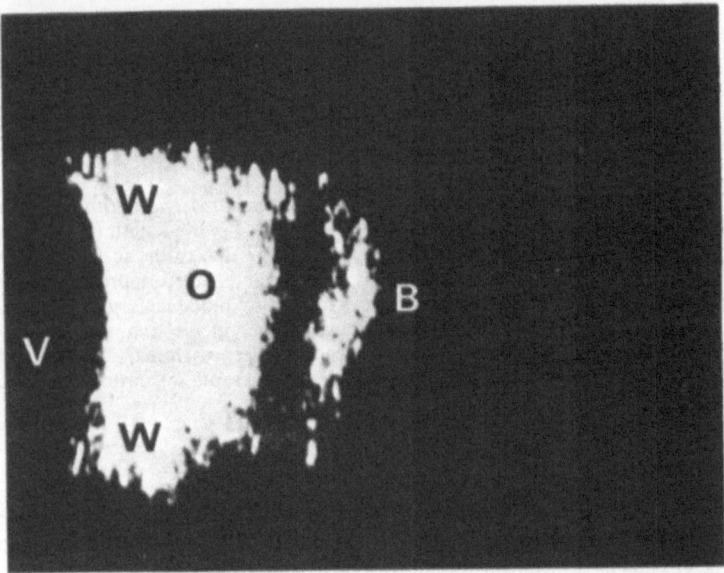

Figure 19: Transocular B-scan echograms from cavernous hemangioma (top) and nor- sues; **H** hemangioma; **B** bony orbital wall. The defect seen next to the bone signal in the normal orbital echogram is due to the strong sound attenuation within the normal orbital tissues (compare angle kappa in A-scan echograms, see *Figure 17*).

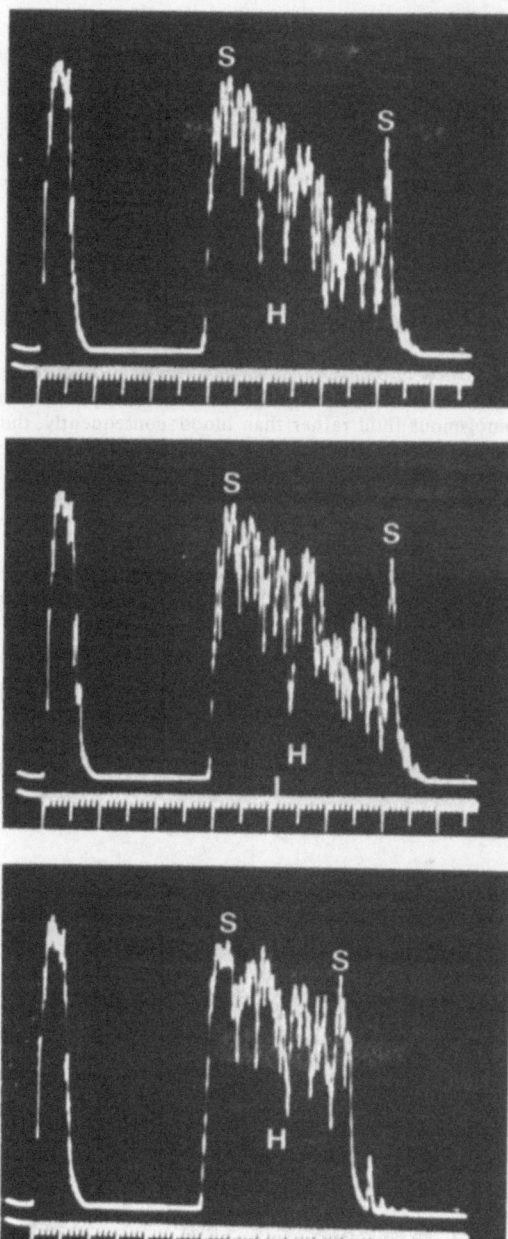

Figure 20: Kinitec A-scan echography demonstrates delayed compressibility of cavernous hemangioma. First the probe is placed on the surface of the globe without significant pressure; the sound beam is directed through the centers of both the globe and the lesion **(top echogram)**. Then the probe is pressed against the globe in order to squeeze the lesion between the globe and bony orbital wall. During the first few seconds of this procedure, the hemangioma pattern maintains its width indicating hard consistency of the lesion **(center echogram)**. However, after more than 20 seconds of exerting pressure, the hemangioma echogram decreases slowly but significantly in width (delayed compressibility, **bottom echogram**). This proves that the content of the lesion to a major part is fluid bloot which is squeezed out by the pressure. **H** cavernous hemangioma; **S** surface signals.

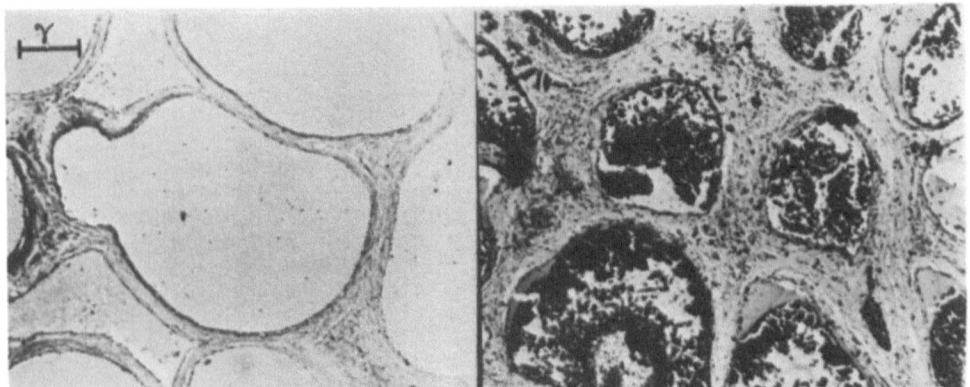

Figure 21: Histological section from lymphangioma **(left)** explaining its acoustic behavior. In contrast to the hemangioma **right)**, the cavernous spaces in the lymphangioma are filled with homogenous fluid rather than blood; consequently, the lower and shorter spikes seen in hemangioma echograms (see *Figure 17*) do not fill the spaces between the higher surface spikes in the lymphangioma pattern (see *Figure 22*).

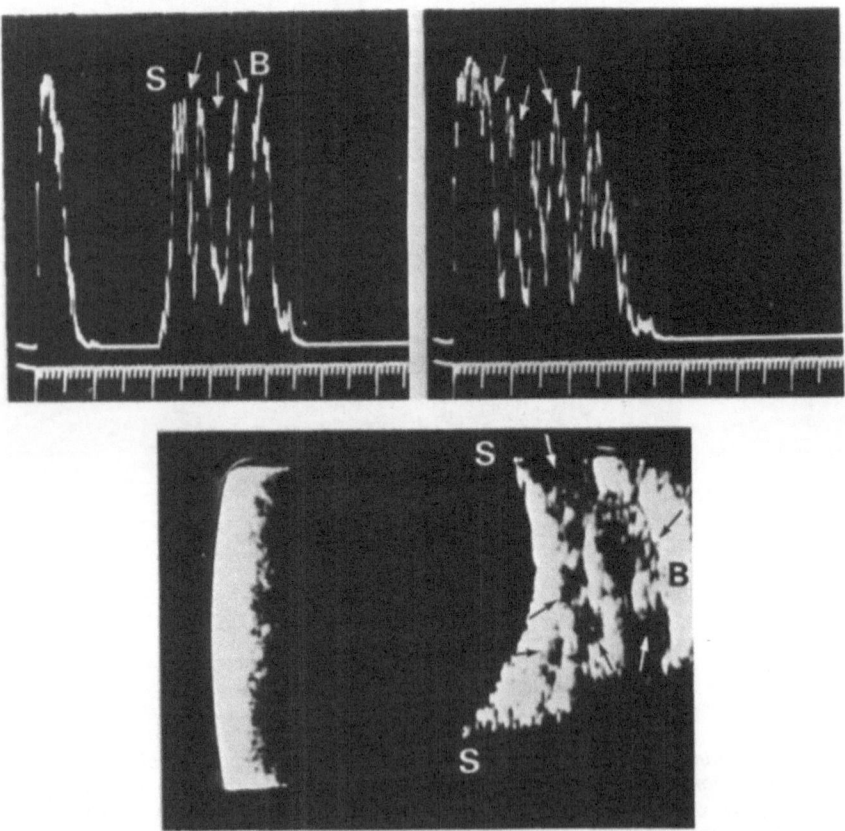

Figure 22: A-scan and B-scan echograms from lymphangioma. The cavernous spaces of this lesion appear in both the A-scan and the B-scan echograms creating an irregular but typical acoustic structure. **S** posterior sclera;

Figure 22 (cont.): **B** orbital bone; **arrows** cavernous spaces of lymphangioma, separated by septa (high, usually double-peaked spikes in the A-scan echograms; thick lines in the B-scan pattern).

large amounts of blood, the sound attenuation and consequently the angle kappa of the echograms are much smaller than in cavernous hemangioma patterns. Lymphangiomas differ also through their often irregular and indistinct borders from cavernous hemangiomas of the adult type.

Cavernous hemangiomas of the infant type differ from the adult type by a markedly irregular internal structure, a soft consistency and signs of pronounced blood flow within the lesion. *Capillary hemangiomas* contain only small acoustic interfaces and are therefore low reflective like lesions of the pseudotumor/lymphoma/sarcoma group. Unlike most pseudotumors and lymphomas, capillary hemangiomas are vascularized which can be documented with Doppler echography.

b) Optic Neuropathy: With standardized A-scan echography, thickening of the optic-nerve structures cannot only be detected but also differentiated into several groups: swelling of the optic nerve (e.g., in ischemic optic neuropathy; *Figure 23*; thickening of the optic-nerve sheaths or separation of the sheaths from the optic nerve by increased fluid (e.g., in Graves' Ophthalmopathy and pseudotumor cerebri, respectively; *Figure 24*). Only when the thickening of the optic nerve amounts to more than 100% as compared to the optic nerve in the fellow orbit can the diagnosis of an optic-nerve tumor (glioma) be made (*Figure 25*). The combination of marked and irregular thickening of the optic-nerve sheaths with progressive, significant loss of vision indicates a meningioma of the optic-nerve sheaths (*Figure 26*). In optic-nerve atrophy, the overall width of the optic-nerve pattern is normal but the nerve itself desplays decreased width (*Figure 27*).

c) Orbital pachymyopathy. As in optic neuropathy, standardized A-scan echography helps to distinguish between thickening of the muscle fibers and thickening of muscle sheaths. Unlike optic neuropathy, most lesions of the

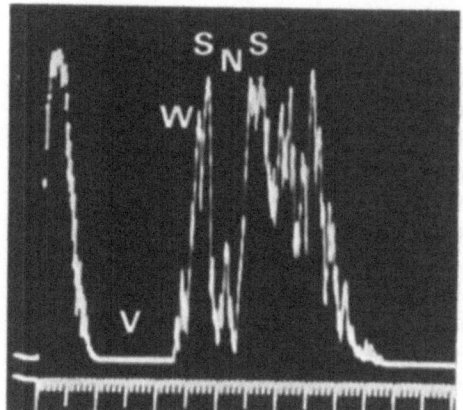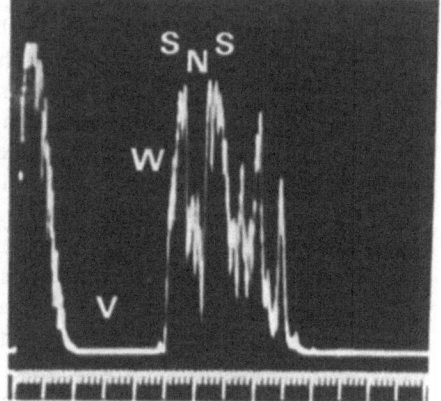

Figure 23. A-scan echograms from *swollen optic nerve* (**left**) and normal optic nerve of the fellow orbit (**right**). V vitreous; W posterior ocular wall; N swollen and normal optic nerves; S optic-nerve sheaths.

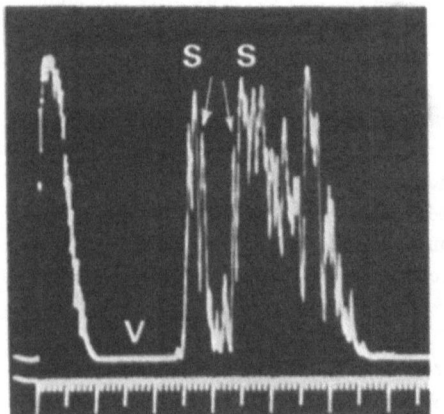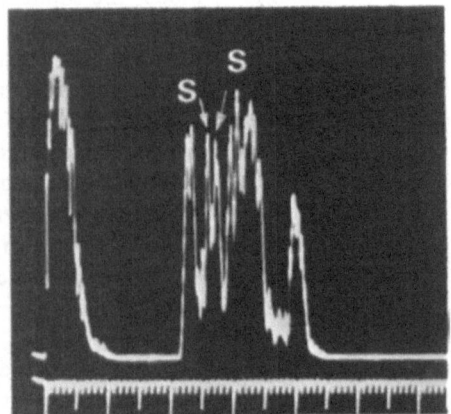

Figure 24: A-scan echograms indicating mildly *thickened optic-nerve sheaths* (together with moderate swelling of the nerve itself in the case of optic neuritis; **left echogram**) and *sheaths markedly elevated from the nerve* (which is atrophic) in a case of pseudo-tumor cerebri (increased subarachnoidal fluid; **right echogram**). V vitreous; S outer surfaces of optic-nerve sheaths; **arrows** surface of optic nerve. Note that both optic nerves are markedly thickened; this increased overall size of the optic nerve is due mainly to swelling of the nerve substance in the first case **(left)**, whereas it is entirely caused by tremendously increased fluid underneath the optic-nerve sheaths in the second **(right)**.

extraocular muscles involve thickening of both the muscle fibers and sheaths. Therefore, the differentiation between the two structures does not usually help in the differential diagnosis of muscle lesions. It is rather the number of muslces involved in one or both orbits and findings of localized and irregular swelling vs. a more diffuse and equally distributed thickening of muscles which helps in the differential diagnosis. *Table 6* lists conditions which so far have been found to cause thickening of one or more extraocular muscles in one or both orbits with and without involvement of the other orbital structures. Diagnosis of Graves' Ophthalmopathy can be made only when several muscles in both orbits appear significantly affected. Frequently, the optic-nerve sheaths are thickened in Graves' disease. Metastatic carcinoma can be identified on the basis of extreme or irregular thickening of primarily one extraocular muscle in cases of known metastatic disease. Mild to moderate diffuse thickening of fellow extraocular muscles in both orbits is a frequent finding in patients with the past history of metastatic carcinoma who have undergone chemotherapy; this thickening of extraocular muscles is comparable to the findings in endocrine orbitopathy, but should not lead t to the diagnosis of carcinoma metastatic to the extraocular muscles. Acute myositis can be diagnosed when associated with echographic signs of episcleritis and the clinical symptom of pain. Hematomas within the muscle sheaths are characterized by sudden onset and rapid decrease of muscla thickening observed during a few days of follow-up. Intracranial arteriovenous fistulas should be suspected when mild thickening of all extraocular muscles in one

526

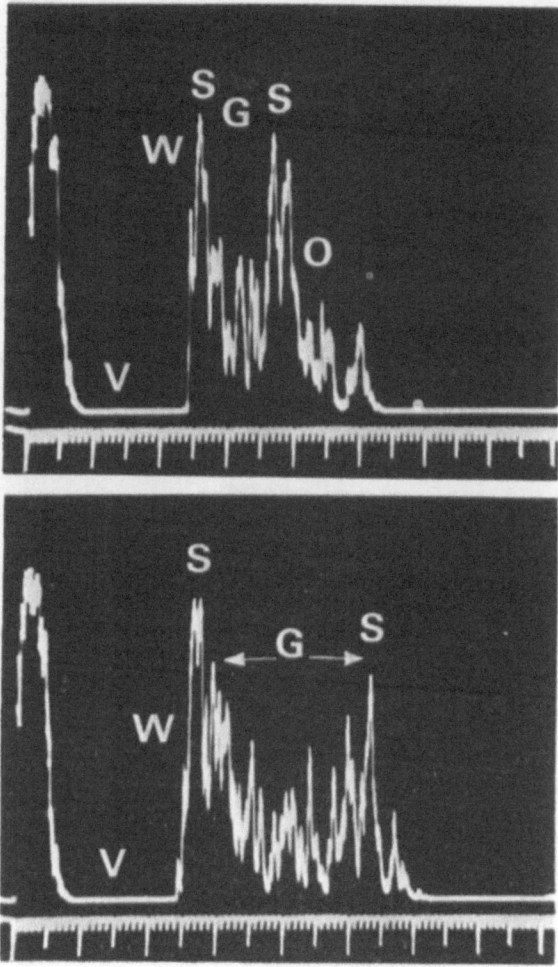

Figure 25: Glioma of optic nerve. **Top** cross section of the tumor; **bottom** long section of the glioma. **V** vitreous; **W** posterior ocular wall; **G** glioma; **S** optic-nerve sheaths; **O** orbital tissues next to glioma. The thickness of this optic nerve exceeds the size of the normal nerve in the fellow orbit by more than 100%; thus, the presence of an optic-nerve tumor (glioma) is diagnosed.

or both orbits is associated with thickening of the optic nerve, mild diffuse widening of all orbital patterns and the clinical sign of congestion of the episcleral veins (increased episcleral venous pressure). Pseudotumors of extraocular muscles can be identified as such only in the presence of more pseudotumors located in other ocular tissues of the same orbit. Frequently the exact cause of thickening of extraocular muscles cannot be identified by echographic examination alone. In these cases, echography is nevertheless extremely helpful by pointing out that a proptosis, lid swelling or

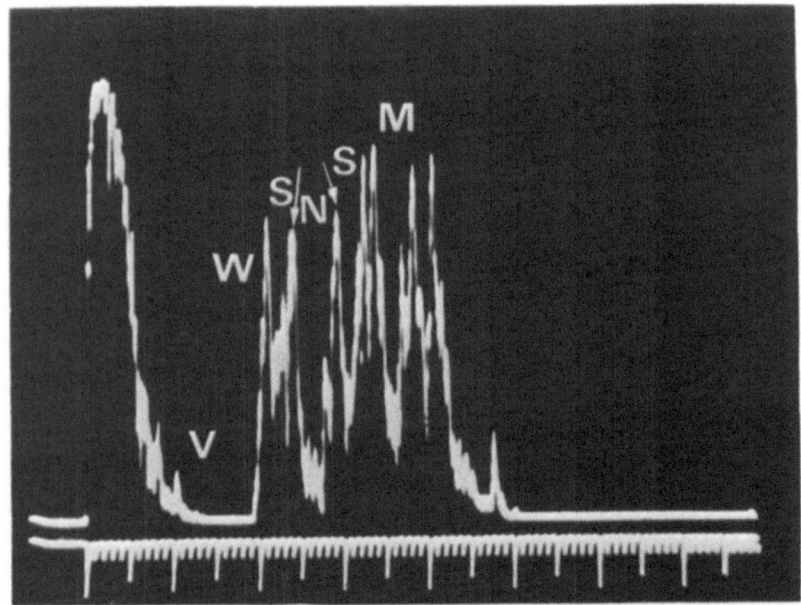

Figure 26: Meningioma of the optic-nerve sheaths. **V** vitreous; **W** posterior ocular wall; **N** optic nerve; **S** markedly thickened optic-nerve sheaths (defects in the echogram on either side of the optic-nerve defect); **arrows** outer surfaces of the optic-nerve sheaths; **M** medial rectus muscle. The overall-width of the optic nerve (nerve and sheaths) in this case exceeds the size of the normal optic nerve in the fellow orbit by more than 100%, thus proving the presence of an optic-nerve tumor; since the optic-nerve sheaths are mainly affected, a meningioma is diagnosed.

Table 6:   Various conditions which have been found to cause thickening of extraocular muscles without significantly involving other orbital tissues.

PRIMARILY UNILATERAL	PRIMARILY BILATERAL
Acute myositis	Endocrine orbitopathy
Chronic myositis	
Pseudotumor	
Metastatic carcinoma	
Hematoma	
Neurofibroma	
Meningioma	
Hypotrophy	

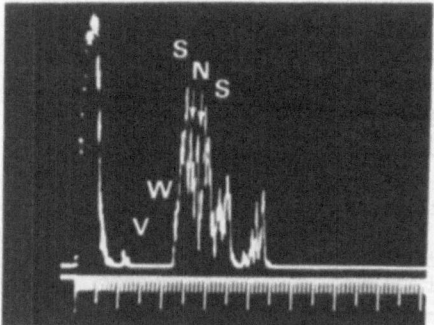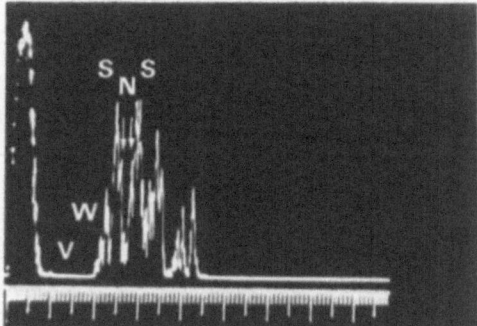

Figure 27: Optic-nerve atrophy (left). **V** vitreous; **W** posterior ocular wall; **N** optic nerve (surrounded by widened subarachnoidal space on either side); **S** outer surfaces of the optic-nerve sheaths (dura and arachnoidea); arrows surface of optic nerve (pia). Note that the thickness of the optic nerve itself appears decreased and the optic-nerve sheaths or the subarachnoidal space is widened; however, the overall-size of the optic nerve is the same as in the fellow orbit **(right)**.

motility problem of an eye are caused by thickening of a specified muslce rather than by an orbital mass lesion.

The accuracy of echographic tissue diagnosis is certainly not comparable to histological examination; nor does echography by any means replace the need for histological proof in many cases. The acoustic differential diagnosis, nevertheless, plays an important role in the management of orbital disorders. The decision of whether to observe the natural course of a lesion or to treat it, whether to do a partial or excisional biopsy prior to treatment, whether invasive diagnostic techniques such as carotid angiography are indicated, and other decisions are heavily influenced by the echographic tissue diagnosis.

3) Measurement and Topographical Mapping

With standardized A-scan echography, the *minimal depth* (distance between the orbital rim or orbital septum and the anterior pole of an orbital mass lesion), the *maximal depth* (distance between the orbital rim or septum and the posterior pole of an orbital lesion) and the *maximal diameters* in both sagittal and frontal directions can be determined accurately by measuring the distances between surface spikes in various sound-beam directions. *Table 7* indicates the accuracy of such measurements which depends on the size, location and outline of the mass lesion. The *border meridians* of an orbital lesion are determined by topographic A-scan echography.

While B-scan echograms may well document the topographic relationship of a tumor with the normal orbital structures (within one or the other a-coustic section), they fail to provide the three-demensional information needed for optimal surgical or radiotherapeutical management of the lesion.

Table 7: ACCURACY OF ECHOGRAPHIC MEASUREMENTS
OF ORBITAL STRUCTURES

		MASS LESION <20 mm	MASS LESION >20 mm	OPTIC NERVE	EXTRA-OCULAR MUSCLES
ANTERIOR ORBIT	well outlined	>± 0.2 mm	>± 0.5 mm		
	poorly outlined	>± 1.0 mm	>± 1.5 mm		
				± 0.5 mm	± 0.75 mm
POSTERIOR ORBIT	well outlined	>± 0.5 mm	>± 1.0 mm		
	poorly outlined	>± 1.5 mm	>± 2.0 mm		

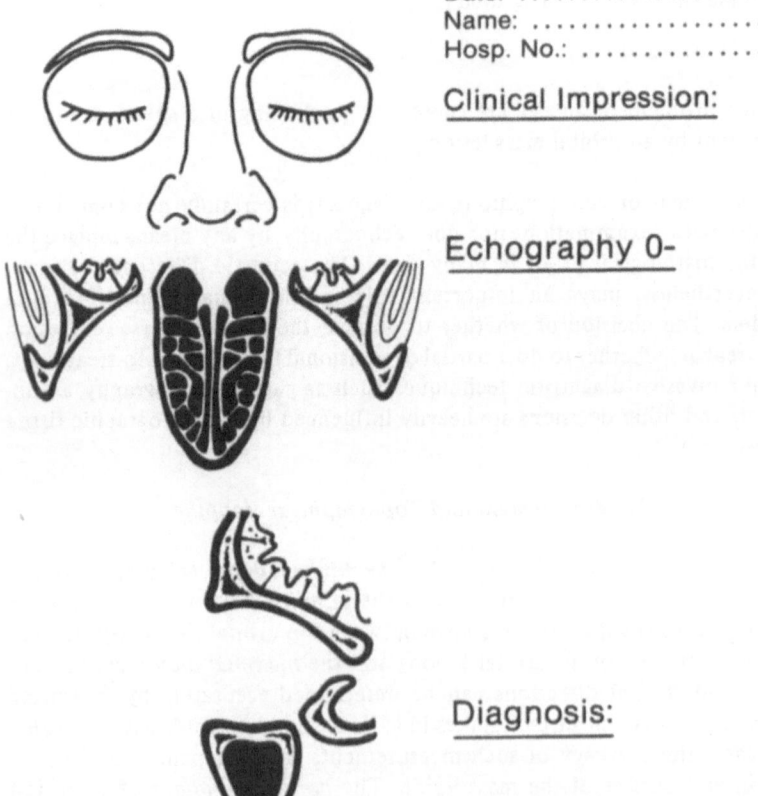

Date: ....
Name: ....
Hosp. No.: ....

Clinical Impression:

Echography 0–

Diagnosis:

Figure 28: Form with schematic drawings representing a frontal view of both orbits (closed lids), a horizontal sagittal section through both orbits and a vertical sagittal section through one orbit. These drawings are used to document the three-dimensional topography of orbital lesions as evaluated with echography.

At this time, the documentation of the three-dimensional situation is best accomplished by drawing the outline of a tumor mass in standard forms (*Figure 28*). The data needed for these drawings are obtained primarily with the standardized A-scan method.

Figure 29 illustrates an example of such a three-dimensional documentation. Such drawings of a tumor mass accompanied by data about the normal orbital structures such as the optic nerve and extraocular muscles help significantly in the following tasks: to establish an *indication* for medical treatment, surgery or radiotherapy: to elect an optimal *surgical*

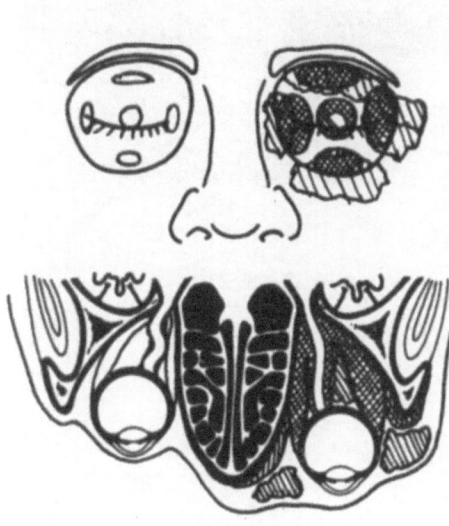

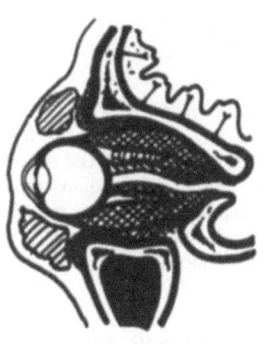

Date: 1-8-75 . . . .
Name: B. K. . . . .
Hosp. No. 75-00439 . . . .

Clinical Impression:

Slowly progressive, painless proptosis, lid swelling and loss of
vision in the left eye over the
past 8 years; neurofibromatosis
suspected.

Echography O- 10036

1. Multiple, solid, low-reflective,
poorly-outlined, mobile lesions in
both lids; the lacrimal-gland area;
near the lateral and medial orbital
rims and in the muscle cone.
Measurements (in mm): inferior
lid lesion 30 x 10 x 6; upper lid
lesion, 25 x 8 x 5; lateral anterior lesion, 10 x 7 x 4; medial
anterior lesion, 6 x 5 x 3; mobile
lesion in anterior muscle cone has
an average diameter of 8 mm.

2. Marked swelling of optic-nerve
sheaths and all extraocular muscles
and their sheaths. The lateral
rectus muscle is the most affected
one; it measures up to 8 mm in
diameter (as compared to the normal 4.2 mm of the right lateral
rectus muscle).

3. Diffuse thickening of periorbit.

4. Diffuse, rock-hard and extremely low-reflective, immobile
mass in the posterior orbit filling it entirely and making it
difficult to distinguish the borders of the various anatomical
structures.

Diagnosis:

Multiple pseudotumors in and around
the left orbit (of the sclerosing
type in the posterior orbit).

Figure 29: Topographic documentation in the case of a massive orbital pseudotumor through one orbit.

531

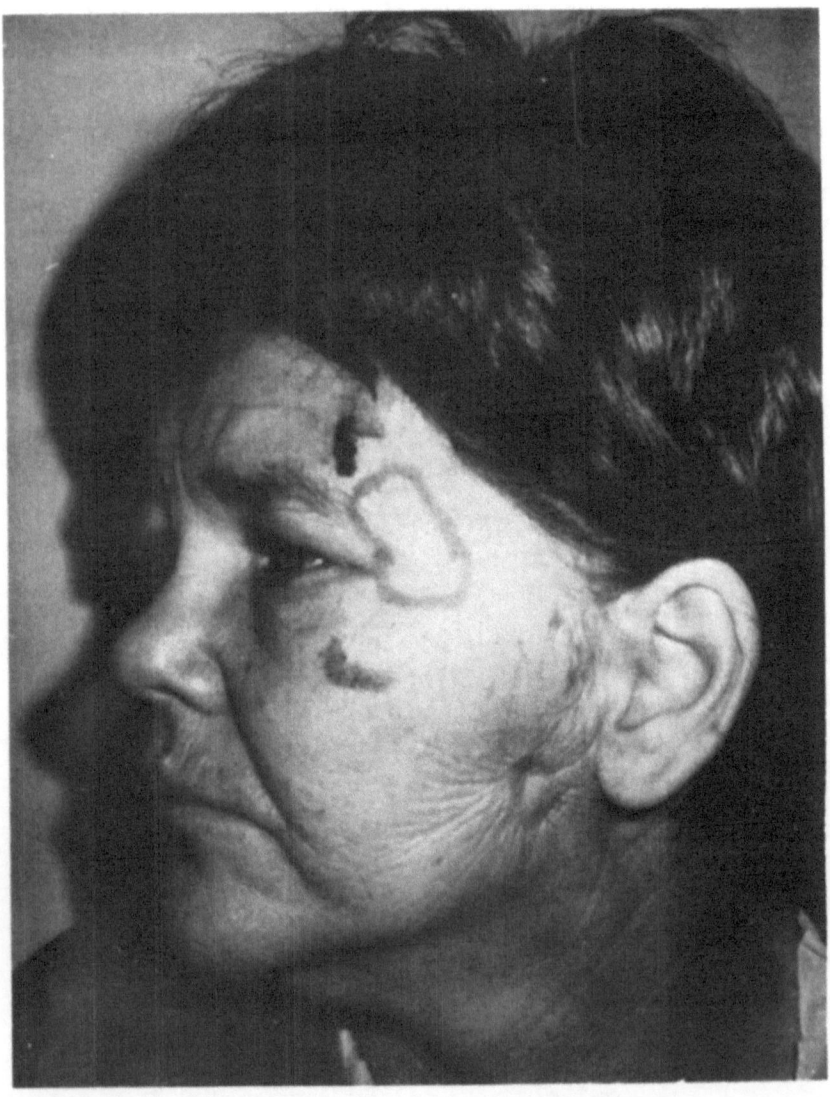

Figure 30: Photographic documentation of the extension of a malignant tumor (scirrhous carcinoma of the breast, metastatic to the left orbit). The borders of the lesion as evaluated with A-scan echography may be drawn directlyon the skin prior to photography or may be drawn on polaroid pictures. This kind of documentation is helpful for radiotherapeutic management; it may also serve to document growth of a lesion in followup examinations. Note that another such metastasis (with typical signs of shrinkage) has affected the patient's pre-auricular region.

approach (e.g., partial vs. excisional biopsies and anterior vs. lateral vs. transfrontal orbitotomies); to provide *guidance during surgery* (e.g., by outlining the topography of a lesion, indicating the tissue type (for instance cysts vs. solid lesions and vascularized vs. nonvascularized lesions; indicating when drainage of an orbital abscess is sufficient, etc.); to plan radiotherapy when drainage of an orbital abscess is sufficient, etc.); to plan *radiotherapy* by indicating the location, shape and size of a tumor mass for optimal dosage and distribution of radiation and by checking the response of a tumor mass to radiation therapy. *Figure 30* illustrates a simple way of marking the borders of a tumor on a photographic picture of the patient's face for the latter indication.

3) Diagnosis of Peri- and Retro-Orbital Lesions

Peri- and retro-orbital lesions, particularly lesions of the peri-orbital sinuses, are diagnosed from the fact that echoes are obtained from these areas. Under normal conditions, the air-filled sinuses and the retro-orbital region do not produce echoes because of the strong sound attenuation in normal bone and due to 100% reflection of ultrasonic energy from air surfaces. The mere fact that echoes are obtained from a sinus indicates that it is not air-filled and therefore is abnormal.

In these presence of bony defects, a differentiation of such pathology is possible. Tumor masses cannot only be detected, but frequently differentiated in various groups (see *Table 4*). Provided such bony defects are present, peri- and retro-orbital lesions can be evaluated with a similar degree of reliability and accuracy as orbital mass lesions.

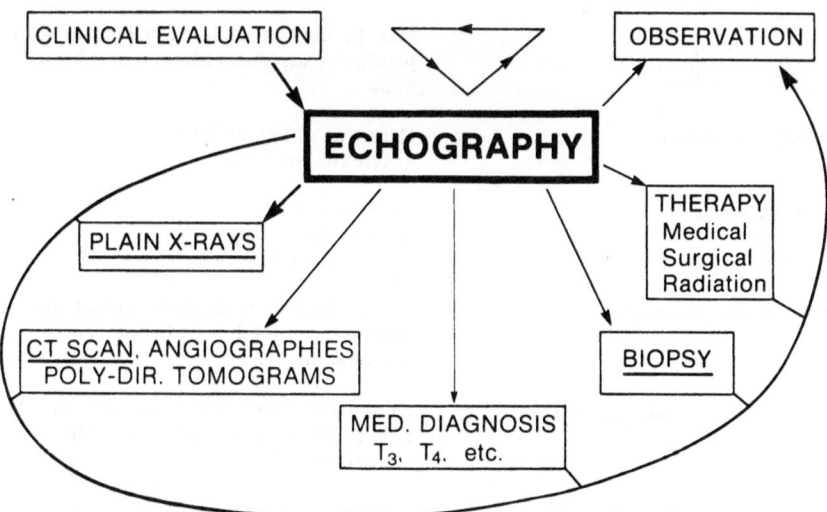

Figure 31: Illustration of the central role echography plays in the diagnosis of orbital lesions: as a routine screening procedure in all cases of suspected orbital pathology in order to detect, differentiate, localize and measure it; as an indicator for other diagnostic tests; as a guidance for medical, surgical and radiation therapy; and as a harmless procedure which may be used frequently in order to to follow up the clinical course or the effectiveness of therapy in cases of orbital lesions.

533

INDICATIONS FOR ORBITAL ECHOGRAPHY

On the basis of the applications and results described in the previous section, clinical echography can be considered as the ideal screening method of the orbit and periorbit; in many instances it will provide the final diagnosis and thus spare the patient the necessity of undergoing other nonconclusive diagnostic tests. On the other hand, echography may indicate the necessity of specific diagnostic procedures such as carotid arteriography. Whenever an orbital lesion is suspected on the basis of proptosis, enophthalmus, lid swelling, pain, unilateral papilledema or optic-nerve atrophy, etc., echography is indicated as the initial diagnostic procedure following clinical evaluation. Although echography is not the primary technique of evaluating peri-orbital sinsues, it will indicate disease in these areas and prompt otolaryngological and radiological examinations. *Figure 31* illustrates the central role clinical echography plays in evaluation of orbital and peri-orbital disorders. The importance of clinical echography as a primary examination technique is emphasized by its various assets listed in *Table 8*.

Table 8:   SOME ASSETS OF ORBITAL ECHOGRAPHY (Particularly
in comparison with X-ray techniques)

● *Harmless procedure*	Echography may be used extensively for meticulous Evaluation and frequently for close Follow-up
	May be used on children or persons with painful conditions without general anesthesia
● *High sensitivity*	Detection of lesions $> 99\%$; differentiation $> 80\%$
● *High accuracy*	Detection $> 99\%$ Differentiation $> 80\%$ Measurement $\pm\ 0.2 - \pm\ 2.0$ mm
● *Real-time technique*	Demonstration of dynamics (blood flow, consistency, mobility of tissues and of extraocular muscles
● *Mobile (portable) equipment*	Examination may be conducted in the office, at the patient's bedside or in the operating room
● *Relatively inexpensive equipment*	as compared to radiological equipment
● *Direct supervision by ophthalmologist*	

REFERENCES

1. Baum G., & I. Greenwood. The Application of Ultrasonic Locating Techniques to Ophthalmology: Theoretic Considerations and Coustic Properties of Ocular Media. I. Reflective Properties. *Am. J. Ophthalmol.* 46: *319-329* (1958).
2. Baum, G. & I. Greenwood. The Application of Ultrasonic Locating Techniques to Ophthalmology. II. Ultrasonic Slit Lamp in the Ultrasonic Visualization of Soft Tisseus. *Arch. Ophthalmol.* 60: *263-279* (1958).
3. Baum, G. & I. Greenwood. Ultrasonography—An Aid in Orbital Tumor Diagnosis. *Arch. Ophthalmol.* 64: *180-194* (1960).
4. Ossoinig, K.C. Zum Problem der akustischen Tumordiagnostik von Auge und Orbita (experimentelle und klinische Untersuchungen mit dem Zeitamplitudenverfahren). Acoustic Diagnosis of Intraocular and Orbital Tumors—Experimental and Clinical Examinations with the A-Scan Technique.)
   In: Diagnostica Ultrasonica in Ophthalmologia (Proc. of SIDUO I, Berlin, 1964, Buschmann W. and Hildebrandt I., eds.). *Wiss. Z. Humboldt-Univ. Berlin, Math.-Nat. R.* 14: *185-191* (1965).
5. Ossoinig, K.C. Die Ultraschalldiagnostik der Orbita (A-Bildverfahren). (Echography of the orbit--A-scan Technique). *Klin. Monatsbl. Augenheilk.* 149: *817-839* (1966).
6. Ossoinig, K.C. & K. Seher. Ergebnisse der Ultraschalldiagnostik orbitaler Tumoren. (Results of Echography in Orbital Tumors). *Klin. Monatsbl. Augenheilk.* 151: ɔ19-524
   519-524 (1967).
7. Hildebrandt, I. Die Lagebeziehungen zwischen Bulbusmittelpunkt und temporalem Obitarand bei Exophthalmus. (Relationship Between the Globe Center and Temporal Orbital Rim in Exophthalmos.)
   In: Diagnostica Ultrasonica in Ophthalmologia (Proc. of SIDUO I, Berlin, 1964, Buschmann W. and Hildebrandt I., eds.). *Wiss Z. Humboldt-Univ. Berlin, Math.-Nat. R.* 14: *213-216* (1965).
8. Ossoinig, K.C. & K. Seher. Einige Erkenntnisse über das histologische Substrat der Echogramme. (Studies of the Histological Basis of Echograms).
   In: Ultrasonics in Ophthalmology (Proc. of the Münster Symposium, 1966, Oksala A. and Gernet H., eds.), 103-109. S. Karger, Basel/New York (1967).
9. Ossoinig, K.C., K. Seher & F. Kaufman. Echographische Untersuchungen feingeweblicher Strukturen. II. Uber ein bei der Ulteaschalluntersuchung von Citrablut beobachtetes Phänomen. (Echographic Studies of Microscopic Structures. II. Phenomena Observed in Echographic Examinations of Citrated Blood). *Graefes Arch. Ophthalmol.* 173: *327-338* (1967).
10. Ossoinig, K.C. Ein neues Ultraschall-Diagnostikgerät für die Augenheilkunde. (A New Ultrasound Apparatus for Echographic Diagnosis in Ophthalmology). *Graefes Arch. Ophthalmol.* 171: *312-317* (1967).
11. Ossoinig, K.C. The Echographic Picture Presented by Healthy Orbita (A-Scan Echograms).
    In: Diagnostica Ultrasonica in Ophthalmologia (Proc. of SIDUO II, Brno, 1967, Vanýsek J., ed.). *Acta Fac. Med. Univ. Brunensis.* 35: *101-107* (1968).
12. Ossoinig, K.C. Grundlagen der echographischen Gewebsdifferenzierung. I. Teil: Experimentelle und klinische Untersuchungen über den Einfluss technischer Faktoren auf den diagnostischen Wert der Echogramme. (Basics of Echographic Tissue Differentiation. I. Experimental and Clinical Examinations of the Influence of System Parameters on the Diagnostic Value of Echograms).
    In: Ultrasonographia Medica (Proc. of the lst World Congress on Ultrasonic Diagnostics in Medicine and SIDUO III, Vienna, 1969, Böck J. and Ossoinig K.C., eds.), 1: 155-168. Verlag Wiener Med. Akademie, Vienna (1971).

13. Ossoinig, K.C. Grundlagen der echographischen Gewebsdifferenzierung. II. Teil: Das akustische Verhalten biologischer Strukturen. (Basics of Echographic Tissue Differentiation. II. Acoustic Behavoir of Biological Structures).
In: Ultrasonographia Medica (Proc. of the lst World Congress on Ultrasonic Diagnostics in Medicine and SIDUO III, Vienna, 1969, Böck J. and Ossoinig K.C., eds.), 1: 419-439. Verlag Wiener Med. Akademie, Vienna (1971).

14. Böck, J. & K.C. Ossoinig. Fundamentals of Non-Traumatic Tissue Differentiation by Ultrasound III. Histological Structures and Ultrasonograms.
In: Ultrasonographia medica (Proc. of the 1st World Congress on Ultrasonic Diagnostics in Medicine and SIDUO III, Vienna, 1969, Böck J. and Ossoinig K.C., eds.), 1: 411-417. Verlag Wiener Med. Akademie, Vienna (1971).

15. Ossoinig, K.C. Grundlagen der klinischen Echo-Ophthalmographie. IV. Teil: Klinische Standardisation der Diagnostikanlage und der Untersuchunstechnik. (Basics of Clinical Echo-Ophthalmography. IV. Clinical Standardization of Equipment and Techniques).
In: Ultrasonographia Medica (Proc. of the lst World Congress on Ultrasonic Diagnostics in Medicine and SIDUO III, Vienna, 1969, Böck J. and Ossoinig K.C., eds.), 2: 83-118. Verlag Wiener Med. Akademie, Vienna (1971).

16. Ossoinig, K.C. Klinische Echo-Ophthalmographic. II. Teil: Echographie bei Erkrankungen der Orbita. (Clinical Echo-Ophthalmography. II. Echography in Orbital Disenses).
In: Ultrasonographia Medica (Proc. of the lst World Congress on Ultrasonic Diagnostics in Medicine and SIDUO III, Vienna, 1969 Böck J. and Ossoinig K.C., eds.), 2: 423-435. Verlag Wiener Med. Akademie, Vienna (1971).

17. Francois, J. & F. Goes. Echographie A et exophthalmies unilaterales. (A-Scan echography and Unilateral Exophthalmos). *Bull. Soc. belge Ophthal.* 155: 475-486 (1970).

18. Ossoinig, K.C. Die Echographie in der Augenheilkunde. (Echography in Ophthalmology). 9 Verhandlungen der Oesterr. Ophthalmol. Ges. (1964), 11-27. Verlag Brüder Hollinek, Wien, (1966).

19. Ossoinig, K.C. Die ultraschalldiagnostik der Tumoren in der Augenhöhle–Untersuchungen mit dem A-Bild und B-Bildverfahren. (Echography of Orbital Tumors–Examinations with A- and B-Scan Techniques). *Graefes Arch. Ophthalmol.* 172: *364-382* (1967).

20. Ossoinig, K.C. Ultrasonic Diagnosis on the Eye–an Aid for the Clinic (Review).
In: Ultrasonics in Ophthalmology (Proc. of the Münster Symposium, 1966, Oksala A. and Gernet H., eds.), 116-133. S. Karger, Basel/New York (1967).

21. Ossoinig K.C. & E. Valencak. L'echotomographie dans le diagnostic des tumeurs orbitaires. (Echo-tomography–a Method for the Diagnosis of Orbital Tumors). *Neuro-Chir.* 13: *899-905* (1967).

22. Ossoinig, K.C. Erste Erfahrungen mit der kombinierten A-Bild- und B-Bildechographie orbitaler Tumoren. (First Experiences with the Combination of A- and B-scan Echography of Orbital Tumors). *Wien. Klin. Wschr.* 80/4: *72-74* (1968).

23. Ossoinig, K.C. Echo-tomography Ultrasonica in Ophtahlmologia (Proc. of SIDUO II, Brno, 1967, Vanýsek J., ed.). *Acta Fac. Med. Univ. Brunnensis.* 35: *117-123* (1968).

24. Ossoinig, K.C. Methodik der Schmittbild-Echographie des Auges und der Augenhöhle. (Techniques of Echo-tomography of the Eye and Orbit).
In: Diagnostica Ultrasonica in Ophthalmologia (Proc. of SIDUO II, Erno, 1967, Vanysek J., ed.). Acta Fac. Med. Univ. Brunensis. 35: 125-132 (1968).

25. Ossoinig, K.C. Routine Ultrasonography of the Orbit.
In: Ultrasonography in Ophthalmology (Wainstock M.A., ed.). Int. Ophthalmol. Clin., 9/3: 613-642. Little, Brown & Co. Boston (1969).

26. Ossoinig, K.C., Massin M. & J. Poujol. L'ultrasonographie, methode de routine pour l'examen de l'orbite. (Echography–a Method for Routine Examinations of the Orbit). *Bull. Soc. Ophthal. Fr.* 69: *1051-1058* (1969).

27. Ossoinig, K.C. Ein neues Gerät für die klinische Echo-Ophthalmographie vorschläge zur Standardisation wichtiger Geräte-Parameter. (The first Standardized System for Echo-Ophthalmography).
In: Diagnostica Ultrasonica in Ophthalmologia (Proc. of SIDUO IV, Paris, 1971, Massin M. and Poujol L., eds.), 131-137. Centre National d'Ophtalmologie des Quinze-Vingts, Paris (1973).

28. Francois, J. & F. Goes. Echographie A et ecophthalmies unilaterales. (A-scan echography and Unilateral Exophthalmos). Bull. Soc. belge Ophthal. 155: 475-486 (1970).

29. Gallenga, P.E.: Diagnostica dei tumori dell'orbita mediante ultrasuoni. (Echography of Orbital Tumors). *Att Soc. It. Canc.*, 7/1: *301* (1970).

30. Tane S. and Horiuchi T.: (Studies on Ultrasonic Diagnosis in Ophthalmology. Report 2: Ultrasonic Diagnosis for Orbital Tumors–Especially Correlations between Histological Structure and the Echogram). *Acta Soc. Ophthalmol. Jap.*, 74: *851-857* (1970).

31. Poujol, J. Possibilites de L'examen echographique de l'orbite en methode A. *Clin. Ophthalmol.*, 3: *85-93* (1971).

32. Sayegh, F., Hallerbach, H., & H.G. Trier. Die Echographie (A- und B- Bildverfahren) im Vergleich mit der Röntgendiagnostik bei raumfordernden Orbitaprozessen. (Comparison between echography (A- and B-scan techniques) and x-ray daignosis in space-occupying lesions of the orbit). In *Ultrasonographia medica* (Proc. of lst World Congress on Ultrasonic Diagnostics in Medicine and SIDUO III, Vienna, 1969, Böck, J., and Ossoinig, K.C., eds.). Vol. 2. pp. 407-422, Verlag Wiener Med. akademie (1971).

33. Sayegh, F., & H.G. Trier. The importance of diagnostic ultrasound (A-and B-mode) of the orbit in cases with suspicious tumors in the paranasal sinus region. *Ophthal. Res.* 2: *183-188* (1971).

34. Soriano H. & Psilas K.: Estudio ecografico de los tumores orbitarios. (Echographic Study of Orbital Tumors). *Arch. Soc. Esp. Oftal.*, 31: *659-66* (1971).

35. Till, P. Echographie nach orbitalen Traumen. (Echography after orbital traumas). In *Ultrasonographia medica* (Proc. of lst World Congress on Ultrasonic Diagnostics in Medicine and SIDUO III, Vienna, 1969, Böck, J., and Ossoinig, K.C. eds.), Vol. 2, pp. 437-441, Verlag Wiener Med. Akademie, Vienna (1971).

36. Till, P. Ultraschalldiagnostik retrobulbärer Hämatome. (Echography of retrobulbar hemantomas). *Klin. Mbl. Augenheilk.* 158: *723-727* (1971).

37. Meyner, E.M. Orbita-Diagnostik mit Ultraschall. (Orbital Diagnosis with Ultrasound). *Klin. Monatsbl. Augenheilkd.*, 160: *507* (1972).

38. Psilas, K. & H. Soriano. Contribution de l'echographie A au diagnostic des tumeurs rétrobulbaires. (Contributions of A-Scan Echography to the Diagnosis of Retrobulbar Tumors). *Rev. Otoneuroophthalmol.*, 44: *359-364* (1972).

39. Schüpbach, M.: Fortschritte in der Ophthalmoechographie mit einem neuen Diagnostikgerät. (Progress in Echo-Ophthalmography for a New Diagnostic Instrument). Ophthalmologica, 165: 245-251 (1972).

40. Till, P., and Ossoinig, K.C.: Die Echographie zur Beureilung des Ubergreifens von Oberkiefertumoren auf die Orbita. (Echographic detection of orbital extension in tumors of the maxillary sinus). *Mschr. Ohrenheilk.* 106: 442-448 (1972).

41. Vogel A. and Buschmann W.: Bisherige Ergebnisse der Ultraschalluntersuchungen der Orbita im A-System. (Results of A-Scan Echography of the Orbit).
In: Fortschritte in Ultraschalldiagnostik und Ophthalmologie. Wiss. Z. Humboldt-Univ. Berlin, Math.-Nat. R., 21: 53-57 (1972).

42. Bellone G. and Gallenga P.E.: Echography of Mixed Tumours of the Lacrimal Gland. Ophthalmologica 166: 156-160 (1973).

43. Meyner, E.M.: Erfahrungen in der klinischen Orbitadiagnosik mit dem A-Bild Verfahren. (Experiences with clinical orbital diagnosis using A-scan echography). In *Diagnostica ultrasonica in ophthalmologia* (Proc. of SIDUO IV, Paris, 1971, Massin, M., and Poujol, J., eds.), pp. 227-231, Centre National d'Ophtalmologie des Quinze-Vingts, Paris (1973).

44. Poujol, J.: L'examen echographique de l'orbite en methode A. (Echographic Examination of the Orbit Using Method A.). Bul. Soc. Ophhal. Fr. No. Special, 115-126 (1973).
45. Tane, S.: The ultrasonic diagnosis of intraorbital tumors. In *Diagnostica ultrasonica is ophthalmologia* (Proc. of SIDUO IV, Paris, 1971, Massin, M., and Poujol, J., eds.) pp. 223-226, Centre National d'Ophthalmologie des Quinze-Vingts, Paris (1973).
46. Bellone G., Gallenga P.E. and Pasquarelli A.: Objective Interpretation of Eye and Orbit Tissue Echograms. Ophthalmologica 169: 290-298 (1974).
47. Ossoinig, K.C. and Blodi, F.C.: Preoperative Differential Diagnosis of Tumors with Echography. IV. Daignosis of Orbital Tumors.
In: Current Concepts in Ophthalmology (Blodi F.C., ed.), 4: 313-341. C.V. Mosby, St. Louis (1974).
48. Söllner, F., Wüstenberg L. and Kohlhase R.: Echographische Differentialdiagnostik des einseitigen Exophthalmus. (Echographic Differential Diagnosis of Unilateral Exophthalmus). Klin. Monatsbl. Augenheilkd., 164: 117-124 (1974).
49. Babel, J., Psilas, K., Soriano, H., & J.P. Houber. Differential diagnosis of orbital tumors by echography A: A clinico-pathological study of 54 cases. In *Modern problems in ophthalmology: Orbital disorders* (Proc. of the 2nd International Symposium on Orbital Disorders, Amsterdam, 1973, Bleeker, G.M., Garston, J.B., Kronenberg, B., and Lyle, T.K., eds.), Vol. 14, pp. 254-264, S. Karger, Basel (1975).
50. Ossoinig, K.C. & P. Till. Klinische Echographie der Tumoren des Auges und der Augenhöhle. (Clinical Echography of Tumors of the Eye and Orbit).
In: Krebsbehandlung als interdisziplinäre Aufgabe–Wiener Arbeitskreis für Geschwulstbehandlung (Kärcher K.H., ed.), 249-270. Springer-Verlag, Berlin/Heidelberg/New York (1975).
51. Frühwald, H. & P. Till. Die Echography in Diseases of the Periorbital Sinuses). *Laryng. Rhinol.* 54: *865-870* (1975).
52. Ossoinig, K.C. A-Scan Echography and Orbital Disease.
In: Proc. 2nd Internatl. Symposium on Orbital Disorders. Mod. Probl. Ophthalmol., 14: 203-235 (1975).
53. Ossoinig, K.C., Keenan T.P. & F. Bigar. Cavernous Hemangioma of teh Orbit (A Differential Diagnosis in Clinical Echography).
In: Ultrasonography in Ophthalmology (Proc. of SIDUO V, Ghent, 1973, Francois J. and Goes F., eds.). Bibl. Ophthalmol., 83: 236-244. S. Harger, Basel/New York (1975).
54. Ossoinig, K.C. & P. Till. Ten-Year Study on Clinical Echography in Orbital Disease.
In: Ultrasonography in Ophthalmology (Proc. of SIDUO V, Ghent, 1973, Francois J. and Goes F., eds.). Bibl. Ophthalmol., 83: 200-216. S. Karger, Basel/New York (1975).
55. Poujol, J. A-scan ultrasound: Accuracy of diagnosis in orbital diseases. In *Modern problems in ophthalmology: Orbital disorders* (Proc. of the 2nd International Symposium on Orbital Disorders, Amsterdam, 1973, Bleeker, G.M., Garston, J.B., Kronenberg, B., and Lyle, T.K., eds.), Vol. 14, pp. 250-253, S. Karger, Basel (1975).
56. Schwab, B. & A. Nover. Ergebnisse der Orbitaechographic im A-Bildverfahren (Results of A-Scan Echography of the Orbit). *Klin. Mbl. Augenheilk.* 166: *758-766* (1975).
57. Thijssen, J.M. & P.A. Gommers. Methodical and Clinical Aspects of Echo-Oculographiy.
In: Ultrasonography in Ophthalmology (Proc. of SIDUO
graphy.
In: Ultrasonography in Ophthalmology (Proc. of SIDUO V, Ghent, 1973, Francois J. and Goes F., eds.). Bibl. Ophthalmol., 83: 25-31. S. Karger, Basel/New York (1975).

58. Till, P. Echography in rhinogenic orbital conditions. In *Modern problems in ophthalmology: Orbital disorders* (Proc. of the 2nd International Symposium on Orbital Disorders, Amsterdam, 1973, Bleekerm G.M., Garston, J.B., Kronenberg, B., Lyle, T.K., eds.), Vol. 14, pp. 273-277, S. Karger, Basel (1975).
59. Till, P. & M.R. Lessel. Doppler-sonography and Echo-ophthalmography of orbital vascular processes. In SIDUO Roundtable (Proc. of the SIDUO Roundtable, Paris, 1974, Massin, M. and Poujol, J., eds.), pp. 51-58. Centre National d'Ophtalmologie Des Quinze-Vingts, Paris (1975).
60. Trier, H.G., Sayegh F. & W. Adler. Results of Orbital Ultrasonography in 200 Clinical Cases. Mod. Probl. Ophthalmol. (Orbital Disorders), 14: 265-272 (1975).
61. Wüstenberg, L. & R. Kohlhase: Echographische Befunde bei eiseitigem Exophthalmus. (Ultrasonic results in unilateral exophthalmos). In *Bibliotheca ophthalmologica: Ultrasonography in ophthalmology* (Proc. of SIDUO V, Ghent, Belgium, 1973, Francois, J., and Goes, F., eds.), Vol. 83, pp. 217-224, S. Karger Basel, 1975.
62. Till,P. Solid tissue model for the standardization of the echoophthalmolograph 7200 MA (Kretztechnik) *Documenta Ophthalm.* 41 (2): *205-240* (1976).
63. Hodes, B.L. Tissue Texture: The Histologic Basis for Standardized A-scan Diagnosis in Ophthalmology.
   In: Ultrasound in Medicine, D. White and R.E. Brown, eds. Vol. 3B, 1895-1916. Plenum Press, London/New York (1977).
64. Ossoinig, K.C. Echography of the Eye, Orbit, and Periorbital Region.
   In: Orbit Roentgenology, Peter H. Arger, M.D., Editor. John Wiley & Sons, Inc. (1977).
65. Till, P. & K.C. Ossoinig: First experiences with a solid tissue model for standardization of A- and B-scan instruments in tissue diagnosis. In *Ultrasound in Medicine* (Proc. of the 3 rd World Congress of Ultrasonics in Medicine, San Francisco, 1976, White, D. N., ed.), pp. 2167-2174. Plemm Press, New York (1977).
66. McNutt, L. Ultrasound of Graves' orbitopathy. Seminar April, 1975, available from Dept. Ophthal., Univ. of Iowa Hospitals, Iowa City, Iowa (1975).
67. McNutt, L., Kaefring S.L. & k.C. Ossoinig. Echographic Measurement of Extraocular Muscles.
   In: Ultrasound in Medicine, Vol. 3A: 927-932, (D. White and R.E. Brown, Eds.) Plenum Press, NY, London (1977).
68. Skalta H.W. Ultrasonography of the Optic Nerve.
   In: Neuro-Ophthalmology Update, J.L. Smith, (Ed.), Masson Publishing USA (1977).
69. Purnell, E.W. Ultrasound in ophthalmological diagnosis. In *Diagnostic Ultrasound* (Proc. of the ist International Conference, University of Pittsburgh, 1965, C.C. Grossmann et al., eds.), pp. 95-110, Plenum Press, New York (1966).
70. Purnell, E.W. Intensity modulated (B-scan) ultrasonography. In *Ultrasonics in ophthalmologny: Diagnostic and therapcutic applications,* Goldberg, R.E. and Sarin, L.K., eds., pp. 102-123, W.B. Saunders, Philadelphia/London (1967).
71. Purnell, E.W.: Ultrasonic interpretation of orbital disease. In *Ophthalmic ultrasound* (Proc. of the 4th International Congress of Ultrasonography in Ophthalmology, Philadelphia, 1968, Gitter, K.A., Kenney, A.H., Sarin L.K., and Meyer, D., eds.), pp. 249-255, C.V. Mosby, St. Louis (1969).
72. Bronson, N.R., Fisher Y.L., Pickering N.C., and Trayner, E.M.: Ophthalmic Contact B-Scan Ultrasonography For the Clinician. Intercontinental Publications, Inc., Westport, CT (1976).
73. Dallow, R.L. Evaluation of Unilateral Exophthalmos with Ultrasonography. Analysis of 258 Consecutive Cases. Laryngoscope, 85: 1905-1919 (1975).
74. Dallow, R. Ultrasonography of the Eye and Orbit. Appl. Radiol., (1975).
75. Coleman, D.J., Jack, R.L., and Franzen, L.A.: High resolution B-scan ultrasonography of the orbit. I. The normal orbit. *Arch. Ophthal.* (Chicago) 88: 358-367 (1972).
76. Coleman, D.J., Jack, R.L., and Franzen, L.A.: High-resolution B-scan ultrasonography of the orbit. II. Hemangioma of the orbit. *Arch. Ophthal.* (Chicago) 88: 368-374 (1972).

77. Coleman, D.J., Jack, R.L., and Franzen, L.A.: High-resolution B-scan ultrasonography of the orbit. III. Lymphomas of the orbit. *Arch. Ophthal.* 88: 375-379 (1972).

78. Coleman, D.J.: Reliability of Ocular and Orbital Diagnosis with B-scan Ultrasound. II. Orbital Diagnosis. Am. J. Ophthalmol., 74: 704-718 (1972).

79. Amramson D.H., Coleman D.J. and Franzen L.A.: Ultrasonography of Optic Nerve Lesions.
    In: Ultrasonography in Ophthalmology (Proc. of SIDUO V, Ghent, 1973, Francois J. and Goes F., eds.). Bibl. Ophthalmol., 83: 231-235. S. Karger, Basel/New York (1975).

80. Coleman, D.J., Lizzi F.L., and Jack R.L.: Ultrasonography of the Eye and Orbit. Lea & Febiger, Philadelphia (1977).

81. Ossoinig, K.C. Die Ultraschalldiagnostik obitaler Gefässprozesse. (Echography of Vascular Tumors of the Orbit). *Klin. Monatsbl. Augenheilk.* 158: *526-533* (1971).

82. Hamard, H., Haye C. & P. Bregeat.: La place de l'échotomographie parmi les explorations complémentaires de l'orbite. (The Role of Echographic Tomography as a Complementary Method in Orbital Diagnosis).
    In: Diagnostica Ultrasonica in Ophthalmologia (Proc. of SIDUO IV, Paris, 1971, Massin M. and Poujol J., eds.), 233-235. Centre National d'Ophthalmologie des Quinze-Vingts, Paris (1973).

83. Hyman, B.N. Doppler sonography – a bedside noninvasive method for assessment of carotid artery disease. *Amer. J. Ophthal.* 77: *227-231*, (1074).

84. Hodes, B.L. & G. Stern. Contact B-Scan Echographic Diagnosis of Ophthalmopathic Graves' Disease. Journal of Clinical Ultrasound, Vol. 3, No. 4: 255-261 (1975).

85. Nover A., Rochels R. & B. Schwab. Eine äquidensitometrische Methode zur objecktiven Auswertung von Ultraschall-B-Bildern. (An Equidensometric Method for Objective Evaluation of Ultrasonic B-Scan Pictures). *Albrecht von Graefes Arch. Klin. Ophthalmol.* 195: *141-148* (1975).

86. Poujol, J. A-scan ultrasound: Accuracy of diagnosis in orbital diseases. In *modern problems in ophthalmology: Orbital disorders* (Proc. of the 2nd International Symposium on Orbital Disorders, Amsterdam, 1973, Bleeker, G.M., Garston, J.B., Kronenberg, B., and Lyle, T.K., eds.), Vol. 14, pp. 250-253, S. Karger, Basel (1975).

87. Hodes, B.L. Edema Fluid as a Contrast Medium in Orbital Echography.
    In: Ultrasound in Medicine, D. White and R.E. Brown, eds., Vol. 3B, 1917-1924. Plenum Press, London/New York (1977).

88. Patel, J.H. & K.C. Ossoinig. A-scan instrumentation for acoustic tissue differentiation. I. Signal processing in the 7200 MA unit of Kretztechnik. In *Ultrasound in medicine* (Proc. of the 3rd World Congress of Ultrasonics in Medicine, San Francisco, 1976, White, D.N., ed.), pp. 1939-1947. Plenum Press, New York (1977).

89. Ossoinig, K.C. & J.H. Patel.: A-scan instrumentation for acoustic tissue differentiation. II. Clinical significance of various technical parameters of the 7200 MA unit of Kretztechnik. *In Ultrasound in medicine* (Proc. of the 3rd World Congress of Ultrasonics in Medicine, San Francisco, 1976, White, D.N., ed.), pp. 1949-1953, Plenum Press, New York (1977).

90. Ossoinig, K.C. & J.H. Patel. A-Scan Instrumentation for Acoustic Tissue Differentiation. III' Testing and Calibration of the 7200 MA Unit of Kretztechnik.
    In: Ultrasound in Medicine, D. White and R.E. Brown, eds. Vol. 3B, 1955-1964. Plenum Press, London/New York (1977).

SUBJECT INDEX